T0177802

OXFORD HANDBOOK OF
Clinical Dentistry

Published and forthcoming Oxford Handbooks

OXFORD HANDBOOK OF
Clinical
Dentistry

SEVENTH EDITION

EDITED BY

Bethany Rushworth

General Dental Practitioner,
Leeds Teaching Hospitals/Leeds Dental Institute,
Leeds, UK

Anastasios Kanatas

Professor of Oral and Maxillofacial Surgery/Consultant Head
and Neck Surgeon, OMFS,
Leeds Teaching Hospitals/University of Leeds,
Leeds, UK

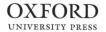

OXFORD
UNIVERSITY PRESS

OXFORD
UNIVERSITY PRESS

Great Clarendon Street, Oxford, OX2 6DP,
United Kingdom

Oxford University Press is a department of the University of Oxford.
It furthers the University's objective of excellence in research, scholarship,
and education by publishing worldwide. Oxford is a registered trade mark of
Oxford University Press in the UK and in certain other countries

© Oxford University Press 2020

The moral rights of the authors have been asserted

First edition 1991 to sixth edition 2014 © David A. and Laura Mitchell

Published in the United States of America by Oxford University Press
198 Madison Avenue, New York, NY 10016, United States of America

British Library Cataloguing in Publication Data
Data available

Library of Congress Control Number: 2020938928

ISBN 978-0-19-883217-1

Printed in China by
C&C Offset Printing Co. Ltd

Preface

In the previous edition's preface, this handbook was described as a mature adult refusing to leave home. However, as it rapidly approaches its 30th birthday the time has now come for this invaluable reference tool to enter a new chapter in its life and move forward, following a substantial update and revision, under new guardianship.

While the format and approach remains the same, all sections have been revised, with the addition of a newly created chapter dedicated solely to implant dentistry, an ever-expanding field with increasing numbers of general dental practitioners now routinely providing this service. With new images, tables, and resources, the text has been brought into line with current evidence and guidelines (at the time of publication), allowing it to serve as an aide-memoire, revision guide, and reference text for dentists and dental students worldwide.

As with all editions of the handbook we are very much indebted to the numerous contributors whose knowledge and expertise over the years have helped to make this book what it is today. However, as with any academic reference book, we would encourage readers to amend or add to the text in response to new evidence, clinical experience, and errors or omissions.

Finally we are hugely grateful to the parents of the book, David and Laura Mitchell, who created, nurtured, and developed the text through six editions into an incredible resource to be used by many generations of dentists over its lifetime. Their encouragement and support has been invaluable as we have endeavoured to make the seventh edition of the *Oxford Handbook of Clinical Dentistry* the most comprehensive and relevant version to date.

BR
AK

Acknowledgements

In addition to those readers whose comments and suggestions have been incorporated into the seventh edition, including P. Clarke, S. Jones, N. Longridge, and J. Humphreys, we would like to thank the following for their time and expertise in updating individual chapters: Dr C. Bates, Dr J. Cairns, Dr H. Gorton, Dr I. Dunn, Dr D. Shah, Dr O. Ikram, Mr P. Rushworth, Dr P. J. Nixon, Dr S. Fayle, and Dr S. Thackeray.

In addition, this book is the sum and distillate of its previous incarnations, which would not have been possible without Mr S. Fayle, Mr A. Graham, Dr H. Gorton, Ms E. McDerra, Dr I. McHenry, Dr L. Middlefell, Mr L. Savarrio, Mr R. Singh KC, Ms J. Smith, Dr I. Suida, Ms Y. Shaw, Mr I. Varley, Mr K. Abdel-Ghalil, Mr B. S. Avery, Mr N. Barnard, Professor P. Brunton, Ms F. Carmichael, Mr N. E. Carter, Mr P. Chambers, Mr M. Chan, Dr A. Dalghous, Mrs J. J. Davison, Dr R. Dookun, Ms S. Dowsett, Dr C. Flynn, Dr I. D. Grime, Mr A. Hall, Mr H. Harvie, Ms V. Hind, Ms J. Hoole, Dr J. Hunton, Mr D. Jacobs, Mr W. Jones, Mr P. J. Knibbs, Ms K. Laidler, Mr C. Lloyd, Mr M. Manogue, Professor J. F. McCabe, Dr L. Middlefell, Dr B. Nattress, Mr R. A. Ord, Dr J. E. Paul, Mr J. Reid, Professor A. Rugg-Gunn, Professor R. A. Seymour, Professor J. V. Soames, Ms A. Tugnait, Dr D. Wood, and Professor R. Yemm. We acknowledge the hard work and expertise of Katherine Grice, the medical artist responsible for some of the excellent drawings throughout the text and would like to thank Mr T. Zoltie and Dr N. Parmar for their contributions of updated photos in this edition. We are grateful to the editor of *The BMJ*, the *British Dental Journal*, and Professor M. Harris, the Royal National Institute of the Deaf, Laerdal, and the Resuscitation Council (UK) for granting permission to use their diagrams, and VUMAN for allowing us to include the Index of Orthodontic Treatment Need.

Once again the staff of OUP deserve thanks for their help and encouragement.

Contents

Contributors *viii*

Symbols and abbreviations *ix*

Contributors

Claire Bates
Consultant Orthodontist and
Head of the Orthodontic
Department
Leeds Teaching Hospitals
NHS Trust
Leeds, UK
Chapter 4: Orthodontics

Ian Dunn
Specialist Periodontist
Rose Lane Dental Practice
Liverpool, UK
*Chapter 5: Restorative dentistry
1: periodontology*

Stephen Fayle
Consultant and Honorary Senior
Clinical Lecturer in Paediatric
Dentistry
Leeds Dental Institute
Leeds, UK
Chapter 3: Paediatric dentistry

Heather Gorton
Consultant Anaesthetist
Leeds Teaching Hospitals
NHS Trust
Leeds, UK
*Chapter 15: Analgesia, anaesthesia,
and sedation*

Omar Ikram
Specialist Endo Crows Nest
Crows Nest NSW 2065, Australia
*Chapter 8: Restorative dentistry
4: endodontics*

Peter J Nixon
Specialist Dentist/Consultant
Clarendon Dental Spa/Leeds
Dental Institute
Leeds, UK
*Chapter 6: Restorative dentistry
2: repairing teeth*
*Chapter 7: Restorative dentistry
3: replacing teeth*
*Chapter 9: Restorative dentistry
5: dental implants*

Dhru Shah
Specialist in Periodontics
Chiswell Green Dental Centre
St Albans, UK
Founder of the Tubules Project at
http://www.dentaltubules.com
*Chapter 5: Restorative dentistry
1: periodontology*

Simon Thackeray
General Dental Practitioner and
Expert Witness
Thackeray Dental Care
Mansfield, UK
Chapter 17: Law and ethics

Symbols and abbreviations

Some of these are included because they are in common usage, others because they are big words and we were trying to save space.

►	this is important	BDA	British Dental Association
⊅	cross-reference	BIPP	bismuth iodoform paraffin paste
Δ	diagnosis	BMA	British Medical Association
$	supernumerary	BNF	British National Formulary
–ve	negative	BOP	bleeding on probing
+ve	positive	BP	blood pressure
&/or	and/or	BPE	Basic Periodontal Examination
↑	increase(d)	BRON(J)	bisphosphonate-related osteonecrosis (of the jaw)
↓	decrease(d)	BSP	British Society of Periodontology
→	leading to	BSS	black silk suture
<	less than	b/w	bitewing
>	greater than	Ca^{2+}	calcium
~	approximately	CAD/CAM	computer-aided design/ computer-aided manufacture
#	fracture	C&S	culture and sensitivity
μ	micro (e.g. μm)	CBCT	cone beam computed tomography
?	question/ask about (when ? appears alone)	CDS	Community Dental Service
∴	therefore	C/I	contraindication/ contraindicated
1°	primary	Class I	Class I relationship
2°	secondary	Class II/1	Class II division 1 relationship
3°	tertiary	Class II/2	Class II division 2 relationship
5; inc	lower second premolar, lower incisor	Class III	Class III relationship
2; inc	upper lateral incisor, upper incisor	CLP	cleft lip and palate
3-D	three dimensional	cm	centimetre
ACS	American College of Surgeons	CMV	cytomegalovirus
ACTH	adrenocorticotrophic hormone	CNS	central nervous system
ADJ	amelo-dentinal junction	CPD	continuing professional development
Ag	antigen	CPITN	Community Periodontal Index of Treatment Needs
AI	amelogenesis imperfecta	CPR	cardiopulmonary resuscitation
AIDS	acquired immune deficiency syndrome	CQC	Care Quality Commission
ALS	advanced life support	CSF	cerebrospinal fluid
AOB	anterior open bite	CT	computed tomography
AP	anteroposterior	CXR	chest X-ray
ASAP	as soon as possible	DCP	dental care professional
ATLS	advanced trauma life support		
BCC	basal cell carcinoma		
bd	twice daily		

dL	decilitre		HAART	highly active antiretroviral therapy
DN	dental nurse		Hb	haemoglobin
DOH/DH	Department of Health		HDU	high dependency unit
DPF	Dental Practitioners' Formulary		Hep B/C	hepatitis B/C
DPT	dental panoramic tomogram/ tomography		Hg	mercury
			HIV	human immunodeficiency virus
DVT	deep venous thrombosis		HLA	human leucocyte antigen
EBA	ethoxy benzoic acid		HPV	human papilloma virus
EBM/D	evidence-based medicine/ dentistry		HSV	herpes simplex virus
			HT	hydroxytryptamine (serotonin)
EBV	Epstein–Barr virus		HU	Hounsfield unit
ECC	early childhood caries		ICP	intercuspal position
ECG	electrocardiograph		ICU	intensive care unit
EDTA	ethylene diamine tetra-acetic acid		ID	inferior dental
			IDB	inferior dental block
e.g.	for example		IDN	inferior dental nerve
EMD	enamel matrix derivative		i.e.	that is
ENT	ear, nose, and throat		Ig	immunoglobulin (e.g. IgA, IgG, etc.)
EO	extra-oral			
ESR	erythrocyte sedimentation rate		IM	intramuscular
F	female		IMF	intermaxillary fixation
F/−	full upper denture (and −/F for lower)		inc	incisor
			INR	international normalized ratio
FA	fixed appliance		IO	intra-oral
FB	foreign body		IOTN	Index of Orthodontic Treatment Need
FBC	full blood count			
FESS	functional endoscopic sinus surgery		IRM	Intermediate Restorative Material®
			ISO	International Organization for Standardization
fL	femtolitre			
FNAC	fine-needle aspiration cytology		ITP	idiopathic thrombocytopenic purpura
f/s	fissure sealant			
FWS	freeway space		IU	international unit(s)
g	gram		IV	intravenous
GA	general anaesthesia/ anaesthetic		K+	potassium
			kg	kilogram
GAP	generalized aggressive periodontitis		kV	kilovolt
			L	litre
GCS	Glasgow Coma Scale		LA	local anaesthesia/anaesthetic
GDC	General Dental Council		LAP	localized aggressive periodontitis
GDP	general dental practitioner			
GDS	General Dental Services		LFH	lower face height
GI	glass ionomer		LFT	liver function test
GIC	glass ionomer cement		LLS	lower labial segment
GKI	glucose, potassium, insulin		LMA	laryngeal mask airway
GMP	general medical practitioner		m	metre
GP	gutta-percha		M	male
GTR	guided tissue regeneration		mand	mandible/mandibular
h	hour			

MAOI	monoamine oxidase inhibitor
max	maxilla/maxillary
MCQ	multiple choice question
MCV	mean corpuscular volume
MEN	multiple endocrine neoplasia
MFDS	Membership of the Faculty of Dental Surgery
mg	milligram
MHRA	Medicines and Healthcare products Regulatory Agency
MHz	megahertz
MI	myocardial infarction
MIH	molar incisor hypomineralization
micromol	micromoles
min	minute
MJDF	Membership of the Joint Dental Faculties
mL	millilitre
mm	millimetre
mmHg	millimetres of mercury
mmol	millimole
MMPA	maxillary mandibular planes angle
MRI	magnetic resonance imaging
MRONJ	medication-related osteonecrosis of the jaw
MSU	mid-stream urine
MTA	mineral trioxide aggregate
NHS	National Health Service
NICE	National Institute for Health and Care Excellence
NiTi	nickel titanium
NLP	neurolinguistic programming
nm	nanometre
nocte	at night
NSAID	non-steroidal anti-inflammatory drug
NUG	necrotizing ulcerative gingivitis
NUP	necrotizing ulcerative periodontitis
O_2	oxygen
o/b	overbite
od	once daily
OD	overdenture
O/E	on examination
OH	oral hygiene
OHI	oral hygiene instruction
OHP	overhead projector/projection
o/j	overjet

OMF	oral and maxillofacial
ORIF	open reduction and internal fixation
OTC	over the counter
OUP	Oxford University Press
OVD	occlusal vertical dimension
P/—	partial upper denture (and —/P for lower)
PA	posteroanterior
PCA	patient-controlled analgesia
PCR	polymerase chain reaction
PDH	past dental history
PDL	periodontal ligament
PEA	pulseless electrical activity
PEG	percutaneous endoscopic gastrostomy
PFM	porcelain fused to metal (crown)
PI	Plaque Index
PJC	porcelain jacket crown
PM	premolar
PMH	past medical history
PMMA	polymethylmethacrylate
PO	per os (orally)
PPD	probing pocket depth
ppm	parts per million
PR	per rectum (rectally)
PRR	preventive resin restoration
qds	four times daily
RA	relative analgesia
RAS	recurrent aphthous stomatitis
RBC	red blood cell count
RCCT	randomized controlled clinical trial
RCF	root canal filling
RCP	retruded contact position
RCT	root canal treatment/therapy
RIG	radiologically inserted gastrostomy
RMGIC	resin-modified glass ionomer cement
Rx	treatment
SC	subcutaneous
SCC	squamous cell carcinoma
SDCEP	Scottish Dental Clinical Effectiveness Programme
sec	second
SF	sugar free
SLE	systemic lupus erythematosus
spp.	species

SS	stainless steel	UK	United Kingdom
STD	sexually transmitted diseases	ULS	upper labial segment
TB	tuberculosis	URA	upper removable appliance
TC	tungsten carbide	US	United States
tds	thrice daily	US(S)	ultrasound (scan)
TENS	transcutaneous electrical nerve stimulation	UTI	urinary tract infection
		VF	ventricular fibrillation
TIBC	total iron binding capacity	WHO	World Health Organization
TMA	titanium molybdenum alloy	Xbite	crossbite
TMD	temporomandibular disorder	X-rays	either X-ray beam or radiographs
TMJ	temporomandibular joint		
TNF	tissue necrosis factor	yr	year
TTP	tender to percussion	ZOE	zinc oxide eugenol
mocw U&Es	urea and electrolytes		

History and examination

Relevant pages in other chapters It could, of course, be said that all pages are relevant to this section, because history and examination are the first steps in the care of any patient. However, as that is hardly helpful, the reader is referred specifically to the following: medical conditions, Chapter 13; the child with toothache, ➜ p. 64; pre-operative management of the dental patient, ➜ Pre-operation, p. 576; cranial nerves, ➜ p. 546; orthodontic assessment, ➜ p. 126; pulpal pain, ➜ p. 230.

Principal sources Experience.

First impressions

Much of what you need to know about any individual patient can be obtained by watching them enter the surgery and sit in the chair, their body language during the interview, and a few well-chosen questions (Chapter 18). One of the great secrets of healthcare is to develop the ability to actually listen to what your patients tell you and to use that information. Doctors and dentists are often concerned that if they allow patients to speak rather than answer questions, history taking will prove inefficient and prolonged. In fact, most patients will give the information necessary to make a provisional diagnosis, and further useful personal information, if allowed to speak uninterrupted. Most will lapse into silence after 2–3min of monologue. History taking should be conducted with the patient sitting comfortably; this rarely equates with supine! In order to produce an all-round history it is, however, customary and frequently necessary to resort to directed questioning. Here are a few hints:

- Always introduce yourself to the patient and any accompanying person and explain what your role is in helping them. It is useful to clarify at this stage the relationship of any chaperones with the patient (e.g. relative, friend, or support worker).
- Remember that patients are (usually) neither medically nor dentally trained, so use plain speech without speaking down to them.
- Questions are a key part of history taking and the manner in which they are asked can lead to a quick diagnosis and a trusting patient, or abject confusion with a potential litigant. Open questions should be used that require more than a simple 'Yes' or 'No' answer, to avoid leading the patient. Be careful of this when the question suggests the answer, e.g. 'Is the pain worse when you drink hot drinks?' However, with the more reticent patient it may be necessary to ask leading questions to elicit relevant information.
- Notwithstanding earlier paragraphs, you will sometimes find it necessary to interrupt patients in full flight during a detailed monologue on their grandmother's sick parrot. Try to do this tactfully, e.g. 'That is a lot of information you are telling me, can we recap how this affects the problem you have come about today?'

Specifics of a medical or dental history are described in ➲ The dental history, p. 4; ➲ The medical history, p. 6. The object is to elicit sufficient information to make a provisional diagnosis for the patient while establishing a mutual rapport, thus facilitating further investigations &/or treatment (Rx).

Presenting complaint

The aim of this part of the history is to establish provisional differential diagnoses even before examining the patient. The following is a suggested outline, which would require modifying according to the circumstances:

Complaining of (C/O) documented in the patient's own words

Use a general introductory question, e.g. 'Why did you come to see us today?' or 'What is the problem?'

If symptoms are present

Onset and pattern When did the problem start? Was it a sudden or gradual onset? Is it getting better, worse, or staying the same?

Frequency How often and how long does it last? Does it occur at any particular time of day or night?

Exacerbating and relieving factors What makes it better? What makes it worse? What started it?

If pain is the main symptom

Origin and radiation Where is the pain and does it spread?

Character and intensity How would you describe the pain: sharp, shooting, dull, aching, etc.? This can be difficult, but patients with specific 'organic' pain will often understand exactly what you mean whereas patients with symptoms with a high behavioural overlay will be vague and prevaricate.

Remember, while 'severity' of pain is subjective this may give an idea of how well a patient is coping.

Associations Is there anything, in your own mind, which you associate with the problem?

The majority of dental problems can quickly be narrowed down using a simple series of questions such as these to create a provisional diagnosis and judge the urgency of the problem.

The dental history

It is important to assess the patient's dental awareness and the likelihood of raising it. A dental history may also provide invaluable clues as to the nature of the presenting complaint and should not be ignored. This can be achieved by some simple general questions:

How often do you go to the dentist? This gives information on motivation, likely attendance patterns, and may indicate patients who change their general dental practitioner (GDP) frequently.

When did you last see a dentist and what did they do? This may give clues as to the diagnosis of the presenting complaint, e.g. a recent root canal treatment (RCT).

How often do you brush your teeth and how long for? Do you use mouthwash, floss, or interdental brushes? This gives information on motivation and likely gingival condition.

Have you ever had any pain or clicking from your jaw joints? This may indicate temporomandibular joint (TMJ) pathology.

Are you aware that you grind your teeth or bite your nails? This may provide information on temporomandibular disorder (TMD) and personality.

How do you feel about dental treatment? This helps in explaining any dental anxiety.

What do you think about the appearance of your teeth? This provides clues about motivation and possible need for orthodontic Rx.

What is your job? This can give indications about socio-economic status, education, availability for attending appointments, possible snacking habits, and frequently changing routines (e.g. night shifts or long-distance driving), that may affect diet (e.g. high-sugar/energy drinks if an athlete).

Where do you live? This gives information on fluoride intake and travelling time to surgery. This question may seem invasive to the patient, so the information can be obtained from their records. Confirm these are up to date and accurate.

What types of dental treatment have you had previously? For example, previous extractions, problems with local anaesthesia (LA) or general anaesthesia (GA), orthodontics, and periodontal Rx.

What are your snacking habits like? For example, types of foods/drinks and frequency. This can give indications about hidden sugars, caries rate, and erosion. It is worth including specific questions as to whether or not they use tobacco, alcohol, or other recreational drugs.

The social history

The patient's social history can give a lot of information about their lifestyle and risk factors for diseases such as periodontal disease and oral cancer. It is important not to be judgemental at this stage; however, these questions can be helpful in getting to know patients and in Rx planning.

Smoking What do they smoke? How long have they smoked for? If they have stopped smoking, when did they stop?

Alcohol The Chief Medical Officer's guidelines now advise no more than 14 units of alcohol per week for both men and women to keep health risks from alcohol to a low level. It is useful to clarify what the patient drinks (spirits, lager, or wine, for example) and often they will need help in calculating the number of units they consume.

Occupation Certain occupations may affect both routine and diet so should be considered when delivering oral health advice and motivating patients.

Diet General information can be gathered regarding a patient's diet; however, a more formal approach is to use a diet sheet. Ideally, this should be completed across a mixture of both working days and non-working days to get an idea what the patient's frequency of sugar intake is. They should include drink as well as food and record if sugar is added to these. It is tempting for patients to change their diet once they know it is being analysed, or to avoid recording things they feel they shouldn't have eaten. It is important to educate patients about hidden sugars and the impact of diet on their dental health regardless of what is recorded, in case there have been any omissions on their completed diet sheets!

Other substances It is useful to know whether patients are using other substances such as gutka, betel nut, or paan (with or without tobacco) as these can lead to staining of teeth and gingival tissues as well as an ↑ risk of oral cancer.

The medical history

There is much to be said for asking patients to complete a medical history questionnaire, as this encourages more accurate responses to sensitive questions. However, it is important to use this as a starting point and clarify the answers with the patient.

Example of a medical questionnaire

QUESTION   YES/NO

Are you fit and well?

Are you seeing a doctor for anything?

Have you ever been admitted to hospital?
• If yes, please give brief details.

Have you ever had an operation?
• If so, were there any problems?

Have you ever had any heart trouble or high blood pressure?

Have you ever had any chest trouble?

Have you ever had any problems with bleeding? Do you bruise easily?

Have you ever had asthma, eczema, or hayfever?

Do you have fits, faints, or headaches?

Do you have any known allergies such as penicillin, latex, or Elastoplast?

Are you allergic to any other drug or substance?

Do you have or ever had:
• Arthritis?
• Diabetes?
• Epilepsy?
• Tuberculosis?
• Jaundice?
• Hepatitis especially B or C?
• Other infectious disease, HIV in particular?

Are you pregnant or breastfeeding?

Are you taking any drugs, medications, or pills?
• If yes, please give details (Chapter 14):
• If a patient cannot recall their regular medications, ask them to bring their prescription to their next appointment or contact their General Medical Practitioner (GMP).

Who is your GMP?

▶ Check the medical history at each recall.
▶ If in any doubt, contact the patient's GMP, or the specialist they are attending, before proceeding.

Screening for medical problems in dental practice

Certain conditions are so commonplace and of such significance that screening (specifically looking for asymptomatic markers of disease) is justifiable. Whether or not it is appropriate to use the dental practice environment to screen for hypertension, smoking, or drug and alcohol abuse is very much a cultural, personal, and pragmatic decision for the dentist.

What is crucial is that if you choose to initiate, say, a screening policy for hypertension in practice (i.e. you measure every adult's blood pressure (BP)), you must ensure you are adequately trained in the technique, are aware of and avoid the risk of inducing disease (people get anxious at the dentist and may have 'white coat hypertension' which is of no significance), and act on significant results in a meaningful way. Generating a cohort of 'worried well' who then overload their GMP is hardly helpful whereas detecting significant hypertension in an unsuspecting middle-aged man who then has this corrected could be.

Medical examination

For the vast majority of dental patients attending as out-patients to a practice, community centre, or hospital, simply recording a medical history should suffice to screen for any potential problems. The exceptions are patients who are to undergo GA and anyone with a positive medical history undergoing extensive Rx under LA or sedation. The aim in these cases is to detect any gross abnormality so that it can be dealt with (by investigation, by getting a more experienced or specialist opinion, or by simple Rx if you are completely familiar with the problem). This is a summary, for more detail see Chapter 13.

General Look at sclera in good light for jaundice and anaemia. Check for cyanosis (peripheral: blue extremities; central: blue tongue) and dehydration (lift skin between thumb and forefinger).

Cardiovascular system Feel and time the pulse. Measure BP. Listen to the heart sounds along the left sternal edge and the apex (normally fifth intercostal space mid-clavicular line on the left), murmurs are whooshing sounds between the 'lub dub' of the normal heart sounds. Palpate peripheral pulses and look at the neck for a prominent jugular venous pulse (this is difficult and takes much practice).

Respiratory system Look at the respiratory rate (12–18/min)—is expansion equal on both sides? Listen to the chest—is air entry equal on both sides? Are there any crackles or wheezes indicating infection, fluid, or asthma? Percuss the back, comparing resonance.

Gastrointestinal system With the patient lying supine and relaxed with hands by their sides, palpate with the edge of your hand for liver (upper right quadrant) and spleen (upper left quadrant). These should be just palpable on inspiration. Also palpate bimanually for both kidneys in the right and left flanks (healthy kidneys are not palpable) and note any masses, scars, or hernia. Listen for bowel sounds and palpate for a full bladder.

Genitourinary system This is mostly covered by the abdominal examination. Patients with genitourinary symptoms are more likely to go into post-operative urinary retention. Pelvic and rectal examinations are neither appropriate nor indicated and should not be conducted by the nonmedically qualified.

Central nervous system Is the patient alert and orientated in time, place, and person? For examination of the cranial nerves see ➔ Cranial nerves, p. 546. Ask the patient to move their limbs through a range of movements, then repeat passively and against resistance to assess tone, power, and mobility. Reflexes—brachioradialis, biceps, triceps, knee, ankle, and plantar—are commonly elicited (stimulation of the sole normally causes plantar flexion of the great toe).

Musculoskeletal system Note limitations in movement and arthritis, especially affecting the cervical spine, which may need to be hyperextended in order to intubate for anaesthesia.

Examination of the head and neck

This is an important aspect of examination that is often undertaught and overlooked in both medical and dental training. In the former, the tendency is to approach the area in a rather cursory manner, partly because it is not well understood. In the latter, it is often forgotten, despite otherwise extensive knowledge of the head and neck, to look beyond the mouth. For this reason, the examination described here is given in some detail, but the depth of examination will vary, dependent on the patient's complaint, risk factors, and clinical suspicion.

Head and facial appearance Look for specific deformities (➲ Cleft lip and palate, p. 170), facial disharmony (➲ Orthodontics and orthognathic surgery, p. 168), syndromes (Chapter 20), traumatic defects (➲ Mandibular fractures, p. 494; ➲ Mid-face fractures, p. 496; ➲ Nasal and malar fractures, p. 498), and facial palsy (➲ Oral manifestations of neurological disease, p. 476).

Assessment of the cranial nerves is covered in ➲ Cranial nerves, p. 546.

Skin Lesions of the face should be examined for colour, scaling, bleeding, and crusting, and palpated for texture and consistency and whether or not they are fixed to, or arising from, surrounding tissues. Those with facial hair who have had radiotherapy may have hairless patches indicating the area which was irradiated.

Eyes Note obvious abnormalities such as proptosis and lid retraction (e.g. hyperthyroidism) and ptosis (drooping eyelid). Examine conjunctiva for chemosis (swelling) and pallor (e.g. anaemia or jaundice). Look at the iris and pupil. Ophthalmoscopy is the examination of the disc and retina via the pupil. It is a specialized skill requiring an adequate ophthalmoscope and is acquired by watching and practising with a skilled supervisor. However, direct and consensual (contralateral eye) light responses of the pupils are straightforward and should always be assessed in suspected head injury (➲ Pupils, p. 492).

Ears Gross abnormalities of the external ear are usually obvious. Further examination requires an auroscope. The secret is to have a good auroscope and straighten the external auditory meatus by pulling upwards, backwards, and outwards using the largest applicable speculum. Look for the pearly grey tympanic membrane; a plug of wax often intervenes.

Mouth See ➲ Examination of the mouth, p. 12.

Oropharynx and tonsils These can easily be seen by depressing the tongue with a spatula, the *hypopharynx* and *larynx* are seen by indirect laryngoscopy, using a head-light and mirror, and the *post-nasal space* is similarly viewed. Skill with a flexible nasendoscope is essential for those (e.g. oral and maxillofacial surgery trainees) who examine this area in detail regularly.

The neck Inspect from in front and palpate from behind. Look for skin changes, scars, swellings, and arterial and venous pulsations. Palpate the neck systematically, starting at a fixed standard point, e.g. beneath the chin, working back to the angle of the mandible and then down the cervical chain, remembering the scalene and supraclavicular nodes. Swellings of the thyroid move with swallowing. Auscultation may reveal bruits over the carotids (usually due to atheroma).

Temporomandibular joint Palpate both joints simultaneously. Have the patient open and close and move joint laterally while feeling for clicking, locking, and crepitus. Palpate the muscles of mastication for spasm and tenderness. Auscultation is not usually used. Clicking can be physiological rather than pathological and in these cases simple reassurance may be required. Examine for diversion of the mandible.

Examination of the mouth

Most dental textbooks, quite rightly, include a very detailed and comprehensive description of how to examine the mouth. Given the constraints imposed by routine clinical practice, this approach needs to be modified to give a somewhat briefer format that is as equally applicable to the routine dental attendee who is symptomless as to the new patient attending with pain of unknown origin.

The key to this is to develop a systematic approach, which becomes almost automatic, so that when you are under pressure there is less likelihood of missing any pathology.

Extra-oral (EO) examination

(➲ Examination of the head and neck, p. 10.) For routine clinical practice this can usually be limited to a visual appraisal, e.g. swellings, asymmetry, patient's colour, etc. More detailed examination can be carried out if indicated by the patient's symptoms. Lymph nodes may be palpated.

Intra-oral (IO) examination

- Oral hygiene. Avoid subjective scores. A validated plaque score is advised, preferably using scores where a higher number is better, to motivate the patient with an objective measurement.
- Soft tissues. The entire oral mucosa should be carefully inspected. Any ulcer of >3 weeks' duration requires further investigation (➲ An approach to oral ulcers, p. 482). Examination should include the tongue, floor of mouth, lips, oropharynx, tonsillar crypt and tonsils, and hard palate. It is important to recognize normal anatomy.
- Periodontal condition. This can be assessed rapidly, using a periodontal probe (➲ Basic Periodontal Examination, p. 178).
- Chart the teeth present (➲ Tooth notation, p. 790).
- Examine each tooth in turn for caries (➲ Caries diagnosis, p. 26) and examine the integrity of any restorations present.
- Occlusion. This should involve not only getting the patient to close together and examining the relationship between the arches (➲ Definitions, p. 124), but also looking at the path of closure for any obvious prematurities and displacements (➲ Crossbites, p. 154). Check for evidence of tooth wear (➲ Tooth wear/tooth surface loss, p. 252).

For those patients complaining of pain, a more thorough examination of the area related to their symptoms should then be carried out, followed by any special investigations (➲ Investigations—specific, p. 16).

Tooth notation

Because of the difficulties of putting the grid notation (Fig. 1.1 and Fig. 1.2) in word processed documents, it is common practice to indicate the quadrant by abbreviating the arch and side. Thus the upper right second premolar is UR5 and the lower left second deciduous molar is LLE.

FDI

Permanent teeth

R $\dfrac{18 \ 17 \ 16 \ 15 \ 14 \ 13 \ 12 \ 11 \ | \ 21 \ 22 \ 23 \ 24 \ 25 \ 26 \ 27 \ 28}{48 \ 47 \ 46 \ 45 \ 44 \ 43 \ 42 \ 41 \ | \ 31 \ 32 \ 33 \ 34 \ 35 \ 36 \ 37 \ 38}$ L

Deciduous teeth

R $\dfrac{55 \ 54 \ 53 \ 52 \ 51 \ | \ 61 \ 62 \ 63 \ 64 \ 65}{85 \ 84 \ 83 \ 82 \ 81 \ | \ 71 \ 72 \ 73 \ 74 \ 75}$ L

Zsigmondy–Palmer, Chevron, or Set Square system

Permanent teeth

R $\dfrac{8 \ 7 \ 6 \ 5 \ 4 \ 3 \ 2 \ 1 \ | \ 1 \ 2 \ 3 \ 4 \ 5 \ 6 \ 7 \ 8}{8 \ 7 \ 6 \ 5 \ 4 \ 3 \ 2 \ 1 \ | \ 1 \ 2 \ 3 \ 4 \ 5 \ 6 \ 7 \ 8}$ L

Deciduous teeth

R $\dfrac{e \ d \ c \ b \ a \ | \ a \ b \ c \ d \ e}{e \ d \ c \ b \ a \ | \ a \ b \ c \ d \ e}$ L

Fig. 1.1 Tooth notation systems.

European

Permanent teeth

R $\dfrac{8+ \ 7+ \ 6+ \ 5+ \ 4+ \ 3+ \ 2+ \ 1+ \ | \ +1 \ +2 \ +3 \ +4 \ +5 \ +6 \ +7 \ +8}{8- \ 7- \ 6- \ 5- \ 4- \ 3- \ 2- \ 1- \ | \ -1 \ -2 \ -3 \ -4 \ -5 \ -6 \ -7 \ -8}$ L

Deciduous teeth

R $\dfrac{05+ \ 04+ \ 03+ \ 02+ \ 01+ \ | \ +01 \ +02 \ +03 \ +04 \ +05}{05- \ 04- \ 03- \ 02- \ 01- \ | \ -01 \ -02 \ -03 \ -04 \ -05}$ L

American

Permanent teeth

R $\dfrac{1 \ 2 \ 3 \ 4 \ 5 \ 6 \ 7 \ 8 \ | \ 9 \ 10 \ 11 \ 12 \ 13 \ 14 \ 15 \ 16}{32 \ 31 \ 30 \ 29 \ 28 \ 27 \ 26 \ 25 \ | \ 24 \ 23 \ 22 \ 21 \ 20 \ 19 \ 18 \ 17}$ L

Deciduous teeth

R $\dfrac{A \ B \ C \ D \ E \ | \ F \ G \ H \ I \ J}{T \ S \ R \ Q \ P \ | \ O \ N \ M \ L \ K}$ L

Fig. 1.2 European and US tooth notation.

Investigations—general

▶ Do not perform or request an investigation you cannot interpret.
▶ Similarly, always look at, interpret, and act on any investigations you have performed.

Temperature, pulse, blood pressure, and respiratory rate You need to be able to interpret the results of these investigations.
- *Temperature* (35.5–37.5°C or 95.9–99.5°F). ↑ physiologically post-operatively for 24h, otherwise may indicate infection or a transfusion reaction. ↓ in hypothermia or shock.
- *Pulse*. Adult (60–80 beats/min); child is higher (up to 140 beats/min in infants). Should be regular.
- *Blood pressure* (120–140/60–90mmHg). ↑ with age. Falling BP may indicate a faint, hypovolaemia, or other form of shock. High BP may place the patient at risk from a GA.
- *Respiratory rate* (12–18 breaths/min). ↑ in chest infections, pulmonary oedema, shock, anxiety, panic attacks, and asthma attacks.

Urinalysis Routinely performed on all patients admitted to hospital. A positive result for:
- *Glucose or ketones* may indicate diabetes.
- *Protein* suggests renal disease especially infection.
- *Blood* suggests infection or tumour.
- *Bilirubin* indicates hepatocellular &/or obstructive jaundice.
- *Urobilinogen* indicates jaundice of any type.

Blood tests (Sampling techniques, ⊃ For sampling, p. 578.) Reference ranges vary.

Full blood count Measures:
- *Haemoglobin* (M 13–18g/dL, F 11.5–16.5g/dL). ↓ in anaemia, ↑ in polycythaemia and myeloproliferative disorders.
- *Haematocrit* (packed cell volume) (M 40–54%, F 37–47%). ↓ in anaemia, ↑ in polycythaemia and dehydration.
- *Mean cell volume* (76–96fL). ↑ in size (macrocytosis) in vitamin B_{12} and folate deficiency, ↓ (microcytosis) iron deficiency.
- *White cell count* (4–11 × 10^9/L). ↑ in infection, leukaemia, and trauma, ↓ in certain infections, early leukaemia, and after cytotoxics.
- *Platelets* (150–400 × 10^9/L). See also ⊃ Platelet disorders, p. 530.

Biochemistry Urea and electrolytes are the most important:
- *Sodium* (135–145mmol/L). Large fall causes fits.
- *Potassium* (3.5–5mmol/L). Must be kept within this narrow range to avoid serious cardiac disturbance. Watch carefully in diabetics, those in IV therapy, and the shocked or dehydrated patient. Suxamethonium (muscle relaxant, used during GA procedures) ↑ potassium.
- *Urea* (2.5–7mmol/L). Rising urea suggests dehydration, renal failure, or blood in the gut.
- *Creatinine* (70–150micromol/L). Rises in renal failure. Various other biochemical tests are available to aid specific diagnoses, e.g. bone, liver function, thyroid function, cardiac enzymes, folic acid, and vitamin B_{12}.

- *Glucose* (fasting 4–6mmol/L). ↑ suspect diabetes, ↓ hypoglycaemic drugs, exercise. Competently interpreted proprietary tests, e.g. 'BMs' equate well to blood glucose (➋ Hypoglycaemia, p. 570).

Virology Viral serology is costly and rarely necessary.

Immunology Similar to virology but more frequently indicated in complex oral medicine patients.

Bacteriology

Sputum and pus swabs Often helpful in dealing with hospital infections. Ensure they are taken with sterile swabs and transported immediately or put in an incubator. May also help to identify appropriate antibiotics for use in persistent infections.

Nasal and axillary swabs Used to screen for methicillin-resistant *Staphylococcus aureus* in all in patients undergoing hospital-based procedures. Stool samples are still generally used to detect *Clostridium difficile* although toxin can be detected in blood.

Blood cultures Useful if the patient has septicaemia.[1] Taken when there is sudden pyrexia and incubated with results available 24–48h later. Take two samples from separate sites and put in paired bottles for aerobic and anaerobic culture (i.e. four bottles, unless your laboratory indicates otherwise). In patients with sepsis there may be an associated tachycardia and hypotension.

Biopsy See ➋ Biopsy, p. 412.

Cytology With the exception of smears for candida and fine-needle aspiration, cytology is little used and not widely applicable in the dental specialties. The diagnosis of premalignant or malignant lesions using cytology only is not widely accepted.

1 ℗ https://www.nice.org.uk/guidance/ng51

Investigations—specific

Sensibility testing It must be borne in mind when vitality testing that it is the integrity of the nerve supply that is being investigated. However, it is the blood supply which is of more relevance to the continued vitality of a pulp. Test the suspect tooth and its neighbours for comparison.

Application of cold This is most practically carried out using Endo-Frost or ethyl chloride on a pledget of cotton wool, held against a dry tooth.

Application of heat Petroleum jelly should be applied first to the tooth being tested to prevent the heated gutta-percha (GP) sticking. No response suggests that the tooth is non-vital, but an ↑ response indicates that the pulp is hyperaemic.

Electric pulp tester The tooth to be tested should be dry, and prophy paste or a proprietary lubricant used as a conductive medium. Most machines ascribe numbers to the patient's reaction, but these should be interpreted with caution as the response can also vary with battery strength or the position of the electrode on the tooth. Table 1.1 lists the misleading results that may occur with the described methods.

Test cavity Drilling into dentine without LA is an accurate diagnostic test, but as tooth tissue is destroyed it should only be used as a last resort. Can be helpful for crowned teeth but should be used with caution.

Percussion This is carried out by gently tapping adjacent and suspect teeth with the end of a mirror handle. A positive response indicates that a tooth is extruded due to exudate in apical or lateral periodontal tissues.

Tooth mobility Tooth mobility is ↑ by ↓ in the bony support (e.g. due to periodontal disease or an apical abscess) and also by a fracture (#) of the root or supporting bone.

Palpation Palpation of the buccal sulcus next to a painful tooth can help to determine if there is an associated apical abscess.

Biting on to a Tooth Slooth, gauze, or rubber This can be used to try and elicit pain due to a cracked tooth.

Local anaesthesia LA can help localize organic pain.

Radiographs (◗ Radiology and radiography, p. 18; ◗ Advanced imaging techniques, p. 20; ◗ Radiographs—practical tips and helpful hints, p. 756.) See Table 1.2.

Table 1.1 Misleading results

False-positive	False-negative
Multi-rooted tooth with vital + non-vital pulp	Nerve supply damaged, blood supply intact
Canal full of pus	Secondary (s) dentine
Apprehensive patient	Large insulating restoration

Table 1.2 Radiographic choice for different areas

Area under investigation	Radiographic view
General scan of teeth and jaws (retained roots, unerupted teeth)	DPT
Localization of unerupted teeth	Parallax periapicals
Crown of tooth and interdental bone (caries, restorations)	Bitewing, periapicals
Root and periapical area	Periapical
Submandibular gland	Lower occlusal view
Sinuses	Occipito-mental, DPT
TMJ	DPT, MRI
Skull and facial bones	Occipito-mental
	PA and lateral skull
	Submento-vertex

Radiology and radiography

Radiography is the taking of radiographs, *radiology* is their interpretation.

Radiographic images are produced by the differential attenuation of X-rays by tissues. Radiographic quality depends on the density of the tissues, intensity of the beam, sensitivity of the emulsion, processing techniques, and viewing conditions.

Intra-oral views

Use a stationary anode (tungsten), direct current ↓ dose of self-rectifying machines. Direct action film (↑ detail) using D or E speed. E speed is double the speed of D hence ↓ dose to patient. Rectangular collimation ↓ unnecessary irradiation of tissues.

Periapical This shows all of the tooth, root, and surrounding periapical tissues. Performed by:
• *Paralleling technique*: film is held in a film holder parallel to the tooth and the beam is directed (using a beam-aligning device) at right angles to the tooth and film. Focus-to-film distance is ↑ to minimize magnification; the optimum distance is 30cm. This is the most accurate and reproducible technique.
• *Bisecting angle technique*: an older technique which can be carried out without film holders. Film is placed close to the tooth and the beam is directed at right angles to the plane bisecting the angle between the tooth and film. Normally held in place by the patient's finger. Not as geometrically accurate a technique as more coning off occurs and needlessly irradiates the patient's finger.

Bitewing This shows crowns and crestal bone levels, and is used to diagnose caries, overhangs, calculus, and bone loss <4mm. Patient bites on wing holding film against the upper and lower teeth and beam is directed between contact points perpendicular to the film in the horizontal plane. A 5° tilt to vertical accommodates the curve of Monson.

Occlusal This demonstrates larger areas. May be oblique, true, or special. Used for localization of impacted teeth and salivary calculi. Film is held parallel to the occlusal plane. Oblique occlusal is similar to a large bisecting angle periapical. True occlusal of the mandible gives a good cross-sectional view.

Key points
• Use paralleling technique.
• Use file holders.
• Rectangular collimation.
• E-speed film.

Extra-oral views

Skull and general facial views use a rotating anode and grid which ↓ scattered radiation reaching the film but ↑ dose to patient. Screen film is used for all EOs (intensifying screens are now rare earth, e.g. gadolinium and lanthanum). X-rays act on the screen which fluoresces and the light interacts with the emulsion. There is loss of detail but a ↓ dose to the patient. Dark-room techniques and film storage are affected due to the properties of the film.

Lateral oblique This has been largely superseded by panoramic views but can use a dental X-ray set.

Posteroanterior (PA) mandible Patient has nose to forehead touching film. Beam is perpendicular to film. Used for diagnosing/assessing # mandible.

Reverse Townes The position is as for PA mandible, but the beam is 30° up to horizontal. Used for condyles.

Occipito-mental Nose/chin touching the film beam parallel to horizontal unless occipito-mental prefixed by, e.g. 10°, 30°, which indicates angle of beam to horizontal.

Submento-vertex Patient flexes neck vertex touching film, and beam is projected menton to vertex. ↓ use due to ↑ radiation and risk to cervical spine.

Cephalometry (➔ Cephalometrics, p. 130; ➔ More cephalometrics, p. 132.) This uses a cephalostat for a reproducible position. Use Frankfort plane or natural head position. Wedge (aluminium or copper and rare earth) to show soft tissues. Lead collimation is used to reduce an unnecessary dose to patient and scatter leading to ↓ contrast. Barium paste can be used to outline soft tissues.

Panoramic Generically referred to as a DPT (dental panoramic tomograph), sometimes by make, e.g. OPT/OPG. The technique is based on tomography (i.e. objects in focal trough are in focus, the rest is blurred). The state-of-the-art machine is a moving centre of rotation (previously two or three centres) which accommodates the horseshoe shape of the jaws. Correct patient positioning is vital. Blurring and ghost shadows can be a problem (ghost shadows appear opposite to and above the real image due to a 5–8° tilt of the beam). This is a relatively low-dose technique and sectional images can be obtained. It is useful for gross pathology but less so for subtle changes such as early caries.

Lead aprons (0.25mm lead equivalent) In well-maintained, well-collimated equipment where the beam does not point to the gonads, the risk of damage is minimal. Apply all normal principles to pregnant women (use a lead apron if the primary (p) beam is directed at the fetus), but otherwise do not treat any differently.

There is no risk in dentistry of deterministic/certainty effects (e.g. radiation burns). Stochastic/change effects are more important (e.g. tumour induction). The thyroid is the principal organ at risk. Follow principles of 'ALARP' (as low as reasonably practicable) (➔ Radiographs—the statutory regulations, p. 754).

Parallax technique This involves two radiographs with a change in position of X-ray tube between them (e.g. DPT and periapical). The object furthest from the X-ray beam will appear to move in the same direction as the tube shift.

Advanced imaging techniques

Computed tomography (CT) Images are formed by scanning a thin cross-section of the body with a narrow X-ray beam (120kV), measuring the transmitted radiation with detectors and obtaining multiple projections, which a computer then processes to reconstruct a cross-sectional image ('slice'). Three-dimensional (3-D) reconstruction is also possible on some machines. Modern scanners consist of either a fan beam with multiple detectors aligned in a circle, both rotating around the patient, or a stationary ring of detectors with the X-ray beam rotating within it. The image is divided into pixels which represent the average attenuation of blocks of tissue (voxels). The CT number (measured in Hounsfield units (HU)) compares the attenuation of the tissue with that of water. Typical values range from air at −1000 to bone at +400 to +1000 units. As the eye can only perceive a limited greyscale, the settings can be adjusted depending on the main tissue of interest (i.e. bone or soft tissues). These 'window levels' are set at the average CT number of the tissue being imaged and the 'window width' is the range selected. The images obtained are very useful for assessing extensive trauma or pathology and planning surgery. The dose is, however, higher compared with conventional films and the National Radiological Protection Board recommends that all radiologists be made aware of the high-dose implications.

Cone beam computed tomography (CBCT) This is a CT technique where the beams are divergent, forming a cone. The scanner rotates around the patient's head creating multiple images (up to 600) which can be reformatted using software into 3-D image reconstructions. The data can also be used to create 3-D models. There are issues around comparability between different machines, distortion due to movement artefact, and bone density determination (as the HU in standard CT and CBCT are not directly comparable). CBCT is helpful for planning implant placement and for assessing teeth undergoing endodontic Rx, in particular if complex root or pulpal anatomy is suspected.

Magnetic resonance imaging (MRI) The patient is placed in a machine which is basically a large magnet. Protons then act like small bar magnets and point 'up' or 'down', with a slightly greater number pointing 'up'. When a radiofrequency pulse is directed across the main magnetic field, the protons 'flip' and align themselves along it. When the pulse ceases, the protons 'relax' and as they realign with the main field they emit a signal. The hydrogen atom is used because of its high natural abundance in the body. The time taken for the protons to 'relax' is measured by values known as T1 and T2. A variety of pulse sequences can be used to give different information. T1 is longer than T2 and times may vary depending on the fluidity of the tissues (e.g. if inflamed). MRI is not good for imaging cortical bone as the protons are held firmly within the bony structure and give a 'signal void', i.e. black, although bone margins are visible. It is useful, however, for the TMJ and facial soft tissues.

Problems These include patient movement, expense, the claustrophobic nature of the machine, noise, magnetizing, and movement of instruments or metal implants and foreign bodies. Cards with magnetic strips (e.g. credit cards) near the machine may also be affected.

Digital imaging This technique has been used extensively in general radiology, where it has great advantages over conventional methods in that there is a marked dose reduction and less concentrated contrast media may be used. The normal X ray source is used but the receptor is a charged coupled device linked to a computer or a photo-stimulable phosphor plate which is scanned by a laser. The image is practically instantaneous and eliminates the problems of processing. However, the sensor is difficult to position and smaller than normal film, which means the dose reduction is not always obtained. Gives ↓ resolution. Now widely used in the UK and European countries.

Ultrasound (US) Ultra-high-frequency sound waves (1–20MHz) are transmitted through the body using a piezoelectric material (i.e. the material distorts if an electric field is placed across it and vice versa). Good probe/skin contact is required (gel) as waves can be absorbed, reflected, or refracted. High-frequency (short wavelength) waves are absorbed more quickly whereas low-frequency waves penetrate further. US is used to image the major salivary glands and soft tissue pathology (cysts/abscesses).

Doppler US is used to assess blood flow as the difference between the transmitted and returning frequency reflects the speed of travel of red cells. Doppler US has also been used to assess the vascularity of lesions and the patency of vessels prior to reconstruction.

Sialography This is the imaging of the major salivary glands after infusion of contrast media under a controlled rate and pressure using either conventional radiographic films or CT scanning. The use of contrast media will reveal the internal architecture of the salivary glands and show up radiolucent obstructions, e.g. calculi within the ducts of the imaged glands. It is particularly useful for inflammatory or obstructive conditions of the salivary glands. Patients allergic to iodine are at risk of anaphylactic reaction if an iodine-based contrast medium is used. Interventional sialography can be used for stone retrieval.

Arthrography Just as the spaces within salivary glands can be outlined using contrast media, so can the upper and lower joint spaces of the TMJ. Although technically difficult, both joint compartments (usually the lower) can be injected with contrast media under fluoroscopic control and the movement of the meniscus can be visualized on video. Stills of the real-time images can be made although interpretation is often unsatisfactory.

Positron emission tomography (PET) This relies on the detection of emitted beta particles. Applications in the head and neck are in tumour detection, particularly when coupled with a metabolite—fluorodeoxyglucose (FDG-PET). Software can allow superimposition of a CT scan onto the FDG-PET image which has a major potential role in the detection of active malignancy after non-surgical Rx or the detection of occult cancers.

Differential diagnosis and treatment plan

Arriving at this stage is the whole point of taking a history and performing an examination, because by narrowing down your patient's symptoms into possible diagnoses you can, in most instances, formulate a series of investigations &/or Rx that will benefit them.

Suggested approach

- History and examination (as shown in → The dental history, p. 4; → The medical history, p. 6; → Medical examination, p. 8; → Examination of the head and neck, p. 10; → Examination of the mouth, p. 12).
- Preliminary investigations.
- Differential diagnosis.
- Specific investigations which will confirm or refute the differential diagnoses.
- Ideally, arrive at the definitive diagnosis/diagnoses.
- List in a logical progression the steps which can be undertaken to take the patient to oral health.
- Then carry them out.

Simple really!

This is the ideal, but life, as you are no doubt well aware, is far from ideal, and it is not always possible to follow this approach from beginning to end. The principles, however, remain valid and this general approach, even if much abbreviated, will help you deal with every new patient safely and sensibly.

Preventive and community dentistry

Relevant pages in other chapters Plaque control, ⊃ Non-surgical treatment—plaque control, p. 204; prevention of secondary caries, ⊃ Principles of operative procedures, p. 242; prevention of trauma to anterior teeth, ⊃ Prevention, p. 99.

Principal sources and further reading British Society for Disability and Oral Health guidelines and policy documents ℘ http://www.bsdh.org.uk. British Society of Paediatric Dentistry guidelines and policy documents ℘ http://www.bspd.co.uk. DOH 2017 *Delivering Better Oral Health—An Evidence-based Toolkit for Prevention* ℘ http://www.dh.gov.uk. J. J. Murray et al. 2003 *Prevention of Oral Disease* (4e), OUP. Scottish Dental Clinical Effectiveness Programme (SCDEP) 2018 *Prevention and Management of Dental Caries in Children* ℘ http://www.sdcep.org.uk. Scottish Intercollegiate Guideline Network (SIGN) guideline 138 (preventing dental caries) ℘ http://www.sign.ac.uk. R. R. Welbury et al. 2018 *Paediatric Dentistry* (5e), OUP.

Dental caries

Dental caries Dental caries is a sugar-dependent infectious disease (Fig. 2.1).[1] Acid is produced as a by-product of the metabolism of fermentable carbohydrate by plaque bacteria, which results in a drop in pH at the tooth surface. In response, calcium and phosphate ions diffuse out of enamel, resulting in demineralization. This process is reversed when the pH rises again. Caries is ∴ a dynamic process characterized by episodic demineralization and remineralization occurring over time. If destruction predominates, disintegration of the mineral component will occur, leading to cavitation.

Enamel caries The initial lesion is visible as a white spot. This appearance is due to demineralization of the prisms in a sub-surface layer, with the surface enamel remaining more mineralized. With continued acid attack the surface changes from being smooth to rough, and may become stained. As the lesion progresses, pitting and eventually cavitation occur. The carious process favours repair, as remineralized enamel concentrates fluoride and has larger crystals, with a ↓ surface area. Fissure caries often starts as two white spot lesions on opposing walls, which coalesce.

Dentine caries Dentine caries comprises demineralization followed by bacterial invasion, but differs from enamel caries in the production of 2° dentine and the proximity of the pulp. Once bacteria reach the amelo-dentinal junction (ADJ), lateral spread occurs, undermining the overlying enamel.

Rate of progression of caries Although it has been suggested that the mean time that lesions remain confined radiographically to the enamel is 3–4yrs,[2] there is great individual variation and lesions may even regress.[3] The rate of progression through dentine is unknown; however, it is likely to be faster than through enamel. Progression of fissure caries is usually rapid due to the morphology of the area. Rapid progression is especially common in 1° molars, with progress from early dentine involvement to pulpal involvement in <1yr in some cases.

Arrested caries Under favourable conditions a lesion may become inactive and even regress. Clinically, arrested dentine caries has a hard or leathery consistency and is darker in colour than soft, yellow, active decay. Arrested enamel caries can be stained dark brown.

Susceptible sites The sites on a tooth which are particularly prone to decay are those where plaque accumulation can occur unhindered, e.g. approximal enamel surfaces, cervical margins, and pits and fissures. Host factors, e.g. the volume and composition of the saliva, can also affect susceptibility.

---

1 E. A. M. Kidd & S. Joyston-Bechal 1987 *Essentials of Dental Caries: The Disease and its Management*, Wright.

2 N. B. Pitts 1983 *Comm Dent Oral Epidemiol* **11** 228.

3 A. Neilson & N. B. Pitts 1991 *Br Dent J* **171** 313.

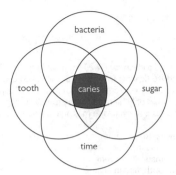

Fig. 2.1 The factors involved in the development of caries.

Saliva and caries Saliva acts as an IO antacid, due to its alkaline pH at high flow rates and buffering capacity. Also:
• ↓ plaque accumulation and aids clearance of foodstuffs.
• Acts as a reservoir of calcium, phosphate, and fluoride ions, thereby favouring remineralization.
• Has an antibacterial action because of its IgA, lysozyme, lactoferrin, and lactoperoxidase content.

An appreciation of the importance of saliva can be gained by examining a patient with a dry mouth.

Chewing sugar-free gum regularly after meals stimulates saliva production and does appear to ↓ caries, but the reduction is small.

Root caries With gingival recession, root dentine is exposed to carious attack. Rx requires, first, control of the aetiological factors and for most patients this involves dietary advice and oral hygiene instruction (OHI). Topical fluoride may aid remineralization and prevent new lesions developing. However, active lesions will require restoration (Ӭ Root surface caries, p. 248).

Caries prevention Classically three main approaches are possible:
• Tooth strengthening or protection.
• Reduction in the availability of microbial substrate.
• Removal of plaque by physical or chemical means.

In practice this means dietary advice, fluoride, fissure sealing, and regular toothbrushing (which is also important in the prevention of periodontal disease). The relative value of these varies with the age of the individual.

Of equal importance with the prevention of new lesions is a preventive philosophy on the part of the dentist, so that early carious lesions are given the chance to arrest and a minimalistic approach is taken to the excision of caries where 1° prevention has failed.

Caries diagnosis

As caries can be arrested or even reversed, early diagnosis is important.

Aids to diagnosis

- Good eyesight (and a clean, dry, well-illuminated tooth). Magnification between ×2 and ×6 (leaning forward with the naked eye magnifies the image but you can only get so close to your patient); loupes are better!
- A blunt probe should only be used to horizontally dredge plaque away from the fissures (as a sharp probe may actually damage an incipient lesion).
- Horizontal bitewing (b/w) radiographs are useful in the detection of approximal caries and in some instances occlusal caries. They are best approached systematically viewing 'approximal–occlusal–approximal' surface for each tooth, first in enamel then dentine, first with the naked eye and then with a viewing box (magnification and external light blackened out or enlargement of digital images). The clinical situation is more advanced than the radiographic appearance. However, it is thought that the probability of cavitation is low when a lesion is confined to enamel on a radiograph.
- Fibreoptic transillumination (FOTI) probes with a 0.5mm tip are useful for detecting dentinal lesions at approximal sites. FOTI is considered to be an adjunct to b/w radiographs.[4]
- Laser-based (e.g. DIAGNOdent®) and impedance-based (e.g. CarieScan PRO®) instruments are available which use properties of the carious lesion to produce a quantitative reading of infected carious tissue, particularly dentine caries.

Diagnosis and its relevance to management

▶ Remember:
- Pre-cavitated lesion—prevention.
- Cavitated lesion—prevention and restoration.

▶ Counsel the patient that if the lesion is not cavitated, it has the potential to arrest. This makes the preventive advice very relevant to the patient, increasing the chance of that patient acting on the advice.

Smooth surface caries This is relatively straightforward to diagnose. The chances of remineralization are ↑ as it is obvious, and accessible for cleaning. Restoration is indicated if prevention has failed and the lesion is cavitated, if the tooth is symptomatic or sensitive, or if aesthetics are poor.

Pit and fissure caries This is difficult to diagnose reliably, especially in the early stages. Testing the suspected cavity with a sharp probe is discouraged as stickiness could be due to the morphology of the fissure and the probe could encourage cavitation. The anatomy of the area also tends to favour spread of the lesion, which often occurs rapidly. As fissure caries is less affected by fluoride and oral hygiene (OH), fissure sealant (f/s) is preferable to watching and waiting particularly in high-risk individuals. Occlusal caries evident on b/w radiographs should not always be excised. If the tooth is

4 Faculty of General Dental Practitioners 2013 *Selection Criteria for Dental Radiography*, RCS (Eng).

fissure sealed or restored, check the margins very carefully, and if intact, monitoring the lesion radiographically is often justified initially. If marginal integrity is not intact, investigate the area with a small round bur. The 'cavity' can be aborted if no caries is found and the surface sealed.

Approximal caries Currently accepted practice:
- If lesion is confined to enamel on b/w radiograph, institute preventive measures and keep under review.
- If lesion has penetrated dentine radiographically, a restoration is indicated unless serial radiographs show that it is static.

If in doubt whether an approximal lesion has cavitated or not, an elastic orthodontic separator may be fitted for 3–7 days to allow surface visualization.

Recall intervals
This subject has evoked considerable controversy, some arguing that regular attendance puts a patient more at risk of receiving replacement fillings, while others contend that regular and frequent check-ups are necessary to monitor prevention.[5] In fact, it would appear that only a minority of the British public attend for 6-monthly check-ups. The available evidence suggests that there is no clear benefit for recall intervals of <1yr for healthy patients, although the at-risk patient often needs to be seen more frequently.[6] In addition, as changing dentist ↑ the likelihood of replacement restorations the profession has to re-examine its criteria for replacement.

In the UK, guidance from the National Institute for Health and Care Excellence (NICE) recommends that dental recall intervals ('oral health review' intervals) should be determined by the needs of the individual patient based on a risk assessment of existing disease progressing or new disease developing. For adult patients this interval can be between 3 and 24 months and for children 3 and 12 months.[5]

A child's first check-up should occur once the first teeth have erupted (i.e. usually between 6 months and 1yr of age).

5 NICE 2004 *Dental Checks: Intervals Between Oral Health Reviews* (CG19) (∽ https://www.nice.org.uk/guidance/CG19).

6 N. B. Pitts & E. A. Kidd 1992 *Br Dent J* **172** 225.

Fluoride

The history of fluoride is covered well in other texts.[7]

Mechanisms of the action of fluoride in reducing dental decay (See Fig. 2.2.)

The concentration of fluoride in enamel ↑ with ↑ fluoride content of water supply and ↑ towards the surface of enamel.

Pre-eruptive effects Enamel formed in the presence of fluoride has:
• Improved crystallinity and ↑ crystal size, and ∴ ↓ acid solubility.
• More rounded cusps and fissure pattern, but the effect is small.

Discontinuation of systemic fluoride results in an ↑ in caries, ∴ pre-eruptive effects must be limited.

Post-eruptive effects NB: newly erupted teeth derive the most benefit.
• Inhibits demineralization and promotes remineralization of early caries. Also enhances the degree and speed of remineralization and renders the remineralized enamel more resistant to further attack.
• ↓ acid production in plaque by inhibiting glycolysis in cariogenic bacteria.
• An ↑ concentration of fluoride in plaque inhibits the synthesis of extracellular polysaccharide.
• It has been suggested that fluoride affects pellicle and plaque formation, but this is unsubstantiated.

At a high pH, fluoride is bound to protein in plaque. A drop in pH results in release of free ionic fluoride, which augments these actions. NB: fluoride is more effective in reducing smooth surface than pit and fissure caries.

Safety and toxicity of fluoride

Fluoride is present in all natural waters to some extent. Many simple chemicals are toxic when consumed in excess, and the same is true of fluoride.

Fluoride is absorbed rapidly, mainly from the stomach. Peak blood levels occur 1h later. It is excreted via the kidneys, but traces are found in breast milk and saliva. The placenta only allows a small amount of fluoride to cross, ∴ prenatal fluoride is relatively ineffective.

Fluorosis Fluorosis (or mottling) occurs due to a long-term excessive consumption of fluoride. It is endemic in areas with a high level of fluoride occurring naturally in the water. Clinically, it can vary from faint white opacities to severe pitting and discoloration. Histologically, it is caused by ↑ porosity in the outer third of the enamel. The degree of mottling/fluorosis ↑ as the concentration of fluoride (parts per million (ppm)) in the water supply ↑.

Toxicity
• Safely tolerated dose (STD). Dose below which symptoms of toxicity are unlikely = 1mg/kg body weight.
• Potentially lethal dose (PLD). Lowest dose associated with a fatality. Patient should be hospitalized = 5mg/kg body weight.
• Certainly lethal dose (CLD). Survival unlikely = 32–64mg/kg body weight.

7 J. J. Murray et al. 2003 *Prevention of Oral Disease* (4e), OUP.

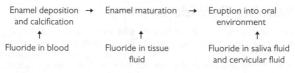

Fig. 2.2 Mechanisms of the action of fluoride.

Fluoride concentration in various products
- Standard fluoride (F) toothpastes:
  - 1000ppm F = 1mg F/mL.
  - 1500ppm F = 1.5mg F/mL.
- Daily fluoride mouthrinse 0.05% NaF = 0.023% F = 0.23mg F/mL.
- Acidulated phosphate fluoride (APF) gel 1.23% F = 12.3mg/mL.
- Fluoride varnish 5% NaF = 2.26% F = 22.6mg/mL.

To reach the 5mg F/kg threshold (requiring hospitalization) a 5yr-old (about 19kg) would have to ingest 95 (1mg F) tablets, 63mL of 1500ppm toothpaste, or 7.6mL of 1.23% of APF gel.

Antidotes <5mg F/kg body weight—large volume of milk. >5mg F/kg body weight—refer to hospital quickly for gastric lavage. If any delay give intravenous (IV) calcium gluconate and an emetic.

▶ For advice about managing fluoride overdose contact the National Poisons Information Service through dialling 111 if in the UK.

Health benefits vs risks of fluoride A number of detailed systematic reviews have been conducted to investigate the efficacy and safety of fluoride, especially in the context of public water fluoridation schemes.[8,9,10] These have all essentially come to the same conclusions:
- Water fluoridation is beneficial in reducing dental caries.
- While a link with cancer (specifically osteosarcoma) has been suggested by some authors, all major systematic reviews have concluded that no conclusive evidence of such a link exists.
- ↑ the level of fluoride in water supplies to optimal levels is accompanied by an ↑ prevalence of dental fluorosis, mostly mild and not considered to be of aesthetic concern.
- Most systematic reviews have concluded that fluoridation has little or no effect on the prevalence of bony fractures.

8 E. G. Knox 1985 *Fluoridation of Water and Cancer: A Review of the Epidemiological Evidence*, HMSO.

9 M. McDonagh et al. 2000 *A Systematic Review of Public Water Fluoridation*, University of York NHS Centre for Reviews and Dissemination.

10 Australian National Health and Medical Research Council 2014, Australian Government.

Planning fluoride therapy

The most important action of fluoride is to favour remineralization of the early carious lesion. Although fluoride incorporated within developing enamel results in a high local concentration following acid attack, the maximum benefit appears to be derived from frequent low-concentration topical administration.[11]

Systemic fluoride

▶ To minimize the risk of mottling, only one systemic measure should be used at a time.

Water fluoridation At 1ppm (1mg F per litre), water fluoridation reduces caries by 50%. The main advantages are systemic and topical effect; no effort is required on the part of the individual; and the low cost. Yet despite this, only 10% of the UK population has fluoridated water. In some countries school water has been fluoridated, but a concentration of 5ppm is required to offset the less frequent intake.

Fluoride drops and tablets The regimen (mg F per day) depends upon drinking water content (Table 2.1). This approach can be almost as effective as fluoridated water, but requires good parental motivation. Unfortunately, compliance is generally poor, so benefit as a public health measure is questionable.

Milk 2.5–7ppm F has been tried successfully.

Salt Cheap and effective for rural communities in developing countries where water fluoridation is not feasible.

Topical fluoride

Professionally applied fluorides Overall, there is a caries ↓ of 20–40%. Gels or foams applied in trays are still popular in some parts of the world, but without adequate suction the systemic dosage can be high and patients may not tolerate these well. Hence, their use in the UK is not extensive. Fluoride varnish (e.g. Duraphat® 5% NaF) is useful for applying directly to individual lesions to aid arrest. Fluoride varnish has been shown to be effective in ↓ caries incidence in children, and regular application (two times per year ↑ to three or four times per year where caries risk is ↑) is now advocated for all children over age 3yrs deemed to be at risk of caries. However, it should be applied carefully and sparingly, especially in young children as it contains 22,600ppm fluoride. Application of Duraphat® varnish is C/I in patients suffering from asthma.

Rinsing solutions C/I in children <7yrs. The concentration depends upon the frequency of use: 0.2% fortnightly/weekly or 0.05% daily. Daily use is the most beneficial. Caries reductions of 16–50% have been reported with rinsing alone. The most widely used solution is sodium fluoride. Should be done at a separate time to brushing.

Toothpastes Aid tooth cleaning, but, most importantly, provide fluoride. In the UK they contain abrasives (to a specified abrasivity standard), detergents, humectants, flavouring, binding agents, preservatives, and active agents, including:

---

11 DOH 2017 *Delivering Better Oral Health—An Evidence-based Toolkit for Prevention* (🖰 http://www.dh.gov.uk).

- Fluoride. Most toothpastes contain sodium monofluorophosphate &/ or NaF, in concentrations of 1000–1500ppm (i.e. 1–1.5mg per 1cm of paste). Caries reductions of 15% (in fluoridated areas) to 30% (in non-fluoridated areas) are reported. Low-dose formulations for children <7yrs containing <500ppm are available, to ↓ risk of mottling, but such low concentrations are unlikely to be effective at significantly reducing caries.
- Anti-calculus agents, e.g. sodium pyrophosphate, can ↓ calculus formation by 50%.
- Desensitizing agents, e.g. 10% strontium or potassium chloride, or 1.4% formaldehyde.
- Antibacterial agents, e.g. triclosan.

Toothbrushing
- Brush twice daily (bd) with a >1000ppm fluoride toothpaste. >3yrs and those at ↑ risk of developing caries use 1350–1500ppm fluoride toothpaste.
- Children <3yrs of age should use a 'smear' and >3yrs a small pea-size blob (<0.3mL) of toothpaste.
- Spit out well, but do not rinse, after brushing.
- Brushing with fluoride toothpaste should start as soon as the first teeth erupt (about 6 months of age). Parents should supervise brushing up to at least 7yrs of age to avoid over-ingestion of toothpaste and ensure adequate plaque removal.

Recommended daily fluoride supplementation (mg F) For children considered to be at high risk of caries and who live in areas with water supplies containing <0.3ppm, see Table 2.1 (see guidelines[12,13]).

Fluoride supplement (drops and tablets) May be prescribed for children deemed to be at risk of developing caries living in areas with less than optimal fluoride in the water supply. Compliance with self-administered fluoride supplements is often poor (i.e. parents often forget to administer them regularly).

Fluoridation of water still remains the most cost-effective method.

Other products
Casein phosphopeptide/amorphous calcium phosphate These components based on concentrated milk proteins show promise for both caries prevention and enamel remineralization.

Chlorhexidine varnish This has also shown some efficacy in preventing approximal caries.

Table 2.1 Daily fluoride supplementation

Age	mg F per day
6 months to 3yrs	0.25
3yrs to 6yrs	0.5
>6yrs	1.0

12 BDA/BSPD/BASCD 1997 *Br Dent J* **182** 6.

13 R. Holt et al. *Int J Paed Dent* 1996 **6** 139.

Bacterial plaque and dental decay

Evidence for role of bacteria in dental caries

- *In vitro*—incubating teeth with plaque and sugar in saliva results in caries.
- Animal experiments, e.g. germ-free rodents fed a cariogenic diet do not develop caries, but following the introduction of *Streptococcus mutans* caries occurs.
- Epidemiological evidence showing that a supply of bacterial substrate results in caries.
- Clinical experiments, e.g. stringent removal of plaque ↓ decay.

A correlation has been found between the presence of *Streptococcus mutans* and caries. This is not surprising, because this organism is acidophilic, can synthesize acid rapidly from sugar, and produces a sticky extracellular polysaccharide which helps bind it to the tooth. However, caries can develop in the absence of *S. mutans*, and its presence does not inevitably lead to decay, e.g. root caries has been associated with *S. salivarius* and *Actinomyces* species. *Lactobacillus* species are also acidophilic and have been implicated in fissure caries. In addition, plaque prevents acid diffusing away from the enamel and hinders the neutralizing effect of salivary buffers.

Methods of preventing caries by bacterial control

Physical removal of plaque

- By a professional. If sufficiently frequent it can ↓ caries,[14] but is impractical as a population-based approach.
- By the individual. The available evidence suggests that toothbrushing alone is not an effective method of caries control. However, a long-term study has demonstrated much less oral disease, including dental caries, in patients who maintain good plaque control over many years.[15] Also ↓ gingivitis.

Chemical removal of plaque To achieve more than a transitory effect, an antiseptic needs to be retained in the mouth. Chlorhexidine, a positively charged bactericidal and fungicidal antiseptic, is capable of this. It is attracted to the negatively charged proteins on the surface of teeth and oral mucosa and in saliva from where it gradually leaches out. It is available as a 0.2% mouthwash and a 1% gel which are cheaper over the counter than by prescription. Although the main application of chlorhexidine is in the management of gingivitis, it has been shown to be effective at ↓ caries when used regularly.[16] While its widespread use for this purpose is not practical, it can be helpful in the management of disabled patients or those with ↓ salivary flow. Unwanted effects include staining, disturbance of taste, and parotid swelling (which is reversible). It is less effective in the presence of a large build-up of plaque and is inactivated by commercial toothpastes.

14 J. Lindhe et al. 1975 *Comm Dent Oral Epidemiol* **3** 150.

15 J. M. Broadbent et al. 2011 *JADA* **142** 415.

16 H. Loe et al. 1972 *Scand J Dent Res* **80** 1.

A variety of pre-brushing rinses are now available. Research suggests that these do have a small beneficial effect if used in conjunction with toothbrushing.[17]

Immunization against caries As no vaccine is completely safe, the ethics of vaccinating against caries, an avoidable non-lethal disease, have been hotly debated.[18] Yet, despite considerable research and efforts to produce one, there is currently no such vaccine commercially available. This may be due to a number of problems:

- Which species of mutans streptococci to target, and whether pathogenicity would then shift to another species.
- Lack of strong economic interests.
- Differing modes of action in monkeys and rodents, ∴ questionable relevance of experiments to humans.
- Cross-reactivity with heart muscle in animal experiments.
- Duration of effect and acceptance by public. Some patients may prefer caries to repeated injections of a vaccine.

17   H. V. Worthington et al. 1993 *Br Dent J* **175** 322.

18   W. Sims 1985 *Comm Dent Health* **2** 129.

Fissure sealants

Pits and fissures provide a sheltered niche for bacterial proliferation. Toothbrush bristles are too wide to fit into these areas, making complete plaque removal impossible. A fissure sealant (f/s) is a material that provides an impervious barrier to the fissure system to prevent the development of caries.

Historical Several approaches to ↓ fissure caries have been tried:
- Chemical Rx of the enamel, e.g. with silver nitrate.
- Prophylactic odontotomy. This involved restoring the fissure with amalgam (hardly a preventive approach!).
- Sealing of the fissures. Several materials have been tried, including black copper cement (not retained), cyanoacrylate (toxic), polyurethane, and resin-modified glass ionomer (GI) cement. The most common type of f/s is a composite resin used with an acid-etch technique. Resin-based sealants show better retention.

Is there a need for sealants? In developed countries, the ↓ in caries seen in recent years has not been uniform for all tooth surfaces. Part of this ↓ is due to an ↑ availability of fluoride, leading to a greater reduction in approximal, rather than in pit and fissure caries. Therefore, the need for a method of preventing occlusal caries is even more pressing.

Are sealants effective? To be effective, f/s need to be carefully applied to susceptible teeth. They are most valuable in recently erupted (especially first) molars, but moisture control may be difficult. Therefore, sealants should be monitored and replaced if lost. For maximum benefit, teeth should be sealed as soon as practicable after eruption and certainly within 2yrs. Guidelines for placement of f/s have been described.[19,20]

Patient selection F/s should be provided for 6s in:
- children with impairments.
- those with extensive caries in the 1° dentition (decayed, missing, filled surfaces index is 2 or more).

Children with caries-free 1° dentitions do not need routine f/s of 6s but should be monitored regularly. F/s of 1° molars is not normally recommended.

Tooth selection For children who fulfil the earlier given criteria:
- All susceptible fissures of permanent teeth should be sealed—occlusal, fissures and cingulum, buccal, and palatal pits. Teeth should be sealed as soon as sufficiently erupted for adequate moisture control.
- Where occlusal caries affects one 6, the remaining caries-free permanent molars (6s and 7s) should be f/s.

19 BSPD 2000 *Int J Paed Dent* **10** 174.

20 Scottish Dental Clinical Effectiveness Programme (SCDEP) 2018 *Prevention and Management of Dental Caries in Children* (⅋ http://www.sdcep.org.uk).

If there is doubt about a stained fissure, a b/w radiograph should be taken. If the lesion is in enamel, f/s and monitor clinically and radiographically. If in doubt, carry out an enamel biopsy. If the lesion extends to dentine place a preventive resin restoration (PRR), providing the cavity does not extend to more than one-third of the occlusal surface, in which case a conventional restoration is required. Composite resin-based sealant retention: >85% after 1yr and >50% after 5yrs.[21]

Discussion of the cost-effectiveness of sealants compared to restoration has been well aired over the years, which is surprising given that the end results are not comparable. A f/s is highly effective and reduces the incidence of dentine caries over 4yrs by >50%.

Types of fissure sealant Sealants can be classified by polymerization method (light- or self-cure), resin system (Bis-GMA or urethane diacrylate), colour (clear or tinted), and whether they are filled or unfilled. The choice is one of personal preference; however, it has been pointed out that coloured/opaque sealants are more readily obvious to the patient and it is more noticeable if the sealant has been lost. An advantage of clear sealants is that they may allow visualization of decay through the resin. The retention rates of the different types are similar: success depends upon maintaining an absolutely dry field during application.

GI sealants do release fluoride but have poorer retention than resin sealants. They are useful for high caries-risk children as a temporary sealant where adequate isolation for successful placement of resin based sealants is not possible, e.g. partially erupted teeth/poor cooperation.

Resin fissure sealant technique
• Prophylaxis (this may be omitted if the tooth is already relatively free from plaque).
• Isolate and dry the tooth.
• Etch for the time recommended by the manufacturer (usually 20–40sec) with 30–50% phosphoric acid.
• Wash thoroughly, re-isolate, and dry well. If salivary contamination occurs or parts of the surface have not etched well, re-etch.
• Application of a suitable enamel bonding agent may improve retention.
• Apply f/s (method depends upon delivery system).
• After polymerization try to remove the sealant. If satisfactory, occlusal adjustment is usually not required unless a large volume has inadvertently been applied or a filled resin is used.

Follow-up F/s should be monitored clinically and where appropriate, radiographically (b/w). Defective sealants should be replenished to maintain their marginal integrity.

21 National Institutes of Health 1984 *J Am Dent Assoc* **108** 233.

Sugar

Sugar is used to refer to the mono- and disaccharide members of the carbo-hydrate family. Monosaccharides include glucose (dextrose or corn sugar), fructose (fruit sugar), galactose, and mannose. Disaccharides include lac-tose (in milk), maltose, and sucrose (cane or beet sugar). Polysaccharides (starch) are chains of glucose molecules and are not readily broken down by the oral flora. Dietary sugars have been classified as intrinsic when they are part of the cells in a food (vegetables and fruit) or extrinsic (milk sugar or, the real baddy, non-milk extrinsic sugar, e.g. table sugar). Both intrinsic and extrinsic sugars may cause decay, although non-milk extrinsic sugars are most cariogenic.

Evidence for the role of sugar in dental caries
- Epidemiological evidence:[22]
  - Worldwide comparison of sugar consumption and caries levels.
  - Low caries experience of people on low-sugar diet, e.g. wartime diet; patients with hereditary fructose intolerance.
  - ↑ caries experience following ↑ availability of sugar, e.g. Inuits.
  - Cross-sectional studies relating caries experience to sugar intake.
- Clinical studies, e.g. Vipeholm study and Turku sugar study (xylitol).
- Plaque pH studies, *in vivo* and *in vitro*. See the Stephan curve in Fig. 2.3.
- Animal experiments, e.g. rats fed by stomach tube do not develop caries.

Sucrose is considered a major culprit—it is the most commonly available sugar and able to facilitate production of extracellular polysaccharide in plaque. However, other sugars can also cause caries, e.g. frequent con-sumption of fruit-based drinks is known to be a key factor in the develop-ment of early childhood caries (ECC). In order of ↓ cariogenicity:
- Sucrose, glucose, fructose, maltose.
- Galactose, lactose.
- Complex carbohydrate (e.g. starch in rice, bread, potatoes).

The frequency of sugary intakes and the interval between them, the total amount of sugar eaten in the diet, and the concentration of sugar and sticki-ness of a food have been shown to be important. The acidogenicity of a sugar-containing food can be modified by other items in the food or meal. Foods that stimulate salivary flow can speed the return of plaque pH to normal (e.g. cheese, sugar-free gum, salted peanuts).

Sugar and health
In 1989, the Committee on Medical Aspects of Food Policy (COMA) Panel on Dietary Sugars and Human Disease reported that dental decay is posi-tively associated with the frequency and amount of non-milk extrinsic sugar consumption. However, while sugar may contribute to the excess calorific intake which causes obesity and predisposes towards diabetes or coronary heart disease, there is no direct evidence linking sugar intake and these medical conditions.[23]

22 A. J. Rugg-Gunn 1993 *Nutrition and Dental Health*, OUP.

23 COMA 1989 *Dietary Sugars and Human Disease*, HMSO.

Prevention of caries by ↓ the availability of microbial substrate in food

This approach aims to take into account the modern habit of 'snacking' (also known as 'grazing'):

- Remove sugar from selected foods.
- Substitute sugar with non-cariogenic sweeteners.
- Modify sugar-containing foods so that they are less cariogenic.

Modification of only a restricted number of snack foods would probably be insufficient to have a significant effect.

Fig. 2.3 is a Stephan curve showing the pH drop that occurs after a sugary drink is consumed (shown by arrow). The dashed line indicates the critical pH; below this pH demineralization will occur. The shape of the curve is affected by a number of factors, including the type of sugary food, buffering potential of the saliva, and foods or drinks ingested after the sugary challenge.

Alternative sweeteners

(In Table 2.2 sweetness of sucrose = 1.)

The bulk sweeteners (largely polyols) can cause osmotic diarrhoea if consumed in large amounts and are ∴ C/I in small children. However, it is probably wise to avoid all artificial sweeteners in pre-school children. The bulk sweeteners are isocalorific with sucrose, whereas the intense sweeteners are low calorie.

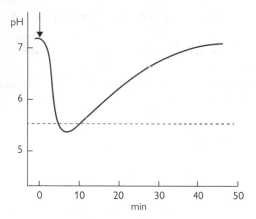

Fig. 2.3 Plaque pH drop after consumption of a sugary drink.

Recommendations for ↓ the risk of caries
- Reduce frequency of consumption of sugar-containing foods and drinks, especially between meals.
- Reduce frequency of consumption of fruit-based drinks, even those labelled 'no added sugar'.
- A few snack foods are 'safe' (e.g. nuts and cheese), and foods containing artificial sweeteners may be less decay-producing.
- Foods containing starch and sugar in combination (e.g. cakes, biscuits) and carbonated sugary drinks are especially decay-producing.

Table 2.2 Comparison of sweeteners

Sweetener	Type	Sweetness	Cariogenicity	Comments
Sorbitol	Bulk sweetener	0.5	Low	Isocalorific to sugar
Mannitol	Bulk sweetener	0.7	Low	
Xylitol	Bulk sweetener	1	None	Diarrhoea
Isomalt	Bulk sweetener	0.5	Low	
Lycasin®a	Bulk sweetener	0.75	Low	
Acesulfame	Intense	130	None	
Aspartame	Intense	200	None	C/I in phenylketonuria
Stevia	Intense	300	Thought to be lowb	Recently approved in EU and USA
Saccharin	Intense	500	None	Bitter aftertaste
Thaumatin	Intense	4000	None	

a Lycasin® is the trade name for hydrogenated glucose syrup (which didn't fit in the table!).

b Currently limited evidence from animal trials.

Dietary analysis and advice

Diet can affect teeth:

- *Pre-eruptively*—fluoride is the most important. The effect of calcium, phosphate, vitamins, and sugar is unclear, but is unlikely to be great.
- *Post-eruptively*—again, fluoride is important, as is sugar. Acidic foods or drinks can cause erosion (➲ Tooth wear/tooth surface loss, p. 252).

Dietary analysis

Aim To ↓ the time for which the teeth are at risk of demineralization and ↑ the potential remineralization period.

Indications (i) High caries activity, (ii) unusual caries pattern, and (iii) suspected dietary erosion.

Dietary advice should be tailored to the individual. This is most easily done after analysing the patient's present eating pattern.

Method A consecutive 3- or 4-day analysis (including at least one weekend day) is the most widely used, with the patient recording the time, content, and quantity of food/drink consumed. In addition, toothbrushing and bedtime should be indicated. When the form is returned, the entries should be checked with the patient.

Analysis

- Ring the main meals. If in any doubt, identify those snacks that contain complex carbohydrate. Assess nutritional value of meals.
- Underline all sugar intakes in red.
- Identify between-meal snacks and note any associations, e.g. following insubstantial meals or at school.
- Decide on a maximum of three recommendations.

Dietary advice This should include an explanation of the effect of between-meals eating and sugary drinks. It must also be personal, practical, and positive! The suggestion that a child should select crisps when friends are buying sweets is more likely to be followed than total abstinence.
Some helpful hints:

- Save sweets to be eaten on 1 day, e.g. Saturday dinnertime, or to be eaten at the end of a meal.
- All-in-one chocolate bars are preferable to packets of individual sweets.
- Foods which ↑ salivary flow (e.g. cheese, sugar-free chewing gum) can help to reverse the pH drop due to sugar if eaten afterwards.
- Treacle, honey, and fruit (especially fruit juice) are cariogenic.
- Artificial sweeteners should be avoided in pre-school children.
- Fibrous foods, e.g. apples, are preferable to a sucrose snack, but they can still cause decay and there is no evidence that they can clean teeth.

Where the nutritional content of meals is inadequate, considerable tact is necessary. It may be possible to suggest that larger meals would reduce the temptation to eat snacks. For children who are 'picky' eaters, snacks and sweets saved until the end of a meal can act as an encouragement to consume more food at mealtimes.
But remember that while cheese, peanuts, and crisps may constitute a safe snack in dental terms, they are all high in fat, and peanuts can be inhaled

by small children. Also, 'diet' cola drinks are sugar free, but can still cause erosion if large quantities are drunk.

Therefore, dental dietary advice should be given in the wider context of the general health of the individual, i.e. ↓ consumption of sugars and fats, and ↑ consumption of fibre-rich starchy foods, fresh fruit, and vegetables. Meals provide a better nutritional balance than snacks. Hence, good eating/drinking at mealtimes and avoiding between-meals snacking is healthy.

Dental health education

What is it? The objective of dental health education is to influence the attitude and behaviour of the individual to maintain oral health for life and prevent oral disease.
- *Primary prevention*—seeks to prevent the initial occurrence of a disease or disorder and is aimed at healthy individuals.
- *Secondary prevention*—aims to arrest disease through early detection and Rx.
- *Tertiary prevention*—helps individuals to deal with the effects of the disease and to prevent further recurrence.

Who should give it? All health professionals. In practice, many patients relate better to advice from a hygienist or nurse.

What information should be given? It is important that the information given is factual and that different sources do not give conflicting advice. In order to unify the profession's approach, the Health Development Agency published a policy document[24] laying out four simple messages which are still recommended:
- Restrict sugar-containing foods to mealtimes.
- Clean teeth and gums thoroughly bd with a fluoride toothpaste.
- Attend the dentist regularly.
- Water fluoridation is beneficial.

How? The way in which the advice is imparted is as important as its content. There are three main routes:
- The mass media. This is an expensive alternative and, while commercial advertisers tempt the consumer, the success of a dental health education message which is exhorting the public to stop doing something they find pleasurable is not guaranteed.
- Community programmes. These need to be carefully planned, targeted, and monitored.
- One-to-one in the clinical environment. This is usually the most successful approach, because the message can be tailored to the individual and reinforcement is facilitated. However, it is expensive in terms of manpower.

Individual dental health education Because many patients find the dental surgery threatening, it may be better to choose a more neutral environment, e.g. a dental health or preventive unit. It is important that the information is given by someone the patient trusts and can relate to—this is not always the dentist! It is important also to have adequate time, as a hurried approach is of dubious value, and to choose words that the patient will understand.

24 R. S. Levine & C. R. Stillman-Lowe 2015 *The Scientific Basis of Oral Health Education* (7e) BDJ/Springer.

The following approach has been used successfully:
- Define the problem and its aetiology. For example, poor OH which has resulted in periodontal disease—is it because the patient lacks motivation or the appropriate skills? This stage includes questioning the patient to discover how often and for how long he or she brushes.
- Set realistic objectives. It is better to start with trying to motivate the patient to brush well once a day rather than teaching them how to floss.
- Demonstrate on the patient, as this makes the advice more relevant, and more likely to be remembered.
- Monitor by comparing plaque scores before and after. This not only enables you to monitor improvement but also allows improvements in the patient's OH behaviour to be reinforced.
- Remember that everyone responds well to praise, so if a patient is doing well, tell them.

Keys to successful dental health education
- Relevant to the individual, their lifestyle and problems.
- Keep the message simple. Too much information may be counter-productive.
- Repetition of message.
- Positive reinforcement.

Where to go for help or information Advice on preparing a talk on dental health education, setting up a preventive unit, or even a health programme can be obtained from Health Education England and more specifically your Local Education and Training Board (🖰 http://www.hee.nhs.uk).

Provision of dental care

Delivery of care

General Dental Service This is the main source of dental care for the majority of the population (whether National Health Service (NHS) or private).

Salaried Dental (Community) Service The Community Dental Service (CDS) was formed from the School Dental Service in 1974.

In 1989, the remit of the CDS was expanded (the guidance being updated in 1997) to cover the following:
• Provision of oral health promotion.
• Rx for patients for whom there is evidence they would not otherwise seek Rx from the GDS, e.g. patients with special needs.
• Rx of patients who have experienced difficulty obtaining Rx from the GDS (normally termed the 'safety net' function).
• Provision of Rx which may not be generally available in the GDS.
• Dental health screening of children in state schools and other vulnerable groups with particular special needs. (This activity has been reduced in recent years.)
• Epidemiology to assist the planning of local health services and as part of coordinated national surveys.

Community Dental Services, Salaried General Dental Services, &/or Emergency Dental Services These services have undergone significant changes in recent years. In many areas of the UK, they have been managerially amalgamated and are now known as *Salaried Primary Dental Care Services*. The range of services provided and patients accepted by such services can vary between localities and many no longer offer 'safety-net' services with more emphasis on care delivery to patients with disability, co-morbidity, and the elderly.

Hospital service The role of the consultant service is to provide specialist advice and Rx, in addition to postgraduate training.

Receipt of care

Two factors are important:
- Availability and accessibility of dental services. Research shows that a greater proportion of the public visit the dentist regularly where the dentist-to-population ratio is high. This ratio tends to follow a geographical pattern, with the greatest number of dentists in the south-east.
- Social class affects both the incidence of dental disease and the uptake of dental care. Interestingly, the differences in caries experience between the social classes are much lower in fluoridated regions.

Because dentists have traditionally preferred to practise in leafy suburbs rather than poor inner-city areas, these effects are often compounded.

Barriers to the uptake of dental care

Aside from the problems experienced by patients accessing NHS dental care, research has shown that the two main barriers to regular uptake of dental care by the general public are anxiety and cost.[25]

Anxiety This manifests as fear of pain or a particular procedure, or a feeling of vulnerability brought about by relinquishing control to the dentist in the sensitive area of the mouth. A patient's first impressions are important as the reception they receive from staff and the environment in which they wait to be seen could either allay or reinforce their anxieties. The attitude of the dentist is also a significant factor: a 'good' dentist has a friendly, personal touch and explains what Rx is going to involve.

Cost The perception still exists that dental Rx is expensive. Patients often find the way in which the charges are calculated confusing but welcome an estimate of the costs prior to Rx.

Furthermore, the pattern of attendance varies throughout life, with children now enjoying a visit to the dentist, but adolescents breaking the habit of regular attendance due to apathy &/or other pressures on their time. A return to the dentist may be triggered by pregnancy and desire to provide a good example to the children, or a need for urgent Rx and a fear of becoming edentulous.

25 K. B. Hill et al. 2003 *Br Dent J* **195** 654.

Dentistry for people with disabilities

A disabled person is someone with a physical or mental impairment which has a substantial and long-term adverse effect on their ability to carry out normal day-to-day activities.

Intellectual impairment (mental disability/learning difficulty) Prevalence 3%. Classified into mild (IQ 50–70) and severe (IQ <50).

Many cases lack a well-defined aetiology but there are some subgroups where the cause/diagnosis is known:
- Down syndrome, fragile-X syndrome.
- Cerebral palsy, birth anoxia.
- Meningitis, rubella.
- Autism, microcephaly.

Physical impairment Most common is cerebral palsy, which is the motor manifestation of cerebral damage. Many patients with cerebral palsy have normal IQs, but ↑ muscle tone and hyperactive reflexes can make Rx difficult. Many can be treated in general dental practice provided there is wheelchair access.

Medical impairment 1% of children have heart disease, bleeding disorders, diabetes, or kidney disease.

Sensory impairment That is, blindness or deafness (Fig. 2.4).

Many have more than one type of impairment.

The described groups are general disabilities. We also need to consider those who are orally disabled, i.e. have a gross oral problem or deficit which necessitates special dental Rx (e.g. cleft lip &/or palate).

Disability Discrimination Act 1995 The Act requires that:
- Employers must not discriminate against disabled employees.
- Service providers (including dentists) have to consider making reasonable adjustments to the way they deliver services so that disabled people can access them.

Problems
It is difficult to generalize, but usually mental disability provides the biggest challenge. Difficulties ↑ in patients with more than one impairment.
- Delivery of care. This has three aspects: (i) ↓ demand, due to low priority placed on dental health; (ii) lack of provision made to provide the necessary care; and (iii) practical difficulties in carrying out dental work.
- In general, disabled patients have ↓ plaque control and ↑ periodontal problems.
- Although caries incidence is not significantly ↑ compared to the normal population, the amount of untreated caries often is.
- Long-term sugared medications.
- Prevalence of hepatitis in institutionalized patients.
- Dentures may be impractical ∴ extractions are not a realistic solution to the problems of providing dental Rx.

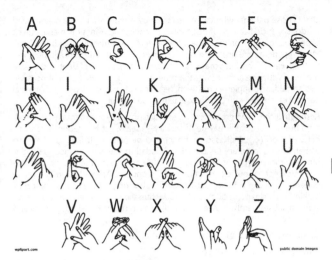

Fig. 2.4 The Standard Manual Alphabet.

Consent See ➔ Consent, p. 135.

Management

This is difficult to generalize. Patients with less severe disabilities can be treated in dental practice. Those with severe medical &/or mental impairments are probably best managed by a specialist who will have ↑ access to specialist facilities.

Rx planning An initial plan should be formulated ignoring the disability. This can then be discussed with the patient, parent, or carer and modified for the individual. Where Rx needs are not urgent, it is advisable to start with OHI and prevention, then reassess Rx requirements in the light of the response. For those patients for whom a satisfactory standard of OH is not possible, restorative Rx should aim to ↓ plaque accumulation. Excellent guidelines for the dental care of patients with disability and impairment have been produced by the British Society for Disability and Oral Health.[26]

26 British Society for Disability and Oral Health (🕮 http://www.bsdh.org.uk).

OHI Those patients who can brush their own teeth should be encouraged to do so. Modification of toothbrush handles (➔ General management problems, p. 330) or purchase of an electric toothbrush may be helpful. Where patients are unable to brush their teeth, instruction should be given to their carer. The best method is to stand behind the patient and cradle the head with one arm, leaving the other free to brush. However, if possible this should be supplemented with regular professional cleaning. Chemical control of plaque with chlorhexidine may be helpful.

Restorative care The greatest problems are posed by the mentally impaired. Kind but firm restraint may be necessary—ideally, get the patient's carer to help. A prop (e.g. McKesson rubber) may be needed. It is often easier to use an intraligamentary LA technique. Sedation may help reduce the spontaneous movements of cerebral palsy. In some cases there is no alternative but to carry out examination and Rx under GA. In addition, for those patients who can tolerate out-patient Rx, but only a little at a time, it may be kinder to clear a backlog under GA, thus allowing concentration on prevention subsequently. However, this approach requires special facilities and no medical C/I.

Down syndrome See ➔ Down syndrome, p. 783.

The Equality Act 2010
This legally protects people from discrimination in the workplace and in wider society by providing a legal framework protecting the rights of individuals while promoting a fair and more equal society. There are nine 'protected characteristics'.
- Age.
- Disability.
- Gender reassignment.
- Marriage and civil partnership.
- Pregnancy and maternity.
- Race.
- Religion or belief.
- Sex.
- Sexual orientation.

Dental care professionals

Dental care professionals (DPCs, previously known as professions complementary to dentistry) are a growth area in dentistry. With ↑ demand for dental Rx and restraints on healthcare costs, the advantages of delegating more routine tasks to dental auxiliaries is obvious. There is also improved job satisfaction for all members of the dental team.

The General Dental Council (GDC) now registers and regulates DCPs. This has resulted in a number of changes:

- Any registrant is able to own a practice and 'carry out the business of dentistry'.
- Registrants have to attain certain skills and competences before registration in a certain group and will be able to develop additional ones during their career. There are, however, some skills which registrants in a particular group would not develop without becoming a different type of registrant because those skills are 'reserved' to other groups.
- All registrants have to undertake verifiable continuing professional development (CPD).
- Dental nurses and technicians have to do 50h, dental therapists, hygienists, orthodontic therapists, and clinical dental technicians have to do 75h, and dentists 100h verifiable CPD in every 5yr cycle (➔ Continuing professional development, p. 772).[27]
- All registrants need to have professional indemnity cover.
- The requirement to carry out certain Rx under prescription from a dentist was removed by the GDC on 1 May 2013.[28]

The following classes of DCP are recognized and regulated by the GDC[29]:

- *Dental nurses*—provide clinical or other support to patients and other registrants. They are not permitted to diagnose disease or plan Rx.
- *Dental hygienists*—help patients maintain their oral health. They are not permitted to undertake any of the skill areas reserved to dental technicians, clinical dental technicians, and dentists.
- *Dental therapists*—carry out certain items of dental Rx under the prescription of a dentist. They are not permitted to undertake any of the skill areas reserved to dental technicians, clinical dental technicians, and dentists.
- *Orthodontic therapists*—carry out certain parts of orthodontic Rx under the prescription of a dentist. They are not permitted to diagnose disease, plan Rx, or activate archwires. This grade of auxiliary is widely employed in many countries, including the US and Scandinavia where their permitted duties may differ.
- *Dental technicians*—make dental devices under prescription from a dentist or clinical dental technician. They may also repair dentures direct to the public. They do not provide Rx or advice for patients as ascribed to hygienist, therapists, orthodontic therapists, or dentists.

27 GDC 2018 *CPD for Dental Professionals* (🖰 https://www.gdc-uk.org/education-cpd/cpd).

28 GDC 2013 *Guidance on Direct Access* (🖰 http://www.gdc-uk.org).

29 GDC 2009 *Scope of Practice* (🖰 http://www.gdc-uk.org).

- *Clinical dental technicians*—provide complete dentures directly to patients and other dental devices on prescription from a dentist. They are also qualified dental technicians. Patients with natural teeth or implants must see a dentist before the clinical dental technician can begin Rx. They do not provide Rx or advice for patients as ascribed to hygienist, therapists, orthodontic therapists, or dentists.

Lies, damn lies, and statistics

Sugar

- The UK per capita consumption of sugar is >0.5kg/week.
- UK children receive about one-fifth to one-quarter of their energy intake from sugars. Of these, two-thirds are added sugars, more than two-thirds of which come from sweets, table sugar, and soft drinks.[30]
- 65% of all soft drink sales are to <15yr-olds.
- Low-income families consume more sugar/person/day than higher-income families.

Fluoride

- Water fluoridation ↓ caries experience and ↑ the proportion of children free of caries by between 5% and 64%.
- A cup of tea may contain up to 6ppm of fluoride. (One in three people in UK take teabags abroad with them on holiday!)
- At equivalent concentrations, there is no difference in the efficacy of sodium fluoride- or sodium monofluorophosphate-containing toothpastes.[31]

Caries

- A reduction of 10–60% in the caries experience of developed countries has been widely reported. This is thought to be due to a variety of factors, including fluoride toothpaste, ↑ public awareness, changes in infant feeding practices, ↓ sugar consumption, and antibiotics in the food chain.
- In addition, there has been a change in the pattern of carious attack, with a greater ↓ in smooth surface than fissure caries (perhaps reflecting the influence of fluoride).
- Small occlusal lesions appear to be becoming the predominant type of lesion.[32]
- *But* there is some evidence to suggest that the ↓ in caries may have slowed down and may have levelled out in young children.[33]

Adult dental health in the UK

The most recent survey showed that across almost all oral health indicators the trend for improvement seen in previous surveys has continued.[34] However, for those with caries or periodontal problems disease can be extensive. In 2009, 94% of adults had at least one natural tooth and 75% of adults said they cleaned their teeth at least once a day (Table 2.3).

30 A. J. Rugg-Gunn et al. 1986 *Hum Nutr Appl Nutr* **40A** 115.

31 *American Journal of Dentistry*, Special Issue, 1993.

32 A. Sheiham 1989 *Br Dent J* **166** 240.

33 R. R. Welbury et al. 2012 *Paediatric Dentistry* (4e), OUP.

34 Health and Social Care Information Centre (ℰ http://www.hscic.gov.uk).

Table 2.3 Survey of adult dental condition

	1978	1988	1998	2009
Proportion of adults edentulous	28%	21%	13%	6%
Average condition of teeth:				
Missing	9 teeth	7.8 teeth	7.2 teeth	6.3 teeth
Decayed	1.9 teeth	1 tooth	1.5 teeth	0.8 teeth
Filled	8.1 teeth	8.4 teeth	7 teeth	6.7 teeth
Sound	13 teeth	14.8 teeth	15.7 teeth	17.9 teeth

Child dental health

- The percentage of 5yr-olds with clinical decay experience in 2013 was 49%, with the mean number of teeth affected being 1.8. The results for 8yr-olds showed 59% and 2.0 affected teeth respectively.[35]
- In 2000/2001, 38% of 12yr-olds in England and Wales had caries experience in the permanent dentition.[36] In 2013, 34% of 12yr-olds and 46% of 15yr-olds in England, Wales, and Northern Ireland combined had obvious decay experience.
- In 2013, nearly a third of 5yr-olds and nearly half of 8yr-olds had obvious decay experience in the 1° dentition.
- Reductions in the extent and severity of tooth decay in permanent teeth of 12 and 15yr-olds was noted in England, Wales, and Northern Ireland between 2003 and 2013.
- 54% of 9yr-old children are in need of orthodontic Rx.

Indices

DMFT	decayed, missing, and filled permanent teeth.
dmft	decayed, missing, and filled deciduous teeth.
deft	decayed, exfoliated, and filled deciduous teeth.
dft	decayed and filled deciduous teeth.
DMFS	decayed, missing, and filled surfaces in permanent teeth.
Care index	Proportion of dmft that has been treated by filling (ft/dmft)

35 NHS Digital *2013 Child Dental Health Survey* (♂ https://digital.nhs.uk).

36 N. B. Pitts et al. 2002 *Comm Dent Health* 19 46.

Paediatric dentistry

Principal sources and further reading J. O. Andreasen et al. 2018 *Textbook and Color Atlas of Traumatic Injuries to the Teeth* (5e), Wiley Blackwell. British Society of Paediatric Dentistry policy documents and clinical guidelines ॐ http://www.bspd.co.uk. COPDEND/DOH 2007 *Child Protection and the Dental Team* ॐ http://www.cpdt.org.uk. M. S. Duggal et al. 2002 *Restorative Techniques in Paediatric Dentistry*, Dunitz. International Association of Dental Traumatology guidelines ॐ http://www.dentaltraumaguide.org. Scottish Dental Clinical Effectiveness Programme (SDCEP) 2018 *Prevention and Management of Dental Caries in Children* ॐ http://www.sdcep.org.uk/published-guidance/caries-in-children/. R. R. Welbury et al. 2018 *Paediatric Dentistry* (5e), OUP.

The child patient

▶ Treat the patient not the tooth.

Principal aims of Rx
- Development and maintenance of healthy, functional, and aesthetic 1° and 2° dentitions.
- Freedom from pain and infection.
- A happy and cooperative patient, if possible.
- Prevention is priority.

Points to remember
- Praise good behaviour (reinforcement ➲ Techniques for behaviour management, p. 60), ignore bad.
- Involve parents (they determine whether the child will return).
- Do not offer choice where there is none. Avoid rhetorical questions ('Would you like to sit on my chair?').
- Children have short attention spans (↑ with age).
- Children have ↓ sensory acuity (may confuse pressure with pain, sensibility tests less reliable).
- Children have ↓ manual dexterity, therefore need help with toothbrushing <7yrs.
- Formulate a comprehensive Rx plan, which should address both operative and preventive care.
- Start with simple procedures (e.g. OHI) and progress, at child's pace, to more complicated Rx.
- Set attainable targets for each visit and attain them.

The first visit
- Children should first visit a dentist as soon as they have teeth (i.e. about 6 months of age, in line with the British Society of Paediatric Dentistry's 'Dental Check by One' initiative). For young children, watching other members of the family receive a check-up prior to their turn may be preferable ('modelling').
- For infants and very young children a full dental examination is not essential if compliance is an issue. The emphasis should be on acclimatization, delivering age-appropriate preventive advice, and establishing rapport and a positive trusting professional relationship with the family.
- Confirm who is with the child and who has parental responsibility: check medical history and reason for attendance.
- Talk to the child: communication is the key to success!
- Show the patient the chair, mirror, and light, and explain their purpose ('Tell, show, do' ➲ Techniques for behaviour management, p. 60).
- Count the patient's teeth.
- If good progress, apply fluoride varnish if appropriate, or polish a few teeth if indicated, but don't tire child by attempting too much.
- Show the parent the child's teeth and what has been done that visit.
- Deal with the patient's complaint. If the child is in pain, the source of this needs to be determined and dealt with as quickly as possible.

- Younger children can sometimes be more successfully examined using the 'knee to knee' examination technique. The parent and dentist should sit facing each other, with their knees touching. The child should be seated on the parent's lap with the child facing them. The parent then lowers the child back on to his/her arm or the dentist's lap. Alternatively, the child can be 'cradled' by the parent, with the child's head toward the dentist, while the parent is sat upright in the dental chair.

Treatment planning for children

Diagnosis

Dental caries is often a rapidly progressing condition in children. It is essential to secure an accurate diagnosis (Δ) before making a Rx plan. This is achieved by taking a history, doing an examination, and, where appropriate, taking b/w radiographs.

▶ Bitewings are important for an accurate Δ unless approximal surfaces of the 1° molars can be visualized (i.e. the dentition is spaced).

Rx plan

The ultimate aim in dentistry for children is for the child to reach adulthood with good dental status and a positive attitude towards dental health and dental Rx. The final Rx plan will take into account the following considerations:

- Behaviour management (⊃ Techniques for behaviour management, p. 60).
- Prevention (Chapter 2).
- Restorative Rx (⊃ Restoration of carious primary teeth, p. 84).

▶ Remember to consider the developing occlusion:

- Long-term prognosis for first permanent molars (⊃ Extraction of poor-quality first permanent molars, p. 140).
- Palpate for 3|3 at 9–10yrs (⊃ Palatally displaced maxillary canines, p. 144).
- Beware disturbances in eruption sequence (⊃ Failure of/delayed eruption, p. 66) and asymmetry.
- Early referral to specialist for skeletal discrepancies, and for any significant abnormal findings.

The Rx plan is drawn up visit by visit. Each visit has both preventive and operative components (optimally aiming to deliver only one key preventive message per visit).

As it is considered to be easier to administer LA for maxillary teeth, these teeth are usually treated before mandibular teeth.

Restorative care (i.e. repair) without prevention is of limited value. Dental caries is treated by 'preventive' measures; 'restoration' primarily repairs the damage caused by the carious process.

In many circumstances, children with caries in 1° molars may be treated by prevention alone if oral hygiene is good.

Other considerations

Pain or evidence of infection may influence the order of the Rx plan.

Temporization (i.e. hand excavation and dressing) of open cavities at the start of Rx:

- Gives a good introduction to dentistry.
- Helps to minimize the risk of pain before Rx is completed.
- Improves comfort (e.g. during brushing and eating).
- Reduces salivary *Streptococcus mutans* count.
- Produces a preliminary coronal seal, enhancing the chances of pulpal recovery and survival.
- May provide slow release of fluoride in the short term if a glass ionomer cement (GIC) is used.

Delivery of care

Once the Rx needs have been decided upon:

- Be aware that Rx plans will change and evolve depending on various factors.
- Discuss with parent and patient the Rx options.
- LA/sedation/GA—consider and discuss risks vs benefits of each (⊃ Sedation, p. 61; ⊃ General anaesthesia, p. 62).
- Plan operative care at a pace appropriate to the child's ability to cope. Be prepared to reconsider method of delivery of care (e.g. sedation/ GA) if patient proves unable to accept Rx using original delivery strategy.
- Where necessary, consider referral to an appropriate service which can provide sedation or GA (e.g. paediatric departments or CDSs).

Look out for any signs of underlying medical or social problems which may modify the Rx plan:

- Systemic disease.
- Failure to thrive.
- Evidence of abuse or neglect (⊃ Safeguarding children, p. 100).
- Small stature.
- Other family circumstances which might affect care, such as home distance from the surgery and other family work or caring commitments.

The anxious child

Techniques for behaviour management

While many of these techniques often come with experience of treating children over a period of time, they can be learnt.

General principles
- Show interest in the child as a person.
- Touch > facial expression > tone of the voice > what is said.
- Don't ignore a child's fears or anxieties.
- Explain—why, how, when.
- Aim to reward behaviour which approximates to positive, desired patterns. Try to ignore inappropriate or negative behaviour.
- Get child involved in Rx, e.g. holding saliva ejector.
- Giving the child some control over the situation will also help them to relax, e.g. a stop signal such as raising their hand if they want you to stop for any reason ('enhancing control').
- The aim is to acclimatize the child to the new experiences associated with dental care, and establish a positive, trusting relationship with the child and family.

Tell, show, do Self-explanatory, but use language the child will understand.

Behaviour shaping Aim to guide and modify the child's responses, selectively reinforcing appropriate behaviour, while discouraging/ignoring inappropriate behaviour.

Reinforcement This is the strengthening of patterns of behaviour, usually by rewarding good behaviour with approval and praise. If a child protests and is uncooperative during Rx, do not immediately abandon the session and return them to the consolation of their parent, as this could inadvertently reinforce the undesirable behaviour. Try to ensure that something is completed (e.g. placing a dressing or even an examination) and focus on the successful completion of this, rather than the failure to complete what might have been originally planned.

Cognitive behavioural therapy A goal-oriented therapy which aims to help the child manage their anxiety by changing how they think and behave in relation to their problems.[1] This can be used with assistance from psychologists and chairside self-help methods.

Modelling Useful for children with little previous dental experience who are apprehensive. Encourage the child to watch other children of similar age or siblings receiving dental Rx happily. Watching a model on a video can also be helpful (e.g. 'my first dental check-up')

Desensitization Used for a child with pre-existing fears or phobias. Involves helping the patient to relax in the dental environment, then constructing a hierarchy of steps which gradually approximate to the fear-provoking stimulus for that patient. These steps are then introduced to the child gradually, with progression on to the next stimulus only when the child is able to cope with previous situation. It is a useful approach for managing needle phobia.

1 Z. Marshman 2017 *BDJ Team* 4 17010.

Should a parent accompany the child into surgery? This is essential on the first visit, and thereafter depends upon the child's age and the clinician's preference. If in doubt, ask about the child's preference. However, if the parent is dental phobic, their anxiety in the dental environment can be detrimental, so in these cases it is worth considering leaving the parent in the waiting room. Younger children are more likely to suffer 'separation anxiety', and many parents nowadays wish to be involved in, and informed about, their child's Rx. In the event of anxiety-related behaviour being encountered, a parental presence in the surgery does enable consent for any adjustment in Rx to be easily maintained. Ideally, parents should be motivated positively and instructed implicitly to act in the role of the 'silent helper'. A 'Parents' Guide' can be downloaded by parents to promote positive language and behaviour even before coming to the dentist for Rx.[2]

Sedation

Sometimes indicated for the genuinely anxious child who wishes to co-operate and also may help children with over-active gag reflexes and those for whom analgesia additional to LA may be needed (e.g. for difficult extractions such as 6s).

Inhalation Uses nitrous oxide/oxygen mixture to produce relative analgesia (RA) and is the most popular technique for use with children. Effective for ↓ anxiety and ↑ tolerance of invasive procedures in children who wish to cooperate but are too anxious to do so without help. It is a good idea not to carry out any Rx during the visit when the child is introduced to 'happy air'. Let the child position the nose piece themselves. See also ➔ Chapter 15.

Intravenous Not commonly used in children <12yrs of age. In the UK, IV sedation for dentistry in children <12yrs of age is considered to be an advanced technique, and should only be administered by staff specifically trained and experienced in use,[3] working in a clinical environment suited to the technique.

Oral Drugs such as midazolam and chloral hydrate have been advocated in the past. Specialized knowledge and skills are required, and midazolam is no longer indicated in the UK.

Intramuscular Rarely used in children.

Per rectum Popular in some countries.
Other options include intranasal sedation, acupuncture, and even acupressure, e.g. to help patients with a particularly severe gag reflex.

Hypnosis

Produces a state of altered consciousness and relaxation, though it cannot be used to make subjects do anything that they do not wish to do.[4] Appropriate training is necessary for those wishing to practise hypnosis. It can be described as either a way of helping the child to relax, or as a special kind of sleep.

2 ⌕ http://www.dental.llttf.com.

3 SDCEP 2018 *Conscious Sedation in Dentistry* (⌕ http://www.sdcep.org.uk/wp-content/uploads/2018/07/SDCEP-Conscious-Sedation-Guidance.pdf).

4 J. Hartland 2001 *Medical and Dental Hypnosis*, Churchill Livingstone.

General anaesthesia

Allows dental rehabilitation &/or dental extractions to be achieved at one visit. GA should only be used for dental Rx when absolutely necessary (i.e. when other methods of management, e.g. LA or sedation, are deemed unsuitable). Alternative strategies and the risks of GA must be discussed to enable parents to make an informed decision. The risk of unexpected death of a healthy person:

• Under GA has been estimated to be about 3 or 4 in 1 million.
• Under sedation has been estimated to be about 1 in 2 million.

Other behaviour problems and their management

• Some children attempt to delay Rx by a barrage of questions. This is usually a sign of anxiety, and firm but gentle handling is needed. Tell the patient that you understand their anxieties and that you will explain as you go along.
• The temper tantrum—try to establish communication. Praise good and ignore bad behaviour. Set an easily achievable goal, e.g. brushing teeth, and make sure it is achieved—comment on the positive outcome, rather than what was not achieved.

The child with toothache

When faced with a child with toothache, pulpal or periodontal pathology are the commonest causes. The dentist has to use clinical acumen to try and determine the state of the affected tooth/teeth, as this will decide the Rx required (Table 3.1). To that end, the following investigations may be used:

History Take a pain history (◑ Dental pain, p. 230) from the child and parent. Beware of variations in accuracy; anxious children may deny being in pain when faced with an eager dentist, whereas parents who feel guilty for delaying seeking dental Rx may exaggerate pain. Remember some pathology is painless, e.g. chronic periradicular periodontitis. Include medical history and confirm who the child has attended with.

Examination Swelling, temperature, lymphadenopathy? Intra-orally look for caries, abscesses, chronic buccal sinuses, mobile teeth (? due to exfoliation or apical infection), and erupting teeth. Colour change may indicate a history of trauma/loss of vitality.

Percussion Can be unreliable in children. Use gentle finger pressure first. Care is needed to establish a consistent response and compare with unaffected 'control' teeth. Consider the tone of the percussive note.

Sensibility testing Using thermal (e.g. ethyl chloride on cotton wool) or electrical stimulation. Again, establish a consistent, reliable response on a 'control' tooth before testing the tooth/teeth in question. Check for false positives, by altering the intensity of stimulus (e.g. cotton ball with ethyl chloride, followed by a dry cotton ball). Less reliable in 1° teeth.

Radiographs Bitewing X-rays may be useful. Not only are they less uncomfortable for small mouths than periapicals, but they also often show the bifurcation area where radiolucency 2° to periodontitis is often first apparent. An upper standard occlusal may be a helpful alternative to periapicals for anterior painful teeth.

Diagnosis Fleeting pain on hot/cold/sweet stimuli = reversible pulpitis. Longer-lasting pain on hot/cold/sweet stimuli &/or spontaneous pain with no initiating factor (? child kept awake) but no mobility, not tender to percussion (TTP) = irreversible pulpitis. Pain on biting and pressure &/or swelling and tenderness of adjacent tissues, mobility = acute periradicular periodontitis. Remember, the only 100% accurate diagnostic method is histological!

With a fractious child, keep examination and operative intervention to a minimum, doing only what is necessary to alleviate pain and win the child's trust.

If extractions under a GA are required, consider carefully the long-term prognosis of remaining teeth to try and avoid a repeat of the anaesthetic in the foreseeable future.

Other common potential causes of toothache include:
• Dentoalveolar trauma (◑ Dental trauma, p. 98).
• Mucosal ulceration (◑ Recurrent aphthous stomatitis (ulcers), p. 440).
• Teething (◑ Abnormalities of tooth eruption and exfoliation, p. 66).
• Mobility prior to exfoliation of deciduous teeth.

Table 3.1 Management of a child with toothache

Diagnosis	Emergency management	Definitive management
Reversible pulpitis	LA Excavate soft caries Restore temporarily with a zinc oxide/eugenol or GIC If exposed and vital—dress polyantibiotic paste (e.g. Ledermix®, Odontopaste®)	Pulpotomy or extraction (if time and cooperation allows, definitive Rx should be completed at the first visit)
Irreversible pulpitis	LA Excavate soft caries Dress polyantibiotic paste Restore temporarily with a zinc oxide/eugenol or GIC	Pulpotomy/pulpectomy or extraction
Acute periradicular periodontitis	LA (may not be necessary if loss of vitality is certain) Excavate soft caries until pulp chamber accessed—dress pulp chamber with polyantibiotic paste on cotton wool Seal with temporary dressing	Pulpotomy/pulpectomy or extraction
Acute periodontitis with facial swelling If: No or mild pyrexia (<38°C) Localized acute erythematous tender soft tissue swelling No significant involvement of 'danger areas' (see below in table) Not otherwise systemically unwell	Antibiotics and analgesics Ensure adequate fluid intake Establish drainage via tooth (and dress) if possible Review every 24h to ensure resolution	Extraction of tooth (or pulpectomy in selected cases) once acute phase has resolved
Acute periodontitis with facial swelling If: Significant pyrexia >38°C Poorly localized, spreading infection Systemically unwell: dehydration, lethargy, nausea, and vomiting Swelling involving a 'danger area', i.e. floor of mouth (inability to feel the lower border of the mandible is a serious sign) Trismus	Immediate referral to specialist centre Aggressive antibiotic Rx (e.g. amoxicillin and metronidazole)	Extraction of tooth &/or IO/EO drainage

Abnormalities of tooth eruption and exfoliation

Natal teeth Usually members of the 1° dentition, can sometimes be supernumerary, and should be retained if possible. Most frequently occur in lower incisor region and because of limited root development at that age, are often mobile. If in danger of being inhaled or causing problems with breastfeeding, they can be removed (usually removed with no LA or some topical LA is applied).

Teething As eruption of the 1° dentition coincides with a diminution in circulating maternal antibodies, teething is often blamed for systemic symptoms. However, local discomfort, and so disturbed sleep, may accompany the actual process of eruption. A number of proprietary 'teething' preparations are available, which usually contain a combination of an analgesic, an antiseptic, and anti-inflammatory agents for topical use. Having something hard to chew may help, e.g. teething ring. Some are designed to be cooled in the fridge, which can enhance their soothing ability.

Eruption cyst This is caused by an accumulation of fluid or blood in the follicular space overlying an erupting tooth. The presence of blood gives a bluish hue. Most rupture spontaneously, allowing eruption to proceed. Rarely, it may be necessary to marsupialize the cyst.

Failure of/delayed eruption

▶ Disruption of normal eruption sequence (Fig. 3.1) and asymmetry in eruption times of contralateral teeth >6 months warrants further investigation.

It must be remembered that there is a wide range of individual variation in eruption times. Developmental age is of more importance in assessing delayed eruption than chronological age.

General causes Hereditary gingival fibromatosis, Down syndrome, Gardner syndrome, hypothyroidism, cleidocranial dysostosis, and rickets.

Local causes
- Congenital absence. Is the most likely cause for failure of appearance of 2 (⊕ Hypodontia (oligodontia), p. 68).
- Crowding. Rx: extractions.
- Retention of 1° tooth. Rx: extraction of 1° tooth (after confirming permanent successor present).
- Supernumerary tooth. Is the most likely reason for failure of eruption of 1 (⊕ Hyperdontia, p. 68).
- Crown or root dilaceration (⊕ Dilaceration, p. 74).
- Dentigerous cyst.
- Trauma to 1° tooth leading to lateral or apical displacement of 2° incisor.
- Abnormal position of crypt. Rx: extraction or orthodontic alignment. See options for palatally displaced 3 (⊕ Palatally displaced maxillary canines, p. 144).
- 1° failure of eruption usually affects molar teeth. The aetiology is not understood. Although bone resorption proceeds above the unerupted tooth, they appear to lack any eruptive potential. Refer for advice, usually extraction is only option.

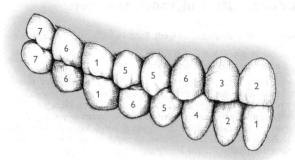

Fig. 3.1 Normal sequence of eruption (permanent dentition).

Infraoccluded (ankylosed) primary molars These occur where the 1° molar has failed to maintain its position relevant to the adjacent teeth in the developing dentition and is therefore below the occlusal level of adjacent teeth. Often due to ankylosis 2° to disruption in normal resorptive/repair cycle of exfoliation. This is usually self-correcting (if the permanent successor is present and not ectopic) and the affected tooth is exfoliated at the normal time. However, where the premolar is missing or ectopic, where the infraoccluded molar moves below the contact of adjacent teeth, or appears in danger of disappearing below the gingival level, extraction may be indicated (monitor carefully and if in doubt get a specialist opinion).

Ectopic eruption of first permanent molars Most commonly occurs in the upper arch—against the distal of E̲ occurs in 2–5% of children. It is an indication of crowding. In younger patients (<8yrs) many self-correct ('jump'). If still present after 4–6 months ('hold') or in older children, insertion of an orthodontic separating spring may allow the 6̲ to jump free. More severe impactions should be kept under observation. If the E̲ becomes abscessed or the 6̲ is in danger of becoming carious then the 1° tooth should be extracted. The resulting space loss can be dealt with later as part of the overall orthodontic Rx plan.

Premature exfoliation The most common reason for early tooth loss is extraction for caries. Traumatic avulsion is less common. More rarely, systemic disease such as neutropenia or leukaemia may result in an abnormal periodontal attachment and thus premature tooth loss. Alveolar bone loss in a young child is a serious finding and warrants urgent referral.

Abnormalities of tooth number

Anodontia
Means complete absence of all teeth. Rare. Partial anodontia is a misnomer.

Hypodontia (oligodontia)
Developmental absence of one or more teeth.

Prevalence 1° dentition: 0.1–0.9%, 2° dentition: 3.5–6.5%.[5] In Caucasians most commonly affected teeth are 8 (25–35%), 2 (2%), lower 5 (3%). Affects F > M and is often associated with smaller than average tooth size in remainder of dentition. Peg-shaped 2 often occurs in conjunction with absence of contralateral 2. NB: 3 migrates down guided by the distal aspect of 2. When 2 is absent, peg-shaped, or small-rooted, it is important to monitor the maxillary canine for signs of ectopic eruption.

Aetiology Often familial—polygenic inheritance. Also associated with ecto-dermal dysplasia and Down syndrome.
- Rx: 1° dentition—none. 2° dentition—depends on crowding and malocclusion.
- 8—none.
- 2—see ➔ Management of missing incisors, p. 114.
- 5 — (NB: 5 sometimes develop late). If patient is crowded, extraction of E, either at around 8yrs for spontaneous space closure or later if space is to be closed as a part of orthodontic Rx. If lower arch is well aligned or spaced, consider preservation of E, and bridgework later (if Es have no pathology and long roots, they can sometimes be maintained into adulthood).

Hyperdontia
Better known as supernumerary teeth.

Prevalence 1° dentition 0.8%, 2° dentition 2%. Occurs most frequently in premaxillary region. Affects M > F. Associated with cleidocranial dysostosis and CLP. Supernumerary ($) in 1° dentition is followed in about 50% of cases by $ in 2° dentition, so warn parent!

Aetiology Theories include offshoot of dental lamina and third dentition.

Classification Classification is either by shape or position (Table 3.2) and orientation (e.g. 'upright', 'inverted', etc.).

Effects on dentition and Rx
- No effect. If unerupted keep watch (radiographic review occasionally to exclude cystic change/damage to adjacent teeth—both relatively rare). If erupts—extract.
- Crowding. Rx: extract; if supplemental, extract tooth with the worse crown or root form, or the tooth with the most displaced apex.
- Displacement. Can cause rotation &/or displacement. Rx: extraction of $ and fixed appliance, but tendency to relapse.

5 A. H. Brooks 1974 *J Int Assoc Dent Child* 5 32.

Table 3.2 Classification of abnormalities by shape and position

Shape	or	Position
Conical (peg-shaped)		Mesiodens
Tuberculate (barrel-shaped)		Distomolar
Supplemental		Paramolar
Odontome		

- Failure of eruption. Most likely cause of <u>1</u> to fail to erupt. Rx: extract $ and ensure sufficient space for unerupted tooth to erupt. May require extraction of 1° teeth &/or permanent teeth and orthodontic appliance. Then *wait*. Average time to eruption in these cases is 18 months.[6] If after 2yrs unerupted tooth fails to erupt despite sufficient space, may require conservative exposure and orthodontic traction.

▶ Children with hypodontia will often benefit from specialist/multidisciplinary management, coordinating paediatric dental, restorative, and orthodontic management.

6 D. D. DiBiase 1971 *Dent Pract Dent Rec* **22** 95.

Abnormalities of tooth structure

Disturbances in structure of enamel

Enamel usually develops in two phases: first, an organic matrix and second, mineralization. Disruption of enamel formation can therefore manifest as follows:

Hypoplasia Caused by disturbance in matrix formation and is characterized by pitted, grooved, or thinned enamel.

Hypomineralization Hypocalcification is a disturbance of calcification. Affected enamel appears white, yellow, or brown and opaque. May become more discoloured post-eruptively. Affected enamel may be weak and prone to breakdown. Most disturbances of enamel formation will produce both hypoplasia and hypomineralization, but clinically one type usually predominates.

Aetiological factors The following is not an exhaustive list:

Localized causes
Infection ('Turner tooth'), trauma, irradiation, and idiopathic (➔ Enamel opacities, p. 76).

Generalized causes
- Environmental (chronological hypoplasia):
  - Prenatal, e.g. rubella, syphilis.
  - Neonatal, e.g. prolonged labour, premature birth.
  - Postnatal, e.g. measles, congenital heart disease, fluoride, nutritional.
- Hereditary:
  - Affecting teeth only—amelogenesis imperfecta.
  - Accompanied by systemic disorder, e.g. Down syndrome, tuberous sclerosis.

Chronological hypoplasia So called because the hypoplastic enamel occurs in a distribution related to the extent of tooth formation at the time of the insult. Characteristically, due to its later formation, $\underline{2}$ is affected nearer to the incisal edge than $\underline{1}$ or $\underline{3}$.

Fluorosis See ➔ Fluoride, p. 28.

Rx of hypomineralization/hypoplasia depends on extent and severity
Posterior teeth
Small areas of hypoplasia can be fissure-sealed or restored conventionally, but more severely affected teeth may require crowning. Stainless steel (SS) crowns (➔ Stainless steel crowns, p. 88) can be used in children as a semi-permanent measure.

Anterior teeth
Small areas of hypoplasia can be restored using composites, microabrasion, or resin infiltration but larger areas may require veneers (➔ Veneers, p. 258) or crowns.

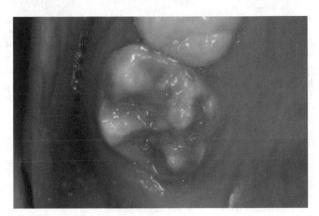

Fig. 3.2 Upper first permanent molar in a patient with molar incisor hypomineralization; the likely Rx would be extraction.

Molar incisor hypomineralization (MIH) See Fig. 3.2.
- Aetiology unknown. Prevalence ↑ over the past two decades in developed countries. Prevalence 14.2%.[7]
- Primarily affects 6s, but ~50% also have defects on permanent incisors.
- Affected 6s have hypomineralized defects of enamel, varying from discoloration to severe enamel dysplasia with post-eruptive breakdown. Sensitivity ↑, 2° caries ↑. Defects may affect anything from one to all 6s.
- Yellow/white opacities on buccal surface of affected incisors. Distribution often asymmetrical. No clear chronological pattern. Incisors less prone to enamel breakdown than 6s.

Rx options include intracoronal restoration, SS crowns, microabrasion, vital bleaching, resin infiltrate, or extraction, depending on aesthetics and prognosis (↪ Extraction of poor-quality first permanent molars, p. 140). Partial composite veneers can be considered to repair post-eruptive breakdown of incisors.

Hypomineralized second primary molars (HSPM) HSPM is a developmental defect of dental enamel that shares features with MIH. Also known as 1° molar hypomineralization. It may lead to post-eruptive breakdown and 2° caries. Recent studies suggest it is a predictor that MIH may be more likely to occur in the permanent dentition.

7 D. Zhao et al. 2018 *Int J Paediatr Dent* **28** 170.

Amelogenesis imperfecta (AI) Many classifications exist, but generally these are classified by the type of enamel defect &/or the mode of inheritance. There are now known to be mutations in at least 15 different genes that are associated with AI[8] (commonly affected genes: *AMELX, ENAM, AMBN, KLK4, MMP20*).

Main types
- *Hypoplastic*—enamel may be thin (smooth or rough) or pitted. Most commonly autosomal dominant inheritance. *Enamel-renal syndrome:* a rare hypoplastic AI associated with the *FAM20A* gene. Clinical features may include severely hypoplasic and discoloured enamel, semi-lunar shape of incisal edges, intra-pulpal calcification, hyperplastic dental follicles, delayed eruption, and gingival hyperplasia.
- *Hypocalcified*—enamel is dull, lustreless, opaque white, honey, or brown coloured. Enamel may breakdown rapidly in severe cases. Sensitivity ↑, calculus ↑ common. May be autosomal dominant or recessive.
- *Hypomaturation*—mottled or frosty-looking white opacities, sometimes confined to incisal third of crown ('snow-capped teeth').

Usually both 1° and 2° dentitions and all the teeth are affected. The different subgroups give rise to a wide variation in clinical presentation, ranging from discoloration to soft &/or deficient enamel. It is therefore difficult to make general recommendations, but it is wise to seek specialist advice for all but the mildest forms. Rx: in more severe cases, SS crowns and composite resin can be used to maintain molars and 2° inc, prior to more permanent restorations when child is older.

▶ *Enamel-renal syndrome*: a rare hypoplastic AI caused by mutation of the *FAM20A* gene and associated with nephrocalcinosis. Suspected individuals should be referred for genetic confirmation, and if confirmed, renal investigation. Clinical features may include severely hypoplasic and discoloured enamel, semi-lunar shape of incisal edges, intra-pulpal calcification, hyperplastic dental follicles, delayed eruption, and gingival hyperplasia.

Disturbances in the structure of dentine
These include dentinogenesis imperfecta, dentinal dysplasias (types I and II), regional odontodysplasia, vitamin D-resistant rickets, and Ehlers–Danlos syndrome—all of which are rare.

Dentinogenesis imperfecta (hereditary opalescent dentine—DI) This is more common, affecting 1 in 8000. Both 1° and 2° dentitions are involved, although later-formed teeth may be less so. Main types:
- I—associated with osteogenesis imperfecta.
- II—teeth only.

Affected teeth have an opalescent brown or blue hue, bulbous crowns, short roots, and narrow flame-shaped pulps. The ADJ is abnormal, which results in the enamel flaking off, leading to rapid wear of the soft dentine. Rx: along similar lines as for severe amelogenesis.

---

8 J. T. Wright *Developmental Defects of the Teeth* (✎ https://www.dentistry.unc.edu/dentalprofessionals/resources/defects/).

▶ Children with opalescent teeth may also have brittle bone disease.
▶ Early recognition and Rx of amelogenesis and dentinogenesis imperfecta is important to prevent rapid tooth wear.

Disturbances in the structure of cementum

Hypoplasia and aplasia of cementum are uncommon. The latter occurs in hypophosphatasia and results in premature exfoliation. Hypercementosis is relatively common and may occur in response to inflammation, mechanical stimulation, or Paget's disease, or be idiopathic. *Concrescence* is the uniting of the roots of two teeth by cementum.

▶ Children with developmental dental anomalies will often benefit from specialist/multidisciplinary management, coordinating paediatric dental, re-storative, and orthodontic management.
▶ Prevention is a priority in children with developmental dental anomalies to minimize the risk of 2° caries, tooth surface loss, and periodontal disease.

Abnormalities of tooth form

Normal width $\underline{1}$ = 8.5mm, $\underline{2}$ = 6.5mm.

Double teeth

Gemination This occurs by partial splitting of a tooth germ.

Fusion Fusion occurs as a result of the fusion of two tooth germs. As fusion can take place between either two teeth of the normal series or, less commonly, with a $ tooth, then counting the number of teeth will not always give the correct aetiology.

As the distinction is really only of academic interest, the term 'double teeth' is to be preferred. Both 1° and 2° teeth may be affected and a wide variation in presentation is seen. The prevalence in the 2° dentition is 0.1–0.2%.

Rx Rx for aesthetics should be delayed to allow pulpal recession. If the tooth has separate pulp chambers and root canals, separation can be considered. If it is due to fusion with a $ tooth, the $ portion can be extracted. Where a single pulp chamber exists, sometimes the tooth can be contoured to resemble two separate teeth or the bulk of the crown reduced.

Macrodontia/megadontia

Generalized macrodontia is rare, but is unilaterally associated with hemifacial hypertrophy. Isolated megadont teeth are seen in 1% of 2° dentitions.

Microdontia

Prevalence 1° dentition <0.5%. In 2° dentition, overall prevalence is 2.5%. Of this figure, 1–2% is accounted for by diminutive $\underline{2}$s. Peg-shaped $\underline{2}$s often have short roots and are thought to be a possible factor in the palatal displacement of $\underline{3}$s (◉ Palatally displaced maxillary canines, p. 144). $\underline{8}$s also commonly affected.

Dens in dente

This is really a marked palatal invagination, which gives the appearance of a tooth within a tooth. Usually affects $\underline{2}$s, but can also affect premolars. Where the invagination is in close proximity to the pulp, early pulp death may ensue. Fissure sealing of the invagination as soon as possible after eruption may prevent this, but is often too late. Extraction may be required, other options include RCT (can be difficult), pulpotomy, and apical Rx.

Dilaceration

This describes a tooth with a distorted crown or root. Usually affects $\underline{1}$s. Two types seen, dependent upon aetiology (Table 3.3).

The traumatically induced type is caused by intrusion of the 1° incisor, resulting in displacement of the developing 2° incisor tooth germ. The effects depend upon the developmental stage at the time of injury.

Rx: depends upon severity and patient cooperation. If mild it may be possible to expose crown and align orthodontically provided the apex will not be positioned against the labial plate of bone at the end of the Rx, otherwise extraction is indicated.

Table 3.3 Types of dilaceration

Developmental	Traumatic
Crown turned upward and labially	Crown turned palatally
Regular enamel and dentine	Disturbed enamel and dentine formation seen
Usually no other affected teeth	
Affects F > M	

Turner tooth

This term is used to describe the effect of a disturbance of enamel and dentine formation by infection from an overlying 1° tooth which therefore usually affects premolar teeth. Rx: as for hypoplasia ⊃ Hypoplasia, p. 70.

Taurodontism

Taurodontism means 'bull-like'. May occur in some types of AI. Radiographically an elongation of the pulp chamber is seen, which resembles a bull's head. Rx: none required, but may complicate endodontic Rx and occasionally extraction.

Abnormalities of tooth colour

Extrinsic staining By definition this is caused by extrinsic agents and can be removed by prophylaxis. Green, black, orange, or brown stains are seen, and may be formed by chromogenic bacteria or be dietary in origin. Chlorhexidine mouthwash causes a brown stain by combining with dietary tannin. Where the staining is associated with poor OH, demineralization and roughening of the underlying enamel may make removal difficult. Rx: a mixture of pumice powder and toothpaste or an abrasive prophylaxis paste together with a bristle brush should remove the stain. Meticulous OHI can help to prevent staining returning, but recurrence is unfortunately relatively common.

Intrinsic staining This can be caused by:
- Changes in the structure or thickness of the dental hard tissues, e.g. enamel opacities.
- Incorporation of pigments during tooth formation, e.g. tetracycline staining (blue/brown), porphyria (red).
- Diffusion of pigment into hard tissues after formation, e.g. pulp necrosis products (grey), root canal medicaments (grey).

Enamel opacities These are localized areas of hypomineralized (or hypoplastic) enamel. Fluoride (↪ Fluoride, p. 28) is only one of a considerable number of possible aetiological agents.

Rx Seven possible approaches:

Approach 1 Acid pumice abrasion technique is effective for some types of diffuse (surface) enamel defects. Two methods available (take pre-operative photos to monitor improvement):

Hydrochloric acid technique (quicker, but great care needed)
A mixture of 18% hydrochloric acid and pumice is applied to the affected area using a wooden stick. Careful isolation with rubber dam, use of a neutralizing agent (e.g. sodium bicarbonate), and protection of the soft tissues/patient is essential. The mixture is rubbed into the surface for 5sec and then rinsed away. These two steps are repeated (max. ten times—removing <0.1mm enamel) until the desired colour change is achieved. The enamel is then polished and a fluoride solution applied.[9] Tell the patient to avoid highly coloured foods for 48h.

Phosphoric acid technique (slower but potentially safer)
A number of variations of this technique are in use. A commonly used method is to etch with 30–50% orthophosphoric acid for 1–2min, wash, then use pumice and water slurry with rubber prophy cup for 1min (take care not to overheat the tooth). Wash. Repeat etch and pumice stage ×2, washing between. Dry tooth and apply topical fluoride solution (avoid pigmented varnishes). May be repeated up to ×2, but leave at least 6 weeks before each repeat to check for improvement.

9 T. P. Croll & R. Cavanaugh 1986 *Quintessence Int* **17** 81.

Approach 2 Resin infiltrate is a valid and well supported approach of treating enamel opacities. There are various systems available but commonly the tooth is etched with hydrochloric acid, dried with ethanol, prior to application of a methacrylate-based resin.

Approach 3 Bleaching (➲ Tooth whitening, p. 256). The patient should be 18yrs or older.

Approach 4 Veneers (➲ Veneers, p. 258). Should not be considered before the gingival position is stable, at least 16yrs old.

Approach 5 Crowns (➲ Anterior crowns, p. 260). Should not be considered before the gingival position is stable, at least 16yrs old.

Approach 6 Localized composite restorations in affected areas including composite veneers.

Approach 7 Resin infiltration is a minimally invasive Rx for hypomineralized areas. The low-viscosity, unfilled resin penetrates areas of demineralization within the enamel and improves the appearance of these. The manufacturer's instructions should be followed for the system being used.

Anatomy of primary teeth (and relevance to cavity design)

1° teeth differ in several respects from permanent teeth, affecting both the sequelae of dental disease and its management (Fig. 3.3). (The following bracketed numbers refer to the numbered features in Fig. 3.3.)

Thinner enamel (1) Enamel in 1° teeth is ~1mm thick, which is half that of 2° teeth.

Larger pulp horns (2) The pulp chamber in 1° teeth is proportionately larger, with more accentuated pulp horns. <u>DE</u>—three pulp horns MB, DB, and palatal. Lower DE—four pulp horns MB, ML, DB, and DL. These features mean that caries will affect the pulp sooner and there is a greater likelihood of pulp exposure during cavity preparation. Aim for only 0.5–1.0mm penetration into dentine, except where caries determines deeper preparation.

Pulpal outline (3) This follows the amelo-dentinal junction more closely in 1° teeth, therefore cavity floor should follow external contour of tooth sinuously to avoid exposure.

Narrower occlusal table Greater convergence of the buccal and lingual walls results in a proportionately narrower occlusal table. This is more pronounced in D than E therefore, over-extension of an occlusal cavity or lock can lead to weakening of the cusps.

Broad and flat contact points (4) This makes detection of interproximal caries more difficult, and means that in 1° molars divergence of the buccal and lingual walls towards the approximal surface is necessary to ensure cavity margins are self-cleansing.

Bulbous crown (5) 1° molars have a more bulbous crown form than 2° molars, making matrix placement more difficult.

Inclination of the enamel prisms (6) In the cervical third of 1° molars the enamel prisms are inclined in an occlusal direction so there is no need to bevel the gingival floor of a proximal box.

Cervical constriction (7) This is more marked in 1° molars, therefore if the base of the proximal box is extended too far gingivally it will be difficult to cut an adequate floor without encroaching on the pulp.

Alveolar bone permeability This is ↑ in younger children, thus it is usually possible to achieve local anaesthesia of 1° mandibular molars by infiltration alone, up to 6yrs of age.

Thin pulpal floor and accessory canals (8) This may explain the greater incidence of inter-radicular involvement following pulp death.

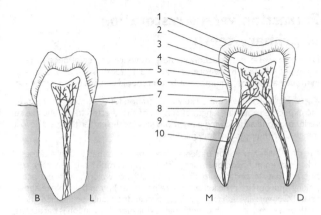

Fig. 3.3 Cross-sections of second deciduous molar showing features of anatomy of primary molars.

Root form (9) 1° molars have proportionately longer roots than their permanent counterparts. They are also more flared to straddle the developing premolar tooth. The roots are flattened mesio-distally, as are canals within.

Radicular pulp (10) This follows a tortuous and branching path, making complete cleansing and preparation of the root canal system almost impossible, although instrumenting canals is often easier than suggested in some texts. In addition, as the roots resorb, a different approach to RCT is needed for the 1° dentition, pure zinc oxide and eugenol being the obturation material of choice.

Extraction versus restoration of primary teeth

Despite a welcome reduction in the prevalence of dental decay, the dilemma of whether to restore or extract a 1° tooth is still all too familiar. In making a decision, a number of factors should be considered, including:

Age This will influence the likely cooperation for restorative procedures, the expected remaining length of service of the affected tooth, and the severity of sequelae following early tooth loss (as the earlier the tooth is lost, the greater the potential for space loss).

Medical history For patients where recurrent bacteraemia carries ↑ risks (e.g. immunocompromised, risk of endocarditis) it is generally considered that 1° tooth pulp therapy should be avoided, with extraction (taking appropriate precautions where necessary) often being more appropriate. Conversely, in haemophiliacs, extractions should be avoided and 1° teeth preserved, if possible, until their exfoliation. Prevention is particularly important in all such patients.

Motivation and cooperation of parents As it is the parents that bring the child to the surgery, we must explain to them the benefits of maintaining the 1° dentition. Unfortunately, a small proportion of the population may regard a dentist that fills 1° teeth with suspicion—after all, everyone knows that baby teeth fall out!

Extent of caries In a child with an otherwise caries-free mouth, every attempt should be made to preserve an intact dentition. Where there is extensive caries, restoration of Es and loss of Ds can be an acceptable compromise.

Pain If a child is suffering pain from one or more teeth, this needs to be alleviated as soon as possible. If symptom free, then the dentist will have more time to explore the extent of the lesion(s) and the child's cooperation.

Extent of lesion(s) In 1° molars destruction of the marginal ridge indicates a high probability of pulpal involvement.[10] If several 1° molars require pulp therapy, and cooperation/motivation is poor, serious thought should be given to extraction rather than restoration.

Position of tooth Although early loss of 1° incisors will have little effect, extraction of C, D, or E will, in a crowded case, lead to localization of the crowding. Extraction of Es, particularly in the upper arch, should be deferred, if possible, until the 6 has erupted.

Presence/absence of permanent successor Bear in mind the amount of crowding present and the likelihood of spontaneous space closure.

10 M. S. Duggal 2002 *Eur J Paed Dent* 3 112.

Malocclusion If still undecided, it is worth considering the occlusion. In a particularly crowded case, restoration of a decayed tooth may be indicated if further space loss would mean that extraction of more than one premolar per quadrant would be required. Much has been written about compensating (same tooth in opposing arch) and balancing (contralateral tooth) extractions, although this is still an area of some controversy.[11] The rationale is that a symmetrical problem is easier to deal with later but if taken to its logical conclusion, gross caries of D| and |E will result in a clearance! In general, loss of Cs in a crowded patient should be balanced to prevent a centre-line shift. Balancing Ds in a child with ↑ risk of caries also has the advantage of removing very caries-prone contacts (i.e. E–D and D–C).

So much for the theory; in practice, it should be remembered that a happy and cooperative patient is more important in the long term. When treating a child under local analgesia, leaving extractions unbalanced and monitoring for centre-line shift may be preferable to prolonging intervention in the dental chair.

11 W. P. Rock & British Society of Paediatric Dentistry 2002 *Int J Paed Dent* **12** 151.

Local analgesia for children

Although there is no scientific evidence to suggest that 1° teeth are less sensitive than 2° teeth, clinically it is sometimes possible to complete cavity preparation of minimal cavities without LA, especially on 1° anterior teeth. Adequate management of approximal caries in 1° molars usually requires LA.

General principles

- Explain to patient in terms they will understand what you are trying to do and why.
- Use flavoured topical anaesthesia (e.g. 20% benzocaine).
- Warm anaesthetic solution to room temperature only.
- Use a fine-gauge (e.g. 30-gauge) disposable needle.
- Always have a dental nurse to assist.
- Hold mucosa taut. Verbal distraction can help at the moment of needle penetration.
- Use slow rate of injection or 'the wand'.
- Warn about post-operative numbness and avoidance of self-inflicted trauma (e.g. lip chewing/sucking).

Choice of anaesthetic agent

First choice Lidocaine 2% with 1:80,000 adrenaline. Maximum dose = 4.4mg/kg.[12]

Second choice Prilocaine 3% with felypressin (0.03IU/mL)—may give slightly less profound anaesthesia. Maximum dose = 6.6mg/kg.

For lidocaine, maximum dosage equates to (i) 2.2mL for a healthy 10kg 1.5yr-old child and (ii) 4.4mL for a healthy 20kg 5yr-old (i.e. 1 × 2.2mL cartridge per 10kg). This may need to be reduced for children with certain medical conditions.

Articaine 4% with adrenaline may be used (maximum dose 7mg/kg) and there is some evidence that lower 1° and 2° molar teeth can be more reliably anaesthetized by infiltration alone. However, articaine is not licensed for children <4yrs of age and greater care is needed to avoid exceeding the maximum dose, as the volume at maximum dosage is less than other LA agents. Some evidence suggests greater risk of prolonged anaesthesia/paraesthesia when articaine is used for ID blocks, so some suggest avoiding the use of articaine for blocks.

Infiltration injection

Can be used in most circumstances. Infiltration technique as for adults (⊖ Local analgesia—techniques, p. 628). In children, the malar buttress overlies <u>6</u>, so it is often advisable to deposit some solution over the more permeable bone mesial and distal to this tooth.

---

12 AAPD 2015 *Guideline on Use of Local Anaesthesia for Paediatric Dental Patients* Clinical guidelines, reference manual, 286 (⌖ www.aapd.org).

Block injection
Inferior dental block Using thumb and forefinger, find the shortest width of the ramus. Penetrate about 1cm into lingual tissues from the internal oblique ridge, on a line between thumb and finger. An aspirating syringe is essential. NB: the mandibular foramen is lower on the ramus in young children (about the same level as the occlusal plane).

Posterior superior alveolar block This is rarely required in children and carries a significant risk of post-injection haematoma. If necessary due to failure of infiltration for 6, the technique should be modified by depositing solution distal to the zygomatic buttress and massaging it backwards towards the posterior superior alveolar foramen (maxillary molar block).[13]

Alternative techniques
Intraligamentary injection These purpose-designed syringes have an ultra-short needle and a 'gun' or 'pen' appearance. This makes it helpful for children with a needle phobia, or as a more acceptable alternative or adjunct to an IDB. In addition, as the lips and tongue are not anaesthetized it is useful for young or disabled children, in whom there is a greater risk of post-operative soft tissue trauma.

Jet injection In this technique, a jet syringe (e.g. Syrijet® or Injex®) is used to inject LA solution under pressure through mucosa and bone to a depth of about 1cm. It is useful for producing soft tissue analgesia prior to conventional LA injection or for infiltration analgesia, and for some patients who will not contemplate LA using a needle, but is not widely used.

Computer-controlled delivery (e.g. The Wand®, Single Tooth Anesthesia (STA®) system) Allows carefully controlled slow delivery via a line and needle resembling an IV-giving set. Especially useful for direct palatal analgesia, intraligamental analgesia, and for anxious patients.

13 A. K. Adatia 1976 *Br Dent J* **140** 87.

Restoration of carious primary teeth

Making an accurate pre-operative Δ (including appropriate radiographs) and Rx plan is essential. This will enable Rx to be provided as efficiently as possible (⊃ Treatment planning for children, p. 58).

Local anaesthesia See ⊃ Local analgesia for children, p. 82.

Isolation Ideally, a rubber dam should be used routinely for restorative procedures. It not only protects the airway, but also improves moisture control and visibility, and aids in patient management. It is essential for all root canal and pulp therapy for permanent teeth, and is advisable for restoration of 1° teeth. If placement of a rubber dam is not possible, plastic disposable salivary ejectors are better tolerated than the metal flange type.

Instruments

Burs High-speed: pear-shaped bur numbers 330 and 525, and short fissure bur number 541. Slow-speed: a selection of pear-shaped and round burs are most useful. For access use a small bur and for caries removal use the largest round bur which fits into the cavity.

Handpiece A miniature-head handpiece is invaluable. Some children are apprehensive of the aspirator tip, making use of a high-speed, water-cooled handpiece difficult; others find the vibration of the slow-speed handpiece distressing, and may confuse it with pain. In these cases distraction or counting (i.e. 'I will count to three each time, then I will stop') can help. Occasionally it is possible, but time-consuming, to complete cavity preparation with hand instruments.

Material selection for intracoronal restorations

GIC This has advantages of adhesion and fluoride release, but is more technique sensitive and less wear resistant than amalgam. Useful in non-load-bearing Class III and V cavities, temporization of 1° teeth in young, pre-cooperative children, or teeth near to exfoliation.

Resin-modified GI cement (RMGIC) This has been demonstrated to have excellent performance in 1° teeth.

Compomer A modified composite-type material with some of the properties of GIC. More technique and moisture sensitive than amalgam, but studies suggest similar longevity.

Composite resin Early studies suggested poor performance in 1° teeth, but modern materials placed with good isolation (i.e. rubber dam) perform as well, or better than amalgam, but take longer to place.

▶ Plastic, intracoronal restorations perform best in 1° molars with small Class I and II cavities. SS crowns (⊃ Stainless steel crowns, p. 88) give superior longevity where lesions are more extensive.

Amalgam Because of concerns about toxicity and environmental pollution, plus the availability of alternative materials, amalgam is less frequently used.

▶ The European Parliament agreed on 14 March 2017 to the final version of its Regulation on Mercury, the EU's instrument to ratify the Minamata Treaty of 2013. This stipulates that amalgam is not to be used for the Rx of

1° teeth, in children <15yrs, or in pregnant or breastfeeding women, except when strictly deemed necessary by the practitioner on the ground of specific medical needs of the patient (from 1 July 2018).

However, many clinicians outside the EU still consider amalgam to be an acceptable and durable material for Class I and II restorations in 1° molars.

Principles of cavity design

Outline form Should include any undermined enamel. Extension for prevention is now outmoded, but any suspect adjacent fissures should be included. Do not cross transverse marginal ridges unless they are undermined.

Caries removal Caries should be excavated from the ADJ first. If necessary, you may need to re-establish outline form to improve access to ensure the ADJ is caries free. Then progress to carefully removing caries from floor.

Resistance form/retention form While not as crucial with adhesive materials, ensuring reasonable resistance form is of value in load-bearing situations.

Reasons for failure of restorations in primary teeth

- Recurrent caries, often due to failure to adequately complete caries removal because of flagging patient cooperation or failure to use adequate LA. If unable to finish cavity it is better to place a temporary dressing (GIC often best) and try again at another visit.
- Cavity preparation does not satisfy the mechanical requirements of the filling material.
- Inadequate moisture control, especially true of GICs, compomers, and composites.
- Presence of occlusal high spot.

There are many others, but these are the most common.

Useful tips

- Let the child participate by 'looking after' the saliva ejector or cotton wool.
- If the child is nervous give them some control by asking them to signal, e.g. by raising their hand, if they want you to stop.
- If the child's cooperation runs out before the cavity is completed, try and ensure all caries is removed from the ADJ and place a dressing of either zinc oxide or GIC. This should suffice for several visits, until you are ready to try again.
- LA is easier to give in the maxilla, so most advocate starting with an upper tooth.
- Don't try to do too much at one visit—plan Rx at a pace the child can accept.

Communication

▶ It is important to explain to the child what you are doing, and why, in terms they can understand.

It may be helpful to describe some of the instruments we use in ways that can make them seem less threatening to a child ('childrenese') (e.g. see Table 3.4).

Table 3.4 Unthreatening alternatives for dental terms ('childrenese')

Slow-speed handpiece	Mr Buzz/buzzy bee/bumble bee
High-speed handpiece	Mr Spray/wizzy brush/tooth tickler
Handpiece and prophylaxis cup	Electric toothbrush/tooth polisher
Aspirator tip	Vacuum cleaner/hoover
Rubber dam	Tooth raincoat
Saliva ejector	Straw
	Curly-wurly (coiled type only)
Air from 3-in-1	Wind
Fissure sealant	Plastic coating
Etchant solution	Tooth shampoo/cleaner
	Lemon juice
Cotton wool roll	Snowman
Dental light	The sun/car light

Plastic restoration in primary molars

See ➲ Anatomy of primary teeth (and relevance to cavity design), p. 78 for anatomy of 1° molars and effect upon cavity design. Have all necessary instruments and filling materials ready so that appointment is kept as short as possible.

- Explain and show child (and parent) what you are going to do.
- Appropriate LA (➲ Local analgesia for children, p. 82). Waiting for the LA to work is sometimes a good opportunity to deliver/reinforce preventive advice,
- In a small cavity, gain access with a high-speed handpiece and pear-shaped bur. The outline can then be established and caries removed.
- *Approximal caries*—cut down through the marginal ridge to allow access for caries removal. Ideally should just extend into embrasures and walls of box should converge occlusally (i.e. the box is wider at the base than at occlusal level) (Fig. 3.4).
- In larger cavities, an excavator or large round bur can be used to start caries removal from the walls. Any undermined enamel should be cut back.
- If caries is deep, stop and re-assess whether pulpotomy (➲ Primary molar pulp therapy, p. 93) is required. If outline form extends beyond acceptable limits, consider an SS crown, especially in Class II cavities.
- Check retention and that walls are caries free.
- Wash and dry cavity.
- Line with hard-setting calcium hydroxide if using amalgam.
- Check occlusion.

▶ Reinforce good aspects of the child's behaviour with praise and possibly a sticker/badge/toothbrush.

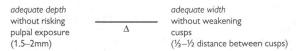

| *adequate depth* without risking pulpal exposure (1.5–2mm) | Δ | *adequate width* without weakening cusps (⅓–½ distance between cusps) |

Fig. 3.4 Adequate depth and width.

Stainless steel crowns

▶ SS crowns are the most durable restoration for 1° molars with extensive caries and those where pulp Rx has been performed.

▶ SS crowns are preformed metal crowns made from high-grade SS and do contain small traces of nickel. They are therefore not suitable for patients with a known nickel allergy.

Indications
- Badly broken down 1° molar.
- After pulp therapy in 1° molars.
- As interim measure for 2° molars, where crowns are required but the patient is too young.
- Temporary coverage during preparation of cast crown for premolar or 2° molar.
- Developmental anomalies.
- Severe tooth loss due to bruxism/erosion.

Instruments High-speed tapered diamond bur and diamond occlusal wheel. Straight handpiece and a stone. Slow-speed handpiece and burs as required. Crown scissors, dividers, selection of suitable crowns, and Adam's pliers. Johnstone contouring pliers (no. 114) and Abel pliers (no. 112) can also be useful, but are not essential.

There are two principal methods for placement:

Conventional technique

SS crowns rely for retention only on a tight adaptation at the gingival margin of the preparation, therefore taper of preparation walls is not critical (Fig. 3.5).
- LA and if possible rubber dam.
- Measure M–D length with dividers to aid crown selection.
- Remove caries.
- Occlusal reduction (~1mm), roughly following cuspal planes.
- Approximal reduction (~20° from vertical) using tapered diamond, without producing a ledge at gingival margin.
- Remove buccal and lingual bulbosities only sufficient to seat crown (often little/no reduction required).
- Select crown. Correct size will be a 'click' fit.
- Check height and occlusion. Minor prematurity is not a problem. If extensive blanching of surrounding tissues or over-extended, trim crown. Usually not necessary.
- Use pliers to adapt contact points and crimp margins. Smooth trimmed margins with stone.
- Cement with zinc polycarboxylate or GIC.

Technique for 2° molars (Fig. 3.6) is similar but more careful adjustment is necessary.

'Hall' technique

Taught as the gold standard for restoring 1° molars with distal or mesial caries. No conventional preparation or caries removal is normally carried out, and is referred to by advocates as a 'biological' technique (as opposed to 'conventional'). After simply removing any loose debris, a crown is cemented over the carious, unprepared molar, with the

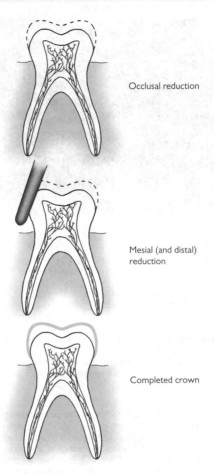

Occlusal reduction

Mesial (and distal) reduction

Completed crown

Fig. 3.5 Preparation for stainless steel crown.

child 'biting' the cement-filled crown down into place. The technique has several potential advantages, and it may allow effective Rx for children who might otherwise be unable to accept 'conventional' interventions. LA is not usually required and it is quicker than conventional SS crown placement. Advocates of the technique suggest that it achieves a coronal seal, cuts off carious lesions from substrate, and protects the pulp from chemical, thermal, and mechanical insults. It is recommended that its use is restricted to asymptomatic teeth with no evidence of pulpal inflammation/necrosis/periodontal involvement.

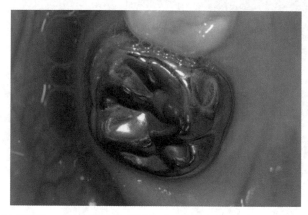

Fig. 3.6 The same tooth as in Fig. 3.2 following placement of a stainless steel crown.

Basic 'Hall' technique
- Separators placed a few days before may aid placement.
- Check carious 1° molar free from obvious pulpal or periradicular pathology.
- Select correct-size crown, fill with a suitable cement (GIC is recommended) and place on tooth.
- Advise child and parent that the patient may feel pushing when seating the crown.
- Get child to bite down on crown, seating it onto the tooth.
- Clear away excess cement.
- Crown is likely to be in premature occlusion, but as long as this is not gross, occlusion usually evens out by dento-alveolar compensation within a few weeks.

Success rates
A number of studies have demonstrated that both conventional and Hall technique crowns have a far superior longevity to conventional restorations in 1° teeth. Initial studies of 'Hall' technique SS crowns have also indicated very favourable results probably due to creation of an effective pericoronal seal.[14] The UK FiCTION (Filling Children's Teeth—Indicated Or Not?) trial is nearing completion and aims to provide more information about the relative merits of 'conventional' vs 'biological' techniques.

14   N. P. Innes et al. 2007 *BMC Oral Health* **7** 18.

Class III, IV, and V in primary teeth

Carious 1° incisors and canines are seen less frequently than molars and are usually indicative of a high caries rate during early infanthood (⊝ Severe early childhood caries, p. 92).

Management Objectives are relief of pain and prevention. Aesthetics are less important.

Rx options Include:
- Extraction.
- Topical 2% sodium fluoride and observation. Intervene if caries progresses.
- Make self-cleansing (with flat fissure no. 1 bur) plus topical fluoride.
- Restoration with adhesive materials.

Class III restoration Similar technique to that used for permanent incisors, but omit incisal retention groove.

Class IV restoration If restoration is essential the greater strength of composite is required. Polycarboxylate (strip) crowns are advocated by some paedodontists, for the well-motivated child.

Class V restoration Remove caries with a small round bur and restore with GIC/composite.

Composite strip crowns Cellulose acetate crown forms for 1° incisors. Enable restoration of 1° incisors using composite resin.

Severe early childhood caries

Aetiology
Frequent ingestion of sugar &/or reduced salivary flow.

Nursing bottle or bottle mouth caries
Terms used to describe patterns of early childhood caries (ECC) associated with frequent consumption of a sugar-containing drink, especially from a feeding-bottle. Commonly the child falls asleep with the bottle of juice or milk and suckles during the night. Possibly related to the relatively high levels of lactose in breast milk.[15] The WHO recommends mothers exclusively breastfeed their child for the first 6 months before introducing nutritious complementary foods.[16] Characteristically, starts with the maxillary 1° incisors, but in more severe cases the first 1° molars are also involved. The mandibular incisors are relatively protected by the tongue and saliva.

Severe ECC may also be associated with the prolonged and frequent intake of sugar-based medications; however, both pharmaceutical companies and doctors are more aware of the problem and the number of alternative sugar-free preparations is ↑. See Table 3.6 for a list (p. 119). Recent studies have confirmed that ECC may be associated with prolonged breastfeeding beyond age 2yrs. Children >1yr old who suckle frequently during the night may be most at risk. Breastfeeding is considered to be optimal for babies and should be encouraged. Counselling about the possible role of on-demand breastfeeding in ECC should be approached with sensitivity and understanding.

Rampant caries
A term with no specific definition, but often used to describe extensive, rapidly progressing caries affecting many teeth in the 1° &/or permanent dentition.

Radiation caries
Radiation for head and neck cancer may result in fibrosis of salivary glands and salivary flow. Patients often resort to sucking sweets to alleviate their dry mouth, which exacerbates the problem. Management of radiation caries requires specialist referral.

---

15 G. J. Roberts 1982 *J Dent* **10** 346.

16 WHO 2011 *Exclusive Breastfeeding for Six Months Best for Babies Everywhere* (℠ https://www. who.int/mediacentre/news/statements/2011/breastfeeding_20110115/en/).

Primary molar pulp therapy

NB: 1° molar roots resorb.

Where the carious process has jeopardized pulpal sensibility there are two alternatives: (i) extraction and (ii) pulp therapy.

Indication and contraindications

See ➔ Extraction versus restoration of primary teeth, p. 80.

- Any medical condition where a focus of infection is potentially dangerous is a C/I to pulp therapy.
- Pulp therapy may be preferable to extraction in children with bleeding disorders.
- Tooth must be restorable following pulp therapy.

The Δ of the state of the pulp can be difficult, as not only is a child's perception of pain less precise than an adult's, but the clinical picture may also be complicated by death of one root canal while the other(s) remain vital.

Indicators of possible pulp involvement

- Breakdown of marginal ridge.
- Symptoms.
- Tenderness to percussion, ↑ mobility, and buccal swelling/sinus.
- Inter-radicular radiolucency seen radiographically (usually on b/w radiographs).

Definitions

- Indirect pulp Rx: Rx without exposure of the pulp.
- Direct pulp capping: management of exposure by direct capping—not usually advocated in 1° molars due to poor outcomes.
- Pulpotomy: removal of coronal pulp and Rx of radicular pulp.
- Pulpectomy: removal of entire coronal and radicular pulp.

Pulp therapy techniques

Indirect pulp Rx

Indicated for asymptomatic, vital 1° molars with no pulp exposure after removal of all soft caries. In common with the Hall crown, this is considered by some as a 'biological' technique and aims to maintain health and vitality of the 1° tooth pulp, which may be more resilient and have greater ability to recover from insult than traditionally thought. Recent studies have shown relatively high rates of success in teeth without evidence of irreversible pulpal damage.

Technique Removal of all soft caries. Leaving carious, but firm, affected dentine in vital, asymptomatic 1° molars has been shown to be reasonably successful. Margins of cavities should be rendered caries free to ensure an adequate coronal seal. Works best in occlusal cavities, less likely to be successful in approximal caries due to early pulpal involvement and difficulty in achieving a good coronal seal. Setting calcium hydroxide can be used in the deepest portion, with GIC, composite, or a SS crown (see ➔ Stainless steel crowns, p. 88). If pulp exposure occurs, pulpotomy/pulpectomy are usually more appropriate restorative techniques.

Pulpotomy (for the vital primary molar pulp)

In 1° molars the relatively larger pulps result in earlier pulpal involvement, therefore amputation of the coronal pulp leaving healthy radicular pulp *in situ* (pulpotomy) gives more consistent results than techniques that attempt to retain vitality of the whole pulp, e.g. indirect pulp capping.

Materials The most commonly used medicaments are:
- *Formocresol*—historically widely used for 1° teeth pulpotomy, because of its ease of use and high success rate (70–90%) However, recent concerns about the toxicity and potential mutagenicity of formalin-containing compounds has led many authorities to advise against its use where suitable alternatives exist.
- *Ferric sulfate*—the technique recommended by many authorities as an alternative to formocresol.[17] Success rates have been shown to nearly match formocresol, but are more technique sensitive.
- *Calcium hydroxide*—very time-consuming and more technique sensitive, but similar success to ferric sulfate in some studies.
- *Mineral trioxide aggregate (MTA)*—recent studies demonstrate similar success to formocresol. Very expensive.
- *Bioactive dentine substitutes*—recent studies show promising results in 1° tooth pulpotomy.
- *Devitalizing paste* (paraformaldehyde)—has fallen out of favour (for the same reasons as formocresol).

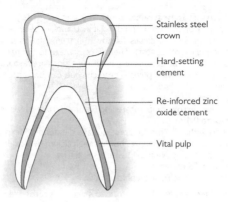

- Stainless steel crown
- Hard-setting cement
- Re-inforced zinc oxide cement
- Vital pulp

Fig. 3.7 Pulpotomy restored with stainless steel crown.

Technique
- Give LA and place rubber dam.
- Complete cavity preparation and excavate caries.
- Remove roof of pulp chamber.
- Amputate coronal pulp with a large excavator or sterile round bur.
- Wash chamber and arrest bleeding with damp cotton wool.
- Place cotton wool pledget dampened with 15.5% ferric sulfate on exposed pulp stumps for at least 1min, then remove. Alternatively, once bleeding arrested, place CaOH or MTA over root stumps.
- Apply dressing of reinforced zinc oxide eugenol (ZOE) cement.
- Restore tooth, usually with a stainless steel crown (Fig. 3.7).

Problems
- *Necrotic pulp (i.e. no bleeding)*—proceed with non-vital technique or extract.
- *Profuse haemorrhage*—indicates more serious inflammation of the radicular pulp. Intermediate dressing with Ledermix® followed by non-vital technique or extraction.

Pulpectomy (for non-vital primary molar pulp)

A pulpectomy is often considered difficult in 1° molars because of the complexity of ribbon-shaped canals (although instrumentation is often easier than some texts might suggest). The risk of damage to the permanent successor also needs to be considered, but if conditions are favourable it is the Rx of choice for non-vital pulps. The technique can be carried out in one or two visits.

- LA and rubber dam.
- Remove the necrotic pulp, locate and file and irrigate canals (sodium hypochlorite 0.1%).
- Cleanse to within 2–3mm of apex, but avoid extending beyond.
- Fill canal with plain ZOE paste, non-setting calcium hydroxide, or iodoform paste (e.g. Vitapex®) with a spiral filler.
- Restore with SS crown.
- Arrange clinical and radiographic review.

If there is evidence of any infection a two-stage Rx is recommended, leaving non-setting calcium hydroxide in the canals for 1–2 weeks prior to filling.

Success rate A success rate of >80% at 3yrs has been reported.

Pulp therapy for primary anterior teeth

Usual Rx is extraction, as A̲ and B̲ are exfoliated before patient is able to cooperate satisfactorily with more complicated Rx. However, C̲ is exfoliated later and unilateral loss may result in centre-line shift, therefore pulp Rx is indicated for some patients. The root canal morphology is amenable to pulpectomy and the canal should be cleaned using files, with care (remember underlying successor). A resorbable filling material, e.g. calcium hydroxide or ZOE, should be used.

Dental trauma

▶ If there is evidence of head injury, transfer patient to hospital immediately.

Note

- By 12yrs of age, 33% of boys and 19% of girls have experienced at least one episode of dental trauma.[18]
- Prognosis ↑ with good immediate Rx, therefore see patient as soon as possible.
- Avulsed permanent teeth should be replanted immediately.
- Child and parent may be upset, therefore handle accordingly and defer any non-urgent Rx.
- Take good notes for future reference and medico-legal purposes.
- If crown # this will have dissipated most of the energy of impact, therefore root # less likely.
- Clinical photos would be beneficial at this stage.

History

Take a structured history as an aide-memoire and for medico-legal purposes.

- Loss of consciousness? Concussion/headache/vomiting (↻ Assessing head injury, p. 492)? Refer immediately to hospital.
- Accompanied by? Parent/teacher? Consider consent issues.
- When? Time interval between injury and Rx affects prognosis.
- Where? Does patient need a tetanus booster? If so, refer to a GMP or hospital.
- How? Be alert to the possibilities of other injuries and child abuse.
- Tooth fragments? These may have been inhaled or embedded in soft tissues (e.g. lip). If fragment/tooth not accounted for &/or loss of consciousness, a chest X-ray (CXR) is mandatory.
- Past dental history (PDH)—previous trauma may affect prognosis and cooperation in the dental setting.
- Past medical history (PMH)—check for bleeding disorder and allergy to penicillin. Ask about immunosuppression, this may impact your decision on whether or not to reimplant a tooth.

Aims of Rx

- 1° dentition: (i) preserve integrity of permanent successor; (ii) preserve 1° tooth if cooperation good and compatible with first aim.
- 2° dentition: (i) preserve vitality of the tooth to allow maturation of the root; (ii) restore the crown to prevent drifting, tilting, and over-eruption.

Principles of Rx

Emergency Rx

- Elimination of pain.
- Protection of pulp.
- Reduction and immobilization of mobile teeth.
- Suturing of soft tissue lacerations (IO—3/0 resorbable suture (Dexon®, Vicryl®); EO—refer to hospital).
- ? Antibiotics, ? tetanus, ? analgesics, ? chlorhexidine mouthwash.

---

18 B. Chadwick 2004 *Children's Dental Health in the UK*, HMSO.

Intermediate Rx
- Pulp therapy.
- Consider orthodontic requirements and long-term prognosis of damaged teeth.
- Semi-permanent restorations.
- Keep under review, usually 1 month, 3 months, and then 6-monthly for 2yrs.

Permanent Rx
- Usually deferred until >16yrs (to allow pulpal and gingival recession and ↓ likelihood of further trauma); e.g. definitive crown.

Classification of tooth injuries

Several exist; some use roman numerals, others describe the injuries sustained (WHO system):
- Complicated #—pulp exposed.
- Uncomplicated #—pulp intact.

Prevention

- Prevalence ↑ as the overjet (o/j) ↑ (>9mm prevalence doubles), ? early orthodontics.
- Mouthguard for sports (vacuum-formed thermoplastic vinyl best, triple thickness).

Be alert for evidence of child abuse (➲ Safeguarding children, p. 100).

Safeguarding children

▶ All professionals involved with children need to be aware of the principles of safeguarding and alert to the possibility of child abuse or neglect.
NB: the term 'child abuse' is now favoured over 'non-accidental injury'.
The following signs are associated with abuse:

- Usually younger children are involved.
- The presenting injuries may not match the parent's account of how they were sustained. The account may change over time.
- Delay attending at a surgery or clinic for Rx of the injury.
- Bruises/injuries of different vintages are found on examination.
- Ear pinches and frenal tears in children <1yr old are highly suspicious.
- 50% of abused children will have signs on the head &/or neck.

'Child Protection and the Dental Team' is a detailed and practical web-based resource developed by COPDEND/DOH aimed specifically at dentists and other DCPs and can be accessed at ℘ http://www.cpdt.org.uk.

Management Local guidelines are produced by Local Safeguarding Children Boards (LSCBs) or Area Child Protection Committees. To find yours, type 'LSCB' followed by your area into an Internet search engine. A copy of the local LSCB guidance should be kept in every practice.

If abuse is suspected

- Take a careful history and keep full records.
- Discuss concerns with an experienced/trusted colleague and decide if further action/referral is justified.
- Provide any urgent/emergency dental care.
- Talk to child and parents—tactfully explain your concerns, seeking consent to sharing of information. Rarely, if you feel informing the parents/carers may put the child or others (including yourself) at risk, you may still share information &/or refer if you believe it is in the child's best interests to do so. Make sure to arrange review with child and parents before they leave the appointment.

Where to get help and advice (Tip: write the telephone numbers of the first three on this list on your copy of the local LSCB guidance.)

- Child protection nurse.
- Local consultant paediatrician.
- Social services.
- Child's health visitor.
- Your defence organization.

Making a referral Referral should be made directly to social services and followed up in writing within 48h. The child's medical practitioner should also be informed. If a child presents with serious injuries which are suspicious, they should be referred to the nearest accident and emergency department, with the department informed of the situation before the child's arrival.

Tact and understanding is required when dealing with the patient's family. Try to avoid making accusations and concentrate on treating the patient's injuries, expressing the need to refer them on to experts who will be able to fully evaluate the situation and offer appropriate help.

Injuries to primary teeth

About 30–40% of 5yr-olds have experienced dental trauma,[19] most frequently at toddler stage. As alveolar bone is more elastic the younger the child, the most common injuries are luxation or avulsion. Crown and root # are relatively rare.

Management

For definitions, see ➲ Definitions, p. 108. If radiographs are required, you may have to get the parent to hold the child and film. Alternatively, try placing a periapical film between the teeth (like an occlusal view) and angle the beam at 45°.

There is a need to consider the effect of any proposed Rx upon the permanent successor.[20] Splinting of 1° incisors is exceedingly difficult and not indicated. When in doubt, extract 1° tooth!

Concussion of tooth Rx: reassurance and soft diet.

Subluxation If tooth near to exfoliation, extract. Otherwise, soft diet (for about 1 week). May become non-vital, therefore keep under observation. Give appropriate advice regarding possible complications.

Lateral luxation/extrusion Extraction if loose and tooth in danger of being inhaled, or if tooth interferes with occlusion. If crown displaced labially, ↑ risk of damage to underlying 2° incisor.

Intrusion Most common injury (>60%). If X-ray confirms that tooth has been forced into follicle of 2° tooth, extract 1° incisor. Otherwise leave tooth and wait to see if spontaneous eruption will occur (between 1 and 6 months). Unfortunately, pulpal necrosis often follows, necessitating either pulp Rx (➲ Pulp therapy for primary anterior teeth, p. 96) or extraction. Should the tooth fail to erupt, then extraction is indicated. It is prudent to warn parents about possible damage to underlying permanent tooth.

Avulsion Replantation not recommended due to risk of damage to permanent successor.

Crown fracture Rare. Minimal # can be smoothed and left under observation. Larger # either restore with composite &/or RCT if pulp involved, or extract.

Root fracture Provided it is not displaced and there is little mobility, advise a soft diet and keep under review. If coronal fragment is displaced or mobile, extract, but leave the apical portion as it will usually resorb.

19 B. Chadwick 2004 *Children's Dental Health in the UK*, HMSO.

20 J. O. Andreasen et al. 2007 *Textbook and Color Atlas of Traumatic Injuries to the Teeth*, Blackwell Publishing.

Sequelae of trauma

Primary dentition

Discoloration

If tooth becomes grey/reddish in early post-trauma period, pulp may be vital and discoloration reversible.

Greying later indicates pulp necrosis. Yellowing of tooth is suggestive of calcification of pulp—no Rx required.

Ankylosis

Rx: extraction to prevent displacement of 2° incisor.

Pulp death

Rx: RCT or extraction.

Permanent dentition In >50% of children <4yrs, trauma to a 1° tooth affects the underlying developing successor.[21] The effect depends upon stage of development, type of injury and severity, Rx, and pulpal sequelae. Trauma can cause hypomineralization, hypoplasia (likelihood ↑ if <4yrs &/ or injury more severe), dilaceration, severe malformation, and arrest of development.

21 G. Roberts 1996 *Oral and Dental Trauma in Children and Adolescents*, OUP.

Injuries to permanent teeth—crown fractures

Prevalence: 26–76% of injuries.

Enamel only

For small enamel #, smooth with white stone.

Enamel and dentine

Need to protect exposed dentine, preferably with a hard-setting calcium hydroxide cement and an acid-etch retained composite. If time permits, this can be done with a crown former to restore tooth contour. Keep under review. Veneer or porcelain jacket crown (PJC) can be considered later. If # near to pulp, treat as for pulp involvement.

Acid-etch composite tip technique
- Place rubber dam, if possible.
- Place hard-setting calcium hydroxide on exposed dentine. No need to bevel enamel.
- Using contralateral tooth as guide, select a cellulose acetate crown former.
- Trim crown former to within 1–2mm of # line.
- Etch enamel for 20sec, wash, and dry.
- Place bonding resin and cure.
- Put sufficient composite and a little extra into crown former and position.
- Allow to cure and remove crown former.
- Trim, using soflex discs.
- Check occlusion.

Enamel, dentine, and pulp

Rx depends upon size of exposure, state of root development (1 root radiographically complete 10–11yrs, histologically 14–15yrs), time since injury, and other injuries (e.g. root #). If apex open, there is an ↑ blood supply to pulp, therefore likelihood of pulp death ↓. This is advantageous as Rx should be directed towards retaining vitality of radicular pulp to allow root closure to continue. If pulp non-vital, see ➲ Root canal treatment—rationale, p. 338. Otherwise, Rx alternatives are as follows:

Pulp cap Indications: exposure <1mm; <24h; complete or incomplete root development; pulp still vital. Cover exposure with calcium hydroxide (e.g. Dycal®), and place composite tip. Review vitality.

Partial (Cvek) pulpotomy Indications: exposure >1mm; >24h; complete or incomplete root development, pulp still vital.
- LA and rubber dam.
- Slightly enlarge access at site of exposure with high speed and amputate pulp to a depth of 2–4mm into healthy pulp tissue.
- Arrest bleeding with sterile, moist cotton wool (usually takes several minutes).
- Cover amputation site with non-setting calcium hydroxide.
- Seal with GIC.
- Restore crown.

Full coronal pulpotomy Indications: large, contaminated exposures; long duration; incomplete root development; coronal pulp demonstrates impaired vascularity.
- LA and rubber dam.
- Open up pulp chamber and amputate coronal pulp to cervical construction with sterile bur/sharp excavator.
- Wash with sterile water.
- Place non-setting calcium hydroxide and restore tooth with polycarboxylate or GIC and composite.
- Leave 6–8 weeks, then review symptoms and vitality. No need to investigate for presence or not of a calcific barrier.
- If tooth becomes non-vital, see ⮎ Root canal treatment—rationale, p. 338.

All pulpotomized teeth should be kept under long-term review as pulp necrosis and calcification are common sequelae. Success rates of 72% for cervical pulpotomies and 96% for minimal (Cvek) pulpotomies have been reported.[22]

22 M. E. J. Curzon 1999 *Handbook of Dental Trauma*, Wright.

Root fractures

Prevalence Account for <10% of injuries to permanent dentition.
- Where root # is suspected, two X-ray views at different angulations in the vertical plane are advisable to improve chances of visualizing the # line.
- The prognosis for this type of injury depends upon whether the # line communicates with the gingival crevice. Actual Rx depends on position of #. The prognosis is also affected by the degree of dislocation of apical and coronal fragments and mobility/displacement.

Apical third Usually no Rx is required unless mobility ↑ significantly. However, the tooth should be kept under observation as death of coronal two-thirds of pulp may occur. Only need to prepare canal to # line as apical third usually retains vitality. Prognosis good. If extraction required, apical third can be left *in situ* to preserve bone.

Middle third In the majority of cases the tooth is loosened, therefore rigid splinting is advisable to attempt to achieve hard-tissue union of # line. 12 weeks of rigid splinting was previously advocated, but recent evidence suggests flexible splinting for 4 weeks may give a similar outcome.[23] If coronal part is not displaced, loss of vitality is unlikely. Where coronal fragment is displaced, re-position, splint, and if loss of vitality occurs, RCT to # line. Calcium hydroxide should be used as an interim dressing to limit inflammation and resorption. Delay in Rx ↓ prognosis. If extraction required, consider leaving apical portion *in situ*.

Coronal third In this group there is a high risk of direct communication with the gingival crevice, allowing ingress of bacteria into pulp. Where no obvious risk, flexible splinting for a prolonged period (up to 4 months) is advocated.[24] Where the # line extends coronally, emergency Rx is either (i) temporary stabilization or (ii) extraction of the coronal fragment. Definitive Rx usually is extraction of both parts of tooth or, preferably, removal of the coronal fragment, and appropriate RCT of remainder, followed by placement of a dressing which will prevent gingival tissues overgrowing root surface. Can use a temporary post-retained crown, but repositioning of the coronal fragment using a dentine-bonding agent and composite has been described. Permanent Rx is post and core crown.

If # extends below alveolar crest, need improved access for crown fabrication. There are two alternatives, shown in Table 3.5.

An orthodontic extrusion will need either an upper removable appliance (URA) or a sectional fixed appliance (FA) with an attachment bonded on to the labial surface of a temporary post and core crown or any available enamel. Gentle forces of 50–100g should be used. When sufficient extrusion has been achieved, retain for at least 3–6 months before fabricating a permanent restoration.

23 IADT 2012 *Treatment Guidelines* (⅋ http://www.dentaltraumaguide.org).

24 M. J. Kinirons (revised 2010) BSPD guideline: *Treatment of Traumatically Intruded Permanent Incisor Teeth in Children* (⅋ http://www.bspd.co.uk).

Table 3.5 Improving access for crown fabrication

Ostectomy/gingivectomy	Orthodontic extrusion
Gives quicker result	Cervical circumference of crown ↓ compared to contralateral tooth
Needs post and diaphragm	Better crown:root ratio
Tend to get perio pocket	Gingival margin migrates with crown
Leads to ↓ gingival width	

Oblique Provided # does not extend above alveolar crest, can treat as coronal #. Otherwise, consider extraction of coronal portion only, leaving apical portion *in situ* to preserve bone.

Vertical Extraction is often the only option.

If tooth extracted, a P/− will need to be fabricated (➲ Treatment planning for patients with missing teeth, p. 274).

Luxation, subluxation, intrusion, and extrusion

Prevalence: 15–40% of injuries.

Definitions

Concussion Injury to supporting tissues of tooth, without displacement.

Lateral luxation Displacement of tooth (laterally, labially, or palatally).

Subluxation Actually means partial displacement, but commonly used to describe loosening of a tooth without displacement.

Intrusive luxation Displacement of tooth into its socket. Often accompanied by # of alveolar bone.

Extrusive luxation Partial displacement of tooth from its socket.

Rx

Concussion Reassurance and soft diet.

Luxation Need to reposition tooth as soon as possible. Give LA and use fingers to push back into place. Then tooth should be splinted flexibly for 2–3 weeks. If there has been a delay of >24h since the injury, manual reduction is unlikely to be successful. In these cases the tooth can be repositioned orthodontically. If the displaced tooth is interfering with the occlusion a URA, with buccal capping, should be fitted as soon as possible. If root development is complete, loss of vitality is a common sequelae following luxation (~70%), leading to inflammatory resorption (⊙ Pulpal sequelae following trauma, p. 112). Teeth with immature apices have a much better chance of pulp survival. External or internal resorption and pulp canal obliteration may also occur, therefore keep under review.

Subluxation If minor, no Rx other than advising a soft diet is necessary. If mobile, splint for 1–2 weeks and watch vitality.

Intrusion Current UK guidelines[25] advise passive repositioning, with commencement of orthodontic repositioning within 3 weeks for all teeth with open apices and for teeth intruded <3mm with closed apices. For intrusions of 3–6mm in teeth with a closed apex, consider orthodontic or surgical repositioning, and if intrusion exceeds 6mm with a closed apex, surgically reposition. Surgically repositioned teeth require flexible splinting for 1–2 weeks. Pulp death &/or root resorption can ensue rapidly after injury and early pulp extirpation and placement of the calcium hydroxide dressing is advisable. Pulp death is virtually certain in teeth with closed apices, and occurs in two-thirds of immature teeth. Replacement resorption is also a common sequel.

Extrusion The affected tooth should be repositioned under LA with digital pressure and splinted for 1–2 weeks. Again, loss of vitality is a common sequel, so the tooth should be observed for any signs of resorption or pulp death.

   If any of these situations occur in conjunction with # of the alveolar bone, the splinting period should be ↑ to 3–4 weeks to aid bony healing. If, however, the socket is comminuted, splinting may need to be extended to 6–8 weeks.

25 S. Albadri et al. 2018 *Int J Paediatr Dent* **20** (Suppl 1) 1.

Splinting

Indications

- To stabilize a loosened tooth to allow periodontal healing and improve patient comfort. In order to promote fibrous rather than bony healing (ankylosis), a short splinting time with a flexible splint is recommended: avulsion 7–10 days; luxation <3 weeks; middle third root # 4 weeks.
- To stabilize a cervical-third root # and encourage healing with calcified tissue, flexible splinting for up to 4 months is indicated.

Methods

Direct Constructed on patient. An almost infinite variety has been described, but the following are the most popular:

- Acid-etch splint with composite/acrylic/epimine resin &/or wire.
- Orthodontic attachments and sectional archwire.
- Preformed metal (titanium trauma splint).
- Lone standing teeth can be supported by sling suture.[26]
- Lead foil &/or cement. Useful in Australian Outback, but better alternatives available in most dental surgeries!

Indirect This type of splint is removable, which can cause trauma with insertion and removal, and therefore less preferable. It does, however, allow an assessment of mobility or firmness, which may be of value in cases of reimplantation. The more common types are:

- URA with cribs 6|6 and occlusal coverage.
- Vacuum-formed thermoplastic polyvinylacetatepolyethylene 'Essix' type. This approach requires an impression of a traumatized mouth and involves some delay (few hours/days) before the splint can be fitted; in practice, direct splinting is preferred.

Factors affecting choice of splint

- Type of injury and therefore length of time splint required. For example, coronal-third root # will need up to 4 months of splinting, therefore composite and wire splint is advisable. For a replanted tooth, prolonged splinting should be avoided as it may lead to ankylosis.
- Number of teeth injured and availability of uninjured adjacent teeth, e.g. if both 1|1 traumatized and no adjacent teeth, a full coverage acrylic splint or sling-suture may be indicated.
- Facilities and time available.

26 M. E. J. Curzon 1999 *Handbook of Dental Trauma*, Wright.

Management of the avulsed tooth

Exarticulation = avulsion. Prevalence: 0–16% of injuries.

Factors affecting prognosis
Success depends upon re-establishment of a normal periodontium.

- *Time from loss to reimplantation*—as PDL cells rarely survive >60min extra-orally, immediate replacement (by whoever is available at the scene) is the Rx of choice.
- *Storage medium*—prognosis saline > milk > water > air (both tap-water and dry storage rapidly damage periodontal cells).
- *Splinting time*—7–10 days flexible splinting. Prolonged splinting may promote ankylosis.
- *Viability of pulp*—seepage of pulp breakdown products into PDL will contribute to the development of inflammatory resorption. Although revascularization is possible in a tooth with an open apex which is replaced within 30min, those teeth with closed apices and longer extra-alveolar times should be considered non-vital.

Immediate Rx (if avulsed tooth not already replaced)
- Avoid handling root surface. If tooth contaminated, hold crown and agitate gently in saline.
- Place tooth in socket. If it does not readily seat, get patient to bite on gauze for 15–20min.
- Compress buccal and lingual alveolar plates.
- Splint a curved piece of light wire (a light twist-flex SS wire is ideal) to acid-etched enamel of affected and adjacent teeth using temporary crown material as this is less traumatic to remove than composite.
- Systemic antibiotics may improve outcomes. Arrange tetanus booster if necessary. Chlorhexidine mouthwash may be useful when OH is compromised.

Intermediate Rx (7–10 days later)
- Review splinting. Stop if tooth appears firm, continue for further week if still mobile. If still mobile after 2 weeks, check nothing has been overlooked, e.g. root # or loss of vitality—in these cases prognosis is poor.
- If apex closed (or tooth with open apex, but extra-alveolar period >30min) extirpate pulp within 7–10 days, clean canal. If an intermediate dressing is required or monitoring inflammatory resorption, place an initial intra-canal dressing of calcium hydroxide. A mineral trioxide aggregate (MTA) plug is the gold standard now. GDPs should always dress a tooth before referring to an appropriate provider to place MTA.
- Keep teeth with open apices under close observation, so that at the first sign of pulp death RCT can be instituted. Waiting for radiographic evidence of inflammatory resorption is too late.
- Keep tooth under review.

Prognosis

If the described procedure is followed, medium-term survival is relatively good[27] but long-term survival is generally poor.

- Incomplete root formation: 60% survive 5yrs.
- Complete root formation: 80% survive 5yrs.

Long-term survival is closely related to extra-alveolar dry-storage time. Teeth stored dry for >30min have a very poor long-term prognosis, but replantation is always preferable, as failure is usually by replacement resorption which is slow (i.e. tooth may last several years) and maintains bulk of alveolus (facilitates future prosthetic replacement). In a patient <10yrs or going through a pubertal growth spurt, ankylosed teeth should be reviewed carefully as alveolar defects can develop as the tooth infra-occludes, and adjacent alveolar bone continues to grow. In this situation a coronectomy may be carried out, allowing the alveolar bone to continue growth over the remaining root dentine. The root will eventually be completely resorbed.

Where prognosis is deemed to be poor, premolar transplant can be considered at 10–12yrs old.

Sequelae

Surface resorption This occurs as a result of minor trauma to PDL cells. Usually is self-limiting and affected areas are repaired by cementum. No Rx.

Replacement resorption (ankylosis) This is caused by damage to PDL cells during the extra-alveolar period and is promoted by prolonged splinting. It appears that the absence of vital periodontal ligament allows resorption of the root and replacement by bone. In the growing child it results in infra-occlusion of the affected tooth. Once started it is usually progressive, resulting in the eventual loss of the tooth. Can also occur due to intrusion, with ↑ severity of intrusion related to ↑ risk of replacement resorption.

Inflammatory resorption Development is dependent upon the presence of both damage to the periodontal ligament and breakdown products from pulp necrosis diffusing through the dentinal tubules to the PDL. Occurs rapidly, as soon as 1–2 weeks after injury. Once evident radiographically, prognosis is poor, as it is progressive and Rx is not always successful. Internal inflammatory resorption can be prevented by extirpation of the pulp as soon as is practicable after injury and placement of non-setting calcium hydroxide. If resorption is halted, a GP root filling can be placed.

Delayed presentation Where viability of PDL cells is doubtful, Andreasen has suggested chemical Rx of the root surface with fluoride to limit resorption. Following RCT with GP, the tooth is immersed in 2.4% sodium fluoride solution for 20min. Then tooth is replanted and splinted for 6 weeks. As some replacement resorption is inevitable, it is best limited to adults. If the extra-alveolar period is >24h, leave and consider instead whether the resulting space should be maintained with a P/− (➲ Treatment planning for patients with missing teeth, p. 274).

27 J. O. Andreaen 1992 *Atlas of Replantation and Transplantation of Teeth*, Mediglobe.

Pulpal sequelae following trauma

Damage to the pulp can occur as a result of disruption of the apical vessels or exposure of the pulp by a crown or root #, or be caused by haemorrhage and inflammation of coronal pulp, resulting in strangulation.

Pulp death

Remember that no response to vitality testing indicates damage to the nerve supply of a tooth, but not necessarily to the blood supply. Therefore, following trauma, you should assess vitality in the light of symptoms, tooth colour, mobility, presence of buccal swelling, and radiographic evidence. Except where a tooth has been replanted, it is best to adopt a 'wait and see' approach if in doubt about vitality. When pulp death has occurred, subsequent Rx depends upon whether the apex is closed or open.

RCT of teeth with immature apices

As achievement of an apical seal is difficult in a tooth with an open apex, Rx should aim to produce apexification (i.e. a hard-tissue barrier across the apex). Under a rubber dam, the necrotic pulp should be extirpated. The working length is set 1–2mm short of the radiographic apex (unless vital pulp tissue is encountered earlier) and narrow files are used in order to negotiate any undercuts. The canal should then be filled with a radiopaque non-setting calcium hydroxide (e.g. Hypocal™ or Ultracal®) to the apex and sealed. The calcium hydroxide should be replaced every 3 months, until a calcific apical barrier is detectable by gentle probing with a paper point. The average time for a calcific barrier to be formed is 9 months.[28] Then the canal can be filled. Usually, because of the width of the canal, a large GP point (a conventional point upside down) can be used. This should be warmed in a flame before pressing into place and then lots of laterally condensed points used to obtain a good seal. Alternatively, thermoplasticized GP (e.g. Obtura®) can be used. A 5yr survival rate of 86% has been reported[29] but many teeth will fail eventually 2° to cervical root fracture. This probably results from weakening of the tooth due to large access cavity and brittleness of dentine which may be associated with long-term dressing with calcium hydroxide. Some now advocate MTA as an alternative to calcium hydroxide, allowing obturation to be achieved more quickly over fewer visits.

Resorption

Commonly seen after avulsion, luxation, intrusion, or extrusion.

Internal resorption This is associated with chronic pulpal inflammation, which results in resorption of dentine from the pulpal surface. It is progressive, therefore the pulp needs to be carefully extirpated. Dressing the tooth with calcium hydroxide appears to help arrest the resorption and once controlled, a GP filling may be placed. If perforation has occurred, the prognosis is ↓ considerably. Raising a flap, removal of granulation tissue, and direct repair can be attempted.

28 I. C. Mackie & V. N. Warren 1988 *Dent Update* **15** 155.

29 I. C. Mackie et al. 1993 *Br Dent J* **175** 99.

External resorption Radiographically, loss of PDL with no radiolucent areas visible. Three types are seen: surface (transient), replacement, and inflammatory. Replacement resorption is usually 2° to irreversible damage to the cementum, leading to ankylosis (usually associated with a high percussion note). Replacement resorption is usually progressive, is not influenced by endodontic therapy, and eventually leads to the root being replaced by bone. Inflammatory resorption is frequently related to pulp necrosis and can often be halted by appropriate endodontic management. Irregular pits are seen on the root with adjacent radiolucency.

Root canal obliteration

Occurs in 6–35% of luxation-type injuries. Prophylactic endodontic Rx is not necessary as pulp necrosis occurs in only 13–16% of cases. A high rate of success (80%) has been reported for subsequent RCT, despite a hairline or no root canal detectable on X-ray.

Management of missing incisors

- 1—rarely congenitally absent; usually lost following trauma or because of dilaceration.
- 2—congenitally absent in ~2% of population (with ↑ likelihood of displacement 3). May also be lost following trauma.

Missing upper anterior teeth are noticed by the general public before other types of malocclusion. The aim of Rx is to provide a 321|123 smile. Although Cary Grant did well enough with a missing upper central incisor, symmetry is usually preferable. The management of missing incisors involves either recovery or maintenance of space for prosthetic replacement, or orthodontic space closure. Previous studies have shown that patients were more satisfied with space closure than prosthetic replacement[30]; however, with the introduction of implants and newer materials this may change.

For each patient a number of factors need to be considered:

Skeletal relationship In a Class III case, space closure in the upper arch could compromise the incisor relationship, whereas in a Class II/1 it would facilitate o/j ↓. Consider also the vertical relationship, as space closure is easier in patients with ↑ lower face height (LFH) and vice versa in ↓ LFH.

Crowding/spacing In a patient with no crowding, space closure is difficult and requires prolonged retention. Before opening a space it is important to ensure that sufficient will be available at the end of Rx for an adequate prosthetic replacement (minimum width for implant to replace 2 is 6.5mm). A Kesling set-up may be useful.

Colour and form of adjacent teeth Although much can be done with veneers, composite additions, and grinding, if 3 is significantly darker &/or caniform in shape, it will be difficult to turn it into a convincing 2 if space closure is planned. 2 can only be used to mimic 1 if root length and circumference at gingival margin are not significantly smaller.

Inclination of adjacent teeth The final axial inclination of the teeth will determine the aesthetics of the finished result.

Buccal occlusion If a good Class I buccal interdigitation exists this may C/I bringing the posterior teeth forward to close space.

Unilateral loss A symmetrical result is more pleasing, therefore maintenance or opening of space is preferable. If a 2 is missing and the contralateral tooth is peg-shaped, thought should be given to extracting this tooth to achieve symmetry.

Smile line If the patient has a high smile line then there is a need to consider gingival level. In some cases, they may need gingival surgery.

30 S. Robertsson & B. Mohlin 2000 *Eur J Orthod* **22** 697.

Patient's wishes and cooperation Only after assessing the earlier listed factors can the patient be given an informed choice. If the patient refuses FAs this may alter the Rx plan.

Kesling set-up This requires duplicate models of both arches, including at least two of the upper arch. Using a small hacksaw, the teeth which will require orthodontic movement are removed from the model and repositioned using wax. As many alternatives as desired can be tried to find the best result.

Space closure In the presence of crowding elsewhere in the arch, this can be facilitated by early extraction of the 1° teeth on the affected side; therefore the earlier the decision is made to close space, the better. Active space closure requires a FA to achieve correct axial inclination. It is sometimes better to carry out any masking procedures before orthodontic Rx, e.g. contouring 3 to resemble 2 (by removal of enamel incisally, interproximally, and from the palatal aspect &/or composite addition) as this will facilitate final positioning and occlusion. Retain with a bonded retainer.

NB: the average difference in width between 3 and 2 is 1.2mm, which can easily be removed mesially and distally from 3.

Space-maintenance/opening If an incisor is selectively extracted and space maintenance is desired, a P/− or acid-etch bridge should be fitted immediately. Where 2 is congenitally missing, space may need to be opened orthodontically with FA. Some advocate encouraging the 3 to erupt adjacent to the 1 and then retracting it to open space to give better bone levels for implant or bridge. Following space opening, retention with a P/− for 3–6 months is advisable to allow the teeth to settle. If an acid-etch retained prosthesis is planned, ensure that there is sufficient room occlusally for the wings.

Resin-bonded bridge See ◑ Resin-bonded bridges, p. 288.

Transplantation Transplantation of a lower premolar into the socket of an extracted incisor can be considered if the lower arch is crowded.

Implant Implant when growth is complete (◑ Introduction to implantology, see p. 362).

Common childhood ailments affecting the mouth

▶ Refer any patient with an ulcer that doesn't heal within 3 weeks or with any soft tissue lesion of unknown aetiology.

See Chapter 11.

Most common disease is gingivitis (see Chapter 5).

Viral

Primary herpetic gingivostomatitis Occurs >6 months of age. Symptoms: febrile, cervical lymphadenitis, vesicles leading to ulcers on gingiva and oral mucosa. Rx: soft diet with plenty of fluids. Self-limiting, lasts for ~10 days. Common in primary school-age children.

Secondary herpes labialis Vesicles form around the lips, and crust. Self-limiting, but 5% aciclovir cream will speed healing.

Hand, foot, and mouth disease Rash on hands and feet plus ulcers on oral mucosa and gingiva. Little systemic upset. Self-limiting.

Herpangina Febrile illness with sore throat due to ulcers on soft palate and throat. Usually lasts about 3–5 days. Rx: soft diet.

Warts Check hands. Usually self-limiting.

Also chickenpox (vesicles leading to ulcers), mumps (inflamed parotid duct), glandular fever (ulcers), and measles.

Bacterial

Impetigo Very infectious staphylococcal (&/or streptococcal) rash. Starts around mouth and may be mistaken for 2° herpes.

Streptococcal sore throat Can contract associated streptococcal gingivitis (as rare as hen's teeth!).

Necrotizing ulcerative gingivitis (NUG) Rare <16yrs (➲ Necrotizing periodontal diseases, p. 199).

Fungal

Candida Commensal of the mouth, which may become pathogenic when oral environment favours its proliferation. Two types of manifestation are seen in children. (i) Acute pseudo-membranous candidiasis (thrush). Seen in newborn, under-nourished infants after prolonged use of antibiotics or steroids. Presents as white patches that rub off. Rx: miconazole (24mg/mL) and correct underlying problem. (ii) Chronic atrophic candidiasis. Most commonly URA and poor OH &/or high sugar intake. Rx: OHI for appliance and teeth. Chlorhexidine mouthwash or miconazole gel.

Miscellaneous

Aphthous ulceration See ➲ Recurrent aphthous stomatitis (ulcers), p. 440.

Orofacial granulomatosis See ➲ Orofacial granulomatosis, p. 470.

Common causes of oral ulceration in children
In order of frequency: aphthous; trauma; acute herpetic gingivostomatitis; herpangina; hand, foot, and mouth disease; glandular fever.

Common causes of soft tissue swellings in children
Abscess; mucocele; eruption cyst; epulides; papilloma.

▶ Oral cancer does occur in children, therefore if in doubt refer for biopsy.

Sugar-free medications

The potential cariogenic effect of long-term medication sweetened with sugar is now well recognized. Therefore sugar-free preparations should be prescribed whenever possible. Unfortunately, there is no evidence that rinsing out or brushing the teeth after use of a sugar-based medicine will significantly ↓ the incidence of caries. Current medical advice is for liquid medicines to be given to children by disposable syringes. This approach has the advantage that an accurate dose can be directed at the back of the mouth.

Table 3.6 is a list of some sugar-free medicines. It is not exhaustive and where required reference should be made to the *British National Formulary (BNF)*.

Table 3.6 Common child medicines available as sugar-free preparations

Analgesics	
Aspirin (>12yrs)	Dispersible aspirin tablets
Paracetamol	Disprol® paediatric Panadol® soluble
Paracetamol and codeine	Paracodol® dispersible tablets Solpadeine®
Ibuprofen	Ibuprofen oral suspension SF
Antacids	
Aluminium and magnesium	Mucogel® Maalox® suspension
Cimetidine	
Ranitidine	Zantac® dispersible tablets Zantac® suspension
Anticonvulsants	
Carbamazepine	Tegretol® liquid
Phenobarbital	Phenobarbital elixir 30mg/10mL
Sodium valproate	Epilim® crushable tablets/elixir
Anti-infectives	
Aciclovir	Zovirax® suspension
Amoxicillin	Amoxil® sachets SF
Amphotericin	
Ampicillin and cloxacillin	
Erythromycin	
Miconazole	Daktarin® oral gel
Respiratory agents	
Salbutamol	Salbutamol syrup Ventolin® syrup
Miscellaneous	
Folic acid	Lexpec® syrup
Iron edetate	Sytron®
Vitamins A, B, C, D, and E	

Orthodontics

Relevant pages in other chapters Surgical management of CLP, ➋ Clefts and craniofacial anomalies, p. 508; abnormalities of eruption, ➋ Abnormalities of tooth eruption and exfoliation, p. 66; supernumerary teeth, ➋ Hyperdontia, p. 68; orthognathic surgery, ➋ p. 510.

Further reading M. T. Cobourne et al. 2015 *Handbook of Orthodontics* (2e), Mosby Elsevier. D. S. Gill 2008 *Orthodontics at a Glance*, Blackwell. D. S. Gill and F. B. Naini 2011 *Orthodontics: Principles and Practice*, Wiley-Blackwell. S. J. Littlewood and L. Mitchell 2019 *An Introduction to Orthodontics* (5e), OUP. See also Cochrane Library ᕦ http://www.thecochranelibrary.com.

What is orthodontics?

Orthodontics has been defined as that branch of dentistry concerned with growth of the face, development of the dentition, and prevention and correction of occlusal anomalies. Ortho (from Greek) = straight. Malocclusion is not a disease—it is variation from ideal occlusion.

Prevalence of malocclusion Crowding ~60%; Class I 60%, Class II/1 20%; Class II/2 10–18%; Class III ~5% (Fig. 4.1).

Why do orthodontics? Research shows that individual motivation has more effect upon the presence of plaque than alignment of the teeth; therefore, the main indications for orthodontic Rx are aesthetics and function. Functional reasons for Rx include deep traumatic overbite, ↑ o/j especially if the lips are incompetent (↑ risk of trauma), and labial crowding of a lower incisor (as this reduces periodontal support labially). While it is accepted that severe malocclusion may affect self-esteem and psychological well-being, the impact of more minor anomalies and, indeed, perceived need are influenced by social and cultural factors. The Index of Orthodontic Treatment Need (IOTN) has been developed to try to standardize and quantify this difficult issue (● The Index of Orthodontic Treatment Need, p. 128). In adults, Rx may be indicated to facilitate restorative management.

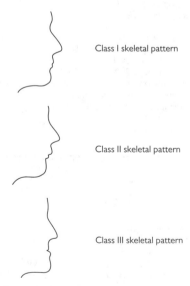

Class I skeletal pattern

Class II skeletal pattern

Class III skeletal pattern

Fig. 4.1 Malocclusion.

Even with good OH, a small loss of periodontal attachment is common and with poor OH this will be ↑. Decalcification will occur if there are frequent sugar intakes between meals. Around 1–2mm of root resorption is associated with FA Rx and in at-risk patients (those with shortened/blunt root shapes) this risk may be ↑. Therefore, the potential benefits of orthodontic Rx must be sufficient to counter-balance these risks.

Who should do orthodontics? All dentists should be concerned with growth and development. Unless anomalies are detected early and any necessary steps taken at the appropriate time, then provision of the best possible outcome for that patient is less likely. Most orthodontic Rx in Europe is now carried out by trained specialist orthodontic practitioners. In the UK, the hospital consultant service acts as a source of advice and a referral point for more complex and multidisciplinary problems.

When should we do orthodontics? Most orthodontic Rx is not started until the early 2° dentition, when the canines and premolars have erupted. At this stage, the response to orthodontic forces is more rapid, appliances are better tolerated, and, most importantly, growth can be utilized to help effect sagittal or vertical change. However, there is some evidence that protraction facemask therapy for Class III malocclusions achieves more skeletal change around age 8–9yrs than in older children.[1]

In adults, lack of growth, ↑ risk of periodontal disease, worn, damaged, and missing teeth, and slower tooth movement will limit the type of malocclusion that can be managed by orthodontics alone.

What to refer and when

Primary dentition
- Cleft lip and/or palate (if patient not under the care of a cleft team).
- Other craniofacial anomalies (if patient not under the care of a multidisciplinary team).

Early mixed dentition
- Delayed eruption of the permanent incisors.
- Impaction or failure of eruption of the 6s.
- 6s of poor long-term prognosis.
- Severe Class III skeletal problems suitable for orthopaedic Rx with protraction facemask.
- Anterior crossbites (Xbites) which compromise periodontal support.
- Ectopic maxillary canines.
- Patients with medical problems where monitoring of the occlusion would be beneficial.
- Pathology, e.g. cysts.

Late mixed dentition
- Growth modification of skeletal Class II malocclusions.
- Hypodontia.
- Most routine problems.

Orthodontics should be involved in the immediate decision-making following repercussions of trauma, particularly following extrusions where orthodontic intrusion may be needed, even if the patient is in the mixed dentition.

---

1 N. Mandall et al. 2016. *J Orthod* **43** 164.

Definitions

Ideal occlusion Anatomically perfect arrangement of the teeth. Rare.

Normal occlusion Acceptable variation from ideal occlusion.

Competent lips Lips meet with minimal or no muscle activity.

Incompetent lips Evident muscle activity is required for lips to meet.

Frankfort plane Line joining porion (superior aspect of external auditory meatus) with orbitale (lowermost point of bony orbit).

Class I The lower incisor edges occlude with, or lie immediately below, the cingulum of upper incisors (Fig. 4.2).

Class II The lower incisor edges lie posterior to the cingulum of the upper incisors. *Division 1*: the upper central incisors are upright or proclined and the o/j is ↑ (Fig. 4.3). *Division 2*: the upper central incisors are retroclined and the o/j is usually ↓ but may be ↑ (Fig. 4.4).

Class III The lower incisor edges lie anterior to the cingulum of the upper incisors and the o/j is ↓ or reversed (Fig. 4.5).

Bimaxillary proclination Both upper and lower incisors are proclined.

Overjet Distance between the upper and lower incisors in the horizontal plane.

Overbite Overlap of the incisors in the vertical plane.

Complete overbite The lower incisors contact the upper incisors or the palatal mucosa.

Incomplete overbite The lower incisors do not contact the upper incisors or the palatal mucosa.

Anterior open bite There is no vertical overlap of the incisors when the buccal segment teeth are in occlusion.

Crossbite A deviation from the normal bucco-lingual relationship. May be anterior/posterior &/or unilateral/bilateral.

Buccal crossbite Buccal cusps of lower premolars or molars occlude buccally to the buccal cusps of the upper premolars or molars.

Lingual crossbite Buccal cusps of lower molars occlude lingually to the lingual cusps of the upper molars.

Dento-alveolar compensation The inclination of the teeth compensates for the underlying skeletal pattern, so that the occlusal relationship between the arches is less severe.

Leeway space The difference in width between C, D, E, and 3, 4, 5. Greater in lower than upper arch.

Mandibular deviation Path of closure starts from a postured position of the mandible.

Mandibular displacement When closing from the rest position, the mandible displaces (either laterally or anteriorly) to avoid a premature contact.

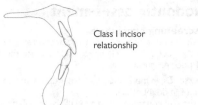

Class I incisor relationship

Fig. 4.2 Class I incisor relationship.

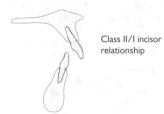

Class II/1 incisor relationship

Fig. 4.3 Class II/1 incisor relationship.

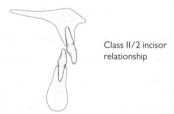

Class II/2 incisor relationship

Fig. 4.4 Class II/2 incisor relationship.

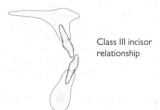

Class III incisor relationship

Fig. 4.5 Class III incisor relationship.

Orthodontic assessment

Brief screening procedure
The purpose of this is to ensure early detection and Rx of any abnormality, prepare the patient for any later Rx, and influence the management of any teeth of poor prognosis.

At every visit Once the 2° incisors have erupted and until 2° dentition is established (if in doubt refer).
- Keep the eruption sequence in mind (➲ Failure of/delayed eruption, p. 66).
- Failure of a tooth to appear >6 months after the contralateral tooth has erupted should ring alarm bells.
- Ask child to close together and look for Xbites, reverse or ↑ o/j.
- Consider the long-term prognosis of the 6s (➲ Extraction of poor-quality first permanent molars, p. 140).

From age 9yrs onwards and until they erupt, palpate for $\underline{3}$ in the buccal sulcus. A definite hollow &/or asymmetry warrants further investigation.

Gathering information
Should be carried out in a logical sequence so that nothing is missed.
- Who wants Rx (patient or parent) and what for?
- Is patient willing to wear braces?
- Enquire about any previous extractions and orthodontic Rx.
- Check medical history.
- Assess growth status.
- Assess suitability for orthodontic Rx including motivation, OH, and commitment.

EO examination (with Frankfort plane horizontal)
- Assess skeletal pattern:
  - Anteroposterior (max = mand—Class I; max > mand—Class II; max < mand—Class III). See Fig. 4.1.
  - Vertically (Frankfort–mandibular planes angle ~25–30°). Lower face height is the distance from the base of the nose (subnasale) to the point of the chin (menton), and in a normally proportioned face is equal to the middle facial third—eyebrow line (glabella) to base of nose (subnasale).
  - Transversely (? asymmetry).
- Soft tissues: can patient achieve lip competence with or without muscle activity? Check the position of the lower lip relative to the inc and how the patient achieves an oral seal (? lip to lip; lip to tongue; or by the lower lip being drawn up behind the incisors). Note also the length of the upper lip, the amount of inc seen, gingival display on smiling, and lip tonicity.
- Check rest position of mandible and for any displacement on closure.
- Habits? Does patient suck a thumb/finger, bite fingernails, or brux?

IO examination
- Record OH, gingival condition, and teeth present. Any teeth of poor prognosis?
- Lower labial segment (LLS): inclination to mandibular base, crowding/spacing, displaced teeth, angulation of lower canines.
- Upper labial segment (ULS): inclination to maxillary base, crowding/spacing, rotations, displaced teeth, presence and angulation of $\underline{3|3}$.
- Measure o/j (mm), overbite (o/b) (↑ or ↓, complete or incomplete) (Fig. 4.6). Check centre lines coincident and correct within face.

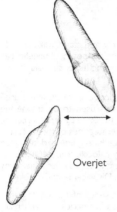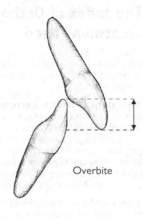

Overjet   Overbite

Fig. 4.6 Overjet and overbite.

- Buccal segments: crowding/spacing, displaced teeth.
- Check molar and canine relationship. Any Xbites?
- Crowding: mild <4mm; moderate 4–8mm; severe >8mm.

Diagnostic records
- To facilitate diagnosis and Rx planning.
- Measuring the progress and outcome of Rx.
- Medico-legal.
- Audit and research.

Radiographs Usually a DPT is taken and, if not clearly visible on the DPT, an intraoral of the inc. A lateral skull view is indicated if the patient has a skeletal discrepancy or AP movement of the incisors is anticipated.
- Look for unerupted, missing, displaced, supernumerary teeth, or other pathology. Check root morphology looking for blunt or pipette-shaped roots.
- Cephalometric analysis, see ➔ Cephalometrics, p. 130.
- An upper standard occlusal may be used in the parallax technique for identifying the position of impacted canines.

Study models Study models should be trimmed so that they occlude correctly on a flat surface. Digital study models are becoming more popular as they are easier to store.

Photographs Good-quality EO and IO colour photos.

Problem list
This information is then collated into a problem list subdivided into:
- *Pathological*—e.g. caries, perio disease, impacted teeth.
- *Developmental*—patient's concerns; skeletal and dental problems in AP, vertical, and transverse; alignment of upper and lower arches including crowding and/or spacing.

The aims of Rx can then be derived from the problem list (➔ Problem list, p. 134).

The Index of Orthodontic Treatment Need

The IOTN (Box 4.1) was developed to quantify and standardize an individual patient's need for orthodontic Rx, so that the potential benefits can be weighed against the possible disadvantages.[2] The Index consists of two components:

The dental health component Developed from an index used by the Swedish Dental Health Board (which was used to determine the amount of financial help that would be given by the State towards Rx costs). The dental health component of IOTN has five categories of Rx need, ranging from little need to very great need. A patient's grade is determined by recording the single worst feature of their malocclusion. 'MOCDO' is helpful when assessing dental health component as it provides a hierarchy of severity—Missing teeth; Overjet; Crossbite; Displacement; Overbite.

The aesthetic component Based on a series of ten photographs of the labial aspect of different Class I or Class II malocclusions, which are ranked according to their attractiveness. A patient's score is determined by the photograph, which is deemed to have an equivalent degree of aesthetic impairment.

Box 4.1 The Index of Orthodontic Treatment Need

Grade 1 (none)
1 Extremely minor malocclusions including displacements less than 1mm.

Grade 2 (little need for treatment)
2a Increased overjet 3.6–6mm with competent lips.
2b Reverse overjet 0.1–1mm.
2c Anterior or posterior crossbite with up to 1mm discrepancy between retruded contact position and intercuspal position.
2d Displacement of teeth 1.1–2mm.
2e Anterior or posterior openbite 1.1–2mm.
2f Increased overbite 3.5mm or more, without gingival contact.
2g Pre-normal or post-normal occlusions with no other anomalies. Includes up to half a unit discrepancy.

Grade 3 (borderline treatment need)
3a Increased overjet 3.5mm ≤ 6mm with incompetent lips.
3b Reverse overjet 1mm ≤ 3.5mm.
3c Anterior or posterior crossbites with 1mm ≤ 2mm discrepancy between retruded contact position and intercuspal position.
3d Contact point displacements 2mm ≤ 4mm.
3e Lateral or anterior open bite 2mm ≤ 4mm.
3f Deep overbite complete to gingival or palatal tissues but no trauma.

---

2 W. C. Shaw 1991 *BDJ* **170** 107.

Grade 4 (need treatment)

4h   Less extensive hypodontia requiring pre-restorative orthodontics or orthodontic space closure to obviate the need for a prosthesis.

4a   Increased overjet 6mm ≤ 9mm.

4b   Reverse overjet >3.5mm with no masticatory or speech difficulties.

4m   Reverse overjet 1mm <3.5mm with recorded masticatory and speech difficulties.

4c   Anterior or posterior crossbites with greater than 2mm discrepancy between retruded contact position and intercuspal position.

4l   Posterior lingual crossbite with no functional occlusal contact in one or both buccal segments.

4d   Severe contact point displacements >4mm.

4e   Extreme lateral or anterior open bites >6mm.

4f   Increased and complete overbite with gingival or palatal trauma.

4t   Partially erupted teeth, tipped and impacted against adjacent teeth.

4x   Presence of supernumerary teeth.

Grade 5 (need treatment)

5i   Impeded eruption of teeth (except for third molars) due to crowding, displacement, the presence of supernumerary teeth, retained deciduous teeth or any pathological cause.

5h   Extensive hypodontia with restorative implications (>1 tooth missing in any quadrant) requiring pre-restorative orthodontics.

5a   Increased overjet >9mm.

5m   Reverse overjet >3.5mm with reported masticatory and speech difficulties.

5p   Defects of cleft lip and palate and other craniofacial anomalies.

5s   Submerged deciduous teeth.

Reproduced from Brook P, et al., The development of an index of orthodontic treatment priority, *Eur J Orthod*, 1989, 11, 309–20, by permission of Oxford University Press on behalf of the European Orthodontic Society.

Cephalometrics

Cephalometric analysis is the interpretation of lateral skull radiographs (Fig. 4.7). They are taken in a cephalostat to standardize position and magnification (usually around 7–8%) so that they are reproducible. It is not obligatory for orthodontic Δ and where the incisor position is not to be changed significantly, the radiographic exposure may not be justified for the information gained. However, where AP movement is required, a lateral skull radiograph will back up the clinical assessment of skeletal pattern and help to determine the degree of difficulty. Serial lateral skulls aid assessment of growth.

Tracing/digitizing

Nowadays, most lateral skull radiographs are digital and can be digitized directly. If a landmark is hard to see, block off the rest of the film so that only that area is illuminated. By convention, the most prominent image should be traced, i.e. the most anterior in the face, so that the difficulty of Rx is not underestimated.

There are many commercial programs of varying complexity and cost to facilitate cephalometric analysis and Rx planning.

Pitfalls

- Consider the cephalometric values for a particular patient in conjunction with their clinical assessment, as variation from the normal in a measurement may be compensated for elsewhere in the face or cranial base.
- Angle ANB varies with the relative prominence of nasion and the lower face. If SNA significantly ↑ or ↓ this could be due to the position of nasion, in which case an additional analysis should be used, e.g. Wits analysis.
- For landmarks which are bilateral (unless superimposed exactly), the midpoint between the two should be taken to correspond with other reference points which are in the midline.
- Tracing errors; with careful technique these should be of the order of ± 0.5° and 0.5mm. Errors are compounded when comparing tracings, therefore changes of only 1° or 2° should be interpreted with caution.

Lower facial height (LFH)

LFH is the distance from anterior nasal spine to menton as a percentage of the total face height (from nasion to menton).

Soft tissue analysis

This is particularly useful in orthognathic patients. The naso-labial angle is the angle between the nose and the upper lip.

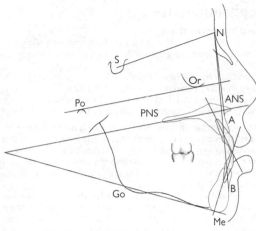

S	= Sella: mid-point of sella turcica.
N	= Nasion: most anterior point on fronto-nasal suture.
Or	= Orbitale: most inferior anterior point on margin of orbit (take average of two images).
Po	= Porion: uppermost outermost point on bony external auditory meatus.
ANS	= Anterior nasal spine.
PNS	= Posterior nasal spine.
Go	= Gonion: most posterior inferior point on angle of mandible.
Me	= Menton: lowermost point on the mandibular symphysis.
A	= A point: position of deepest concavity on anterior profile of maxilla.
B	= B point: position of deepest concavity on anterior profile of mandibular sympshysis.
Frankfort plane	= Po–Or.
Maxillary plane	= PNS–ANS.
Mandibular plane	= Go–Me.

Fig. 4.7 Most commonly used cephalometric points.

More cephalometrics

Analysis and interpretation

The analysis of lateral skull tracings is carried out by comparing a number of angular measurements and proportions with average values for the population as a whole (Table 4.1).

When interpreting a tracing, bear in mind:

- 68% of values lie within 1 standard deviation of the mean.
- 95% of values lie within 2 standard deviations of the mean.
- >99% of values lie within 3 standard deviations of the mean.

It is important to remember that the ANB difference is not an infallible assessment of skeletal pattern as it assumes (incorrectly in some cases) that there is no discrepancy in the cranial base and that A and B are indicative of basal bone position. When a cephalometric tracing seems at odds with your clinical impression it is worth doing another analysis which avoids reliance on the cranial base, such as a Wits analysis.

Before deciding on a Rx plan it is helpful to consider what factors have contributed to a particular malocclusion, e.g. in a patient with a Class II/1 incisor relationship on a Class I skeletal pattern, the prognosis for Rx is much better if the ↑ o/j is due to proclination of the upper rather than retroclination of the lower incisors. The relative contribution of the maxilla and mandible to the skeletal pattern may indicate possible lines of Rx; e.g. if an ↑ o/j is due to a retrusive mandible, a better aesthetic result may be achieved by use of a functional appliance.

As a rough guide, one can assume that there is 5° of angular movement for every millimetre of linear movement of the incisor edge.

CBCT scans are increasingly available and used instead of radiographs in many cases. 3-D analyses are being developed but the main value of this technique is the additional spatial dimension for assessing asymmetry, tooth position, pathology, etc. For a good discussion of the pros and cons see reference.[3]

Table 4.1 Analysis of lateral skull tracings (normal values for Caucasians (UK), standard deviations in parentheses)

SNA	= 81° (±3)
SNB	= 78°(±3)
ANB	= 3°(±2)
1–Max	= 109°(±6)
1–Mand	= 93°(±6) or 120 minus MMPA
MMPA	= 27°(±4)
Facial proportion	= 55% (±2)
Inter-incisal angle	= 135°(±10)

3 A. Abdelkarim 2012 *J World Fed Orthod* 1 e3.

Wits analysis
Used to assess AP skeletal pattern (Fig. 4.8).

Method
- Construct the functional occlusal plane (FOP) by drawing a line through the cusp tips of the molars and premolars or 1° molars.
- Drop perpendiculars to the FOP from A point (to give AO) and B point (to give BO).
- Measure the distance from AO to BO.

In Class I AP relationship
- Males: BO is 1mm (±1.9mm) ahead of AO.
- Females: BO = AO (±1.77mm).

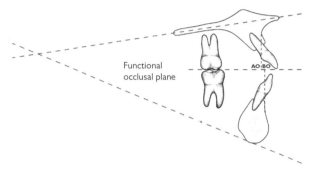

Functional occlusal plane

AO BO

Fig. 4.8 Wits analysis.

Treatment planning

Problem list

The problem list is a logical summary of the main features of a malocclusion, i.e. the diagnosis. It is usually subdivided into pathological and developmental features (◆ Orthodontic assessment, p. 126).

Aims of Rx

The next step is to work through these and decide which problems will be accepted and which corrected—the latter are the aims of Rx. Then possible solutions and their relative risks and benefits can be considered. These should be discussed with the patient (along with the option of no Rx) before informed consent is obtained for the definitive Rx plan.

Basic Rx planning principles

The lower arch This lies in a zone of relative stability between the lips, cheeks, and tongue; therefore, in most cases it is advisable to maintain its current position. This gives a starting point around which to plan Rx. The first step is to decide if the lower arch is sufficiently crowded to warrant extractions. If the crowding is moderate to severe and likely to ↑, then extractions are probably indicated (◆ Extractions, p. 138). In some cases, movement of the LLS is indicated but these are the province of the specialist, e.g. Class III where retroclination of the LLS is required for camouflage; Class II/2 cases where it may be advisable to accept a little proclination to help ↓ o/b and improve aesthetics.

   If in doubt, refer for advice.

The upper arch Next, the position of the upper arch can be planned to achieve a Class I incisor relationship. This usually requires positioning, in the mind's eye, the $\underline{3}$ into a Class I relationship with $\overline{3}$ (in corrected position if LLS crowded). This will give an indication of the space required and the amount and type of movement necessary. In the upper arch, space for retraction of $\underline{3}$ can be gained by: (i) extractions, (ii) expansion (only indicated if a Xbite exists), (iii) distal movement of the upper buccal segments (◆ Distal movement of the upper buccal segments, p. 142), or (iv) a combination of these. Should extractions be indicated in both arches, mechanics are often easier if the same tooth is extracted in the upper as in the lower. However, in Class II cases it may be advantageous to extract further forward in the upper arch and vice versa in Class III cases.

Buccal segments It is not always necessary to plan to a Class I buccal segment relationship. If only upper arch extractions are required to gain space to ↓ an o/j, then the final molar relationship will be Class II. Likewise, if only lower teeth are extracted, the molar relationship will be Class III at the end of Rx.

Rx mechanics The next step is to plan what tooth movements need to be carried out, including which appliances are to be used and in what sequence. These decisions should be made based on available evidence of efficiency, predictability, minimal risks, and minimal patient cooperation.

Anchorage To every force there is an equal and opposite reaction. In orthodontic Rx, the resistance to unwanted tooth movement is called anchorage and also needs to be considered when planning Rx. *Retention* of the final result should be included in the Rx plan and the need for compliance with wearing retention appliances explained to the patient. Many orthodontists now plan for long-term retention.

Consent

In some cases, more than one Rx plan can be offered to the patient, with a hierarchy of complexity and finished result. The risks and benefits of each option (including no Rx) should be carefully explained to the patient/parent so they can make an informed choice. If a compromise plan is chosen by the patient, this should be recorded in the consent process. It is advisable to get written consent, including specific details of the Rx and associated risks.

Refer for advice if the malocclusion under consideration contains one of the following features:

- Marked skeletal discrepancy, AP (II or III), or vertically.
- If the o/j is ↑ and the upper incisors are upright.
- If the o/j is reversed and there is no o/b to hold the corrected incisor relationship.
- Severe Class II/2 malocclusions.
- Class II/I incisor relationship, with molars a full unit Class II and a crowded lower arch.

Rx planning is the most important, and most difficult, part of orthodontics.

Further reading

S. J. Littlewood et al. 2016 Retention procedures for stabilising tooth position after treatment with orthodontic braces. *Cochrane Database Syst Rev* 1 CD002283.

Management of the developing dentition

See also delayed eruption, ➲ Failure of/delayed eruption, p. 66.

The way in which mixed dentition problems are approached will often affect the ease or difficulty of subsequent Rx.

Normal development of dentition The 1° incisors are usually upright and spaced. If there is no spacing, warn the parents that the 2° incisors will probably be crowded. Overbite reduces throughout the 1° dentition until the incisors are edge to edge. All 2° incisors develop lingual to their predecessors, erupt into a wider arc, and are more proclined. It is normal for 1|1 to erupt with a median diastema which reduces as 2|2 erupt. Later, pressure from the developing canines on the roots of 2|2 results in their being tilted distally and spaced. This has been called the 'ugly duckling stage', but it is better to describe it as normal development to parents. As the 3 erupts, the 2 upright and the spaces usually close.

The majority of Es erupt so that their distal edges are flush. The transition to the normal stepped (Class I) molar relationship usually occurs during the 2° dentition as a result of greater mandibular growth &/or the leeway space.

Development of dental arches In the average (!) child, the size of the dental arch is more or less established once the 1° dentition has erupted, except for an ↑ in inter-canine width (2–3mm up to age 9yrs) which results in a modification of arch shape.

Retained primary teeth If deflecting eruption of 2° tooth, extract.

Infraoccluded primary molars Prevalence 8–14%. Provided there is a successor, an infraoccluded 1° molar will probably be exfoliated at the same time as the contralateral tooth.[4] However, even if there is a successor tooth, the fact that the tooth is infraoccluded is a good indicator for extraction. Often, infraocclusion can impede eruption or cause palatal eruption of the successor tooth. It is wise to seek an orthodontic opinion in this instance.

Impacted upper first permanent molars Prevalence 2–6%. Indicative of crowding. Spontaneous disimpaction rare after 8yrs. Can try dislodging 6 by tightening a piece of brass wire round the contact point with E over several visits. Otherwise just observe, extracting E if unavoidable and dealing with resultant space loss in 2° dentition.

Habits Effects produced depend upon duration of habit and intensity. It is best not to make a great fuss of a finger-sucking habit. If parents are concerned, reassure them (in the presence of the child) not to worry, as only little girls/boys suck their fingers. Appliances to break the habit may help, but most children will stop when they are ready. However, this is no reason to delay the start of Rx for other aspects of the malocclusion.

4 J. Kurol 1985 *Am J Orthod* **87** 46.

Effects of premature loss of primary teeth Unfortunately, when a child attends with toothache, in the rush to relieve pain it is all too easy to extract the offending tooth without consideration of the consequences. The major effect of early 1° tooth loss is localization of crowding, in crowded mouths. The extent to which this occurs depends upon the patient's age, the degree of crowding, and the site. In a crowded mouth, the adjacent teeth will move round into the extraction space, therefore, unilateral loss of a C (and to a lesser degree a D) will result in a centre-line shift. This is also seen when a C is prematurely exfoliated by an erupting 2. As correction of a centre-line discrepancy often involves FAs, prevention is better than cure, so loss of Cs should always be balanced. If Es are lost, the 6 will migrate forward. This is particularly marked if it occurs before eruption of the permanent tooth, so if extraction of an E is unavoidable try to defer until after the 6s are in occlusion and do not balance or compensate.

The effect of early loss of 1° teeth on the eruption of the permanent successor is variable.

Timely loss of Cs is indicated for:
• 2 erupting palatally due to crowding. Extraction of C|C as the 2 is erupting may allow the tooth to escape labially and prevent a Xbite.
• Extraction of lower Cs when a lower incisor is being crowded labially will help to ↓ loss of periodontal support.

Balancing extraction Extraction of the same (or adjacent) tooth on the opposite side of the arch to preserve symmetry.

Compensating extraction Extraction of the same tooth in the opposing arch.

Further reading
M. Cobourne 2014 *Guideline for Extraction of First Permanent Molars in Children* (✎ http://www.rcseng.ac.uk).
O. Yaqoob 2016 *Management of Unerupted Maxillary Incisors Guideline* (✎ http://www.rcseng.ac.uk).

Extractions

In orthodontics, teeth are extracted to relieve crowding, level and align, and to provide space to compensate for a skeletal discrepancy.
* Before planning the extraction of any permanent teeth a thorough orthodontic and radiographic examination should be carried out.
* In a Class I or II, it is advisable to extract at least as far forward in the upper arch as the lower; vice versa in a Class III.

Lower incisors These are rarely the teeth of choice as it is difficult to arrange 6 ULS teeth around 5 LLS teeth. Indications: ↓ prognosis or perio support, Class I buccal segments and LLS crowding, mild Class III with well-aligned buccal segments.

Upper incisors If traumatized or dilacerated, there may be no alternative (➲ Management of missing incisors, p. 114). A peg-shaped $\underline{2}$ may be extracted if the contralateral $\underline{2}$ is absent.

Lower canines Usually only extracted if severely displaced.

Upper canines See ➲ Buccally displaced maxillary canines, p. 143.

First premolars These are a popular choice in moderate to severe crowding because of their position in the arch. They also give best chance of spontaneous improvement especially if extracted just as the 3s are appearing, but if appliance therapy is planned, defer until the canines have erupted.

Second premolars These are preferred in cases with mild crowding, as their extraction alters the anchorage balance, favouring space closure by forward movement of the molars. FAs are required, especially in the lower arch. If 5s are hypoplastic or missing there may be no choice. Early loss of an E will often lead to forward movement of the 6 and lack of space for 5s. In the upper arch this results in $\underline{5}$ being displaced palatally and provided $\underline{4}$ is in a satisfactory position, extraction of $\underline{5}$ on eruption is advisable. In the lower arch, 5s are usually crowded lingually. Extraction of lower 4 is easier and will give lower 5 space to upright spontaneously.

First permanent molars See ➲ Extraction of poor-quality first permanent molars, p. 140.

Second permanent molars Extraction of $\overline{7}$ will not alleviate incisor crowding but may relieve mild lower premolar crowding and avoid difficult extraction of impacted $\overline{8}$.

To ↑ likelihood of $\overline{8}$ erupting successfully to replace $\overline{7}$, need: posterior crowding and 8 formed to bifurcation and at an angle of between 15° and 30° to long axis $\overline{6}$. Even so, may still require appliance therapy to align 8 on eruption.

In the upper arch, extraction of $\underline{7}$ is often limited to facilitating distal movement of the upper buccal segments.

Third permanent molars Early extraction of lower 8s is no longer advocated to prevent LLS crowding (as now thought to be due to late facial growth and soft tissue change).

Space can also be provided in selected cases by:
- Expansion (only in upper arch with a Xbite, otherwise not stable).
- Distal movement of the upper buccal segments (→ Distal movement of the upper buccal segments, p. 142).
- Reducing the width of the teeth interproximally (usually limited to LLS in selected cases).

Extraction of poor-quality first permanent molars

First permanent molars are never the first choice for extraction, as even if they are removed at the optimal time, a good spontaneous alignment of the remaining teeth is unlikely. However, if there is hypoplasia or a large restoration is required in a molar tooth for a child, the long-term prognosis should be considered. A well-timed extraction may be better for the child (and your BP) than heroic attempts to restore hopeless molars. Equally well, placing a dressing and maintaining a poor-quality 6 until the 7 has erupted and the extraction can be incorporated into an orthodontic plan, may keep you on the specialist orthodontists' Christmas card list. Points to note[5]:

- Check the remaining teeth are present and in a good position. If not, avoid extraction of 6 in affected quadrant.
- Timing of loss of a $\overline{6}$ is critical. There is a greater tendency for mesial drift in the maxilla, therefore, the timing of loss of $\underline{6}$ is less important.
- In the lower arch, good spsontaneous alignment is more likely following extraction $\overline{6}$ if: (i) lower second permanent molar development has reached bifurcation, (ii) angulation between crypt $\overline{7}$ and $\overline{6}$ is <30°, (iii) lower second permanent molar crypts overlap lower first permanent molar roots.
- If the $\underline{6}$ is extracted after eruption of the $\overline{7}$ little space closure will occur and the $\overline{7}$ will tilt and roll lingually.
- Assess the prognosis for remaining 6s. If they are all restored then extraction of all four is probably indicated. If only one poor $\underline{6}$, do not extract corresponding lower tooth. If $\overline{6}$ of poor prognosis it is advisable to extract opposing $\underline{6}$ as otherwise this tooth will over-erupt and prevent $\overline{7}$ moving forward. Balancing with extraction of a corresponding sound $\overline{6}$ is inadvisable; better to deal with other side of arch on its merit.
- In Class I with anterior crowding and Class II malocclusions, $6|6$ should, if possible, be preserved until $7|7$ have erupted, and can be held back by an appliance and the extraction space utilized for relief of crowding and/or o/j reduction.
- In Class III, if $6|6$ of poor prognosis try to preserve until incisor relationship corrected (to provide retention for appliance). In cases with poor-quality lower first permanent molars, extract at optimal time to aid space closure.
- If the dentition is uncrowded, avoid extraction of 6s as space closure will be difficult.
- Extraction of 6s will relieve buccal segment crowding, but will have little effect on labial segment crowding. Impaction of 8s less likely but not impossible.

▶ In a child with poor-quality 6s, remember that the premolars may well be in a similar condition 6yrs on unless the caries rate is stabilized.

---

5 M. T. Cobourne 2014 *A Guideline for the Extraction of First Permanent Molars in Children*, Royal College of Surgeons (ℛ https://www.rcseng.ac.uk/dental-faculties/fds/publications-guidelines).

Spacing

Uncommon in the UK; crowding is the norm.

Generalized spacing

This is due either to hypodontia or small teeth &/or large jaws. Note that hypodontia is associated with small teeth (➔ Hypodontia (oligodontia), p. 68). Rx of spacing is problematic; a purely orthodontic approach is liable to relapse and requires prolonged retention. In milder cases, it may be wiser to build up the teeth if small or accept the spacing. In more severe cases, a combined restorative/orthodontic approach to localize space for the provision of prostheses or implants may be required.

Median diastema

Prevalence 6yr-olds = 98%, 11yr-olds = 49%, 12–18yr-olds = 7%.

Aetiology Small teeth in large jaws; absent or peg-shaped 2|2; midline $; proclination of ULS; physiological (caused by pressure of developing teeth on upper incisor roots which reduces as 3 erupts), or due to a fraenum.

The upper incisive fraenum is attached to the incisive papilla at birth. As 1|1 erupt the fraenum recedes, but this is less likely if the arch is spaced. A fraenum contributes to a diastema in a small number of cases and is associated with the following features:

- Blanching of incisive papilla when fraenum put under tension.
- Radiographically there is a V-shaped notch in the interdental bone between 1|1 indicating the attachment of the fraenum.
- Anterior teeth may be crowded.

Management Take a periapical radiograph to exclude presence of a $.

- Before 3 erupted: if diastema <3mm—review after eruption of canines as will probably ↓ unaided. If >3mm—may need to approximate incisors to provide space for canines to erupt, but care is required not to resorb roots of 2|2 against crowns of 3|3. Requires FA and prolonged retention.
- After 3 erupted: orthodontic closure will require prolonged retention as has high tendency to relapse. If fraenum an aetiological factor, consider doing a fraenectomy. There is no evidence to indicate whether this should be done before or during FA Rx. Long-term retention still required. Alternatively, measure width of 1 and 2, and if they are narrower than average (1 = 8.5mm, 2 = 6.5mm) consider composite additions or veneers to close space. If teeth of normal width and no other orthodontic Rx required, you could try and talk the patient into accepting their diastema (currently very fashionable!).

Distal movement of the upper buccal segments

This is usually thought of as an alternative to extraction, but in practice often results in the crowding being shifted distally, requiring the loss of 7̲ or 8̲. It is only applicable to the upper arch. Indications:

- Either Class I with mild upper-arch crowding, or Class II/1 with well-aligned lower arch and molars <1 unit Class II.
- High anchorage case where extraction of one tooth per quadrant does not provide sufficient space to align upper arch.

Can be achieved either using a temporary anchorage device (TAD) (Ɔ Temporary anchorage devices, p. 158) or more usually by headgear to molar bands on 6̲|6̲. As 6̲|6̲ move distally, they will need some expansion to keep the roots in cancellous bone. The chances of success are greater in a growing child. Can expect 1/2 unit change in 3–4 months with good cooperation. If need unilateral distal movement, extraction of 7̲ on that side can be considered (provided 8̲ present and in good position). To facilitate distal movement, a direction of pull parallel to the occlusal plane is advisable.

Headgear safety

Cases have been reported where damage to the eye as a result of headgear has resulted in loss of vision. For this reason, headgear should only be used by those who have received training and to avoid injury to the face, it should only be used in conjunction with two safety mechanisms which prevent displacement &/or recoil of the facebow. If eye injury should occur, immediate referral to an ophthalmologist is required. Patient information leaflets are available for more information via the British Orthodontic Society.[6]

6 ℘ https://www.bos.org.uk.

Buccally displaced maxillary canines

▶ Width $\underline{3}$ > width $\underline{4}$ > width $\underline{C}$.

$\underline{3}$ is usually the last tooth to erupt anterior to $\underline{6}$. If the upper arch is crowded, $\underline{3}$ may be squeezed buccal to its normal position, in which case space needs to be created for its alignment. Usually $\underline{4}$ is the tooth of choice for extraction and, if so, this should be carried out just as $\underline{3}$ is about to erupt. If space is critical, an appliance should be fitted first.

Where $\underline{2}$ and $\underline{4}$ are in contact, extraction of $\underline{4}$ alone will not provide sufficient space to accommodate $\underline{3}$ so consider extracting $\underline{3}$. Less commonly, $\underline{3}$ may develop well forward over the root of $\underline{2}$. In this case, orthodontic Rx to align $\underline{3}$ will be prolonged. If the arch is crowded, it may be simpler to extract $\underline{3}$ and align remaining teeth. If $\underline{3}$ has been extracted, there is a need to rotate $\underline{4}$ slightly mesio-palatally with a FA to hide the palatal cusp.

Transposition

This almost exclusively involves a canine tooth. In the maxilla, $\underline{3}$ is usually transposed with $\underline{4}$, and in the mandible, the lateral incisor is more commonly involved. Rx options include alignment of teeth in transposed position, extraction of the most displaced tooth, or correction if transposition of root apices is not complete.

Palatally displaced maxillary canines

▶ Early detection is essential.
Width $\underline{3}$ > width $\underline{4}$ > width $\underline{C}$.

Prevalence Up to 2%. Occurs bilaterally in 17–25% of cases. F > M.

Aetiology In normal development, the maxillary canine develops palatal to $\underline{C}$ and then migrates labially to erupt down the distal aspect of the root of $\underline{2}$. The aetiology of palatal displacement is not fully understood, but some suggest a lack of guidance is the reason behind the association with missing or short-rooted $\underline{2}$[7] (~6% of palatal $\underline{3}$ associated with small $\underline{2}$). Others argue that it is an inherited polygenic trait and that the link with missing or short-rooted $\underline{2}$ is part of an association with other dental anomalies including microdontia and hypodontia.[8] Others have noted that palatal displacement of $\underline{3}$ is evident radiographically as early as age 5yrs.

Assessment Clinically by palpation and from inclination of $\underline{2}$; and by radiographs. A DPT and an IO view or two IO views with tube shift can be used to assess the position of the canine by parallax (➲ Parallax technique, p. 19; remember, your 'pal' goes with you!). Consider also position and prognosis of adjacent teeth (including $\underline{C}$), the malocclusion, and available space.

Management Early detection is key, therefore when examining any child >9yrs, palpate for unerupted $\underline{3}$. If there is a definite hollow &/or asymmetry between sides, further investigation is warranted.

Interceptive extraction of $\underline{C}$ has long been advocated to facilitate an improvement of a displaced $\underline{3}$ but there is currently no robust evidence to support this approach.[9] Nevertheless most orthodontists continue provided:
• The $\underline{3}$ is not too far displaced.
• The pros and cons have been discussed with the patient and informed consent obtained.
• The patient is willing to commit to exposure and alignment if the $\underline{3}$ does not erupt unaided.
• Recent evidence has suggested the chances of success are ↑ if space is created.

If the canine is only very slightly palatally displaced or impacted between $\underline{2}$ and $\underline{4}$, provision of space should result in eruption. The majority of palatally displaced canines, however, do not erupt spontaneously, so hopeful watching and waiting may only result in an older patient who is less willing to undergo the prolonged Rx required to align the displaced tooth.
Rx alternatives available:
• Maintain $\underline{C}$ and keep unerupted canine under radiographic review. Provided no evidence of cystic change or resorption, removal of $\underline{3}$ can be left until GA required, e.g. for extraction of 8s. Patient must understand that $\underline{C}$ will eventually be lost, necessitating a prosthesis.

7 A. Becker et al. 1981 *Angle Orthod* **51** 24.

8 S. Peck et al. 1994 *Angle Orthod* **64** 249.

9 N. Parkin et al. 2012 *Cochrane Database Syst Rev* **12** CD004621.

- No Rx, if $\underline{2}$ and $\underline{4}$ are in contact and appearance is satisfactory, or if patient refuses other options. Again, $\underline{3}$ will require removal in due course.
- Exposure and orthodontic alignment only feasible if: (i) canine in favourable position for orthodontic alignment; (ii) sufficient space available for $\underline{3}$, or can be created; (iii) patient willing to undergo surgery and prolonged orthodontic Rx (usually 2+yrs). Sequence is to arrange exposure, and allow tooth to erupt for 3 months, and then commence orthodontic traction to move tooth towards arch. FAs are required.
- Autotransplantation is not an instant solution, as space is needed to accommodate $\underline{3}$, which may involve appliances &/or extractions. Prognosis is ↑ by avoiding damage to PDL and if root formation is not complete. If apex not open, should root fill <10 days. Immature apex may revascularize.

Resorption Unerupted and impacted canines can cause resorption of incisor roots. For this to occur, a 'head-on' collision between the two seems to be required. If detected on a radiograph, a specialist opinion should be sought, quickly. Extraction of the canine may be necessary to limit resorption, but if extensive, removal of the affected incisor may be preferable, thus allowing the canine to erupt.

Further reading

Cochrane Library (✒ https://www.cochranelibrary.com).

Faculty of Dental Surgery clinical guidelines (✒ http://www.rcseng.ac.uk).

Increased overjet

The 'normal' range for o/j is 2–4mm. The risk of trauma to the <u>inc</u> ↑ as the o/j ↑ especially if the lips are grossly incompetent.

Aetiology

Skeletal pattern ↑ o/j can occur in association with Class I, II, or even III skeletal patterns. If Class II (~75%), often due to a normally sized mandible being positioned posteriorly on the cranial base. Be wary of patients with vertical proportions at either extreme of the range, as they are difficult to treat.

Soft tissues The effects of the soft tissues are usually determined by the skeletal pattern, as the greater the discrepancy, the less likely it is that the patient will have competent lips. Where the lips are incompetent, the way an anterior oral seal is achieved will influence incisor position; e.g. if the lower lip is drawn up behind the upper incisors this may have contributed to the ↑ o/j, but if the incisors can be retracted within control of the lower lip at the end of Rx the prognosis for stability is ↑. The soft tissues can also help to compensate for the skeletal pattern by proclining the lower &/or retroclining the upper incisors.

Dental Crowding may contribute to an ↑ o/j. Digit-sucking can cause proclination of the upper and retroclination of the lower incisors. The effects are related to frequency, intensity, and duration. Steps should be taken to stop the habit before active o/j ↓ is started.

▶ In the majority of cases, the skeletal pattern will determine the difficulty of Rx and the soft tissues will influence stability of the end result.

Management of increased overjet

See also ➋ Functional appliances—rationale and mode of action, p. 164.

Class I or mild Class II skeletal pattern The majority of patients in this category are managed using FA to retract the upper incisors. Extractions are often required to relieve crowding and provide space for o/j ↓. Anchorage requirements should be assessed and if required reinforced (➋ Reinforcing anchorage, p. 156).

  If the skeletal pattern is more Class II then a functional appliance can be used for growth modification prior to FA.

Moderate to severe Class II skeletal pattern Approaches available:
- Modification of growth—either by restraint of maxillary growth with headgear, or by encouraging mandibular growth with a functional appliance.
- Orthodontic camouflage—by extractions in upper arch and bodily movement of <u>inc</u> with FAs.
- Surgical correction.

Because mandibular growth predominates during the teenage years, a greater proportion of Class II than Class III skeletal problems is amenable to orthodontic correction. Research would suggest that the amount of growth modification that can be achieved is limited, but every little helps and in practice the majority of growing children in this category are treated by a combination of growth modification and camouflage. This usually takes the form of an initial phase of functional appliance therapy in the early permanent dentition, followed by FA ± extractions.

Adults whose skeletal pattern is not too severe may be treated by orthodontic camouflage, but in cases with a more severe skeletal problem &/or an ↑ o/b, a surgical correction may be the only option.

Retention This should be planned and presented to the patient as part of the overall Rx package.

Beware:
• Obtuse naso-labial angle as o/j ↓ will further reduce lip support.
• Grossly incompetent lips as stability is compromised.
• Significantly ↑ or ↓ vertical proportions.

Further reading
K. B. Batista et al. 2018 Orthodontic treatment for prominent upper front teeth in children. *Cochrane Database Syst Rev* 3 CD003452.

Increased overbite

Normal o/b is between one-third and one-half overlap of the lower incisors. It is usual to record o/b in terms of whether it is ↑, ↓, or normal,
rather than to try to measure it with a ruler. ↑ o/b is associated with
Class II/2 incisor relationship, where typically 1|1 are retroclined and 2|2 are
proclined, reflecting their relationship to the lower lip. But the o/b can also
be ↑ in Class III and II/1 malocclusions. ↑ o/b per se is not an indication for
Rx, unless it is traumatic and this is relatively rare, but o/b reduction may
be necessary before correction of other anomalies. In Class III cases an ↑
o/b is advantageous as this will help to retain the corrected incisor position.

Aetiology

The lower incisors usually erupt until they contact the upper incisors, the
palatal mucosa, or are prevented by the tongue or a habit. An ↑ o/b occurs
because the incisors are able to erupt past each other due to a combination
of some or all of the following interrelated factors: ↓ LFH; high lower lip
line; retroclined incisors; ↑ inter-incisal angle.

Normal inter-incisal angle is 135°. Highest acceptable angle is 145°.
Above this value the tendency for the lower incisors to erupt may be inadequately resisted.

In some Class II/2 cases, the LLS teeth are trapped by the ↑ o/b behind
the ULS. Freeing them by, e.g. provision of an upper removable appliance
(URA) with a biteplane, may allow the lower incisors to spontaneously
procline to a new stable position. This is one of the few situations where
proclination (within reason!) of the LLS is stable.

Approaches to reducing overbite

- *Extrusion/eruption of molars.* Passive eruption of lower molars occurs
  when a URA incorporating a bite plane is worn. Active extrusion of
  molars in either arch is possible using FAs. However, unless the patient
  grows vertically to accommodate this ↑ dimension, the molars will re-
  intrude under the forces of occlusion once appliances are withdrawn.
  This approach is of limited value in adults.
- *Intrusion of incisors.* This is difficult, requires FAs, and in most cases the
  major effect is extrusion of the buccal segments. More successful in
  growing patients.
- *Proclination of lower incisors.* Movement of the lower incisors from their
  position of stability within the soft tissue envelope is unstable in most
  cases. Active proclination should only be attempted by the experienced
  orthodontist, who will be better able to judge those cases where this is
  indicated.
- *Surgery.* Indicated in severe cases especially if associated with AP skeletal
  discrepancy, and in adults.

Management of increased overbite

Class II/2 It is often prudent to avoid extractions when the lower arch is mildly crowded in a Class II/2, to avoid moving the lower incisors lingually during space closure as this will ↑ o/b. Cases with sufficient crowding to warrant premolar extractions in the lower arch and moderately to severely ↑ overbite are best treated with FA to close space by forward movement of the buccal segments and to correct the incisor relationship.

Where o/b ↓ is required, the inter-incisal angle will need to be reduced in order to achieve a stable result. Usually this necessitates FAs. However, in growing patients with a skeletal II pattern, an alternative approach is to procline ULS to convert to a Class II/1 and use a functional appliance to reduce the resultant o/j. Proclination can be done either with a URA first, or with a sectional FA on ULS, or by incorporating a spring in the functional appliance.

Class II/1 o/b ↓ is required before o/j ↓. If a functional appliance is indicated for AP correction then some o/b reduction can often be achieved during this phase by trimming the appliance to allow eruption of the lower molars. If headgear is being used then it may be helpful to commence o/b ↓ with a URA with a flat anterior bite plane, clipped over the bands on the upper molars. Rx of most II/1 will need FA either as the sole Rx or following a functional appliance or headgear. Including lower second molars in the FA will aid intrusion of the LLS (by ↑ vertical anchorage), but inevitably some extrusion of the molars will occur.

Class III See ➲ Reverse overjet, p. 152.

Avoid reducing o/b as it will aid retention of the corrected incisor position.

Stability of overbite reduction Stability of o/b ↓ is enhanced by:
- Reducing the inter-incisal angle and creating an occlusal stop to prevent the lower incisors over-erupting.
- Favourable growth as this compensates for molar extrusion.
- Eliminating or reducing the aetiological factors but ↓ LFH and high lower lip line can only be altered if growth is favourable.

Further reading
W. J. B. Houston 1989 Incisor edge-centroid relationships and overbite depth. *Eur J Orthod* **11** 139.
D. T. Millett et al. 2018 Orthodontic treatment for deep bite and retroclined upper front teeth in children. *Cochrane Database Syst Rev* **2** CD005972.

Anterior open bite

Anterior open bite (AOB) can occur in Class I, II, and III malocclusions.

Aetiology Either *skeletal*—vertical > horizontal growth (↑ LFH &/or ↑ MMPA), or *environmental*—habits, tongue thrust, or iatrogenic, or a combination of these. If the distance between the maxilla and the mandible is sufficiently ↑ such that even if incisors erupt to their full potential they do not meet, an AOB will result (Fig. 4.9). This is often associated with incompetent lips and a lip-to-tongue anterior oral seal, which may exacerbate the AOB. Tongue thrusts are usually adaptive and can maintain an AOB due to a habit even after the habit has stopped.

Localized failure of maxillary dento-alveolar development resulting in an open bite is seen in CLP.

Rx Rx is generally difficult, except where due mainly to a habit, therefore it is wise to refer the patient to a specialist for advice.

Skeletal In milder cases can align arches and accept, or try to restrain vertical development of the maxilla &/or upper molars with headgear &/or a functional appliance with posterior bite blocks. TADs can be used to facilitate molar intrusion in the management of AOB. Most operators leave the TADs *in situ* during initial months of retention to continue intrusive forces and offset relapse. Extrusion of the incisors is unstable. For more severe cases, the only alternative is surgery.

Habits It is better to await the natural cessation of a habit. Once the habit stops, o/b should re-establish within 3yrs, unless perpetuated by soft tissues or because it is skeletal in origin.

Tongue thrust None.

Hints Hints for cases with ↑ vertical dimensions and ↓ o/b or AOB:
• Avoid extruding molars, e.g. cervical pull headgear to 6|6, URA with a bite plane.
• Avoid upper arch expansion as this will tip down the palatal cusps of buccal segment teeth, reducing o/b.
• Extraction of molars will not 'close down bite'.
• Space closure is said to occur more readily in patients with ↑ vertical skeletal proportions.

Further reading
D. A. Lentini-Oliveira et al. 2014 Orthodontic and orthopaedic treatment for anterior open bite in children. *Cochrane Database Syst Rev* 9 CD005515.

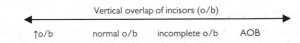

Fig. 4.9 Anterior open bite diagram.

Reverse overjet

This will include only those cases with more than two teeth in linguo-occlusion, i.e. Class III cases. For management of one or two teeth in Xbite, see ➲ Crossbites p. 154.

Aetiology

Skeletal Reverse o/j is usually associated with an underlying Class III skeletal pattern. This is most commonly due to either a large mandible &/or a retrusive maxilla &/or a forward position of glenoid fossa. Class III malocclusions occur in association with the whole range of vertical patterns. Xbites are a common feature, due to the more forward position of the mandible relative to the maxilla.

Soft tissues A patient's efforts to achieve an anterior oral seal often result in dento-alveolar compensation, i.e. retroclination of the lower and proclination of the upper incisors, therefore the incisor relationship is often less severe than underlying skeletal pattern.

Growth Growth is often unfavourable in Class III malocclusions.

Dental crowding This is usually greater in the upper than the lower arch.

Assessment See ➲ Orthodontic assessment, p. 126.
Consider also the following:
• Patient's opinion about their facial appearance (be tactful!).
• Severity of skeletal discrepancy.
• Amount and anticipated pattern of facial growth.
• Amount of dento-alveolar compensation as if this marked will limit further decompensation for orthodontic camouflage.
• Amount of overbite. Need a positive o/b to retain corrected incisor position at the end of Rx. Remember that proclination of ULS will ↓ o/b and retroclination of LLS will ↑ o/b.
• Can patient achieve an edge-to-edge contact of the incisors? If so this ↑ prognosis for correction of incisor relationship.

Rx approaches
▶ Class III malocclusions tend to become worse with growth.

Accept Accept in mild cases particularly with ↓ o/b. Some patients with more severe skeletal Class III opt for alignment, accepting incisor relationship rather than proceeding with surgery.

Early orthopaedic Rx There is some evidence to show that in <10yr-olds one can use a protraction face-mask or bone-anchored screws or miniplates in the maxilla to enhance forward growth of the maxilla. But this approach still needs to be evaluated in the longer term.

Camouflage This involves proclining the ULS &/or retroclining the lower incisors with FAs (Fig. 4.10 and Fig. 4.11).

Surgery Surgery is for more severe cases, particularly with ↑ vertical skeletal proportions &/or asymmetry. It is difficult to produce hard and fast rules, but two predictors from a cephalometric analysis which have been suggested are:
• ANB value below –4°.
• Lower incisor angle to the mandibular plane of <80°.

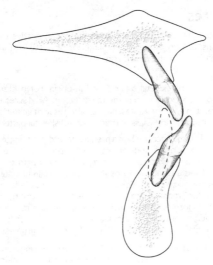

Fig. 4.10 Correction of a Class III incisor relationship by retroclination of the lower incisors increases overbite.

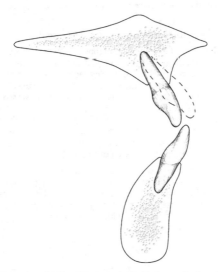

Fig. 4.11 Correction of a Class III incisor relationship by proclination of the upper incisors alone reduces overbite.

Crossbites

By convention, the lower teeth should be described relative to the upper (➔ Definitions, p. 124). Xbites can be anterior or posterior (unilateral/bilateral), with displacement, or with no displacement.

Aetiology

Xbites Xbites can be skeletal &/or dental in origin. For posterior Xbites, the skeletal component is usually the major factor. AP discrepancies obviously play a part in anterior Xbites, but can also result in posterior Xbites in Class II (lingual Xbite) and Class III (buccal Xbite) skeletal patterns.

Displacement This may occur when a premature or deflecting cuspal contact is encountered on closure and the mandible is postured either anteriorly or laterally to achieve better interdigitation. This new path of closure becomes learned and the patient closes straight into maximum interdigitation. To help detect displacement on closure, try to get the patient to close on a hinge axis by asking them to curl their tongue back to touch the back of the palate and then close together slowly, while guiding the mandible back via the chin. In addition, look for other clues like a centre-line shift (of lower in direction of displacement) in association with a posterior unilateral Xbite.

Anterior crossbites For Class III see ➔ Reverse overjet, p. 152.

Anterior Xbites can be treated interceptively in mixed dentition if associated with a displacement, provided sufficient o/b exists to retain the result. If not, it is probably best to defer until the 2° dentition and use FAs. Upper lateral incisors that are displaced bodily will require buccal root torque for correction.

Posterior crossbites For review, see reference.[10]

Unilateral Generally, the greater the number of teeth involved, the greater the skeletal contribution to the aetiology. If only one or two teeth in each arch are affected, movement of opposing teeth in opposite directions can be achieved by cross-elastics attached to attachments on the affected teeth. Unilateral Xbite from the canine region distally is usually associated with a displacement, as true skeletal asymmetry is rare. If the arches are of a similar width when the patient closes, the cusps will meet so the patient displaces laterally to achieve a better interdigitation. In these cases, Rx should be directed towards expanding the upper arch so that it fits around the lower, provided the upper teeth are not already buccally tilted.

Bilateral buccal crossbite This suggests a greater underlying transverse skeletal discrepancy. It is less commonly associated with displacement.

Correction of a bilateral Xbite should be approached with caution, because partial relapse may result in the teeth occluding cusp to cusp and development of a unilateral Xbite with displacement.

10 P. Agostino 2014 *Cochrane Database Syst Rev* **8** CD000979.

Bilateral lingual crossbite (or scissor bite) This occurs due to either a narrow mandible or a wide maxilla. In milder cases, only 4|4 may be involved, and if these teeth are extracted to relieve crowding or for retraction of 3|3, so much the better. Where the whole buccal segments are involved, Rx will probably involve expansion of the lower &/or contraction of the upper, therefore refer to a specialist.

Rapid maxillary expansion This involves a screw appliance comprising bands attached to 64|46 and connected to a midline screw. The object is to expand the maxilla by opening the midline suture and is therefore more successful in younger patients. Large forces are required to accomplish this—the screw is turned 0.2mm twice a day for about 2 weeks. Overexpansion is necessary as the teeth relapse about 50% under soft tissue pressure. Not to be attempted by the inexperienced!

Quad helix appliance This is a very efficient fixed, slow expansion appliance. It is made of 1mm SS attached to bands on 6|6 and is W-shaped. Activated by expanding 1/2 tooth width per side before placement (Fig. 4.12).

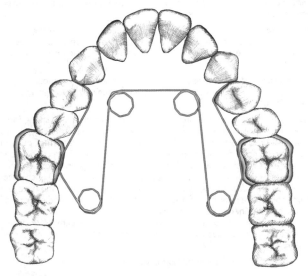

Fig. 4.12 Quad helix appliance.

Anchorage

Anchorage is defined as the source of resistance to the reaction from the active component(s) in an appliance. In practice, it is the balance between the applied force and the available space, e.g. in a case where 3|3 are being retracted following extraction of 4|4, an equal, but opposite force will also be acting on 65|56. The amount of forward movement of these anchor teeth will depend largely upon their root surface area and the force used.

Anchorage loss can be minimized by limiting the number of teeth being moved at any one time, applying the correct force for the movement required, and ↑ the resistance of the anchor teeth (e.g. by permitting only bodily movement). In some situations, movement of the anchor teeth is desirable, e.g. in a Class III where space is being opened up for an unerupted 3. However, it is important to assess the anchorage requirements of a particular malocclusion before embarking on Rx. If no or little movement of the anchor teeth is desirable, then anchorage should be reinforced from the start.

Reinforcing anchorage

Intra-maxillary (teeth in same arch) This is achieved by including the maximum number of teeth in the anchorage unit.

Inter-maxillary (teeth in opposing arch) This is achieved by running elastics from one arch to the other during FA Rx. The direction of elastic pull is described according to the type of malocclusion to which it is applicable (Fig. 4.13).

Transpalatal and lingual arches By virtue of linking the upper molars, a palatal arch limits their forward movement and thereby ↑ anchorage, and vice versa for the lingual arch.

Extra-oral A force is transmitted to the teeth by an elastic or spring force from a head or neck strap. This involves a facebow, which engages tubes soldered onto molar cribs (URA) or bands (FA). The direction of pull can be selected according to the malocclusion with an overall direction of pull above the occlusal plane for patients with ↑ vertical proportions (hi-pull) and vice versa for ↓ vertical proportions (cervical pull). For EO anchorage, 250g for 10h/day should suffice. For EO traction (i.e. using the headgear force to achieve movement rather than just resist it), forces in the region of 500g for 14–16h/day are necessary.

Following reports of a number of cases where eye damage (including blindness) occurred due to headgear, the use of at least two safety mechanisms is advised.

TADs See ➔ Temporary anchorage devices, p. 158.

Anchorage loss

This may occur because of:
- Failure to appreciate fully the anchorage requirements at Rx planning stage (generally if 75–100% of space generated from extractions is required for planned tooth movement, anchorage requirements are high).
- Active force exceeding available anchorage (often due to over-activation or too many teeth being moved at a time).
- Poor patient compliance.

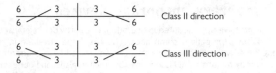

Fig. 4.13 Reinforcing anchorage.

Temporary anchorage devices

Implants have been adopted in orthodontics to provide skeletal anchorage, to ↓ need for patient compliance. This has ↑ the envelope in terms of the severity of malocclusions that can be treated by orthodontics alone. Currently the term TAD is in vogue, but mini-implants and bone anchorage devices (BADs) are also used (Table 4.2). Success rates of 86.5% have been reported.[11]

A screw design with no osseointegration is now the most widely used in orthodontics, because it is easy to place and remove. It is typically 1–2mm wide and 6–15mm in length with a neck that protrudes through the mucosa and a head designed for attaching an orthodontic force system (e.g. elastic or coil spring).

There are two sub-divisions:
- Self-tapping—site is pre-drilled with a specially designed handpiece prior to insertion of the screw.
- Self-drilling—implant is screwed directly into bone. It gives better results as it causes less thermal damage to bone.

Site selection
- Rx mechanics—including direction of desired force.
- Anatomy—tooth roots, other structures.
- Depth of available bone including thickness of cortical plate.
- Bone quality.
- Access for placement.
- Gingival health and quality—good OH. Attached gingiva is better.
- Need good radiographs.

Local anaesthesia is used by most operators. A stent can be used to guide placement. Screws can be inserted with a hand (screw) driver or using an engine driver, i.e. a speed reduction (<30rpm) contra-angle handpiece.

Table 4.2 Types of implant

Osseointegrated	No osseointegration
Designed to maximize surface contact for integration	Designed for ease of placement and removal
Short body length and large diameter	Screw or plate
Surface coating	No surface coating
More difficult to place. ↑ morbidity at removal due to osseointegration	Plate design more difficult to place and remove than screw
Usually used in edentulous, retromolar, palatal areas	Can be placed in dento-alveolar bone between tooth roots
Useful when wish to replace a missing tooth after orthodontic Rx	

11 F. Alharbi et al. 2018. *Eur J Orthod* 40 519.

Loading Most operators load the screws immediately. The osseointegrated type requires a latent period for integration. Need to avoid excess force levels (<250g).

Removal For osseointegrated types, need to raise a flap and cut out implant. Screw designs can usually be removed without LA by unscrewing.

Problems Success is a screw that is functional for the duration the orthodontic force is required. A screw that is slightly mobile may still be functional. If a screw contacts a root then this usually results in the screw becoming loose &/or some patient discomfort.
- Screw becomes loose—remove and replace in another site.
- Breakage—about 3–4%.
- Root damage—evidence suggests that if the root is perforated, then healing by cementum occurs.
- Mucosal discomfort—check OH.

Further reading
R. R. J. Cousley 2015 Mini-implants in contemporary orthodontics part 1: recent evidence on factors affecting clinical success. *Orthodontic Update* **8** 6.
R. R. J. Cousley 2015 Mini-implants in contemporary orthodontics part 2: clinical applications and optimal biomechanics. *Orthodontic Update* **8** 56.
S. Jambi et al. 2014 Reinforcement of anchorage during orthodontic brace treatment with implants or other surgical methods. *Cochrane Database Syst Rev* **8** CD005098.

Removable appliances

Removable appliances are single-arch appliances that can be taken out of the mouth by the patient. They are only capable of tilting movements of individual teeth, but can be used for moving blocks of teeth. In addition, they can be used to allow differential eruption of teeth via bite planes or buccal capping. Now used more as an adjunct to comprehensive FA Rx and for retention after FAs.

Indications

Active

- Movement of blocks of teeth, e.g. correction of a buccal Xbite by expansion of upper arch (Fig. 4.14).
- As an interceptive Rx in the mixed dentition, e.g. correction of an upper incisor in Xbite.
- o/b reduction.
- In conjunction with other appliance, e.g. to facilitate distal movement of upper molar(s) with headgear.
- Elimination of occlusal interferences by addition of bite plane or buccal capping. Useful for movement of a tooth over the bite during FA Rx.

Passive

- Space maintainer, e.g. following loss of an upper central incisor due to trauma.
- Retaining appliance, e.g. following FA Rx.
- Habit deterrent.

Practical points

Active components

- Springs (made in SS wire) are the most commonly used active component because they are versatile and cheap to construct.
- Screws are useful when the teeth to be moved need to be clasped for retention (Fig. 4.14).

Retention This is the means by which the appliance is retained in the mouth. The best retention posteriorly is provided by the Adams crib (Fig. 4.15), which is made in SS wire in either 0.7mm (for permanent molars) or 0.6mm (for premolars and 1° molars). Anterior retention can be gained by a labial bow or a clasp—these components are usually constructed in 0.7mm wire.

Baseplate Holds other elements together and may also itself be active. Heat-cure acrylic is more robust than self-cure.

- A flat anterior bite plane will allow the lower molars to erupt and will if worn well result in o/b ↓.
- Buccal capping frees the occlusion on the tooth being moved and allows further relative eruption of the incisors (therefore is C/I if o/b is already ↑).

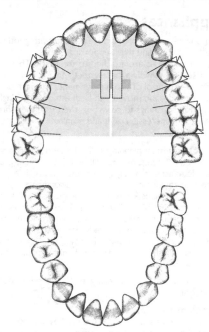

Fig. 4.14 Upper removable appliance to expand upper arch with midline screw. Cribs 6|6 0.7mm SS; 4|4 0.6mm SS; buccal capping or flat anterior bite plane.

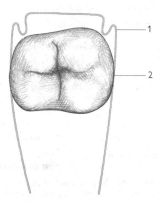

Fig. 4.15 Adjustment of Adams crib. 1. Arrowhead moves horizontally towards tooth. 2. Arrowhead moves towards tooth and also vertically towards gingival crevice.

Fixed appliances

▶ FAs should only be used in cooperative patients with good OH, to minimize damage to the teeth and their supporting tissues.

As the name implies, FAs are attached to the teeth. They vary in complexity, from a sectional involving a few teeth to full FAs in both arches. FAs give precise 3-D control of tooth movement. They can be used to tilt, rotate, intrude, extrude, and move teeth bodily. Not surprisingly, FAs have a greater propensity for things to go wrong, therefore they should only be used by those with the necessary skills and training.

Principles

- Rx planning (➋ Treatment planning, p. 134). Need particular attention to anchorage requirements, especially if apical movement is planned.
- As FAs are able to achieve bodily movement, it is possible (within limits) to move teeth to compensate for a skeletal discrepancy.
- FAs can be used in conjunction with other appliances &/or headgear.
- For initial alignment, flexible archwires are used, but to minimize unwanted movements, progressively more rigid archwires are necessary.
- Archwires should be based on the pre-Rx lower arch-form for stability.
- Mesio-distal movement is achieved either by: (i) sliding the teeth along the archwire with elastic force (sliding mechanics), or (ii) moving the teeth with the archwire.

Intermaxillary traction (➋ Inter-maxillary, p. 156) is often used to aid AP correction and ↑ anchorage.

Components of fixed appliances

Bands Bands are usually used on molar teeth. They are indicated for other teeth if bonds fail or lingual attachment is required for de-rotation. If tooth contacts are tight, these will need to be separated prior to band placement using an elastic doughnut stretched around the contact point for 1–7 days. Use of GI cements helps to ↓ decalcification.

Bonds Bonds are attached to enamel with (acid-etch) composite. There are two commonly used types: (i) metal (poor aesthetics) and (ii) ceramic (prone to # and can cause enamel wear). There is a wide variety of designs (see ➋ Types of fixed appliance, p. 162).

Archwires Flexible nickel titanium archwires are used in the initial stages of Rx and more rigid SS wires used in the later stages for the planned tooth movements. Tungsten molybdenum and cobalt chromium alloys are also popular.

Auxiliaries Elastic rings or wire ligatures are used to tie the archwire to the brackets. Forces can be applied to the teeth by auxiliary springs or elastics.

Types of fixed appliance

There is an almost infinite variety, but the most well-known are as follows:

Standard edgewise Historical. Brackets are rectangular and wide mesio-distally for rotational control. The intended final 3-D position of each tooth had to be built into rectangular SS archwires by bends placed in all three planes of space.

Pre-adjusted systems These 'pre-programmed' brackets are designed with the average values for the intended final 3-D position built into the archwire slot. Thus the amount of archwire bending required is reduced. As each tooth has its own individual bracket with a built-in prescription for that tooth, these systems are more expensive, but that is offset by savings in operator time. A number of different prescriptions are available.

Self-ligating systems These have a clip mechanism incorporated into the bracket to hold the archwire in place (rather than elastic or wire tie) which is said to ↓ friction, theoretically making tooth movement quicker, there is, however, no evidence to support this claim.[12] Examples include Damon®, SmartClip™, and Innovation®.

Tip edge This appliance was based on the Begg philosophy which used round wires which fitted loosely into a vertical slot in the bracket, thus allowing the teeth to tip freely. Auxiliaries were required to achieve apical and rotational movements. Tip-edge brackets also have pre-adjusted values incorporated to give the 'finish' produced by using a straight wire appliance.

Lingual appliances These are popular with patients, but not widely available as access for placement and adjustment are more challenging! Expensive.

Clear plastic aligners. These are vacuum-formed thermoplastic appliances which look like a thin mouthguard. Although strictly not a FA they are included here as they are popular with patients as a more aesthetic alternative to FA. Study models are scanned digitally and then the computer program designs a sequence of models with increment changes in tooth position. A series of clear plastic aligners are then made which move teeth to the desired final result. The rate of tooth movement is 0.25 to 0.33mm/aligner. Best suited to mild malocclusions treated without extractions.

▶ FAs should only be used by clinicians trained in their use and management of the problems that can arise.

12 S. S. H. Chen et al. 2010 *Am J Orthod Dentofacial Orthop* **137** 726.

Functional appliances—rationale and mode of action

Definition Functional appliances utilize, eliminate, or guide the forces of muscle function, tooth eruption, and growth to correct a malocclusion.

Philosophy Functional appliances are so called because it was thought that by eliminating abnormal muscle function, normal growth and development would follow. Nowadays, the importance of both genetic and environmental factors in the aetiology of malocclusion is acknowledged, but functional appliances are still successfully used in the Rx of Class II malocclusions by a combination of skeletal and dental effects. Functional appliances (or just 'functionals') can also be used in the management of AOB and Class III, but those approaches are beyond the scope of this text.

Mode of action In the average child, the face grows forward relative to the cranial base and mandibular growth predominates. Functional appliances help to harness this change to correct Class II malocclusions by a restraining effect on the maxilla and maxillary teeth and a forward pressure on the mandible and mandibular teeth. A similar effect is produced with Class II elastics (→ Reinforcing anchorage, p. 156). Functional appliances are ineffective for individual tooth movement.

Indications To achieve some AP correction for a Class II malocclusion prior to FA ± extractions. Ideally: Class II/1 with mandibular retrusion, average or reduced LFH, or upright or retroclined LLS. A useful test is to examine the profile with the patient postured forward to a Class I incisor relationship, and if not improved consider another appliance. Can also use for Class II/2 but need to procline ULS, e.g. with sectional FAs.

Changes produced by functional appliances
Skeletal
- Research would suggest that changes seen are 25% skeletal and 75% dental.
- Optimizing of mandibular growth. The evidence would suggest that in the short term an extra 1–2mm mandibular growth results, however, in the long term that overall gain is small.
- Restraint of forward maxillary growth.
- Forward movement of the glenoid fossa.
- ↑ LFH.

Dental
- Palatal tipping of the upper incisors.
- Labial tipping of the lower incisors (not a consistent finding).
- Inhibition of forward movement of the maxillary molars.
- Mesial and vertical eruption of the mandibular molars.

Keys to success with functional appliances
- Cooperative and keen patient. Remember cooperation is finite.
- Favourable growth; therefore should coincide Rx with pubertal growth spurt.
- Confident operator, so that the child believes the appliance will work and will persevere with wearing it.

Further reading

K. B. Batista 2018 Orthodontic treatment for prominent upper front teeth in children. *Cochrane Database Syst Rev* **3** CD003452.

K. D. O'Brien et al. 2003 Effectiveness of treatment for Class II malocclusion with the herbst or twin-block appliances: a RCCT. *Am J Orthod Dentofac Orthop* **124** 128.

K. D. O'Brien et al. 2009 Early treatment for Class II divisions 1 malocclusion with the Twin-Block appliance: a multi-center randomized controlled trial. *Am J Orthod Dentofac Orthop* **135** 573.

Types of functional appliance and practical tips

Choice of appliance

Some of the more popular types include:

Twin block This is the most commonly used design in the UK. It comprises separate upper and lower removable appliances which by means of sloping buccal blocks help to posture the mandible forward. Because they are individual upper and lower appliances and are retained by clasping the teeth, they are well tolerated by patients and can be worn for meals. In addition, a screw can be incorporated in the upper twin block if expansion is required, as well as springs (e.g. to procline ULS or align 2). Need a wax bite recorded with the mandible postured forwards 7–10mm so that blocks are >5mm height (Fig. 4.16 and Fig. 4.17).

Medium opening activator (MOA) This is useful in cases with ↓ LFH as the design allows eruption of lower molars. It is a one-piece functional therefore a preliminary phase of upper arch expansion prior to fitting the MOA is required in most patients to coordinate arch widths. Must be made in heat-cure acrylic as extensions to lower arch are prone to fracture. Worn full-time except during eating.

Herbst This is a fixed functional appliance. It comprises metal cast splints cemented onto the buccal segment teeth which are connected by metal arms in a piston arrangement which hold the mandible forward. Achieves rapid AP correction. Expensive to make.

Practical tips

- Advise the patient to wear the appliance full-time. Only Herbst and twin-block appliances can be worn for eating. See every 2 months.
- Problems with appliances that fall out in bed at night are often cured by ↑ wear during the day.
- Expect at least 1mm o/j reduction per month (more with Herbst).
- If no progress or progress stalls, this may be due to poor wear (most likely), lack of growth, &/or problems with fit or design of appliance.
- Functional appliances are successful in around 80% of growing patients.

End-point of functional appliance Rx

In most patients it is wise to slightly over-correct AP to an edge-to-edge incisor relationship. Most operators then get the patient to wear at nights only for 3 months before making the transition to FAs ± extractions. The buccal blocks of a twin block can be reduced to encourage molar eruption during this phase.

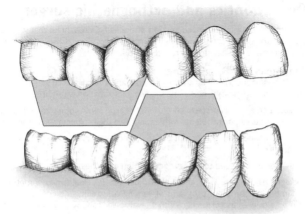

Fig. 4.16 Demonstrating how the inclined bite blocks of the twin-block appliance hold the mandible forward in a postured position.

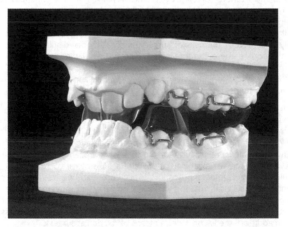

Fig. 4.17 Twin-block appliance. A spring positioned behind the ULS or a sectional fixed appliance can be used to procline 1|1.

Orthodontics and orthognathic surgery

Orthognathic surgery is the correction of skeletal discrepancies that, due to their severity, lie outside the scope of orthodontics alone. Usually deferred until active growth has slowed to adult levels.

Diagnosis and Rx planning

This is best done jointly by an orthodontist and a maxillofacial surgeon and ideally with psychology input. The following information is required:

Patient's perception of problem Are they concerned with appearance of jaws or teeth, speech, or problems with eating? Are their expectations realistic?

Clinical examination Assessment of the balance and proportions of full face and profile.[13]

Study models Needed to assess coordination of arches.

Radiographs Require DPT and lateral skull, plus PA skull for asymmetries. A number of computer programs of varying complexity and cost are available to aid in Δ and planning. With ↑ availability of CBCT, 3-D programs are now in use. However, these should not supersede clinical assessment.

Photographs Required as pre-Rx record and can also be manipulated with lateral skull for visual computer predictions.

It is important to correlate desired facial changes with the patient's occlusion. Pre-surgical orthodontics will be required to decompensate teeth so that a full surgical correction is possible.

It is important (in order to obtain informed consent) that patients are fully informed of the risks of surgery, particularly mandibular procedures, in addition to the orthodontic risks. The British Orthodontic Society has produced an excellent DVD and an online resource 'Your Jaw Surgery' (℘ http://www.bos.org.uk) which provides a well-balanced overview for prospective patients.

Sequence of Rx

Pre-surgical orthodontics The aim of this phase is to align and coordinate the arches so that the teeth will not interfere when the jaws are placed in their correct position. This usually involves decompensation, i.e. removal of any dento-alveolar compensation for the skeletal discrepancy so that the teeth are at their correct axial inclinations and a full surgical correction can be achieved. If a segmental procedure is planned, space will be needed interdentally for surgical cuts. It is inefficient to carry out movements that can be accomplished more readily at surgery (e.g. expansion of upper arch if Le Fort 1 planned), or following surgery (e.g. levelling of lower arch in Class II/2). In addition, the FA provides a means of fixation at surgery.

Surgery (➔ Orthognathic surgery, p. 510.) Full records should be taken for final planning. For bimaxillary procedure, study models mounted on semi- or fully adjustable articulator are needed.

13 N. P. Hunt & S. J. Rudge 1984 *Br J Orthod* **11** 126.

Table 4.3 Hierarchy of stability

Very stable	Max up
	Mand forward
	Chin—any direction
Stable	Max forward
	Max asymmetry
Stable with rigid fixation	Max up & mand forward
	Max forward and mand back
	Mand asymmetry
Least stable	Mand back
	Max down
	Widening of max

Post-surgical orthodontics Lighter round wires and inter-maxillary traction are used to detail occlusion.

Retention This is the same as after conventional FA Rx.

Relapse This can be surgical or orthodontic, or both. Relapse is more likely in Rx of deficiencies as soft tissues are under greater tension post-operatively. Research[14] has shown the hierarchy of stability in Table 4.3.

Distraction osteogenesis A proportion of severe cases (particularly congenital craniofacial deformity) require movements beyond the scope of conventional orthognathic surgery—principally due to soft tissue restriction. Distraction osteogenesis is useful in the management of these cases as it involves slow distraction across the osteotomized bones, which stretches the surrounding soft tissues. The surgical cuts for an osteotomy are made in the usual way, but then after allowing a few days for initial callus formation, traction is applied across the bone cuts via a distractor. The healing callus is put under tension and bone is laid down in the direction of force. A period of consolidation is required after the desired surgical movements are achieved.

Further reading
S. Cunningham et al. 1998 Psychological assessment of patients requiring orthognathic surgery and the relevance of body dysmorphic disorder. *Br J Orthod* 25 293.

14 W. R. Proffit et al. 2007 *Head Face Med* 3 21.

Cleft lip and palate

Prevalence CLP varies with racial group and geographically. Occurs in ~1:1000 Caucasian births, but prevalence ↑. M > F. If unilateral L > R. Family history in 40% of cases.

Isolated cleft palate occurs in 1:2000 births. F > M. Family history in 20%.

Aetiology Multifactorial with both genetic and environmental factors (including maternal smoking, alcohol, and phenytoin intake) involved. Can occur in isolation or as part of a syndrome.

Classification Many exist, but the best approach is to describe cleft: 1° &/or 2° palate; complete or incomplete; unilateral or bilateral. Submucous cleft of the palate is often missed until poor speech noticed, as overlying mucosa is intact.

Problems

Embryological anomalies Tissue deficit, displacement of segments, and abnormal muscle attachments.

Post-surgical distortions Unrepaired clefts show normal growth. In repaired clefts maxillary growth is ↓ AP, transversely, and vertically. Mandibular growth also ↓.

Hearing and speech These are impaired.

Other congenital anomalies These occur in up to 20% of cases with CLP and are more likely in association with isolated clefts of palate than lip.

Dental anomalies In CLP, ↑ prevalence of hypodontia and $ teeth (especially in region of cleft). Teeth adjacent to cleft are often displaced. Also ↑ incidence of hypoplasia and delayed eruption.

Management (of unilateral complete CLP) Team usually includes cleft surgeon, ear, nose, and throat (ENT) surgeon, health visitors, orthodontist, speech therapist, clinical psychologist, and central coordinator. Centralization of care and audit of outcome gives better results.

Prenatally/birth Parents need explanation, reassurance, and help with feeding. Pre-surgical orthopaedics is now out of vogue as benefits are not proven.

Lip closure Usually between 3 and 6 months of age. Delaire or Millard &/or modifications are the most popular. Some surgeons do a Vomer flap at same time. Bilateral lips are closed in either one or two operations.

Palatal closure Usually between 9 and 12 months. Delaire or Von Langenbeck ± modifications are the most popular. Deferring repair until patient is older ↓ growth disturbance, but speech development is adversely affected.

Primary dentition Speech and hearing assessments. Establishment of good dental care.

Mixed dentition In most cases any orthodontic Rx is better deferred until just prior to 2° bone grafting at 8–10yrs.

Alveolar bone graft If an alveolar cleft is present then this should be grafted when the canine root is half to two-thirds formed (around age 8½ to 10½yrs) with cancellous bone. Advantages:
- Provides bone for 3 to erupt through.
- Allows tooth movement into cleft site, may avoid prosthesis.
- ↑ bony support for alar base.
- Aids closure of oro-nasal fistulae.
- Also helps to stabilize mobile premaxillary segment in bilateral cases.

To aid surgical access and improve outcome, usually need to expand collapsed arches and align the upper incisors prior to grafting. FAs are usually used and care is required not to move roots of adjacent teeth into cleft. Bone usually harvested from the iliac crest.

Permanent dentition Because of the restraining effects of 1° surgery upon facial growth, cleft patients often have a Class III malocclusion. If this is not significant (and/or patient doesn't want orthognathic surgery) then definitive Rx for alignment and space closure with FA can be carried out. Ideally, if 2 missing, Rx should aim to bring 3 forward to replace it, thus avoiding a prosthesis.

Late teens If orthognathic surgery is indicated (➲ Orthognathic surgery, p. 510) then this should be deferred until active growth has slowed to adult levels. Pre-surgical orthodontic alignment with FAs will be required. If nasal revision surgery is planned then this should be carried out after bony surgery.

  A proportion of cleft patients will have a skeletal discrepancy that is too severe for conventional surgical movements. In addition, advancement of the maxilla may, by bringing forward the soft palate, adversely affect speech. In these cases distraction osteogenesis (➲ Distraction osteogenesis, p. 169) can be considered.

  See also ➲ Clefts and craniofacial anomalies, p. 508.

Limited treatment orthodontics

Limited treatment orthodontics or short-term orthodontic treatments have gained popularity in recent years, with many GDPs training as providers and a significant number of systems are available. In these cases, anterior teeth are aligned using either brackets and wires on the teeth or with clear aligners. This Rx is generally for adults wanting to improve the appearance of teeth in the aesthetic zone.

Restorative dentistry 1: periodontology

Principal sources and further reading T. Dietrich
et al. 2019 Periodontal diagnosis in the context of the 2017
classification system of periodontal diseases and conditions—
implementation in clinical practice. *Br Dent J* **226** 16–22. K. S.
Kornman & M. S. Tonetti (eds) Special issue: Proceedings of
the World Workshop on the 2017 Classification of periodontal
and peri-implant diseases and conditions. *J Periodontol* **89** S1–
318. J. Lindhe et al. 2008 *Clinical Periodontology and Implant
Dentistry* (5e), Blackwell Munksgaard. See also *Journal of Clinical
Periodontology*.

Classification of periodontal disease

The classification of periodontal and peri-implant diseases was revisited in 2017/2018. In November 2017, the American Academy of Periodontology (AAP) and the European Federation of Periodontology (EFP), together with members from other countries around the world, met in Chicago to discuss the reclassification of periodontal health, periodontal disease, and peri-implant disease. This was presented at EuroPerio9 in Amsterdam in June 2018. This document is now referred to as the 2017 World Workshop on the Classification of Periodontal and Peri-Implant Diseases and Conditions (see Box 5.1) and supersedes the previous classification system (1999 International Workshop for a Classification of Periodontal Diseases and Conditions (Box 5.2)).

The 2017 classification consisted of four working groups and within those groups there were further subgroups (Box 5.1).

Box 5.1 2017 classification of periodontal and peri-implant diseases and conditions

I. Periodontal health, gingival diseases, and conditions
Periodontal and gingival health.
Gingivitis: dental biofilm induced.
Gingival diseases: non-dental biofilm induced.

II. Periodontitis
Necrotizing periodontal diseases.
Periodontitis.
Periodontitis as a manifestation of systemic disease.

III. Other conditions affecting the periodontium
Systemic diseases or conditions affecting the periodontal supporting tissues.
Periodontal abscesses and endodontic-periodontal lesions.
Mucogingival deformities and conditions.
Traumatic occlusal forces.
Tooth and prosthesis-related factors.

IV. Peri-implant diseases and conditions
Peri-implant health.
Peri-implant mucositis.
Peri-implantitis.
Peri-implant soft and hard tissue deficiencies.

Box 5.2 1999 classification of periodontal diseases and conditions

I. Gingival diseases

A. Plaque induced

1. *Gingivitis associated with plaque only.*
   a. Without local contributing factors.
   b. With other local contributing factors.
2. *Gingival disease modified by systemic factors.*
   a. Endocrine system: puberty-associated gingivitis, menstrual cycle-associated gingivitis, pregnancy-associated gingivitis, pyogenic granuloma, diabetes mellitus-associated gingivitis.
   b. Gingivitis associated with blood dyscrasias, e.g. leukaemia-associated gingivitis.
3. *Gingivitis modified by medications.* These would include drug-influenced gingival enlargement and drug-induced gingivitis, e.g. oral contraceptive-associated gingivitis and drug-induced gingival overgrowth due to phenytoin or ciclosporin.
4. *Gingival disease modified by malnutrition.* These would include ascorbic acid-deficiency gingivitis (scurvy) and gingivitis due to protein deficiency.

B. Non-plaque induced

These include gingival lesions of specific bacterial, viral, or fungal origin (e.g. 1° herpetic gingivostomatitis, ➲ Herpes simplex virus, p. 434), lesions of genetic origin (e.g. hereditary gingival fibromatosis), gingival manifestations of systemic conditions (mucocutaneous disorders, allergic reactions), traumatic lesions, and foreign body reactions.

II. Chronic periodontitis
Localized.
Generalized.

III. Aggressive periodontitis
Localized.
Generalized.

IV. Periodontitis as a manifestation of systemic disease

V. Necrotizing periodontal diseases
Necrotizing ulcerative gingivitis (NUG).
Necrotizing ulcerative periodontitis (NUP).

VI. Abscesses of the periodontium

VII. Periodontitis associated with endodontic lesions

VIII. Developmental or acquired deformities and conditions

1999 International Workshop for a Classification of Periodontal Diseases and Conditions.

The largest change in the reclassification was undoubtedly in the working group relating to the diagnosis of periodontitis. The new classification system requires the clinician to not only diagnose periodontitis and whether it is localized or generalized (there is an added distribution category of molar/incisor relationship), but to also comment on the stage and grade of the disease, to reflect on whether the disease is stable, in remission, or active (Box 5.3), and finally to list the identified risk factors. The distribution of localized or generalized is still based on <30% of sites affected or >30% of sites affected. The only risk factors included in the World Workshop paper were diabetes, specifically unstable diabetes, and smoking.

While the 2017 World Workshop on the Classification of Periodontal Diseases has been widely accepted, the British Society of Periodontology (BSP) felt that it was too complicated to be used in its raw form in general practice in the UK and set up a working group to look at how this new system could be implemented in UK general practice. In early 2019, the BSP published their document 'Periodontal diagnosis in the context of the 2017 classification system of periodontal diseases and conditions— implementation in clinical practice'. This simpler system mirrors the style of the original document but simplifies the staging and grading elements of the diagnosis to allow for easier use in general practice (Box 5.4 and Box 5.5).

Box 5.3 2017 assessment of current periodontal status

I. Currently stable
Bleeding on probing (BOP) <10%.
Probing pocket depth (PPD) ≤4mm.
No BoP at 4mm sites.

II. Currently in remission
BOP ≥10%.
PPD ≤4mm.
No BoP at 4mm sites.

III. Currently unstable
PPD ≥5mm or
PPD ≥4mm and BOP.

It should be noted that in the BSP implementation document they make the point that a 5mm or 6mm pocket that does not bleed may not be unstable.

Box 5.4 British Society of Periodontology UK implementation (gingivitis)

Clinical gingival health
BPE code 0/1/2 with <10% bleeding on probing.

Localized gingivitis
BPE code 0/1/2 with 10–30% bleeding on probing.

Generalized gingivitis
BPE code 0/1/2 with >30% bleeding on probing.
For BPE code 2, diagnosis should also include a comment on plaque retentive factors.

Box 5.5 British Society of Periodontology UK implementation (periodontitis)

I. Distribution
Molar–incisor pattern.
Localized <30% of teeth.
Generalized ≥30% of teeth.

II. Staging
Stage I (early/mild): <15% bone loss or up to 2mm bone loss.
Stage II (moderate): bone level in coronal third of root.
Stage III (severe): bone level in mid third of root.
Stage IV (very severe): bone level in apical third of root.
Stage is assessed on the worst affected tooth.

III. Grading—% bone loss/patient's age
Grade A (slow): <0.5.
Grade B (moderate): 0.5–1.0.
Grade C (rapid): >1.0.
Grade is assessed on the worst affected tooth.

IV. Assessment of current periodontal status
Currently stable: BOP <10%, PPD <4mm, no BOP at 4mm sites.
Currently in remission: BOP >10%, PPD <4mm, no BOP at 4mm sites.
Currently unstable: PPD >5mm or PPD >4mm and BOP.
It should be noted that in the BSP implementation document they make the point that a 5mm or 6mm pocket that does not bleed may not be unstable.

V. Risk factors
Smoking.
Sub-optimally controlled diabetes.

Example of a diagnosis statement
Generalized periodontitis stage III grade B currently unstable with smoking as a risk factor.

We have included the 1999 classification, the 2017 World Workshop classification, and the BSP's implementation document in this section. We believe that it is important for dentists and dental students to be familiar with the 1999 classification, be up to date with the 2017 classification, and, if practising in the UK, should know the BSP's 2019 document as this will be the referred-to document in the UK when diagnosing periodontitis.

Further reading

G. C. Armitage 2002 Classifying periodontal diseases—a long-standing dilemma. *Periodontol 2000* **30** 9.
T. Dietrich et al. 2019 Periodontal diagnosis in the context of the 2017 classification system of periodontal diseases and conditions—implementation in clinical practice. *Br Dent J* **226** 16.
K. S. Kornman & M. S. Tonetti (eds) 2018 Special issue: Proceedings of the World Workshop on the 2017 classification of periodontal and peri-implant diseases and conditions. *J Periodontol* **89** S1.

Epidemiology of periodontal disease

Epidemiology is the study of the presence, severity, and effect of disease on a population. This helps identify aetiological and risk factors and effectiveness of preventive and therapeutic measures at a population level. Various scoring systems such as gingival, plaque, and periodontal indices for measuring periodontal disease have been developed,[1,2] some for use at a population level (e.g. Community Periodontal Index, Community Periodontal Index of Treatment Needs (CPITN)) and some for screening and management of individual patients (e.g. BPE). There is no single ideal index. Full mouth recording gives the most information but is time-consuming. Partial recording systems have been used in large-scale epidemiological studies but tend to underestimate disease. Operator measurement errors may occur and there may be inter-observer variation.

The direct association between the presence of tooth surface plaque and gingivitis has been confirmed. Gingivitis precedes periodontitis but there is no evidence to suggest that periodontitis develops in the absence of gingivitis.

In epidemiological studies, there is a lack of consensus on the definition of periodontitis.[3] Although mild to moderate periodontitis is common, severe periodontitis affects a relatively small subset of the population. Certain risk factors such as smoking, poorly controlled diabetes, and colonization by specific bacteria at high levels have been identified.

Localized aggressive periodontitis (LAP) affects <0.1–0.2% of Caucasians and up to 22% of Afro-Caribbeans. Generalized aggressive periodontitis (GAP) affects <5%.

Further longitudinal prospective studies are needed to analyse emerging hypotheses.

Basic Periodontal Examination

The BPE was developed from the CPITN.[4] The BPE is a simple screening tool that will be used to determine what further examination is needed and therefore provides a direction of the next phase of Rx. This technique is used to screen for those patients requiring more detailed periodontal examination in the dental practice setting. It examines every tooth in the mouth (except third molars), thus taking into account the site-specific nature of periodontal disease. A World Health Organization (WHO) periodontal probe is used. It has a ball end which is 0.5mm, then a coloured (normally black) band from 3.5 to 5.5mm (Fig. 5.1). The mouth is divided into sextants, i.e. two buccal and one labial segment per arch. All teeth in each segment are explored and the highest score per sextant recorded, usually in a simple six-box chart. The probe is 'walked' around the sulcus in each sextant with a light probing force (20–25g) and the highest score is recorded in each sextant. For a sextant to qualify for recording, it must contain at least two teeth.

1 G. Barnes et al. 1986 *J Periodontol* **57** 643.

2 E. D. Beltrán-Aguilar et al. 2012 *Periodontol 2000* **60** 40.

3 L. Borrell & P. N. Papapanou 2005 *J Clin Periodontol* **32** (Suppl 6) 132.

4 J. Ainamo et al. 1982 *Int Dent J* **32** 281.

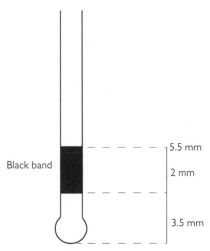

Fig. 5.1 WHO probe for use in BPE/CPITN.

When to record the Basic Periodontal Examination
- All new patients should have a BPE recording including children and adults.
- For patients with BPE code 0, 1, or 2 on a previous BPE recording, the BPE should be followed up at each follow-up examination.
- For patients with BPE codes 3 and 4, further detailed periodontal charting would be needed and further Rx as indicated in the following sections.
- BPE should not be used around implants. Six-point pocket charting is recommended instead.

0 = pockets <3.5mm and the first black band is completely visible
- Healthy periodontal tissues.
- No bleeding after gentle probing.
- No calculus and no overhangs on restorations.
Rx: no need for periodontal Rx.

1 = pockets <3.5mm and the first black band is completely visible
- Gingival bleeding after gentle probing.
- No pockets >3mm.
- No calculus.
- No plaque retaining factors (e.g. overhanging restoration).
- Special investigations would not be needed; however, it is important to note that any recession would be unaccounted for.
Rx: OHIs.

2 = pockets <3.5mm. First black band is visible but plaque retention factors present (e.g. calculus/overhang)
• Plaque and bleeding charts can be recorded as part of special investigations.
Rx: OHIs plus removal of plaque retentive factors including sub- and supragingival calculus.

3 = coloured area of probe remains partly visible in deepest pocket in sextant → deepest pocket 4 or 5mm
• More detailed periodontal charting required.
• Plaque and bleeding charts can be recorded as part of special investigations.
• Radiographs should be considered to assess bone levels and to establish true attachment loss.
Rx: initial therapy including self-care advice (OHIs and risk factor control), record six-point periodontal pocket chart of involved sextants at a review 3 months post initial therapy. If pocket depths persist despite initial therapy and excellent OH, root surface instrumentation would be required.

4 = coloured area of probe disappears into pocket → one or more teeth in sextant has a pocket >6mm
• More detailed periodontal charting required for the entire dentition.
• Plaque and bleeding charts can be recorded as part of special investigations.
• Special investigations would include radiographs to assess bone levels and to establish true attachment loss.
Rx: OHIs, six-point periodontal pocket chart, root surface debridement, and referral to a specialist may be indicated.

* = furcation involvement
• More detailed periodontal charting required for the entire dentition.
• Plaque and bleeding charts can be recorded as part of special investigations.
• Special investigations would include radiographs.
Rx: treat according to BPE code. More complex Rx and referral to a specialist may be necessary.

Patients with a sextant code of 4 or * will require a full probing depth chart, plus recordings of mobility, recession, and furcation involvement, and radiographs. The BPE cannot be used for close monitoring of the progress of Rx.

If the black band disappears on probing a pocket, perform a full periodontal examination in that sextant.

BPE probing is not appropriate for implants sites. The soft tissue connection to implants is not the same as teeth, therefore peri-implant soft tissues are less resistant to probing. In addition, the position of the implant in relation to the bone and soft tissues may present deeper probing depths.

The BPE cannot be used to monitor the response to periodontal Rx because it cannot provide information on how sites change within a sextant, after Rx. The BPE is a screening tool.

Oral microbiology

The mouth is colonized by microorganisms a few hours after birth, mainly by aerobic and facultative anaerobic organisms. The eruption of teeth allows the development of a complex ecosystem of microorganisms. More than 700 different species can colonize the mouth and >400 species may be found in periodontal pockets. Resident oral microflora form multi-species biofilms on oral surfaces. In health there is a balanced relationship between oral microflora and the host which is mutually beneficial. The resident microflora are important in preventing colonization by exogenous microbes. Some resident oral bacteria can reduce dietary nitrate to nitrite which confers benefits on the host cardiovascular and gastrointestinal systems. Microbial composition alters with health and disease.

The composition of the biofilms varies with the site: biofilms in occlusal fissures are mainly Gram +ve and facultatively anaerobic. They metabolize host and dietary sugars. Biofilms in periodontal pockets have large amounts of obligately anaerobic Gram −ve rods and cocci and are proteolytic in metabolism.

Microorganisms worth noting

Streptococcus mutans group Several species are recognized within this group, including S. mutans and S. sobrinus. Facultative anaerobe. Synthesizes dextrans, → plaque formation. Colony density rises to >50% in presence of high dietary sucrose. Able to produce acid from most sugars. Most important organisms in the aetiology of caries.

S. oralis group Includes S. sanguinis, S. mitis, and S. oralis. Account for up to 50% of streptococci in plaque. Heavily implicated in 50% of cases of infective endocarditis. These are pioneer species.

S. salivarius group Accounts for about half the streptococci in saliva. Inconsistent producer of dextran.

S. intermedius, S. anginosus, S. constellatus (Formerly S. milleri group.) Common isolates from abscesses in the mouth and at distant sites. Believed to contribute to periodontal disease progression.

Lactobacillus $2°$ colonizer in caries. Very acidogenic. Often found in dentine caries.

Porphyromonas gingivalis Obligate anaerobe associated with chronic periodontitis and aggressive periodontitis.

Aggregatibacter actinomycetemcomitans Microaerophilic, capnophilic, Gram −ve rod. Particular pathogen in aggressive periodontitis.

Tannerella forsythia Anaerobic, Gram −ve. Implicated in periodontal diseases.

Prevotella intermedia Found in chronic periodontitis, LAP, necrotizing periodontal disease, and areas of severe gingival inflammation without attachment loss.

P. nigrescens New, possibly more virulent.

Fusobacterium Obligate anaerobes. Originally thought to be principal pathogens in necrotizing periodontal disease. Remain a significant periodontal pathogen. Within the symbiosis dysbiosis theory (➲ Symbiosis dysbiosis, p. 185) these species are known to be 'quorum sensing' organisms that are capable of sensing and influencing their environments via chemical cues. This can elicit a stronger host response.

Spirochaetes Obligate anaerobes implicated in periodontal disease; present in most adult mouths. *Borrelia*, *Treponema*, and *Leptospira* belong to this family.

Borrelia vincenti (refringens) Large oral spirochaete; probably only a co-pathogen.

Actinomyces israelii Filamentous organism; major cause of actinomycosis. A persistent rare infection which occurs predominantly in the mouth and jaws and the female reproductive tract. Implicated in root caries.

Candida albicans Yeast-like fungus, famous as an opportunistic oral pathogen; probably carried as a commensal by most people.

Aetiology of periodontal disease

The 1° aetiology of virtually all forms of periodontal disease is plaque. It exists in a biofilm at the supragingival margin and can progress subgingivally.

Microbiology Plaque biofilm causes gingivitis by inducing an inflammatory host response. The inflammatory response of gingiva to the presence of initial young plaque creates gingival inflammatory changes and a minute gingival pocket which serves as an ideal environment for further bacterial colonization, providing all the nutrients required for the growth of numerous fastidious organisms. In addition, there is an extremely low oxygen level within gingival pockets, which favours the development of obligate anaerobes, several of which are closely associated with the progression of periodontal disease. High levels of carbon dioxide favour the establishment of the capnophilic organisms, some of which are associated with LAP.

Clinically healthy gingivae are associated with a high proportion of Gram +ve rods and cocci which are facultatively anaerobic or aerobic. Gingivitis is associated with an ↑ number of facultative anaerobes, strict anaerobes, and an ↑ number of Gram –ve rods. Established periodontitis is associated with a majority presence of anaerobic Gram –ve rods.

The 1996 World Workshop in Periodontics identified three species as causative factors for periodontitis. These are *Aggregatibacter actinomycetemcomitans* (Aa) (previously called *Actinobacillus actinomycetemcomitans*), *Porphyromonas gingivalis*, and *Tannerella forsythia*. However, these are not the only causative pathogens and there are other putative pathogens for which there is evidence. These are *Prevotella intermedia, P. nigrescens, P. melaninogenica, Fusobacterium nucleatum, Peptostreptococcus micros, Eubacterium* spp., *Eikenella corrodens, Selenomonas* spp., *Treponema denticola*, and *Campylobacter rectus*. There is a strong association between Aa and LAP.

Some studies have suggested that specific viruses may be responsible for the aetiology and progression of periodontal lesions.[5]

Complexes of organisms, associated in a structured way, have been identified.[6]

The role of plaque in aetiology There are four hypotheses. They are inter-related and concepts for Rx are derived from them.

Non-specific plaque hypothesis This is the theory that the disease is the outcome of the overall activity of the total plaque microflora → rationale for surgical and non-surgical Rx.

Specific plaque hypothesis Only a few species in the plaque microflora are actively involved in the disease → rationale for use of antimicrobials.

Ecological plaque hypothesis Takes elements of both the first two hypotheses. Local environmental changes arising from inflammation due to plaque accumulation causes an ecological shift in the microflora likely to produce

---

5 J. Slots 2005 *Periodontology 2000* 33 33.

6 S. S. Socransky et al. 1998 *J Clin Perio* 25 134.

more inflammation → rationale for interfering with environmental factors that drive changes in host/microflora balance. Plaque removal or altering pocket environment to suppress growth.

Symbiosis dysbiosis This considers the previous three hypotheses and develops it further. While the ecological plaque hypothesis takes into account that a shift in the microflora, towards a more pathogenic biofilm, produces more inflammation, this in itself is not sufficient to cause the periodontitis. The periodontitis results from more complex interactions between the biofilm and inflammatory immune response from the host. A health-promoting biofilm would trigger a host response that is more resolving and thus the symbiotic relationship between the biofilm and host promotes health. However, if the biofilm is not disrupted regularly, certain species such as *Fusobacterium nucleatum* are favoured. These enable a stronger host response and thus create the conditions that promote the development and growth of traditional pathogens such as *P. gingivalis*. This is known as incipient dysbiosis because in non-susceptible individuals the inflammation does not progress beyond gingivitis. However, in susceptible individuals incipient dysbiosis can trigger a host response that is excessive, resulting in collateral periodontal tissue damage.

Virulence factors Pathogens use a number of mechanisms to exert damage on host tissue: adherence, proteases, bone resorption factors, cytotoxic metabolites, leucotoxins, and induction of the inflammatory response via cytokines and chemotaxins.

Host defences The host response to the biofilm is meant to be protective but can also cause local tissue damage. Both inflammatory and immunologically mediated pathways can contribute to periodontal damage.

Innate host defences Intact epithelium acts as a physical barrier. If junctional epithelium develops into pocket epithelium its protective function is due to its permeable structure. Supragingivally, saliva prevents drying of the oral tissues and has antimicrobial effects via salivary IgA, salivary peroxidase, lysozyme, and lactoferrin. The inflammatory response is relatively non-specific. There is a fluid component in the form of gingival crevicular fluid. This washes out non-adherent bacteria from the crevice and contains inflammatory mediators (cytokines, prostaglandins, and matrix metalloproteinases). The cellular component includes neutrophils and macrophages.

Specific immune response
- Humoral response: involves antibody production.
- Cell-mediated response: T-helper cells produce cytokines, assist in the differentiation of B cells to plasma cells, and activate neutrophils and macrophages.

Systemic risk factors can modify this host response.

Plaque biofilm

Dental plaque, which is a biofilm, is an adherent mass of diverse microorganisms in a muco-polysaccharide matrix.[7] It cannot be rinsed off but can be removed by brushing.

Biofilms are made up of symbiotic communities of different microorganisms. They develop in a structured way and are spatially and functionally organized.[8] The species within communicate with each other. They are less susceptible to host defences and antimicrobial agents than planktonic bacteria. Resident bacteria can dampen the immune response via communication with mucosal cells. If this balanced coexistence breaks down, disease can occur. It forms in stages:

Biofilm formation Although it is possible for plaque to collect on irregular surfaces in the mouth, to colonize smooth tooth surfaces it needs the presence of *acquired pellicle*. This is a thin layer of salivary glycoproteins, formed on the tooth surface within minutes of polishing. The pellicle has an ion-regulating function between tooth and saliva and contains immunoglobulins, complement, and lysozyme. Up to 10^6 viable bacteria per mm^2 of tooth surface can be recovered 1h after cleaning;[7] these are selectively adsorbed streptococci (pioneer species ➔ S. *oralis* group, p. 182). Bacteria recolonize the tooth surface in a predictable sequence. The pioneer species are attached by weak van der Waals forces (reversible adhesion). It leads to a stronger, irreversible attachment. Co-adhesion of the new colonizers to the already attached bacteria → diversity. Attached organisms multiply and biofilm forms. Bacteria synthesize extracellular matrix. Detachment of cells from the biofilm allows colonization of new surfaces.

Cocci predominate in plaque for the first 2 days, following which rods and filamentous organisms become involved. This is associated with ↑ numbers of leucocytes at the gingival margin. Between 6 and 10 days, if no cleaning has taken place, vibrios and spirochaetes appear in plaque and this is associated with clinical gingivitis. It is generally felt that the move towards a more Gram −ve anaerobe-dense plaque is associated with the progression of gingivitis and periodontal disease.

Plaque and caries (➔ Dental caries, p. 24.) As several oral streptococci, most notably mutans streptococci, secrete acids and the matrix component of plaque, there is a clear relationship between the two. However, various other factors complicate the picture, including saliva, other microorganisms, and the structure of the tooth surface.

7 P. Marsh 2005 *J Clin Periodontol* **32** (Suppl 6) 7.

8 A. Haffajee & S. S. Socransky 2006 *Periodontol 2000* **42** 7.

Plaque and periodontal disease There is a direct correlation between the amount of plaque at the cervical margin of teeth and the severity of gingivitis, and experimental gingivitis can be produced and abolished by suspending and reintroducing OH.[9] It is commonly accepted that plaque accumulation causes gingivitis, the major variable being host susceptibility. While there are numerous interacting components which determine the progression of chronic gingivitis to periodontitis, particularly host susceptibility, the presence of plaque, particularly 'old' plaque with its high anaerobe content, is widely held to be crucial, and most Rx is based on the meticulous, regular removal of plaque.

Summary points for plaque biofilm
- Plaque biofilm develops in a structured manner.
- It starts by development and formation of the acquired pellicle.
- Streptococci are the earlier species to develop.
- Formation of a biofilm and the presence of plaque has a direct correlation with gingivitis.
- *Fusobacterium nucleatum* are quorum sensing species that can initiate an environmental change towards the more pathogenic species.
- Incipient dysbiosis may occur.
- If the host response is such that there is resulting periodontal tissue damage, frank dysbiosis will occur.

9 H. Loe et al. 1965 *J Periodont* **36** 177.

Calculus

Calculus (tartar) is a calcified deposit found on teeth (and other solid oral structures) and is formed by mineralization of plaque deposits. The mineral content of supragingival calculus derives from saliva, that for subgingival is from gingival crevicular fluid.

Supragingival calculus This is most often found opposite the openings of the salivary ducts, i.e. 76|67 opposite the parotid (Stensen's) duct and on the lingual surface of the lower anterior teeth opposite the submandibular/sublingual (Wharton's) duct. It is usually creamy-coloured but can become stained a variety of colours.

Subgingival calculus This is found (not surprisingly) underneath the gingival margin and is firmly attached to tooth roots. It tends to be brown or black, is extremely tenacious, and is most often found on interproximal and lingual surfaces. It may be identified visually, detected by touch using a BPE or CPITN or any periodontal probe, or on radiographs. It is associated with subsequent periodontitis in some cases. With gingival recession it can become supragingival.

Composition It consists of up to 80% inorganic salts, mostly crystalline, the major components being calcium and phosphorus. The microscopic structure is basically that of a randomly orientated crystal formation. There are different morphological types (octacalcium phosphate, hydroxyapatite, whitlocktite, brushite).

Formation Calculus is always preceded by plaque deposition, the plaque serving as an organic matrix for subsequent mineralization. Initially, the matrix between organisms becomes calcified with, eventually, the organisms themselves becoming mineralized. Subgingival calculus usually takes many months to form, whereas friable supragingival calculus may form within 2 weeks.

Pathological effect Calculus (particularly subgingival calculus), is associated with periodontal disease. This may be because it is invariably covered by a layer of plaque. Its principal detrimental effect is probably that it acts as a retention site for plaque and bacterial toxins. The presence of calculus makes it difficult to implement adequate OH.

Anti-calculus dentifrices Contain crystal growth inhibitors, e.g. triclosan, zinc citrate, to prevent formation of supragingival calculus. They have not been shown to be effective against subgingival deposits.

Progression and risk factors

Progression from gingivitis to periodontitis can occur as there is a shift from 'friendly' commensal bacteria to periodontopathic bacteria and their products and the host response that ensues. The way in which plaque does this is complex. It involves the oral environment, the pathogenicity of organisms, host defence, and plaque maturity. Some individuals may have large amounts of plaque without developing periodontitis, others may have periodontal destruction with relatively small amounts of plaque.

The shift of microbial species in the gingival sulcus from Gram +ve facultative fermentative organisms to predominantly Gram –ve anaerobic and proteolytic organisms has been strongly associated with periodontal breakdown previously and the associated changes in the host response have also been associated. There are various risk factors.

Risk factors

Local factors Those which predispose to plaque accumulation, e.g. tooth position and morphology, calculus (➲ Calculus, p. 188), overhangs and appliances, occlusal trauma, and mucogingival state.

Systemic factors Those which modify the host response, e.g. smoking, diabetes, obesity, genetic factors, immune status, stress, age, and nutrition. Modifiable risk factors such as smoking are important in managing periodontal disease.

Periodontal disease and risk for systemic disease

There is a growing body of evidence suggesting an association between periodontal disease and atherosclerotic cardiovascular disease, pregnancy complications, diabetes, respiratory disease, kidney disease, and certain cancers. No conclusions can yet be drawn as to whether these are causal associations; however, it highlights the importance of oral health as part of a generally healthy lifestyle.[10] There is a stronger association and possible causation associated with type 1 diabetes.

Further reading

M. Tonetti & K. S. Kornman (eds) 2013 Special issue: Periodontitis and systemic disease—proceedings of a workshop jointly held by the European Federation of Periodontology and American Academy of Periodontology. *J Clin Periodontol* **40** (Suppl 14).

10 R. C. Williams et al. 2008 *Curr Med Res Opin* **24** 1635.

Pathogenesis of gingivitis and periodontitis

Overall, gingivitis and periodontitis are a continuum of the same condition but gingivitis does not always progress to periodontitis.

Initial lesion At 24h there is vasodilation in the adjacent gingival tissues. At 2–4 days: ↑ intercellular gaps therefore gingival crevicular fluid flow flushes noxious substances away and releases antibodies, complement, and protease inhibitors. Neutrophils and a few lymphocytes and macrophages appear. Gingiva appears clinically healthy.

Early lesion After about 1 week there are ↑ numbers of vascular units therefore clinically there is erythema. Lymphocytes and neutrophils predominate with very few plasma cells. Fibroblasts degenerate and collagen fibres break down. The basal cells of the junctional epithelium and sulcular epithelium proliferate to form rete pegs in the adjacent connective tissue. Subgingival biofilm develops as junctional epithelium loses contact with enamel. May persist for a long time without shifting to established lesion.

Established lesion Gingival crevicular fluid flow ↑. Neutrophils predominate. There are ↑ numbers of lymphocytes and plasma cells in the connective tissue and junctional epithelium. The junctional epithelium converts to pocket epithelium. Clinically the gingival is red, swollen, and bleeds easily. The established lesion may remain stable with no progression for months or years or may convert to a destructive advanced lesion.

Advanced lesion As the pocket deepens the biofilm continues to develop apically. Apical migration of the JE occurs → formation of a true pocket lined with pocket epithelium. Inflammatory cell infiltrate extends further apically into the connective tissues. Plasma cells dominate and now constitute >50% of the cellular infiltrate. There is loss of connective tissue attachment and alveolar bone which represents the onset of periodontitis.

The disease is initiated and maintained by substances produced by the biofilm. Some (such as proteases) cause direct injury to host cells; some cause tissue injury by activation of host inflammatory and immune responses.

Initially, pockets will be shallow (4–5mm) representing 1–2mm of clinical attachment loss (❯ Clinical attachment levels (CALs), p. 195). Bone loss is likely to be horizontal with suprabony pockets. As disease progresses and pockets deepen, CALs ↑. Bone loss may be vertical with infrabony pockets.

The transition from gingivitis to periodontitis is difficult to predict and susceptibility varies from site to site. Disease progression is traditionally measured by CAL or probing pocket depth measurements. Linear and burst models for progression have been proposed.

Clinical features of gingivitis and periodontitis

Gingivitis The classic triad of redness, swelling, and bleeding on gentle probing are diagnostic and are usually associated with a complaint by the patient that their 'gums bleed on brushing'. The 'knife-edge' margins and stippled appearance associated with health disappear and are replaced by a more rounded, shiny appearance. Pain is not usually a feature. Halitosis may be present. Affects gingiva only.

It is *not* associated with alveolar bone resorption or apical migration of the junctional epithelium. Probing depths >3mm can occur in chronic gingivitis due to an ↑ in gingival size because of oedema or hyperplasia (false pockets).

The recent 2017 World Workshop on the Classification of Periodontal Diseases came up with working definitions of health and gingivitis (Box 5.6).

They also defined a patient who had a reduced periodontium but not through periodontitis, e.g. a patient who had crown lengthening or the distal aspect of a second molar where there had been an impacted third molar removed (Box 5.7).

Chronic periodontitis Clinical signs may include gingival inflammation and bleeding, pocketing, gingival recession, tooth mobility, tooth migration, discomfort, and halitosis (Fig. 5.2). It affects gingiva, PDL, cementum, and alveolar bone. At earlier stages there is usually very little in the way of obvious signs or symptoms therefore probing is essential. It can be regarded as a progression of the combination of infection and inflammation of gingivitis into the deep tissues of the periodontal membrane. All periodontitis develops out of gingivitis but not all gingivitis progresses to periodontitis. Some people with poor OH may develop gingivitis but not periodontitis. Some people with good OH and little in the way of gingivitis may develop periodontitis. The proportion of sites that do progress in a subject or population is not known and the factors → progression are not well understood. Periodontitis is classified as localized when <30% of sites are affected and as generalized when >30% of sites are affected.

Stage As previously discussed, the staging of the disease describes the degree of attachment loss.

Grade The grade describes the rate of progression of the disease to date.

Box 5.6 Patients with an intact periodontium

I. Health
- Probing attachment loss: no.
- PPD: ≤3mm.
- BOP: <10%.
- Radiographic bone loss: no.

II. Gingivitis
- Probing attachment loss: no.
- PD: <3mm.
- BOP: ≥10%.
- Radiographic bone loss: no.

Box 5.7 Patients with a reduced periodontium

I. Health
- Probing attachment loss: yes.
- PPD: ≤3mm.
- BOP: <10%.
- Radiographic bone loss: possible.

II. Gingivitis
- Probing attachment loss: yes.
- PPD: <3mm.
- BOP: ≥10%.
- Radiographic bone loss: possible.

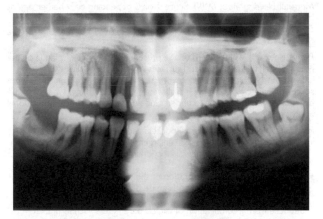

Fig. 5.2 DPT showing the typical appearance of established periodontitis; the patient was a diabetic who smoked.

Diagnosis and monitoring

Diagnosis of periodontal diseases is arrived at by thorough history taking, clinical and X-ray examination, and special investigations.

History

Achieving a periodontal diagnosis is a process of collecting all the information including obtaining a good history. Identify the patient's presenting complaint which may include bleeding, drifted teeth, abscesses, mobile teeth, loss of some teeth, receding gums, etc. It is important to identify the reason and also the patient's concerns and main aims.

It is important at this point to elicit the patient's attitude to Rx, previous Rx experience, and systemic risk factors (e.g. smoking, poorly controlled diabetes) and medical factors relevant to safe Rx (e.g. anticoagulants).

Clinical examination

There is a need to assess plaque control, presence of supra- and subgingival calculus, loss of gingival contour, swelling, suppuration, recession of periodontal tissues, periodontal pocketing, furcation lesions, local risk factors, and tooth mobility. The BPE (● Basic Periodontal Examination, p. 178) provides an overview of the periodontal status. For scores of 1 and 2, marginal gingival bleeding-free and plaque-free scores are recorded. For sextants with scores of 3, initial therapy is conducted and then probing depths and bleeding on probing are recorded if the BPE does not change. For sextants with scores of 4 or * probing pocket depths, recession, clinical attachment levels, bleeding on probing, suppuration, furcation (● Furcation involvement, p. 220), and mobility (● Tooth mobility, p. 222) are recorded noting six sites per tooth.

Marginal bleeding index (MBI) Score 1 or 0 depending on whether or not bleeding occurs after a probe is gently run around the gingival sulcus. A percentage score is obtained by dividing by the number of teeth and multiplying the result by 100.

Plaque index (PI) This is based on the presence or absence of plaque on the mesial, distal, lingual, and buccal surfaces revealed by disclosing.

Both the MBI and PI can be expressed as bleeding-free or plaque-free scores. In this way obtaining a high score is a good thing, which may be both easier for the patient to understand and a more positive motivational approach.

Periodontal pocketing Periodontal pockets can be divided as follows:
- *False pockets* are due to gingival enlargement with the pocket epithelium at or above the amelocemental junction in cases such as altered active eruption.
- *True pockets* imply apical migration of the junctional epithelium beyond the amelocemental junction and can be divided into suprabony and intrabony pockets. Suprabony or intrabony defects are normally deduced from a combination of clinical parameters such as pocket depths and from radiographic intervention. Suprabony defects may be described as horizontal bone loss and intrabony as vertical bone loss.

Intrabony defects are described according to the number of bony walls:
- A three-walled defect is the most favourable, as it is surrounded on three sides by cancellous bone and on one side by the cementum of the root surface.
- A two-walled defect may be either a crater between teeth having bone on two walls and cementum on the other two, or have two bony walls, the root cementum, and an open aspect to the overlying soft tissues.
- A one-walled defect may be a hemiseptal through-and-through defect, or have one bony wall, two root cementum, and one soft tissue.

Probing pocket depths Measured from the gingival margin to the estimated base of the pocket.

Clinical attachment levels (CALs) Measured from a fixed reference point: the cementoenamel junction (CEJ) or margin of a restoration to the base of the pocket. Pockets are therefore dependent on the position of the gingival margin. If recession is present CAL = recession + periodontal probing depth.

Periodontal probes The key instruments in detecting pockets. Numerous designs exist, and while individual preference will influence choice, it is sensible to reduce variability by selecting a single type of probe and using that type of probe throughout any one individual's Rx. The use of the WHO probe for screening is described in the BPE section (◐ Basic Periodontal Examination, p. 178). Patients who are identified as having periodontitis should then be investigated further, including probing around each tooth. The main other indicator of periodontal disease, bleeding, is also detected using a probe (gently), and again consistency with a single type of probe is necessary.

Probing variables The depth of penetration depends upon:
- Type of probe and its position.
- Amount of pressure used.
- Degree of inflammation.[11]

It is now apparent that the measurement obtained with a probe does not correspond to sulcus or pocket depth. In the presence of inflammation, a probe tip can pass through the inflamed tissues until it reaches the most coronal dento-gingival fibres, about 0.5mm apical to the apical extent of the junctional epithelium, i.e. an overestimation of the problem. The amount of penetration into the tissues varies directly with the degree of inflammation, so that, following resolution of inflammation, an underestimate of attachment levels may be given. Formation of a tight, long junctional epithelium following Rx may also give a false sense of security if probing measurements are not interpreted with a degree of caution. For this reason, the term 'probing pocket depth' is preferred to pocket depth.

Mobility Assessed using instrument handles:
- Grade I: <1mm horizontal mobility.
- Grade II: >1mm horizontal mobility. No vertical displacement possible.
- Grade III: vertical displacement of tooth in its socket is possible.

11 M. A. Listgarten 1980 *J Clin Periodontol* **7** 165.

Radiographic examination

Used to support clinical diagnosis in cases with BPE scores of 3, 4, or *, in monitoring the bone levels and in monitoring stability of periodontal health. Standardized sequential radiographs allow monitoring of disease.

Radiographs can be used to aid diagnosis and help determine the prognosis of specific teeth when combined with the clinical examination, patient history, and risk factors. All radiographs should be able to view crestal bone levels for initial assessment and also for long-term review to track changes in bone level over time.

Care should be taken to ensure that each exposure is suitably justified and provides clear benefit to the patient. The number and type of radiographs will depend on findings during the clinical examination.

- Horizontal b/ws provide a good view of interproximal bone, and are useful for relatively minor degrees of bone loss (pocketing <5mm) and to detect calculus deposits. Horizontal b/ws are routinely taken in practice to assess caries and thus they can give an indication of the interproximal bone loss and also any plaque retentive factors such as poorly contoured restorations. Subgingival calculus would be detected in such radiographs too.
- Vertical b/ws may be indicated when there are relatively mild degrees of bone loss (where pocketing is <5mm). Vertical b/ws provide a view of the crestal bone levels in relation to the CEJ in opposing arches. Vertical b/ws are difficult to take in patients with shallow palatal arches &/or shallow floor of mouth, and periapical radiographs may be more suited. In addition, vertical b/ws may not show the full root length hence making it difficult to assess the percentage of bone loss in relation to the root length.
- Full mouth periapicals (preferably of the long cone parallel technique), have been the radiographs of choice for patients with severe periodontal disease. They can clearly demonstrate root surface deposits, furcation involvement, extensive bone loss, intrabony pocketing, and periodontal–endodontic lesions. Periapical radiographs also allow for assessment of the root morphology.
- Full mouth periapical radiographs also allow for assessment of the extent of bone loss in relation to the root length and thus can provide a more accurate way to classify the grading according to the new periodontal classification.
- There is no indication for DPT for routine screening purposes; however, if the patient is not able to tolerate IO radiographs due to reasons such as gagging, then an OPT may be considered to assess bone levels in periodontitis patients.

Making records

Assessment of radiographs should be recorded in the notes including:
- Degree of bone loss (as a % of root length if apex visible as should be in periapical radiographs).
- Pattern of bone loss (angular vs horizontal, furcation involvement) and any other pathology noted.
- Presence of furcations.
- Subgingival deposits.

- Any other features, e.g. periodontal–endodontic lesions, widened periodontal ligament spaces, overhanging restorations, abnormalities in root length or morphology.

Diagnosis

Based on the new classification system, if there is any sign of bone loss radiographically or signs of interdental attachment loss clinically, a diagnosis of periodontitis can be made with the additional recording of the distribution, stage, and grade of the disease and additional comment on if it is stable, in remission, or unstable together with identified risk factors.

As such, an example of a contemporary diagnosis would be 'generalized periodontitis stage III grade B that is currently unstable with smoking as a risk factor'.

Monitoring

The results of radiographs, clinical assessment, and assessment of pocket depth can all be marked on an updatable periodontal chart to monitor progress with Rx.

It is widely accepted that disease active and inactive pockets exist. Progression is episodic and more likely in susceptible patients. Bleeding on probing has traditionally been the most useful indicator of disease activity; however, only 30% of sites which bleed will go on to lose attachment.[12] Absence of bleeding on probing is an indicator of periodontal stability.

With ↑ emphasis on specific periodontopathic bacteria (➜ Microorganisms worth noting, p. 182) and availability of assays for components of immunological response, chair-side diagnostic tests using gingival crevicular fluid have been developed. Although these are aimed to predict sites of future and actual disease progression, this is not as specific or sensitive as initially thought. Research in this area continues and therefore these diagnostic tests have a greater use in research as opposed to clinical practice.

There is a huge amount of ongoing research into improving and refining these tests, but evidence is still required to demonstrate predictive ability and a higher level of accuracy than bleeding on probing.

Summary points for diagnosis and monitoring

- Take a good history.
- Consider any medical or systemic factors and any other risk factors such as smoking.
- Conduct a BPE recording and a more advanced six-point periodontal charting for the greater BPE scores.
- Take appropriate radiographs for monitoring.
- Consider your diagnosis from a periodontal perspective based on the classification system and any other associated diagnosis (e.g. periodontal–endodontic lesions, caries, etc.).

12 N. Lang 1986 J Clin Periodont 13 590.

Aggressive periodontitis

Aggressive periodontitis described a type of periodontitis in the 1999 classification and replaced disease terminology like early-onset periodontitis in previous classification systems.

The new, 2017 classification does not recognize aggressive periodontitis as a separate disease entity and comments that it is merely an extreme presentation of the same disease, periodontitis.

The authors felt it was appropriate to leave this information here for historical perspective and as clinicians may come across these patients with a more rapid form of periodontitis, they should be aware of the appropriate management.

Aggressive periodontitis historically described a group of rare and often severe, rapidly progressive forms of periodontitis. Often characterized by an early age of onset and tending to occur in families and with non-contributory medical history. The amounts of plaque are out of proportion with the severity of periodontal destruction. Often associated with *Aggregatibacter actinomycetemcomitans. Porphyromonas gingivalis* may also be associated. Hyper-responsive macrophage phenotype. Phagocyte abnormalities are found. Progression of attachment loss may be self-arresting.

Two main forms

- *Generalized aggressive periodontitis* (GAP): previously known as generalized juvenile periodontitis.
- *Localized aggressive periodontitis* (LAP): previously known as localized juvenile periodontitis.

GAP A severe form of generalized periodontitis affecting young adults (<30yrs). Generalized interproximal attachment loss affecting at least three permanent teeth other than first molars and incisors. Pronounced episodic nature of the destruction of attachment and alveolar bone. Poor serum antibody response to infecting agents. Affects 1–2% of the Western population with an ↑ in Afro-Caribbeans.

LAP A severe form of localized periodontitis with onset around puberty. Localized attachment loss of at least two permanent teeth one of which is a first molar and involving no more than two teeth other than first molars and incisors. Robust serum antibody response to infecting agents.

Rx

- Achievement of adequate supragingival plaque control.
- Subgingival instrumentation to disrupt biofilm but this may not eradicate virulent organisms.
- Non-surgical approach with adjunctive use of systemic antibiotics is the preferred Rx option. Amoxicillin/metronidazole combination seems to provide additional benefit to non-surgical management. In the situation where amoxicillin or metronidazole cannot be prescribed, azithromycin has a good evidence base.
- Surgery has a role but there is no consensus regarding the use of systemic antibiotics for this approach.
- ↑ evidence that regenerative surgical techniques are a suitable option for defects associated with aggressive periodontitis.
- Regular supportive care is important.

Necrotizing periodontal diseases

This destructive, painful, inflammatory condition is rapid, debilitating, and usually runs an acute course. Includes:
- Necrotizing ulcerative gingivitis (NUG).
- Necrotizing ulcerative periodontitis (NUP).
- Necrotizing stomatitis: where the necrotizing lesion has spread to include tissue beyond the mucogingival junction.

NUG Painful, ulcerated, necrotic papillae and gingival margins with a punched-out appearance. The ulcers are covered by a pseudomembranous grey slough. Associated with a metallic taste and sensation of teeth being wedged apart and foetor oris. Interproximal craters develop with loss of crestal bone and in some cases bony sequestra. Loss of attachment and development of NUP may occur. Regional lymphadenitis, fever, and malaise feature in some cases. Can be confused with 1° herpetic gingivostomatitis. Rarely occurs in children in Northern Europe and the US. Prevalence is ↑ in developing countries. NUG is associated with poor OH, but stress and smoking act as co-factors. Immune suppression, including HIV, also predisposes to NUG. It is usually a limited gingival condition, but a rare and more serious form known as cancrum oris or noma is found in patients who are malnourished, and in this form can lead to extensive destruction of the jaws and face.

Microbiology Specific fusiform/spirochaete bacterial aetiology. *Prevotella intermedia*, *Fusobacteria* spp., *Selenomonas* spp., and *Treponema* spp. The crucial aspect of NUG is that it is a Gram –ve anaerobic infection which has been shown to actually invade the tissues but usually responds to local debridement. The association with HIV and severe NUG, sometimes with bone necrosis, has renewed interest in it. Remember that NUG in an otherwise apparently healthy young adult may be a presenting sign of HIV infection. Consider examining the mouth for other signs of infection (➔ Oral manifestations of HIV infection and AIDS, p. 478), and directing the patient to appropriate counselling &/or HIV testing.

Initial Rx Removal of gross deposits of plaque and calculus ± LA. Ultrasonics are useful due to their flushing action. Chlorhexidine rinses (0.2% × 10mL twice daily) may also be prescribed as an adjunct to brushing, which is painful initially. Usually local measures will suffice; however, if systemic upset (lymphadenopathy), metronidazole 200mg tds for 3 days is indicated. Penicillins are also effective. Once the ulcers have healed, non-surgical periodontal Rx can be carried out and smoking cessation advice given. Later Rx, e.g. gingivectomy for persistent craters, is only rarely required.

Periodontal abscess

This is a localized collection of pus within the tissues adjacent to a peri-odontal pocket. It occurs either due to the introduction of virulent organisms into an existing pocket or ↓ drainage potential. The latter classically occurs during Rx as reduction of inflammation in the coronal gingival tissues occludes drainage by a tighter adaptation to the tooth. It may also occur due to impaction of a foreign body such as a fishbone in a pre-existing pocket or even in an otherwise healthy periodontal membrane. Commonly occurs in furcations. May get super-infection with opportunistic organisms following systemic antibiotics in patients with untreated periodontal disease. Multiple or recurrent abscesses may indicate underlying immunocompromise, e.g. poorly controlled diabetes.

Clinically there may be swelling, pus from a pocket or sinus, pain, tenderness to percussion, and signs of periodontitis. There may be systemic involvement.

Differential diagnosis Gingival abscess, pericoronal abscess, periapical abscess, combined periodontal/endodontic lesion (→ Periodontitis associated with endodontic lesions, p. 201), or other (e.g. cyst/tumour) (Table 5.1).

Insertion of a GP point into an associated sinus and a radiograph may be helpful in tracking the infection source.

Emergency Rx Incision and drainage under LA; systemic antibiotic, e.g. metronidazole 200–400mg tds &/or amoxicillin 250–500mg tds for 5 days if systemic involvement.

Further Rx Mechanical debridement after the acute problem has settled to avoid iatrogenic damage to healthy periodontal tissues adjacent to the lesion.

Follow-up Conventional Rx for periodontal pockets (→ Principles of treatment, p. 202), combined periodontal–endodontic lesion (→ Rx of combined lesion, p. 201).

Table 5.1 Features of periapical vs periodontal abscess

Periapical abscess	Periodontal abscess
Non-vital	Usually vital
TTP vertically	Pain on lateral movements
May be mobile	Usually mobile
Loss of lamina dura on X-ray	Loss of alveolar crest on X-ray

Periodontitis associated with endodontic lesions

▶ It is essential to sensibility test any heavily restored tooth with periodontal involvement.

A combined periodontal–endodontic lesion is where both lesions coalesce regardless of whether the origin is primarily periodontal (necrotic pulp due to periodontal involvement) or primarily endodontic (periodontal tissues involved after pulp necrosis). Given the relative frequency of both periodontal disease and periapical pathology, it is not surprising that both may occur together, which can result in diagnostic confusion. In fact, there is little evidence to support the popular notion that periodontitis leads to pulp necrosis. However, there is no doubt that pulp pathology can exacerbate periodontal problems.

Rx of combined lesion

First, resolve the acute infection and inflammation by drainage (&/or antibiotics), then treat with orthograde RCT (the greater the pulpal component, the better the prognosis).

The apparent periodontal lesion will often be seen to resolve to a substantial degree over a period of months, therefore, the decision to carry out surgery should be deferred. Combined apical surgery and periodontal surgery is quite feasible but carries a poorer long-term prognosis. The worst prognosis applies to those teeth where the periapical/pulpal pathology has been due entirely to apical extension of the periodontal pocket. These are often diagnosed after the fact, when endodontics completely fails to resolve the lesion.

Principles of treatment

- Establish diagnosis, based on current classification (➲ Classification of periodontal disease, p. 174).
- Record location, extent, and severity (➲ Diagnosis and monitoring, p. 194) and any associated risk factors (➲ Risk factors, p. 189).
- The overall aim could be summarized as the creation of a healthy periodontium which the patient is both capable of, and willing to, maintain.

It is often convenient to divide the principles of periodontal therapy into three phases:

The *initial* (cause-related) phase This is where the aim is to control plaque and address modifiable risk factors (e.g. smoking cessation counselling, liaise with GMP if poorly controlled diabetes). Periodontal disease is an infection due to the presence of plaque biofilm, therefore, disruption of the plaque biofilm and control of plaque is the key to success. More complex Rx will always fail in the absence of effective plaque control. Includes recording of baseline indices, OHI, scaling and root surface debridement, and elimination of plaque retention factors. Response is monitored 8–12 weeks after Rx and a further plan made. If successful, can move to supportive phase. If residual disease, then move to corrective phase.

The *corrective* phase This is designed principally to restore function and, where relevant, aesthetics. Corrective techniques include further non-surgical therapy, periodontal access surgery, regenerative surgery, mucogingival surgery, resective surgery (e.g. gingivectomy), selected use of local and systemic antibiotics where indicated (➲ Treatment with antimicrobials, p. 208), Rx of furcation lesions, restorative work, endodontics, and occlusal adjustment.
   The aims of this phase are to:
- Eliminate pathological periodontal pockets, or to create a tight epithelial attachment where the pocket once existed.
- Arrest loss of, and in some cases improve, the alveolar bone support.
- Create an oral environment which is relatively simple for the patient to keep plaque free.

The *supportive* phase This aims to reinforce a patient's motivation so that their OH is adequate to prevent recurrence of disease. This phase is receiving ↑ attention due to the relative ease with which disease activity can be monitored by probing and chair-side diagnostic assays (➲ Supportive periodontal therapy, p. 224).

Non-surgical treatment—plaque control

Following the comments in the sections covering the aetiology and epidemiology of periodontal disease, it is quite clear that dental plaque is the cause of the problem and its elimination will prevent periodontal diseases. This is easier said than done—remember, most of the world's population has gingivitis and/or periodontitis. The key to prevention is regular and thorough plaque removal, therefore, OHI is probably the most useful advice you can give to your patients. The aim is to maintain dental biofilms at a level compatible with health so that the beneficial properties of resident microflora are ↑ and the risk of dental disease is minimized. Smoking exacerbates periodontal disease and adversely affects Rx outcome. Patients should be advised of this.

Oral hygiene instruction

OHI should include an explanation of the nature of the patient's disease and hence the reasons for good OH. Identify and demonstrate to the patient the disease (swollen gingivae, bleeding on probing) using a hand mirror, then demonstrate the cause (plaque), either directly, by scraping off a deposit, or by disclosing. The use of disclosing solution to visually demonstrate the areas of plaque deposits are very useful and can be used to show the specific sites that need particular attention during home care. Explain how plaque starts to grow immediately after toothbrushing, so that regular removal is necessary, and that it cannot be rinsed away. Then demonstrate how to remove it, avoiding overt criticism of the patient's present efforts, as this is often counter-productive. Scaling may be done during this visit.

Mechanical plaque control

Toothbrushing Toothbrushing requires a brush, ideally with a small head and even nylon bristles (3–4 tufts across by 10–12 lengthways), which should be renewed at least monthly. Numerous methods can be described, based on the movement of the brush stroke: rolling, vibratory, circular, vertical, horizontal. The best is the one which works for that patient (as demonstrated by absence of plaque on disclosing after brushing) and does no harm to tooth or gingivae. The horizontal scrub is notorious for possibly exacerbating gingival recession. Modifications to toothbrushes and brushing technique are often required in children, the elderly, and those with disabling diseases. Oscillating, rotating powered toothbrushes are effective. Toothpaste makes the process more pleasant and is a useful medium for topical fluoride and other agents. Anticalculus pastes ↓ plaque formation by about 50%. Chlorhexidine-containing toothpastes are active against plaque microorganisms.

Interdental cleaning Brushing alone will not clean the interdental spaces adequately; interdental cleaning is also necessary. The European Federation of Periodontology workshop in November 2014 focused on the best methods of interdental cleaning to reduce gingivitis and plaque levels between teeth when used in addition to mechanical tooth brushing. The workshop concluded that cleaning between the teeth on a daily basis is essential to maintain gum health. Flossing, mini interdental brushes (particularly good for concave root surfaces), and interspace brushes are available for cleaning interproximally. The use of dental floss is something of an art form and must be learned by demonstration. The 2014 European workshop also concluded that there is reduced efficacy of flossing in removing plaque between the teeth and this is mainly because patients find flossing difficult to perform and it is frequently performed incorrectly. In that respect, interdental brushes are the most efficient in removing interdental plaque if there is space to accommodate them. There was a moderate evidence base noted in the European workshop that supported the use of interdental brushes as being effective in removing plaque between the teeth. These brushes are thus recommended as the method of choice for interdental cleaning where spaces between teeth allow their insertion without causing trauma.

Chemical plaque control

Mouthwashes may help patients who struggle with mechanical methods. This may be because of a lack of dexterity, disability, or due to mucosal conditions (e.g. aphthae, benign mucous membrane pemphigoid) or following periodontal surgery. The anti-septic of greatest proven antiplaque/antigingivitis value is chlorhexidine gluconate. It exhibits substantivity. It is commonly used in a 0.2% mouthwash or gel, although 0.12% mouthwash is also available. A standard regimen is 10mL of solution rinsed for 1min bd (or 15mL of 0.12% for 30sec bd). The gel can be used instead of toothpaste. Chlorhexidine causes staining and altered taste. NB: an interaction between conventional toothpaste and chlorhexidine reduces the antiseptic's efficacy. Other proprietary antiseptic rinses have yet to meet this 'gold standard'.

It is also important to note that in patients who do have good manual dexterity for mechanical cleaning, mouthwashes have a very limited adjunctive effect.

Further reading
P. D. Marsh 2012 Contemporary perspective on plaque control. *Br Dent J* **212** 601.

Non-surgical periodontal therapy— scaling and root surface debridement

Non-surgical periodontal therapy consists of scaling, root surface debridement, restorative Rx (to correct coexisting or exacerbating factors, e.g. periapical infection, overhanging margins), and the possible use of adjunctive antibiotics in very specific cases. The aim is to remove supra- and subgingival plaque and calculus deposits and local plaque retention factors.

Scaling   Scaling is the removal of plaque and calculus from the tooth surface, either with hand instruments (e.g. sickles, curettes, and hoes) or mechanically (e.g. Cavitron®). Scaling can be sub- or supragingival depending upon the site of the deposits. Supragingival scaling is usually completed first as part of initial therapy. LA is not usually necessary. Supragingival scaling is often done together with OHIs.

Root surface instrumentation most likely requires LA and involves the removal of subgingival root deposits. It is no longer considered necessary to remove endotoxin-loaded cementum as it is weakly bound and easily removed by scalers. Historically, an ultrasonic scaler has been used for the bulk of the work to disrupt the biofilm and remove the subgingival deposits, then Rx is finished off with hand instruments. However, there is no direct evidence for this. Some clinicians simply use ultrasonics for removal of subgingival deposits. Evidence shows both to have no significant difference in Rx outcomes. The precise use of hand instruments is largely a matter of personal preference; Langer curettes are commonly used, however, it is essential to use controlled force and a secure finger-rest. Hand instruments must be sharp. Ultrasonic instruments are quicker, but they can be uncomfortable and leave an uneven root surface (though the significance of the latter is controversial). They can generate a contaminated aerosol. Ultrasonic scaling employs a frequency of 25,000–40,000 cycles/sec.

Traditionally one quadrant at a time is treated under LA, partly because it is painful and partly because it is tedious when performed meticulously, which is the only worthwhile way to do it. It has been suggested, however, that a full mouth approach is preferable. This means completion of root debridement within 24h, with concurrent use of a chlorhexidine mouthwash. The aim is to reduce the bacterial load and minimize chance of reinfection by reducing bacterial load in pockets and IO niches. More recently, comparison of full mouth disinfection and the quadrant approach has failed to demonstrate a clinically significant difference in outcomes although there is statistical significance.[13,14] Success will allow tight adaptation of the pocket epithelium to the root, creating a *long junctional epithelium*. Wennström et al.[15] concluded that their results demonstrated that a single session of full mouth ultrasonic debridement is a justified initial Rx approach that offers tangible benefits for the chronic periodontitis patient.

13   N. Lang et al. 2008 *J Clin Periodontol* **35** 8.

14   J. Eberhard et al. 2008 *Cochrane Database Syst Rev* **1** CD004622.

15   J. L. Wennström et al. 2005 *J Clin Periodontol* **32** 851.

The teeth are usually polished after scaling, preferably using a rubber cup and a fluoride-containing paste (e.g. toothpaste). Patients can then appreciate the feeling of a clean mouth, which they must then maintain. Other than this it offers no clinical benefits.

Summary points for non-surgical treatment
- Non-surgical Rx is best done after good OHIs have been provided and techniques demonstrated.
- Non-surgical Rx is normally done under LA at one quadrant per visit.
- Ultrasonics are used to disrupt the biofilm and mechanically remove supra- and subgingival deposits and these can be supplemented with hand instruments.
- There is limited evidence to show the difference between a quadrant approach and full mouth disinfection; however, both offer tangible benefits to patients.

Treatment with antimicrobials

There are few reasons to use antimicrobials in periodontal therapy. The plaque biofilm affects the response, concentration in gingival crevicular fluid is low, antibiotics have side effects, and there is the growing problem of antibiotic resistance. Antibiotics are not really justified for use in chronic periodontitis. There are, however, a few indications for the use of systemic and local antimicrobials.[16,17,18,19,20]

Systemic antimicrobials

Periodontal abscess The first line of Rx is always drainage either by subgingival debridement or by incision. If there is systemic involvement antimicrobials may be used (amoxicillin/metronidazole).

Necrotizing periodontal diseases Fusospirochaetal anaerobes are involved. Management involves removal of risk factors (e.g. poor OH, smoking) and use of metronidazole 200mg tds for 3 days in combination with non-surgical debridement.

Aggressive periodontitis Antimicrobials can be used in combination with conventional subgingival debridement. Amoxicillin 500mg tds and metronidazole 400mg tds are used in combination for 7–10 days starting on the first day of Rx.

Chronic periodontitis Tetracyclines have been advocated as an adjunct in Rx of chronic periodontitis. In addition to being antibacterial they have a number of non-antibiotic properties: tetracyclines ↓ host and neutrophil collagenases and ↓ bone loss. Crevicular fluid concentrations are high. CollaGenex Pharmaceuticals Periostat® (doxycycline 20mg bd for 3 months) makes use of these non-antibiotic properties. At this dose it has no detrimental effect on the periodontal microflora and its action is mainly to reduce collagenolytic metalloproteinases. Clinical benefits need further investigation.

Local delivery of medicaments

Due to controversy over the efficacy and unwanted effects of systemic antibiotics, methods of direct delivery into the pocket have been explored. These have included using injected pastes or gels, or by impregnated fibre. This gives a high local dose, low systemic uptake, and prolonged exposure of the pathogens to the drug. The rate of crevicular fluid turnover is such that the substantivity of these agents is low.

16 J. Slots & T. E. Rams 1990 *J Clin Periodontol* **17** 479.

17 W. J. Loesche et al. 1984 *J Clin Periodontol* **55** 325.

18 D. Herrera et al. 2012 *J Evid Based Dent Pract* **12** 50.

19 D. Herrera et al. 2002 *J Clin Periodontol* **29** 136.

20 A. Haffajee et al. 2003 *Ann Perio* **8** 182.

Indications Chronic periodontitis where isolated recurrent or residual pockets of >5mm persist after conventional Rx and good plaque control. Root debridement must be carried out prior to placement to disrupt the biofilm. They may be used if surgery is not appropriate (e.g. severe systemic illness). They are *not* indicated in aggressive periodontitis.

Outcome Only small ↑ in attachment levels have been reported.

Examples Blackwell Dentomycin® (minocycline gel), Colgate-Palmolive Elyzol® (metronidazole gel), Atrix Laboratories Inc. Atridox® (doxycycline hyclate gel) and PerioChip® (chlorhexidine).

   Photodynamic disinfection systems have been developed. These combine non-thermal laser light with a photosensitizing solution used against periodontal pathogens remaining after conventional instrumentation.

Periodontal surgery—principles

Non-surgical root surface instrumentation can be very effective and there is no absolute maximum depth of pocket where it is ineffective. However, it is less effective in deeper pockets (>6mm). Non-surgical Rx should always be carried out first but where pockets fail to respond (as evidenced by bleeding, loss of attachment, or suppuration) surgical Rx may be considered.

Applications of periodontal surgery
- Provide access for root surface instrumentation. Direct vision of the root surface is possible. This is particularly helpful with furcation defects.
- Result in a site which is accessible for cleaning.
- Correction of gingival overgrowth by gingivectomy.
- Create new periodontal attachment in the case of regenerative procedures.
- Improved aesthetics and function following gingival recession by root coverage techniques.

Contraindications
- Poor plaque control.
- Systemic disease, e.g. uncontrolled diabetes, severe cardiovascular problems, bleeding disorders. Liaise with GMP and specialist.
- As smoking ↓ outcome of Rx, some periodontists have limited Rx in those continuing to smoke. While periodontal surgery hardly has the public impact of cardiac surgery, the ethical problem is the same.
- Teeth with poor long-term prognosis.

Choice of surgical procedure
The choice of the surgical procedure is dependent on the desired outcome and whether the aim is to reduce the pocket, to eliminate the pocket, to regenerate lost attachment, to cover root surfaces affected by gingival recession, or to crown lengthen for restorative or aesthetic reasons.

General principles
LA The infiltration, block, &/or lingual/palatal injections required will be determined by the site of surgery. Both LA and haemostasis are improved by injecting directly into the gingival margin and interdental papillae until blanching is seen.

Flaps Some procedures involve the raising of flaps. These should be large enough to provide good access and clear vision. Most flaps are full thickness, lifting all soft tissue off the underlying bone. Some techniques involve a split thickness flap where the mucoperiosteum remains on bone (◑ The apically repositioned flap, p. 212).

Suturing techniques Interrupted interproximal sutures are used when buccal and lingual flaps are being re-apposed at the same level. When flaps are re-positioned at different levels, a suspensory suture is used where the suture only passes through the buccal flap and is suspended around the cervical margins of the teeth.

Periodontal packs These are essential after gingivectomy to ↓ post-operative discomfort. Many favour them after all periodontal surgery to help re-oppose the flap to bone. Classified:

- Eugenol dressings, e.g. ZOE, have the advantage of being mildly analgesic but can cause sensitivity reactions.
- Eugenol-free dressings, e.g. Coe-Pak™, are more popular.

Summary points for periodontal surgery

- Periodontal surgery is contraindicated in the presence of plaque and poor plaque control by the patient.
- Periodontal surgery is mostly considered after a course of non-surgical debridement.
- Periodontal surgery may be indicated for a variety of reasons and the choice of the surgical procedure is dependent on the desired outcome.
- A very brief overview of the main steps is given.

Periodontal surgery—types of surgery

The modified Widman flap

This is a technique which enables open debridement of the root surface, with a minimal amount of trauma.[21] There is no attempt to excise the pocket, although a superficial collar of tissue is removed. This has the advantage of allowing close adaptation of the soft tissues to the root surface with minimal trauma to, and exposure of, underlying bone and connective tissue, thus causing fewer problems with post-operative sensitivity and aesthetics (Fig. 5.3).

Technique (after Ramfjord and Nissle 1974) A scalloped incision is made parallel to the long axis of the teeth involved 1mm from the crevicular margin. This incision is extended interproximally as far as possible, separating the pocket epithelium from the flap to be raised, and then extended mesially and distally, allowing the flap to be raised as an envelope without relieving incisions. The flap should be as conservative as possible and only a few millimetres of alveolar bone exposed by a second incision intercrevicularly to release the collar of pocket epithelium and granulation tissue. A third incision at 90° to the tooth separates the pocket epithelium, and this is removed along with accompanying granulation tissue with curettes and hoes. The root surface is then thoroughly debrided. Although bony defects can be curetted *no* osseous surgery is carried out. The flaps are then repositioned close to the original position to cover all exposed alveolar bone and sutured into position. Post-operatively, chlorhexidine 0.2% 10mL rinse bd is given. As healing occurs, pocket reduction is achieved by a long junctional epithelial attachment to the root surface.

The apically repositioned flap

This procedure is used to expose alveolar bone and includes the option for osseous surgery to correct infrabony defects. It allows excellent access to the root surface for debridement (Fig. 5.4). The principal difference between this procedure and the modified Widman flap is the deliberate exposure of alveolar bone, and the apical repositioning of the flap with post-operative exposure of the root surfaces. This is primarily a buccal procedure, and although it can be performed on lingual pockets, it is obviously impossible on the palate where a conventional or reverse bevel gingivectomy approach has to be used.

Technique A reverse bevel incision is made in the attached gingiva angled to excise the periodontal pocket in a scalloped outline with vertical relieving incisions at either end. A split thickness flap is made down to bone and then converted to full thickness, leaving a residual collar of tissue around the root surfaces. This combination of pocket epithelium and granulation tissue is removed with a curette. If indicated, the alveolar crest can be remodelled. The flaps are displaced apically and sutured.

21 S. Ramfjord & R. R. Nissle 1974 *J Periodont* **45** 601.

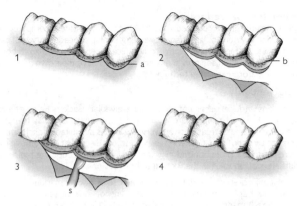

Fig. 5.3 Modified Widman flap. 1. Design of flap; a, incision. 2. Flap elevated; b, gingival cuff to be discarded. 3. Excision of supra-alveolar pocket; s, scalpel blade. 4. Flap repositioned and sutured in place.

Advantages These include exposure of alveolar bone with controlled bone loss; exposure of furcation area; minimal post-operative pocket depth; ability to reposition the flap; and 1° closure of the wound. In addition, keratinized gingiva is preserved.

Disadvantages These include exposure of root surface (leading to ↑ susceptibility to caries and sensitivity) and loss of alveolar bone height, which accompanies full exposure of the bone at operation. Not suitable for the aesthetic zone.

Osseous surgery
Bone recontouring has become less popular as it is always accompanied by some degree of alveolar resorption and therefore ↓ support for the tooth.
- *Osteoplasty* is conservative recontouring of the bone margin that is non-supporting bone.
- *Ostectomy* is excision of bone aimed at eliminating infra-alveolar pocketing, but unfortunately it also ↓ alveolar support.

The aim of osseous surgery should be to establish a more anatomically correct relationship between bone and tooth while maintaining as much alveolar support as possible.

Other flap procedures

These include simple replaced flaps which give bony access compared to the modified Widman flap. Also crown-lengthening procedures, which can range from a simple gingivectomy to an apically repositioned flap ± bone removal (Fig. 5.4). In addition, many periodontists have their own modification of the aforementioned techniques.

Gingivectomy

Indications include persistent deep supra-alveolar pockets (e.g. gingival hypertrophy), reshaping severely damaged gingivae into an easily manageable contour, and to treat gingival overgrowth. It is *not* suitable for the management of deep 'true' pocketing as excision of the pocket will remove the entire thickness of keratinized gingivae and possibly disrupt the biological width. It is of no value in the Rx of intrabony lesions.

Technique Pockets can be delineated by the use of pocket marking forceps, e.g. Crane–Kaplan forceps, marking out a line of incision (either smooth or scalloped) made with a blade angled at 100–110° to the long axis of the tooth. This bevelled incision excises supragingival pockets and allows for gingival recontouring. Once the incision has been made, the strip of gingiva remaining is released by an intercrevicular incision. The root surfaces are then curetted and an open area of freshly cut granulation tissue left to heal under a periodontal pack for about 1 week. Chlorhexidine mouthwash 10mL bd.

Disadvantages These include loss of attached gingiva, raw wound, and exposed root surface (which ↑ likelihood of sensitivity and caries). Some remodelling of alveolar bone occurs, despite there being no operative interference.

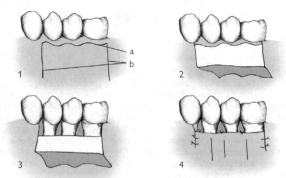

Fig. 5.4 Apically repositioned flap. 1. Design of flap; a, reverse bevel incision; b, relieving incisions. 2. Elevating the flap. Tissue enclosing pocketing is discarded. 3. Flap elevated, pockets excised. Osseous surgery can be performed at this stage. 4. Flap apically repositioned and sutured in position.

Periodontal surgery—regenerative techniques

Guided tissue regeneration (GTR)

The recognition that epithelium migrated along the root surface before any other cell type, after periodontal surgery, and created the *long junctional epithelium* which prevented new attachment, created the possibility that prevention of migration of epithelium would allow new connective tissue attachment. In the first reported case in 1982, Nyman placed a barrier membrane in the pocket of a tooth that was planned for extraction. Histological analysis of the tooth after extraction showed that the barrier membrane prevented apical migration of the epithelium and true regeneration was achieved. True regeneration involves a whole new cementum, periodontal ligament, and bone.

True regeneration can only be determined by histological analysis. This is not possible in real-life cases (unless you extract the tooth—which would in effect defeat the purpose of periodontal surgery). Therefore, surrogate measures such radiographic evidence of bony infill are used to assess the success of any regenerative procedures.

GTR is essentially interposing a barrier to epithelial migration prior to completion of surgical or non-surgical therapy. Original barriers were non-resorbable. More recently, resorbable membranes (e.g. Bio-Gide®) have been developed. These eliminate the need for a second stage of surgery. Bio-absorbable flowable polymer (Atrisorb® FreeFlow) has also been developed. GTR can be used alone or with bone grafts or enamel matrix derivatives.

Bone grafts These may be used in combination with a barrier membrane. Grafts are autogenous, allografts (such as demineralized freeze-dried bone), or xenografts such as grafts from inorganic bovine bone matrix (Bio-Oss®). These are in widespread use. Patients may have religious, cultural, or personal beliefs that may impact upon the choice of graft material. Synthetic bone substitutes are also used (e.g. PerioGlas®) in some cases.

Enamel matrix derivatives (EMDs) Emdogain® is a product containing porcine EMD proteins in a propylene glycol alginate gel. Enamel matrix proteins (e.g. amelogenin) are found in Hertwig's sheath and induce root formation in the developing tooth. Locally applied enamel matrix proteins may help form acellular cementum, the key tissue in the development of a functional periodontium.

Indications Case selection is important in success of regeneration techniques. They work best in cases with three-walled defects or grade I furcations. GTR is useful for Rx of two- or three-walled intrabony defects and furcation defects. Other regenerative procedures are also similar in terms of outcome predictability. Three-walled defects have a better chance of regeneration compared to two-walled defects which in turn have a better chance of regeneration than one-walled defects. Horizontal defects are very unpredictable and the chances of regeneration are very poor. Similarly, grade 1 furcation defects have greater predictability compared to grade 2 furcation defects. Regeneration in grade 3 furcation defects is very poor.

The shape and depth of the three-walled defect also determines predictability. Narrower and deeper defects have better predictability compared to shallower and wider defects.

There is limited use in generation of new bone for implant placement. Good OH is essential. Smoking has an adverse effect on outcomes. It requires careful and meticulous surgical technique.[22]

Technique Access to the root surface is gained surgically, the cementum is mechanically cleaned, and EMD solution is applied to the root surfaces following conditioning with ethylene diamine tetraacetic acid (EDTA) to remove the smear layer after instrumentation. The access flaps are then repositioned and sutured.

Outcome Regeneration of cementum, periodontal ligament, and alveolar bone appears to be possible. A Cochrane review of the use of EMD to regenerate periodontal tissue in intrabony defects has shown it to be effective.[23]

However, the predictability of these is unknown. Future developments in tissue engineering may allow the possibility of regeneration of replacement teeth and periodontal tissues in humans.[24]

22 G. Sharpe et al. 2008 *Dental Update* **35** 304.

23 M. Esposito et al. 2004 *J Dent Educ* **68** 834.

24 H. C. Slavkin & P. M. Bartold 2006 *Periodontology 2000* **41** 9.

Periodontal surgery—mucogingival surgery

Mucogingival surgery encompasses those techniques aimed at the correction of local gingival defects. The rationale for this type of surgery has been hotly debated over many years. Initially, it was felt that a margin of attached gingiva of around 3mm was required to protect the periodontium during mastication and to dissipate the pull to the gingival margin from fraenal attachments. In fact, data from properly conducted experimental work have demonstrated that the width of attached gingiva and the presence or absence of an attached portion is not of decisive importance for the maintenance of gingival health.[25] As a result of this, the indications for mucogingival surgery have been rationalized:

• Where a change in the morphology of the gingival margin would improve plaque control, e.g. the presence of high fraenal attachments or deep areas of recession.
• Areas where recession creates root sensitivity or aesthetic problems.
• A very thin layer of attached gingiva overlying a tooth which is to be moved orthodontically: the evidence for this is somewhat anecdotal.

Gingival recession The two commonest causes are plaque-induced gingival inflammation and toothbrush trauma, revealing dehiscences in alveolar bone. Therefore, basic periodontal care and correction of faulty toothbrushing technique are the first lines of Rx. While anatomical features may contribute, these and trauma from occlusion, high fraenal attachments, and impingement from restorations are 2° considerations.

Classification of gingival recession The most commonly used classification system is Miller's classification (1985) which looks at the recession defect and the interproximal attachment levels. There are many other recession classifications as well.

Mucogingival surgery Grafting is subdivided into:

Free grafts Free grafts are completely removed from their donor area. *Free gingival grafts*, commonly of palatal mucosa and connective tissue, are taken and grafted to donor sites prepared by incising between attached and alveolar mucosa. A template may be used to harvest the correct amount of tissue. Mucoperiosteum is exposed at the recipient site and the harvested tissue is sutured carefully over this. Free grafts are normally thicker and normally retain the colour of the donor area. A *subepithelial connective tissue graft* from the palate gives a better aesthetic result. At the recipient site it is covered by a coronally advanced flap.

25 J. Wennström 1987 *J Clin Periodontol* **14** 181.

Pedicle grafts Pedicle grafts are not separated from their blood supply. Commonly used pedicle grafts are the laterally repositioned flap, coronally repositioned flap, and the double papilla flap. These techniques may be of some value in very narrow areas of isolated gingival recession. Technically, of course, these are flaps *not* grafts.

Recession coverage can be used in conjunction with EMD although the improvement is not always clinically significant.

Furcation involvement

The extension of periodontal disease into the bi- or trifurcation of multirooted teeth is known as furcation involvement.

Diagnosis This is established by probing into the furcation and by radiographs. The possibility of pulpal pathology is ↑ in teeth with furcation involvement and sensibility testing is essential. Radiographs give a guide to the degree of alveolar bone loss both mesially and distally, and in the furcation area.

Classification

Class 1 Probe can be inserted <3mm between the roots. Requires scaling and root planing, possibly with furcation plasty.

Class 2 Horizontal probing depth exceeding 3mm but not extending fully through the width of the furcation area. GTR together with graft materials and EMD can be used to treat class 2 furcations.

Class 3 Horizontal through-and-through destruction in the furcation area. May require tunnel preparation, &/or root resection, &/or extraction. GTR less predictable with Class 3 defects.

Rx techniques

Scaling and root debridement (➲ Non-surgical periodontal therapy—scaling and root surface debridement, p. 216.) Unless the post-Rx morphology can be kept clean by the patient it will not be successful.

Furcation plasty An open procedure involving a muco-periosteal flap to allow root debridement and scaling, followed by the removal of tooth structure in the furcation area to achieve a widened entrance to give access for cleaning. Osseous recontouring may be used if indicated. The flap is repositioned and sutured to ↑ access post-operatively. There is an obvious risk of pulpal damage and post-operative dentine sensitivity/caries.

Tunnel preparation This is a similar procedure to furcation plasty using buccal and lingual flaps, the main difference being that the entire furcation area is exposed and the flaps are sutured together intra-radicularly to leave a large exposed furcation. There is a high risk of post-operative caries, dentine sensitivity, and pulpal exposure, making this a method to be used with caution. It is of most value for mandibular molars in patients with optimal OH. In many cases considered for furcation plasty or tunnelling, it may be more sensible to proceed to a more radical approach such as root resection.

Root resection This involves amputation of one (or even two) of the roots of a multirooted tooth, leaving the crown and the root stump. It is important to ensure that the root to be retained can be treated endodontically, is in sound periodontal state with good bony support, is restorable, and will be a viable tooth in the long term. At operation it is wise to raise a flap to enable direct visualization of the root surface. Resection of the root with a high-speed bur is followed by smoothing, recontouring, and restoration of any residual pulp cavity. It is sometimes not possible to proceed with root resection, despite apparently favourable radiographs, especially in maxillary molars, so warn patient pre-operatively.

Hemisection This involves dividing lower molars in half to give two smaller units each with a single root. One is extracted and the other retained. Again, RCT is necessary pre-operatively and restoration of the divided crown is required post-operatively.

Extraction This ensures removal of periodontal disease but carries its own problems.

Guided tissue regeneration (See reference[26].) See ➲ Guided tissue regeneration (GTR), p. 216.

Enamel matrix derivatives See ➲ Enamel matrix derivatives (EMD), p. 216.

It is important to note that the techniques described here are of less significance to long-term outcome than the degree of plaque control that can be achieved and maintained by the patient. Mini interproximal brushes are a valuable aid in cleaning furcation defects and are available in a variety of sizes and shapes.

26 R. Ponteriero et al. 1989 *J Clin Periodont* **16** 170.

Occlusion and splinting

If occlusal load is excessive or the periodontium is reduced in height, tissue changes may be seen. Occlusal trauma cannot induce periodontal tissue breakdown but may enhance the rate of progression of disease. Periodontal tissues can adapt to occlusal loading but where forces are too great for adaptation, teeth may become mobile or drift.

Tooth mobility ↑ tooth mobility may simply be a result of loss of periodontal attachment and bony support. It may also result purely as a localized effect due to a heavy occlusal loading, causing a widening of the periodontal membrane space, though this is usually iatrogenic in origin. It is now felt that the Δ of occlusal trauma should only be made where progressive ↑ tooth mobility is observed, but in order to do this it is necessary to have an objective method of measuring tooth mobility. This can be done using a Mobility Index:

- Grade 1 = mobility <1mm buccolingually.
- Grade 2 = mobility 1–2mm buccolingually.
- Grade 3 = mobility of >2mm buccolingually &/or vertical mobility.

Occlusal analysis can be carried out clinically and on study models mounted in RCP on a semi-adjustable articulator.

Rx The first priority should be to diagnose and treat any existing periodontal disease and correct any pre-existing iatrogenic causes (e.g. poor crowns or bridges, high restorations). If tooth mobility persists as a direct result of diagnosable occlusal trauma, occlusal adjustment is a sensible Rx modality. If the tooth is mobile as a result of lack of alveolar bone support, this is not automatically an indication for splinting.

Splinting Splinting is indicated in the following situations:

- A tooth with healthy but ↓ periodontium where mobility is progressive.
- A tooth with ↑ mobility which the patient finds uncomfortable during function.

It is very easy to design splints which are impossible for the patient to keep clean as all additions to the natural tooth surface will ↑ plaque retention. A wide range of different techniques and materials have been described, including orthodontic wire fastened to teeth by resin-composite, resin-composite alone, fixed bridges, partial prostheses, acid-etch retained splints, and more recently, fibre-reinforced resin-composite splinting.

Peri-implant mucositis and peri-implantitis

Following implant placement and connection of the transmucosal abutment, a soft tissue cuff develops. This is attached to the implant via an epithelial zone of about 2mm in depth. There is an underlying connective tissue layer of about 1.5mm. The fibres in this layer run parallel to the implant surface and do not attach directly to the implant. Plaque formation around the implant can lead to inflammation of the periodontal tissues. This is called peri-implant mucositis which is reversible. If the inflammation spreads to the supporting tissues it is called peri-implantitis. This can lead to bone loss and ↑ probing depths. Crater-like defects in the bone around the implant can be seen on a radiograph. If bone loss progresses, implants can become mobile.

Implant salvage in the failing stage consists of the entire arsenal of periodontal therapies. Local antibiotics and bone-supplemented GTR may be particularly useful.

Tissue transformation using bone morphogenetic protein may also prove useful in the future.

Implant surfaces can be easily damaged, so plastic or carbon fibre scaling instruments are used.

Supportive periodontal therapy

The success of Rx is characterized by a reduction in bleeding on probing and on brushing/flossing, a reduction in probing pocket depths, and a change in gingival contour. Once the corrective phase is complete, a programme of supportive therapy begins. To avoid further attachment loss and to maintain the therapeutic benefits, long-term patients require monitoring and sometimes Rx to support their own home care. Maintenance visits will involve re-evaluation of plaque control, bleeding on probing, pus and furcation lesions, and radiographs if required. Rx of persistent bleeding pockets and a full mouth polish should be carried out. The first 6 months after completion of corrective Rx is the healing phase and regular professional tooth cleaning should take place. Then maintenance visits begin at 3–4-monthly intervals and may be lengthened up to 6 months if appropriate although there is no good evidence for the ideal frequency of maintenance visits. Various aspects such as plaque control, bleeding on probing, and alveolar bone heights are considered and frequency decided on accordingly.

Restorative dentistry 2: repairing teeth

Relevant pages in other chapters Caries diagnosis,
⊃ p. 26; amalgam, ⊃ p. 650; resin composite, ⊃ Composite
resins—constituents and properties, p. 652; the acid-etch technique, ⊃ Enamel and dentine bonding, p. 656; dentine adhesive
systems (dentine bonding agents), ⊃ p. 658; glass ionomers, ⊃
p. 660; cements, ⊃ p. 664.

Principal sources and further reading
A. Banerjee & T. F. Watson 2015 *Pickard's Guide to Minimally
Invasive Operative Dentistry* (10e), OUP. P. A. Brunton &
N. H. F. Wilson 2002 *Decision-Making in Operative Dentistry*,
Quintessence. S. J. Davies & R. J. Gray 2002 *A Clinical Guide
to Occlusion*, British Dental Association. B. G. N. Smith & L. C.
Howe 2007 *Planning and Making Crowns and Bridges* (4e),
Dunitz. See also *Operative Dentistry*, *Dental Update*, and the
British Dental Journal.

To attempt to resolve the problem of caries by preparing and
restoring teeth is comparable to trying to resolve the problem
of poliomyelitis by manufacturing more attractive and better
quality crutches, more quickly and more cheaply.

Repair and replacement of teeth

Dental tissue may be damaged by caries (⊙ Dental caries, p. 24), trauma (⊙ Dental trauma, p. 98) or tooth wear/tooth surface loss (⊙ Tooth wear/tooth surface loss, p. 252), or may be developmentally defective (⊙ Abnormalities of tooth structure, p. 70). Patients may present C/O pain/ sensitivity (⊙ Dental pain, p. 230), dissatisfaction with dental aesthetics, or fractured teeth, or may not be aware of any problems. In order to main- tain structure, function, and aesthetics, the resultant lesions may be helped to repair biologically or may be repaired technically by direct and indirect restorations within a context of careful diagnosis, prevention, control, and holistic patient care.

Increasingly, the approach is tending towards a biological concept of man- agement rather than a mechanistic 'drill and fill' philosophy.

This is important as the population lives longer and teeth are retained longer. As soon as a restoration is placed, there is entry into a 'cycle of replacement' with ever more destructive restorations inevitable over a lifetime. This is sometimes referred to as the 'restorative escalator', with the patient moving closer to losing the tooth with each restoration (how- ever, it should be borne in mind that without appropriate restoration the tooth would be lost much sooner!). A minimally invasive approach wher- ever possible is, therefore, important in extending the longevity of an individual tooth.

Where there is total loss of tooth/teeth then replacement with fixed or removable prosthodontics, incorporating indirect, laboratory-made pros- theses (e.g. fixed partial dentures (bridges)/removable partial dentures/ complete dentures) may be required (see Chapter 7). These may be im- plant retained.

Management planning

Management planning is dependent on a thorough information gathering process. This includes a history of the presenting complaint, medical history (⊇ The medical history, p. 6), dental history (⊇ The dental history, p. 4), and social history (⊇ The social history, p. 5). This is followed by examination: general (e.g. pallor, disability), EO (e.g. facial asymmetry, swelling ⊇ Examination of the head and neck, p. 10), and IO examinations (⊇ Examination of the mouth, p. 12). IO examination includes soft tissues, periodontal tissues, teeth, occlusion (⊇ Occlusion—1, p. 234), and any existing prostheses. For complex cases, mounted study models and diagnostic wax-up should be considered. In some cases, a facebow record may be required, particularly if there is not a reproducible occlusion, or the occlusion is to be reorganized. Relevant special investigations (e.g. radiographs/ sensibility testing) complete the process and allow a diagnosis and risk assessment to be made.

Risk/susceptibility for caries and tooth wear can be identified by gathering information from a *targeted verbal history* (e.g. irregular attender/frequent sugar intake, eating disorder/clenching grinding habits) and *clinical evidence* (e.g. poor OH/new lesions, masseteric hypertrophy).

Staging of carious lesions with an index (e.g. ICDAS: International Caries Detection and Assessment System) and consideration of caries risk and radiographic examination allow the best management option to be chosen. Caries cannot solely be diagnosed from a radiograph however, this is a clinical diagnosis. Caries may also be deeper than suggested by a radiograph, or artefact/burnout may lead to false positive diagnoses.

Under ideal circumstances, an integrated management plan is formulated for each patient at the start of every course of Rx. Very often, however, the plan will need to be revised in the light of clinical findings as care progresses (e.g. patient cooperation, response to periodontal therapy, investigation of teeth of doubtful prognosis, etc.). When dealing with patients with a range of problems it is therefore wise to formulate a plan which has a number of achievable goals, and then on completion of this to reassess the patient to decide on what further management is necessary. Contemporaneous, accurate notes must be kept at all times and written information given to the patient.

Sequence of Rx

The following list is obviously an oversimplification but should serve as a general guide to the order in which Rx should be carried out:

- Relief of pain.
- Control of active disease and achievement of stability:
  - Low caries risk: OHI, dietary modification, and topical fluoride.
  - High caries risk: as for low risk with the addition of professional tooth cleaning, stabilizing restorations, high-concentration toothpaste (2800/5000ppm fluoride), fluoride mouthwash in patients ≥8yrs, professionally applied fluoride varnish, topical remineralizing agents, management of hyposalivation, fissure sealants, and sealant restoration. There is evidence for sealing of non-cavitated occlusal

carious lesions even when there is radiolucency extending up to one-third of the way into dentine.[1]

- Patients with risk of tooth wear: modification of behaviour to remove aetiological factors. Consider provision of protective splint.
- Initial periodontal therapy.
- Extraction of unsaveable teeth.
- In patients with multiple carious lesions it may take several weeks/months to complete the permanent restorations necessary to secure oral health. In these cases, it may be advisable to prevent any symptomless large lesions ↑ in size by placing temporary dressings. The cavities should be rendered caries free at the margins, and temporarily restored with a cement (e.g. GIC).
- Consideration of definitive denture design.
- Remaining simple restorations.
- RCT (see Chapter 8).
- Reassessment of success of initial Rx, OH, periodontal condition, and prognosis of teeth.
- Definitive Rx: crowns, bridgework, dentures, and implants (➔ Introduction to implantology, p. 361).
- Monitoring at intervals appropriate to level of risk.

Practical points

- *Listen* to patients and enquire as to their expectations and priorities. Discuss the management plan with them and the role they will have to play in controlling their dental disease. Success is dependent upon patient compliance, therefore time spent actively discussing their expectations, Rx options, time involved, cost implications present and future, and their role in maintenance is invaluable. Without such a discussion, consent may not be deemed to be valid.
- It is important to bear in mind subsequent items on a Rx plan, e.g. the design of a partial upper denture (P/−) may influence the choice of material and contour of direct/indirect restorations.
- For complex cases, several short Rx plans, each ending with a reassessment, are more logical and efficient than one long one that keeps changing.
- When formulating a Rx plan, group items together into appointments to form a visit plan. Consider the time needed for each visit and anaesthetic requirements, if relevant.
- Although it is usually advantageous to complete as much work as possible at each visit, this can be counter-productive. If in doubt about how much Rx to do at a visit, discuss this with the patient.
- Record-keeping is very important. At the end of each appointment carefully note what has been done and the materials used (including sizes and shades). Do not wait until the end of the day to document this information as important details may be confused or forgotten. Cross that item off the Rx plan and adjust the patient's chart. Note what is to be done next visit: this will save time.
- It is important to recognize your own limitations and, where appropriate, refer a patient for advice or Rx.

1 C. Deery 2013 *Br Dent J* **214** 551.

Dental pain

When a patient attends the surgery and complains of toothache, pain may be arising from a variety of different structures and may be classified as follows:

- Pulpal pain.
- Periapical/periradicular pain.
- Non-dental pain/non-odontogenic pain.

Dental pain can be very difficult to diagnose, and the clinician must first gather as much information as possible from the history, clinical and radiographic examinations, and other special tests (see Chapter 1).

Pulpal pain

The pulp may be subject to a wide variety of insults (e.g. bacterial, thermal, chemical, traumatic), the effects of which are cumulative and can ultimately lead to inflammation in the pulp (pulpitis) and pain. The dental pulp does not contain any proprioceptive nerve endings, therefore a characteristic of pulpal pain is that the patient is unable to localize the affected tooth but the pain does not cross the midline. The ability of the pulp to recover from injury depends upon its blood supply, not the nerve supply, which must be borne in mind when vitality (sensibility) testing is carried out (→ Sensibility testing, p. 16).[2] It is impossible to reliably achieve an accurate Δ of the state of the pulp on clinical grounds alone; the only 100% accurate method is histological section.

Although numerous classifications of pulpal disease exist, only a limited number of clinical diagnostic situations require identification before effective Rx can be given.

Reversible pulpitis

Symptoms

Fleeting sensitivity/pain to hot, cold, or sweet with immediate onset. Pain is usually sharp and may be difficult to locate. Quickly subsides after removal of the stimulus.

Signs

Exaggerated response to pulp testing. Carious cavity/leaking restoration. Tooth not tender to percussion.

Rx

Remove any caries present and restore or place a sedative dressing (e.g. ZOE) or permanent restoration with suitable pulp protection.

Irreversible pulpitis

Symptoms

Spontaneous dull, throbbing pain which may last several minutes or hours, be worse at night, and is often pulsatile in nature. Pain exacerbated by hot and cold. In later stages, cold may actually ease symptoms. A characteristic feature is that the pain remains after the removal of the stimulus. Localization of pain may be difficult initially, but as the inflammation spreads to the periapical tissues the tooth will become more sensitive to pressure. Application of heat (e.g. warm GP) elicits pain.

Signs

The affected tooth may give exaggerated or reduced or no response to an electric pulp tester. In later stages it may become TTP.

Rx

Extirpation of the pulp and RCT (see Chapter 8) is the Rx of choice (assuming the tooth is to be saved). If time is short or if anaesthesia proves elusive then removal of the coronal pulp and an Odontopaste® or LEDERMIX® dressing can often control the symptoms until the remaining pulp can be extirpated under LA at the next appointment.[3]

Dentine hypersensitivity This is pain arising from exposed dentine in response to a thermal, tactile, or osmotic stimulus (not all exposed dentine gives rise to symptoms). It is thought to be due to dentinal fluid movement stimulating pulpal pain receptors. Prevalence is ~1:7 adults, with peaks reported in young adults (due to erosions with dentine exposure)[4] and at 30–40yrs. About 25–30% of the adult population report dentine hypersensitivity.[5] Δ is by elimination of other possible causes and by evoking symptoms.

Rx

Involves ↓ aetiological factors (i.e. OHI, possibly including toothbrushing technique and intrinsic and extrinsic dental erosion) and by ↓ permeability of dentinal tubules (e.g. by toothpaste containing strontium and potassium salts &/or fluoride; placement of varnishes, dentine desensitizers, dentine adhesive systems, or, if indicated, a restoration).

Cracked tooth syndrome

Symptoms

Sharp pain on biting (e.g. cotton-wool roll or a 'Tooth Slooth®')—short duration, pain may cease on release of bite/pressure, and possible cold sensitivity. Some patients find pain elicited on sudden release of bite.

Signs

Often relatively few, therefore Δ difficult. Tooth often has a large restoration. Crack may not be apparent at first but transillumination and possibly removal of the restoration may aid visualization. There is a positive response to vitality (sensibility) testing. May be associated with bruxing habit. Similar symptoms can be caused by bruxism/clenching a particular tooth which may not be fractured.

Rx

An adhesive resin composite restoration with cuspal coverage may be appropriate in teeth which are minimally restored, but in some cases an indirect restoration with full occlusal coverage will be needed. Occasionally RCT may be required, or as a last resort, extraction. Placement of an orthodontic band around a tooth can relieve symptoms and help with diagnosis.

3 Scottish Dental Clinical Effectiveness Programme 2007 *Emergency Dental Care* (⅏ http://www. sdcep.org.uk).

4 P. Dowell et al. 1985 *Br Dent J* **158** 92.

5 C. H. Splieth & A. Tachou 2013 *Clin Oral Investig* **17** (Suppl 1) 3.

Occlusal overload
Symptoms
Pain on biting which can be sharp, short duration but can linger as an ache. Often combined with instantaneous hot and cold sensitivity. Tooth may become mobile.

Signs
Often relatively few, therefore Δ difficult. Check excursive movements of the occlusion to see if tooth is taking guidance or where there are few remaining occluding units. Look for wear facets indicating bruxism (note these may not be present if patient tends to clench.)

Rx
Soft splint for nocturnal use initially—pain may take some time to settle. If pain persists, check tooth is not cracked or another diagnosis (as previously described). A Michigan splint should be considered in these patients.

Periapical/periradicular pain
Progression of irreversible pulpitis ultimately leads to death of the pulp (pulpal necrosis). At this stage, the patient may experience relief from pain and thus may not seek attention. If neglected, however, the bacteria and pulpal breakdown products leave the root canal system via the apical foramen or lateral canals and lead to inflammatory changes and possibly pain. Characteristically, the patient can precisely identify the affected tooth, as the periodontal ligament, which is well supplied with proprioceptive nerve endings, is inflamed.

Pulpal necrosis with periapical periodontitis
Symptoms
Variable, but patients generally describe a dull ache exacerbated by biting on the tooth.

Signs
Usually no response to sensibility (vitality) testing, unless one canal of a multirooted tooth is still vital. The tooth will be TTP. Radiographically there may be loss of lamina dura in the periapical region, the apical PDL may be widened, or there may be a periapical radiolucency (granuloma or cyst).

Rx
RCT or extraction.

Acute periapical abscess
Symptoms
Severe pain which will disturb sleep. Tooth is exquisitely tender to touch.

Signs
Affected tooth is usually extruded, mobile, and TTP. May be associated with IO and facial swelling or with a more localized IO swelling. Sensibility testing may be misleading as pus may conduct stimulus to apical tissues. Radiographic changes can range from a widening of the apical PDL space to an obvious radiolucency. It is important to differentiate this condition from a periodontal abscess.

Rx
Drain pus and, if indicated, relieve occlusion. Drainage of pus can often be achieved by entering the pulp chamber with a high-speed diamond bur, steadying the tooth with a finger to prevent excessive vibration. After drainage has been achieved it is preferable to prepare the canal and place a temporary dressing. Avoid 'open drainage' if possible, but if absolutely necessary for <24h, as after this time further bacterial contamination of the root canal makes subsequent RCT very difficult. If a fluctuant soft tissue swelling is present, this should be incised to achieve drainage. Antibiotics should be prescribed if there is systemic involvement or if the infection is spreading significantly along tissue planes. When the acute symptoms have subsided, RCT must be performed or the tooth extracted.

Chronic periapical periodontitis Often symptomless. Possibly associated with persistent sinus. Presentation may be a coincidental finding or acute exacerbation. Radiographs show well-demarcated periapical radiolucency (granuloma or cyst).

Lateral periodontal abscess
Symptoms Similar to periapical abscess with acute pain and tenderness, and often an associated bad taste.

Signs Tooth is usually mobile and TTP, with associated localized or diffuse swelling of the adjacent periodontium. A deep periodontal pocket is usually associated, which will exude pus on probing. Radiographs normally show vertical or horizontal bone loss, and vitality (sensibility) testing is usually positive, unless there is an associated endodontic problem (periodontal–endodontic lesion).

Rx Achieve drainage of pus. Irrigate with a chlorhexidine solution. If there is systemic involvement or it is a recurrent problem, prescribe antibiotics (metronidazole or amoxicillin). Debride the pocket once acute symptoms have settled. In the case of a periodontal–endodontic lesion (1° endodontic disease) this may make reattachment of the periodontal tissues less likely, so this is an exception to the rule. Extraction may be indicated if prognosis of the tooth is poor.

Non-dental pain
When no signs of dental or periradicular pathology can be detected then non-dental causes must be considered. Other causes of pain that can present as toothache include:
- TMD (→ Temporomandibular pain—dysfunction/facial arthromyalgia, p. 484).
- Maxillary sinusitis (→ Maxillary sinusitis, p. 422).
- Psychological disorders (atypical odontalgia) (→ Atypical facial pain, p. 465).
- Tumours (→ Benign tumours of the mouth, p. 420; → Oral cancer, p. 451).
- Fibromyalgia, trigeminal neuralgia.

Occlusion—1

In a book of this size it is not possible to consider all aspects of occlusion, therefore the focus will be on the practical aspects and the more esoteric considerations are left to other texts. Significant occlusal adjustment is rarely indicated and should only be attempted by a specialist.

Definitions

Ideal occlusion Anatomically perfect occlusion—rare.

Functional occlusion An occlusion that is free of interferences to smooth gliding movements of the mandible, with absence of pathology.

Balanced occlusion Balancing contacts in all excursions of the mandible to provide ↑ stability of F/F dentures; not applicable to natural dentition (except rarely in full mouth reconstruction).

Group function Multiple tooth contacts on working side during lateral excursions, but no contact on non-working side.

Canine-guided occlusion During lateral excursions there is disclusion of all the teeth on the working side except for the canine, and no contacts on the non-working side.

Hinge axis The axis of rotation of the condyles during the first few millimetres of mandibular opening.

Terminal hinge axis The axis of rotation of the mandible when the condyles are in their most superior position in the glenoid fossa.

Retruded arc of closure The arc of closure of the mandible with the condyles rotating about the terminal hinge axis.

Anterior guidance A functional relationship between the maxillary and mandibular anterior teeth. It consists of the horizontal overlaps of anterior teeth (overjet) and the vertical overlap of anterior teeth (overbite).

Intercuspal position (ICP) or centric occlusion Position of maximum interdigitation.

Retruded contact position (RCP) or centric relation Position of the mandible where initial tooth contact occurs on the retruded arc of closure. Occurs when condyles are fully seated in the glenoid fossa. In ~10% of patients RCP and ICP are coincident; the remainder have forward slide from RCP to ICP.

Rest position The habitual postural position of the mandible when the patient is relaxed with the condyles in a neutral position.

Freeway space The difference between the rest and intercuspal positions.

Centric stops The points on the occlusal surface which meet with the opposing tooth in ICP. These are normally the cusp tips, marginal ridges, and central fossae.

Supporting or functional cusps The cusps that occlude with the centric stops on the opposing tooth. Usually palatal on upper and buccal on lower.

Non-supporting cusps The cusps that do not occlude with the opposing teeth. Usually buccal on upper and lingual on lower.

Deflective contacts Deflect mandible from natural path of closure.

Interferences Contacts that hinder smooth excursive movements of mandible.

Occlusal vertical dimension (OVD) Relationship between maxilla and mandible in ICP, i.e. face height.

Do occlusal factors play a role in TMDs? TMD is recognized as being of multifactorial aetiology (⊕ Temporomandibular pain—dysfunction/facial arthromyalgia, p. 484). The evidence would suggest that occlusal interferences usually cause either subclinical or no dysfunction because they lie within the adaptive capacity of the patient's neuromusculature. However, this may be lowered by stress and emotional problems so that in susceptible patients occlusal interferences can result in muscle hyperactivity at certain times. It is important therefore to ensure that iatrogenic interferences are not introduced during restorative procedures.

Occlusion—2

Occlusal examination

Prior to carrying out restorative Rx it is important to examine the patient's occlusion. Occlusal contacts can be identified with 8µm metal foil (Shimstock™) and marked using thin articulating paper (20µm). Important features to look for are:

- Number and distribution of occluding teeth.
- Over-eruption, tilting, rotation, etc.
- Presence or absence of centric stops.
- The RCP and any slide between RCP and ICP.
- Anterior guidance—look for disclusion of posterior teeth on protrusion.
- Lateral excursions—? group function, ? canine guidance. Check for non-working interferences.
- TMJs and muscles of mastication.

The clinical examination can only reveal a limited amount of information and in some circumstances (such as prior to crown and bridgework or in patients with a TMD) a more detailed occlusal examination is required. This is called an *occlusal analysis* or a *diagnostic mounting*, and is done by mounting study models on a semi-adjustable articulator to facilitate the examination of the features.

Occlusal considerations for restorative procedures

In most situations, restorations are made to conform to the patient's existing occlusion and the main consideration is to prevent the introduction of iatrogenic occlusal interferences. This approach to Rx is known as the *conformative approach*.

In some circumstances, the conformative approach is not appropriate and a new occlusal scheme must be planned. This is often the case when extensive crown and bridgework is required, such that the patient's existing occlusion will be effectively destroyed by the preparations. A new occlusion is established, free of interferences and with the patient occluding in retruded contact position, which is the only reproducible position. This approach to Rx is called the *reorganized* approach and further consideration of this line of Rx is beyond the scope of this book.

Generally, for simple intracoronal restorations complex methods are not needed, but care must be taken to ensure the correct occlusal scheme is reproduced. Before preparing a tooth it is worthwhile marking the centric stops with articulating paper and trying to preserve them if possible. On completion of the restoration it must be checked in intercuspal position to ensure that it is not high, but also to ensure that it has recreated the centric stops, as if it is out of occlusion then over-eruption will occur (which may produce interferences). The restoration should then be checked in all mandibular excursions to ensure that no interferences have been introduced.

One or two units of extracoronal restorations can again be constructed in a relatively simple manner. This is usually done in the laboratory using hand-held models to reproduce the occlusion. Again, great care must be taken at the try-in stage to check the occlusion. Care is also required when restoring the most distal tooth in the arch as it is very easy to introduce errors in this situation; it may be more appropriate to use an occlusal record (transfer coping technique) and mount the models on an articulator.

More complex laboratory-made restorations may need to be constructed with the models mounted on an articulator. This allows the restorations to be constructed in harmony with the patient's occlusion in all mandibular positions, which should minimize the amount of time spent adjusting the restoration at the try-in stage. Also, if any changes to the patient's occlusion are planned, then they can be made on the articulator in a controlled fashion.

An articulator is a device which holds the models in a particular relationship and simulates jaw movements. Numerous types of articulators are available but only certain types are appropriate for use in crown and bridge-work, e.g. the Denar® Mark II which is a semi-adjustable articulator. The articulator must accurately reproduce mandibular movements and to do this the casts must be mounted in the correct relationship to the TMJs; this is achieved by taking a facebow record. In a conformative approach, casts should be related in ICP for restoration.

Occlusal records

Occlusal records are required to mount the models on an articulator in a particular position. Two positions are commonly used for the mounting, the ICP and the RCP.

A wax 'squash bite' has commonly been used to record ICP; however, it is inaccurate as the mandible can be deviated as the teeth 'bite' through the wax. For ICP, it is better not to use any record and to mount the models to the position of 'best fit'.

After the preparations have been carried out it can be difficult to locate the working model to this position of best fit; in this situation the *transfer coping technique* can be used. In this technique, DuraLay® copings are constructed on the working dies, which are taken to the clinic and seated in place on the preparations; they are then adjusted to ensure they are clear of the occlusion. A further mix of DuraLay® is applied to the occlusal surface of the coping and the patient is asked to close their teeth together; this produces an indent of the opposing tooth in the resin and provides a very accurate occlusal registration.

When the models are to be mounted in RCP, this is achieved by recording the position of the mandible on the retruded arc of closure just before tooth contact occurs. This is termed the *pre-centric record* and is generally registered with a relatively hard wax (Moyco® Dental Wax). The record is constructed on the maxillary model and trimmed flush with the buccal surfaces of the teeth. It is then softened and seated on the maxillary teeth and the mandible manipulated onto the retruded arc of closure to indent the wax, without allowing tooth contact to take place. The registration can be refined by using a low-viscosity material (e.g. TempBond®) in the wax record.

Alternatively, a proprietary inter-occlusal registration material (e.g. Jet Bite™, Blu-Mousse®) may be used to record the space between prepared teeth and their opponents.

Teamworking

It is essential for the whole dental team (dentist, dental nurse, hygienist/therapist, dental technician, and receptionist) to work together and communicate well for optimum outcomes for the patient and optimum use of individual skills. Referral to a specialist may sometimes be required.

Four-handed dentistry

The dental nurse usually takes an active role by working closely with the dentist.

Advantages
- ↑ comfort for dentist and nurse.
- ↑ efficiency.
- ↑ patient comfort.
- ↑ operator visibility.
- ↓ backache.
- ↑ professional satisfaction for the dentist and dental nurse.

Seating the patient Except for the old, infirm, or pregnant patient, a totally supine position is preferable for most examinations and Rx. However, for some procedures such as those in oral surgery, clinicians may prefer to stand with the patient sat more upright. Remember to warn the patient before reclining the chair.

Seating the dentist The aim is a relaxed, undistorted, and comfortable posture, with good vision of the teeth to be treated. Adjust the stool so that the top of the dentist's thighs slope at 15° to the floor. Position the dental chair so that, with the operator's back straight, the patient's mouth is at the dentist's focal distance (mid-sternal level). Forearms should slope upwards to this point. The operator's location is between 10 and 11 o'clock relative to the patient's head. Ensure the patient's head is at the top of the headrest.

Seating the dental nurse The dental nurse must also be seated comfortably with a straight back, with their eye level 10cm higher than the dentist's for maximum vision. The dental nurse's normal working environment is at between 2 and 3 o'clock, within easy reach of the instruments and equipment to be used.

Instrument transfer The transfer zone is just in front of, and slightly below the patient's mouth, not over their eyes. There are several techniques which enable the dental nurse to pass and receive instruments effectively from the dentist. Each dental team needs to choose, adapt, practise, and perfect a system that safely achieves instrument transfer.

Role of the dental nurse
- Assisting the dentist by preparing and maintaining the clinical environment, carrying out infection control procedures, handling dental materials, recording notes, and processing radiographs.
- Supporting the patient by monitoring and providing support, advice, and reassurance. Providing support if a medical emergency occurs.

Dental nurses can develop additional skills such as oral health promotion, fluoride application, and taking impressions/radiographs at the prescription of a dentist.

Isolation and moisture control

Isolation and moisture control is required to protect the patient from caustic materials or aspiration of foreign material, aid visibility, prevent contamination during moisture-sensitive techniques, and maintain a relatively aseptic environment.

Aspiration

High-volume suction Such as an aspirator.

Low-volume suction Such as a saliva ejector.

Compressed air This tends to redistribute the moisture to somewhere else (e.g. your eye) rather than remove it. It should be used with care in deep preparations as prolonged use can cause pulpal damage, let alone displace adhesive materials when the solvent is being evaporated prior to curing.

Absorbents

- Cotton-wool rolls. Insert with a rolling action away from the alveolus. Moisten before removal to prevent tearing mucosa.
- Paper pads.
- Carboxymethylcellulose pads (Dry Tips®). Very effective if inserted the correct way round with the impermeable plastic against the tooth.

Rubber dam

This provides effective isolation and also improves access to the operating site. It is indicated where airway protection and moisture control are essential, e.g. RCT (RCT without rubber dam is considered negligent), bonding. With practice, a rubber dam can be applied quickly and often saves time in the long run. The dam must be secured to the teeth; several methods are available:

- Rubber dam clamps. These consist of two metal jaws linked by one or more bows. Commonly used for posterior teeth.
- Floss ligatures.
- Wedges.
- Proprietary rubber bands (Wedjets®) or pieces of dam, worked through contact points.
- By pinching the dam between a tight contact point.

Types of dam

- Sheet grade, 6-inch square (15cm), which is supported with a frame. Moderate to thicker gauges are preferable.
- Mask type or 'dry dam', which is supported by a paper margin and looped over ears with elastic. Increasingly, latex-free rubber dam is available and arguably should be used routinely.
- OptraGate® lip and cheek retractors.
- More anatomically shaped rubber dams (OptiDam™).

Placement Several regimens have been described; the following is popular:
- Punch holes, which correspond to tooth size, cleanly in the rubber dam at the centre of each tooth to be included.
- Try in clamp (with floss tied to it—to retrieve clamp if dropped).
- Fit clamp into appropriate hole punched in dam, with bridge distally, and using forceps place clamp and dam on to tooth (winged technique). Alternatively, the clamp may be placed first and the dam pulled over (wingless). The latter is especially useful for broken down teeth or poor access.
- Position dam on other teeth, using floss to ease through contact points.
- Secure dam anteriorly using one of the methods described earlier in this section.
- If a frame is required, position.
- Put a gauze, swab, or napkin on the patient's chin under the dam to prevent the frame digging in. A saliva ejector will add to the patient's comfort.

If using caustic materials, a rubber dam sealer (e.g. OraSeal®) should be used.

Removal
- Take away clamps/ligatures, etc.
- Stretch dam, carefully cut interdental septa with scissors, and remove.

Protection of the airway
A rubber dam should be used when fitting crowns, bridges, inlays/onlays, and carrying out RCT. With the exception of during RCT, if it is not possible to place a rubber dam a butterfly sponge or gauze may be used, but airway protection should always be considered.

Gingival retraction
↓ gingival exudate and exposes subgingival preparations prior to impression-taking. Some retraction cords are impregnated with substances such as adrenaline to ↓ bleeding. The cord should be gently placed into the gingival crevice with a cord packing instrument (leaving no tag hanging out) prior to impression-taking and temporization. Braided cords are better than twisted. Bleeding from the gingival margin can be ↓ by applying an astringent (e.g. ferric sulfate). A paste (Expasyl™) which contains aluminium chloride provides for retraction and haemorrhage control. Expasyl™ is useful for preparations finished within or just below the level of the gingival crevice, otherwise retraction cord is more appropriate.

Electrosurgery
May be indicated where a margin extends subgingivally and gingival over-growth is hampering restoration placement or impression-taking. Also for crown-lengthening procedures, although bone removal is required too. (See ◐ Coronal third, p. 106 on crown lengthening.)

Principles of operative procedures

Why restore?

- To allow for daily self-, mechanical debridement of dental biofilm.
- For pain relief in reversible pulpitis.
- To allow the pulpodentinal complex to respond and heal.
- To restore function, form, and aesthetics.
- To prevent further spread of an active lesion which is not amenable to preventive measures or where preventive measures have failed.

However, these reasons need to be evaluated with regard to the patient and the rest of the dentition (➲ Management planning, p. 228).

Minimally invasive dentistry

Tooth preparation should be minimally invasive. It should be based on:

- *The morphology of the carious lesion.* Cavities should be kept as small as possible by excavation of only diseased enamel and dentine.
- *The requirements of the restorative material being used.* The remaining cavity walls are prepared chemically and physically in a manner appropriate to the material.

The final restoration should support and strengthen the remaining tooth tissue, promote remineralization, seal any remaining bacteria and deprive them of their nutritional supply, and predictably restore form, function, and aesthetics.

General principles of tooth preparation

- Gain or widen access to caries through enamel using rotary instruments or hand chisels.
- Cut away all significantly unsupported enamel and demineralized enamel margins creating a sound enamel margin.
- Caries-infected (dark brown, soft, wet) dentine should be removed using low-speed rose head burs or hand excavators or chemo-mechanical gels.
- In smaller lesions with optimal moisture control, some peripheral caries-affected (light brown, sticky, scratchy) dentine can be left at the ADJ provided there are no aesthetic concerns.
- In larger lesions or where moisture control is not optimal, then sound dentine at the ADJ is essential to maximize bonding.
- A small amount of caries-affected dentine can be left overlying the pulp in a symptomless tooth with an achievable peripheral seal if there is a risk of pulpal exposure (➲ Management of the deep carious lesion, p. 249).
- Where endodontics is planned, all carious dentine should be removed.
- Once caries has been removed, further modifications should be made according to the restorative material chosen.
- For all materials, all internal line angles should be rounded to ↓ internal stresses.
- Removing caries with a large-diameter round bur automatically produces the desired shape internally.

Resin composite (See also ➔ Composite resins—constituents and properties, p. 652.)
- Bevel enamel margin; ↑ surface area for bond.
- Need to acid-etch enamel (± dentine) with 37% orthophosphoric acid.

Amalgam (See also ➔ Amalgam, p. 650.)
- Amalgam is brittle, therefore an amalgam cavo-surface margin of at least 70°, preferably 90°, is required to prevent ditching. Also avoid leaving amalgam overlying cavity margins and overcarving.[6]
- Accepted minimal dimensions for amalgam are 2mm occlusally and 1mm elsewhere.
- Undercuts are required for retention unless the amalgam is bonded.
- In deep preparations, sealers and/or liners can be used to seal the dentine and prevent ingress of bacteria.

Glass ionomer (See also ➔ Glass ionomers, p. 660.)
- Wear precludes use in load-bearing situations except for 1° teeth.
- Management of root caries, temporary restorations, and the atraumatic restorative technique.
- Use 10% polyacrylic/citric acids to condition dentine and prepare the surface for chemical adhesion.

Helpful hints
- Mark centric stops with articulating paper prior to tooth preparation and try to preserve if possible, or place the preparation margins past the occlusal contact areas.
- Avoid crossing marginal ridges if possible.
- When removing caries mechanically, a tactile appreciation of the hardness of dentine is important, therefore use slow-speed instruments or excavators.
- Margins should be supragingival where possible.

Nomenclature
Cavities should not be cut to a predetermined design dictated by a classification but by the biological extent of the caries, the material chosen, and the remaining tooth structure. Experience in tooth preparation cannot possibly be adequately assimilated from the written text. For classification of cavities, see Table 6.1. The purpose of the following sections is to give the reader some practical tips on how to do the procedures considered, as well as to describe recent innovations and techniques.

Table 6.1 Classification of cavities

Class	Black's class	Site
Occlusal	Class I	Pits and fissures
Proximal	Class II	Proximal surface(s) of posterior tooth
Proximal	Class III	Proximal surface(s) of anterior tooth
Incisal	Class IV	Anterior incisal edge
Cervical	Class V	Cervical third of buccal or lingual surface of any tooth

6 P. B. Robinson 1985 *Dent Update* **12** 357.

Posterior composite restorations

Although amalgam is inexpensive, durable, easy to handle and is still widely used, there is ongoing debate regarding its use in patients and the environmental issues around production/disposal. The Control of Mercury (Enforcement) Regulations 2017 stipulate there should be no use of amalgam in the Rx of deciduous teeth, in children <15yrs, or pregnant or breast-feeding women, except when strictly deemed necessary by the practitioner on the grounds of specific medical needs of the patient.[7] It is likely further phasing down will occur (possibly to a full ban!) over the years worldwide. Additionally, patient expectations increasingly include tooth-coloured restorations. Posterior composite restorations are an established feature of contemporary dental practice. Many dental educators no longer consider amalgam the 'material of choice' for restoring posterior teeth. There is ↑ evidence to justify the use of composite in the restoration of posterior teeth. National remuneration systems, however, do not always support best practice. All new dental graduates should be competent in providing posterior composite restorations but there is still some inconsistency in how they are taught.[8]

Indications for posterior composite restorations
- 1° carious lesions in occlusal or proximal surfaces.
- Core build-ups.
- Restoration of endodontically treated teeth.
- Restoration of worn teeth.
- Repair/replacement of failed restorations.
- Restorations extending onto root surface (may require RMGIC layer in 'open sandwich' technique).

Manipulation
- Success depends on effective isolation, preferably with a rubber dam.
- Outline form is determined by the extent of the caries and undercuts are not necessary for retention.
- Bevelling of occlusal surface is C/I as it would result in a thin composite layer in a load-bearing area which would be prone to fracture.
- Bevelling of margin of proximal box is indicated to ↑ surface area for bond, except when little enamel bulk remains or if restoration finishes on dentine or cementum.
- Linings/bonding: there is a wide range of commercially available techniques for bonding or basing deeper cavities and a lack of consensus as to the most suitable technique.
- Can use three-step total etch or two-step or self-etching.
- Many different matrix systems are available including metal (single use and traditional), transparent matrix bands, and sectional matrices.
- Finishing with discs, polishing burs, and interproximal finishing strips is necessary to achieve excellent marginal adaptation, especially proximally and cervically.

Occlusal (Class I) Resin composite.

---

7 ♂ https://www.legislation.gov.uk/uksi/2017/1200/contents/made.

8 C. D. Lynch et al. 2007 *Br Dent J* **203** 183.

Technique for small cavitated lesions

Known as *preventive resin restoration* or *partial resin restoration*. Preparation is limited to caries removal and the resultant preparation restored using fissure sealant alone if small, or resin composite followed by sealant if larger. The rationale of this approach is that adjacent fissures are sealed for prevention. If the preparation extends significantly into load-bearing areas, conventional tooth preparation should be carried out and the tooth restored with resin composite or other suitable material.

Technique for medium-sized lesions

Following tooth preparation:
- Etch enamel margins and occlusal surface for 15–20sec. Wash and dry.
- Apply a dentine adhesive system, taking 20sec to do so.
- Restore preparation with resin composite placed and cured in increments.
- Polish with discs/points/cups/strips.
- Remove rubber dam and check occlusion.
- Remove any high spots.

Proximal (Class II) Following tooth preparation:
- Place pre-curved metal matrix band and wooden or plastic wedge.
- Etch enamel margins and occlusal surface for 15sec. Wash and dry.
- Apply a dentine adhesive system, taking 20sec to do so.
- Restore preparation with resin composite placed and cured in increments.
- Polish with discs/points/cups/strips.
- Remove rubber dam and check occlusion.
- Remove any high spots.

Hints for resin composite restorations
- Use etchant gel in a syringe to aid placement. Many newer adhesive systems do not have a separate etch stage, however, and rely on the use of acidic primers often used in conjunction with bonding resins or as a separate stage (➲ Dentine adhesive systems (dentine bonding agents), p. 658).
- Additions are generally easy as new resin composite will bond to old.
- Avoid eugenol-containing cements with resin composite restorations.
- Resin composite must be cured incrementally, with increments being no deeper than 2mm.
- Pre-wedging one but not both proximal contacts aids creation of a contact point.
- If possible, centric stops should be preserved on sound tooth tissue or the restorative material, but never on the marginal interface of the restoration.

Direct posterior resin composites may not perform so well in the following situations:
- Cusp replacements.
- Poor moisture control.
- Restorations with deep gingival extensions, although a bonded base approach can be adopted.
- Bruxism or heavy occlusion.

Use of indirect composite or porcelain inlays/onlays may combat some of these problems (➲ Indirect resin composite or porcelain inlays/onlays, p. 246).

Indirect resin composite or porcelain inlays/onlays

These inlay/onlay techniques appear to overcome some of the problems associated with direct resin composite restorations. Onlays provide cuspal coverage whereas inlays do not. As inlays are wedge-shaped preparations, they do not resist tooth fracture but may in fact predispose to fracture. Curing resin composite outside the mouth (in the manufacture of resin onlays/inlays) with the addition of heat (110° for 5min) or pressure overcomes polymerization shrinkage and possibly ↑ strength. As the inlays are bonded to the tooth with an adhesive, parallel walls are less important, but undercuts must be removed or blocked out. In general, porcelain inlays offer improved aesthetics, surface finish, and bond in comparison to resin composite inlays; however, placement and adjustment can be more difficult.

Technique: preparation
- The preparation should have slightly divergent walls, rounded line angles, and a slight bevel of the enamel margins, but not occlusally. For onlays, a minimum 1.5mm reduction of cusps is necessary.
- Block out any undercuts.
- Take an impression of the preparation and opposing arch, and if necessary make an inter-occlusal record.
- Choose shade.
- Make and place temporary with a proprietary resin-based temporary material (e.g. Fermit™, Clip™, Telio™).

Technique: cementation
- Place rubber dam.
- Remove temporary restoration and clean tooth. Be careful not to alter prep during removal of temporary and cleaning.
- Try-in inlay/onlay, and carefully check marginal fit and adjust as necessary.
- Polish any adjusted areas.
- Remove inlay/onlay and clean with alcohol. For porcelain only, place layer of silane coupling agent on fitting surface.
- Etch enamel and dentine (total etch concept). Wash and remove excess moisture, but do not over-dry.
- Place dentine adhesive system to moist surface, taking 20sec to do so. Also apply to restoration fit surface if recommended.
- Apply dual-cure resin composite luting cement to prep and inlay and carefully seat.
- Remove gross excess cement, then cure for 10sec and then remove any further excess resin composite.
- Complete light-curing (dual-cure resin composite will finish setting chemically under inlay in ~6min).
- Trim any excess cement (especially interdentally) and polish.
- Remove rubber dam, check occlusion, and adjust.

Posterior amalgam restorations

In practice, preparation size is determined by the size of the carious lesion and extension beyond this should be minimal. If enamel margins are cut to an angle of 90° (or, if cusps steeply inclined, >70°) the resultant preparation will be adequately retentive. Proximal preparations comprise a proximal box with vertical grooves. The preparation should only extend occlusally if there is evidence of caries in the occlusal fissures. Retention from occlusal forces is derived from a 2–5° divergence of the walls towards the floor in both parts of the preparation. Amalgam restorations are prone to # at the isthmus in restorations extended occlusally, therefore sufficient depth must be provided in this area. The width of the isthmus should not be overcut (ideally one-quarter to one-fifth intercuspal width). If the cusps are extensively undermined or missing they should be replaced with a bonded restoration (⊙ Indirect resin composite or porcelain inlays/onlays, p. 246). A chisel or bur can be used to plane away unsupported enamel from the margins of the completed preparation to produce a 90° butt joint. In molar teeth with mesial and distal caries, it is preferable to try and cut two separate cavities, but often a confluent mesio-occlusal-distal preparation is unavoidable. Increasingly, the use of resin composite placed in conjunction with a dentine adhesive system is advocated for the restoration of premolar and molar teeth.

Lining

Recently, emphasis has changed, with linings being used to seal the underlying dentine for moderate to deep cavities. Light-cured RMGICs (e.g. Vitrebond™) are now recommended. A preparation sealer (Gluma® Desensitizer) can be used in minimal preparations.

▶ Avoid the creation of an overhang at the cervical margin and ensure a good contact point with adjacent tooth with a well-contoured matrix band and wedges.

Anterior proximal (Class III), incisal (Class IV), cervical (Class V), and root surface caries

Anterior proximal Resin composite is the most widely used material for anterior proximal restorations.

Access should be gained from either the buccal or lingual aspect, depending on the position of the lesion. As resin composite is adhesive, the preparation is just extended sufficiently to remove all peripheral caries. Some unsupported enamel can be retained labially, but the margins should be planed with chisels or burs to remove any grossly weakened tooth structure. Tooth preparation can be almost entirely completed with slow-speed burs and hand instruments. Ideally the margins are bevelled. A slight excess of material should be moulded into the preparation with a mylar strip, wedged cervically. Once the material is set, the excess can be removed. After checking the occlusion the restoration can be polished using one of the proprietary products (e.g. Sof-Lex™ discs, Enhance®) if necessary.

Incisal The restoration of choice is resin composite, the so-called acid-etch tip (◆ Acid-etch composite tip technique, p. 104); however, for very large incisal/proximal cavities in the adult patient, a dentine-bonded crown or porcelain veneer may give better retention and aesthetics.

Cervical Although cervical cavities are seen less frequently in younger patients, they are an ↑ problem in older age groups with gingival recession. Resin composite (e.g. flowable, compomer, or RMGIC) are the preferred materials in this situation.

Once caries has been removed, the occlusal margin should be bevelled. The cervical margin should not be bevelled as it has been shown to ↑ microleakage. The materials are ideally placed incrementally under rubber dam isolation.

Root surface caries As gingival recession is a prerequisite to root caries, it occurs predominantly in the >40yrs age group. Dentine, which has a critical pH below that of enamel, is thus directly exposed to carious attack. It is sometimes seen 2° to ↓ saliva flow (which reduces buffering capacity and may alter dietary habits) caused by salivary gland disease, drugs, or radiotherapy. Long-term sugar-based medication may also be a factor. Rx requires, first, control of the aetiological factors, and for most patients this involves dietary advice and OHI. Topical fluoride varnishes, high-fluoride toothpastes, and mouthrinses may aid remineralization and prevent new lesions developing. However, active lesions require restoration, typically with composite or a traditional/RMGIC. See also ◆ Severe early childhood caries, p. 92.

Management of extensive/ deep restorations

Extensive loss of coronal tooth tissue leads to problems with retention of subsequent restorations, weakening of tooth structure, and challenges of obtaining a coronal seal. In the past, dentine pins were used to improve retention but now their use is ↓. Where amalgam is used, pins have largely been replaced by bonding techniques coupled with the use of auxiliary forms of retention such as boxes and slots, circumferential grooves, and the use of amalgam cores in the Rx of non-vital teeth. Dentine pins can produce stresses within the teeth while weakening restorative materials and there are few indications for their continued use. Where composite is used, a good seal can be achieved where enamel is present but if restorations cover a large surface area, bonded indirect restorations in composite, ceramic, or gold should be considered.

Management of the deep carious lesion
Assessment
- Is the tooth restorable and is restoration preferable to extraction?
- Is the tooth symptomless? If not, what is the character and duration of the pain?
- Sensibility test and percuss the tooth (before LA!).
- Take radiographs to check extent of lesion and if there is apical pathology.

Management
Depends upon an assessment of pulpal condition (◑ Pulpal pain, p. 230).
- Irreversible pulpitis/necrotic pulp—Rx: RCT (◑ Root canal treatment— rationale, p. 338) or extraction.
- Reversible pulpitis/healthy pulp—aim to maintain pulp vitality by selective removal of carious dentine without pulp exposure. See ◑ Pulp-preserving therapies, p. 334.

If in doubt, treat as for reversible pulpitis. Can always institute RCT later; however, be sure to warn the patient of a possible further need for Rx.

Rationale
Bacteria sealed under a restoration that provides a good peripheral seal are denied substrate, therefore lesion arrests. This allows the pulpodential complex to lay down reparative dentine.[9]

9 D. Rickets et al. 2013 *Cochrane Database Syst Rev* 3 CD003808.

Survival and failure of restorations

Survival of restorations

Patients who change dentists frequently are more at risk of replacement restorations than those who are loyal to the same GDP.[10] In order to ↑ longevity we need to consider the reasons and types of failure of restorations.

Reasons for failure of restorations

- Further caries, tooth fracture, or material fracture.
- Aesthetic deterioration due to staining.
- Poor understanding of the occlusion.
- Incorrect preparation, e.g. insufficient caries removal, incorrect margin preparation, inadequate retention, preparation too shallow, or weakened tooth tissue left unprotected.
- Incorrect choice of restorative material, e.g. inadequate strength or resistance to wear for situation.
- Incorrect manipulation of material, e.g. inadequate moisture control, or over- or under-contouring.
- Patient factors, e.g. bruxism, using teeth to open beer bottles, or biting on something hard.

Before replacing a failed restoration, it is important to identify the cause of failure and decide whether this can be dealt with by repair rather than replacement. Keep in mind that cavity size is ↑ on average by 0.6mm each time a restoration is removed.

Types of failure

Failed aesthetics This may be due to underlying discoloration from stained dentine or corrosion products or superficial from surface staining. Patients may not be concerned so it is worth checking before replacing.

Failed marginal integrity This can be due to creep/corrosion and ditching of amalgams or shrinkage of composites/GIC or marginal chipping.

If the patient can keep the margin plaque free and there is no recurrent caries then it may not be necessary to replace the restoration. If not, 2° or recurrent caries may be a risk. 2° caries is difficult to diagnose, but careful observation (clinically and radiographically) rather than intervention, is now advocated. Intervention is only indicated when the lesion is in dentine, and there is evidence of progression &/or cavitation is present. To prevent 2° caries it is important not only to educate the patient to reduce their caries rate but also to use an excellent restorative technique to ensure good long term-restorations.

Bulk fracture Can be due to heavy occlusal loading, poor cavity design, or poor bonding.

10   J. A. Davies 1984 *Br Dent J* **157** 322.

Tooth wear/tooth surface loss

Definition

This is the irreversible loss of tooth substance by factors other than trauma or caries. Usually caused by combinations of erosion, attrition, abrasion, and possibly abfraction.

Some tooth wear during life is inevitable (physiological), but where it has resulted in an unsatisfactory appearance, sensitivity, loss of vitality, or mechanical problems (pathological), the condition warrants investigation and Rx. Differentiating between these can be difficult. Wear that might be considered normal in a 70yr-old would not be normal in a 20yr-old.

Epidemiology

The Adult Dental Health Survey 2009 showed that 77% of people in the UK have at least one tooth worn to dentine. By the age of 75 about 40% of people have moderate tooth wear but severe wear only affects a small proportion of the population. Identifying what proportion of the population have problematic wear and what Rx they might need is very difficult.

Erosion Loss of tooth substance from non-bacterial chemical attack. Enamel initially becomes smooth and shiny then eventually dentine is exposed. This leads to cup-shaped lesions on the occlusal and incisal surfaces and proud amalgams. Once erosion is through to dentine it can accelerate. Sources of acid may be intrinsic or extrinsic. Patients with xerostomia are at ↑ risk.

Intrinsic

Acid from stomach due to gastro-oesophageal reflux, vomiting in relation to eating disorder (➲ Anorexia nervosa/bulimia nervosa, p. 555), pregnancy, stress, or rumination. Such conditions warrant referral. Affects palatal surfaces of ULS and occlusal/buccal of lower molars.

Extrinsic

- *Dietary* (e.g. citric, phosphoric, acetic acid)—found in carbonated drinks, fruit/citrus juices, and pickles. Labial surfaces of ULS teeth classically affected.
- *Environmental*—occurred historically in industrial areas (e.g. battery manufacture). Rare now due to health and safety laws. Pitting on labial surfaces of ULS. Competitive swimmers and professional wine tasters have ↑ risk.
- *Medication*—iron tonics, vitamin C, acidic salivary flow stimulants and substitutes, and nutritional supplements.

Attrition Physical wear caused by tooth to tooth contact. It can affect interproximal but mainly occlusal surfaces. ↑ in more abrasive diets and in bruxism. Occlusal wear facets match with opposing teeth. Often occurs in combination with erosion.

Abrasion Physical wear of a tooth caused by objects other than teeth. Hard toothbrushing and abrasive toothpastes can result in dished or V-shaped cervical lesions. Habits such as pipe smoking or nail-biting may also produce incisal wear/grooves.

Abfraction Stresses produced by clenching may concentrate at cervical margins and result in V-shaped cervical lesions. Can occur just subgingivally and on teeth involved in guidance. This is still controversial.

Diagnosis

This is made from the history, clinical picture, and special investigations. As tooth wear may be due to a factor which no longer operates, it may be necessary (tactfully) to delve into the patient's past. Targeted questions (e.g. diet, digestion disorders, eating disorders, pregnancy sickness, alcohol intake, stress, habits) help to assess the aetiology. In a proportion of cases, the aetiology will remain obscure and this will complicate prevention. It is important to establish whether the tooth wear is ongoing. Staining of worn surfaces can indicate historic or slowly progressing wear. Sensitivity is suggestive of progression. Monitoring is useful before operative intervention.

Basic Erosive Wear Examination (BEWE)

This is becoming a commonly used objective measure of wear with the most severely affected surface in each sextant recorded using a four-level score and the cumulative score classified and matched to risk levels which guide the management of the condition (Table 6.2).[11] All teeth excluding the third molars in a sextant are examined. Note this is not useful to monitor for progression.

Table 6.2 Basic Erosive Wear Examination scores

Score	Site
0	No erosive tooth wear
1	Initial loss of surface texture
2	Distinct defect, hard tissue loss <50% of the surface area
3	Hard tissue loss ≥50% of the surface area

Reproduced from Bartlett, D et al., *Clin Oral Invest* (2008) 12 (Suppl 1): 65. ⚲ https://doi.org/10.1007/s00784-007-0181-5 © Springer-Verlag 2007.

11   D. Bartlett et al. 2008 *Clin Oral Investig* **12** (Suppl 1) 65.

Management

- Focus should be on removal of aetiological factors, prevention, and monitoring.
- Dietary and oral hygiene advice, supplemental fluoride.
- Prevention requires an understanding of the aetiology. However, an explanation of possible exacerbating factors to the patient may help to limit loss even if the exact aetiology is unknown.
- For patients where parafunction is thought to be a factor, a splint may be provided for night wear. Hypnotherapy may also be useful.
- Referral to a physician (gastrointestinal problems), psychiatrist (bulimic patient), or restorative specialist (complicated restorative problem).
- Monitoring. Take study models, silicone indices, and photos to allow the rate of wear to be monitored. Intervention is indicated in cases with an unsatisfactory appearance, sensitivity, or functional problems.
- If restorative Rx is required, GI or resin composite restorations may help improve appearance and ↓ sensitivity.
- If there has been compensatory over-eruption it may not be possible to provide an aesthetic result without ↑ OVD or carrying out surgical crown lengthening. Generally, if ULS teeth are not seen when the patient is smiling then an ↑ in incisal length is required. If excessive gingiva shows when smiling or there is insufficient coronal structure to retain restorations, then surgical crown lengthening is required. For localized anterior tooth wear, use of the 'Dahl' approach can create space by a combination of anterior tooth intrusion and posterior tooth eruption.[12] Composite is added to the palatal surfaces of the anteriors (minimum thickness 1.5mm palatally). Warn the patient that the posterior teeth will be out of contact but will come together again in 3–6 months. The predictability of this method ↓ with ↑ age.
- Restoration can be achieved by direct composite restorations or by indirect restorations. These may be full coverage crowns or bonded onlays.
- Overdentures may be indicated in cases of excessive tooth wear, but are aesthetically less satisfactory.
- Sensitivity is a frequent problem in tooth wear. There may be pulpal involvement in 9–12% of cases.[13,14] If pulps are exposed, root canal Rx may be indicated.

12 A. B. Gulamali et al. 2011 *Br Dent J* **211** E9.

13 J. S. Rees et al. 2011 *Dent Update* **38** 24.

14 K. Simvasithamparan et al. 2003 *Aus Dent J* **48** 97.

'Cosmetic' dentistry

All procedures carried out in the anterior region have an integral aesthetic element as Rx is intended to restore appearance as well as function. 'Cosmetic' Rx is Rx intended to 'improve' a person's appearance. There is a huge market in procedures aimed at 'enhancing' or 'improving' natural aesthetics. Some of these procedures are relatively non-invasive: tooth whitening/bonding procedures/orthodontics. Some, however, can be highly destructive and risk doing harm.

While there may undoubtedly be a psychological benefit to enhancing personal appearance, all patients need to be fully informed of the risks involved in preparing sound, healthy tooth tissue, the irreversible nature of the procedure, the risks of sensitivity and marginal failure, and the inevitable need for replacement over a lifetime. Management of expectations is essential and can be challenging.

Tooth whitening

Tooth whitening (bleaching) provides a non-invasive solution for mild to moderately discoloured vital or root-filled teeth. It is safe and effective provided it is used properly. Potential local adverse effects include gingival irritation and tooth sensitivity. Some shade rebound may occur shortly after Rx.

Following amendment in 2012, the current European Directive position is as follows:

- Whitening is the practice of dentistry and that it should only be undertaken by regulated dental professionals.
- Products containing or releasing between 0.1% and 6% hydrogen peroxide cannot be used on any person under 18yrs of age.
- Products containing between 0.1% and 6% hydrogen peroxide should only be used after appropriate clinical examination to ensure there are no risk factors or oral pathology concerns.
- Products should be available only via a dentist/hygienist or dental therapist.
- For each cycle of use, the first use must be carried out by dental practitioners or under their direct supervision.
- After that, the product may be provided by the dental practitioner to the consumer to complete the cycle of use.

Vital bleaching

Two methods have been described. Take photos as a pre-operative record or alternatively note shade of tooth using a porcelain shade-guide.

Home bleaching technique A gel of 10–15% carbamide peroxide in a soft splint has also been advocated for 'home bleaching'. 10% carbamide peroxide provides around 3% hydrogen peroxide. This is worn for a few hours, up to 8h each day for several weeks, usually 2 weeks, and is the preferred technique.

- Take an alginate impression.
- Ask the laboratory to make a bleaching splint.
- Fit the splint, dispense the carbamide peroxide (10%), and give instructions.
- Advise 6–8h Rx per day.
- Review weekly.

'In-office' bleaching technique This uses gels of high concentration which can cause tissue burns (hydrogen peroxide 25–40%). Gingival barrier protection must be used and checked for signs of leakage. Dental curing lights are commonly used to activate the bleaching agent.[15] However, usually no activation is necessary.

- Apply Orabase® to gingivae prior to placing rubber dam over teeth to be treated.
- Polish teeth with pumice.
- Apply the bleaching agent according to the manufacturer's instructions.
- Wash teeth with copious amounts of water.

15   R. A. Howell 1980 *Br Dent J* **148** 159.

- Remove rubber dam and polish teeth.
- Advise patient to avoid tea, coffee, red wine, cigarettes, etc., for 1 week and that some sensitivity may occur.
- Can repeat as required.

Non-vital bleaching

This provides a conservative alternative to a post-retained crown for the discoloured root-filled tooth. However, it usually only achieves an improvement in shade. There is a tendency for the discoloration to recur over time, therefore warn the patient and over-bleach. Interestingly, it has been shown that the degree and duration of discoloration and the age of the patient do not affect the prognosis for a successful result.[16]

Walking bleach technique

- Place Orabase® around gingivae of tooth to be treated and isolate with rubber dam.
- Open access cavity and remove root filling to 2mm below gingival margin (a perio probe is a useful guide).
- Place thin layer of GI over root filling to prevent root resorption.
- Remove any stained dentine within pulp chamber.
- Clean access cavity with etchant on a pledget of cotton wool and then repeat with alcohol. Wash and dry.
- Place 35% carbamide peroxide.
- Seal with a pledget of cotton wool and GI.
- Review after 1–2 weeks and repeat (up to 2×) if necessary.
- Seal access cavity permanently with a light shade of resin composite.
- Alternatively, after sealing and cleaning access cavity, place 10% carbamide peroxide into pulp chamber and ask patient to change the material regularly through the open access cavity over a 24h period combined with wearing a tray for simultaneous external bleaching of the tooth (inside/outside bleaching). The tooth is sealed coronally when the patient returns.

Thermocatalytic techniques, where the hydrogen peroxide is heated within the pulp chamber, should no longer be used, as they are associated with the development of cervical resorption lesions.

Microabrasion

This is indicated for fluorosis, post-orthodontic demineralization, localized hypoplasia due to infection or trauma, and idiopathic hypoplasia where discoloration is limited to the outer enamel layer. Affected teeth are carefully isolated, cleaned, and dried before 'polishing' the teeth with a slurry of either phosphoric acid (etch) mixed with pumice or a similar commercially available product (usually based on hydrochloric acid). Teeth treated in this way should be reviewed at 1–4 weeks for effect once teeth have re-hydrated and photographs taken.

16 P. J. Nixon et al. 2007 *Dent Update* 34 2.

Veneers

Indications These include where teeth are fundamentally sound but discoloured. Mild discolation (can ↑ success by bleaching first), hypoplasia, fractured teeth, tooth wear lesions, closing space, or modifying shape (within limits).

Contraindications Contraindications include large existing restorations, severe discoloration, insufficient tooth substance to bond restoration to, and severe parafunction. Overlapping teeth, pencil-chewing, or nail-biting are relative C/I.

As whitening becomes more common the need for veneers is less but they still provide the least destructive restoration for anterior teeth compared to crowns. On the other hand, survival rate at 10yrs is almost 20% lower than crowns.[17]

Types
Resin composite Useful for the Rx of adolescent patients. Can be made directly (less destructive) or, more commonly, indirectly (due to processing they have improved properties). Problems are shrinkage, staining, and wear. Surface quality changes and temporary post-operative sensitivity are more frequent in composite than ceramic veneers; however, they cost less and are easier to repair. Average lifespan ~4yrs.[18]

Porcelain Better performance and aesthetics than resin composite and long-term follow-up now available.[19] In addition, porcelain is less plaque retentive. They are made indirectly in the laboratory and roughened on their fitting surface by etching and sandblasting. This surface is treated with a silane coupling agent prior to bonding to the etched tooth enamel with resin composite luting cement. Porcelain laminate veneers have an estimated survival of 93.5% over 10yrs.[20]

Technique for porcelain veneers
Tooth preparation Veneers are usually 0.5–0.7mm thick, therefore unless deliberate overbuilding is required (in which case a no-preparation veneer may be possible), the tooth needs to be reduced labially. To guide reduction depth, cuts of 0.5mm are advisable. A definite chamfered finishing line will make the technician's job considerably easier and this should be established first. If the tooth is discoloured the margin should be subgingival (but still in enamel), otherwise keep slightly supragingival. The finishing line is extended into the embrasures, but kept short of the contact points. Incisally, the veneer can be finished to a chamfer at the incisal edge or wrapped over onto the palatal surface (Fig. 6.1).

17 P. S. Lucarotti & T. Burke 2018 *Br Dent J* 223 9.

18 J. S. Clyde & A. Gilmour 1988 *Br Dent J* 164 9.

19 F. J. Shaini et al. 1997 *J Oral Rehabil* 24 553.

20 U. S. Beier et al. 2012 *Int J Prosthodont* 25 79.

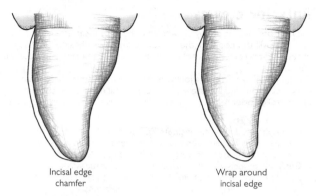

Incisal edge
chamfer

Wrap around
incisal edge

Fig. 6.1 Porcelain veneer preparations.

An impression of the preparation is taken digitally or using an elastomeric impression material in a stock tray and the shade taken with a porcelain shade-guide. Temporary coverage is not usually required (➲ Temporary restorations, p. 270).

Try-in Careful handling is necessary so as not to contaminate the fitting surface of the veneer. Do not check the fit of the veneer on the stone cast. The prepared tooth should be cleaned and isolated and then the veneer tried in wet (to ↑ translucency). Minor adjustments are best deferred until after cementation to ↓ risk of #. The effect of different shades of resin composite &/or opaquers and tints can be tried prior to etching to get the best colour match. If several veneers are to be fitted, check them individually and then together to work out the order of placement.

Placement The fitting surface of the veneer is cleaned with alcohol, dried, and then coated with a thin layer of silane coupling agent followed by bonding resin. The tooth is re-isolated and cellulose acetate strips used to separate from adjacent teeth. After etching, washing, and flash drying, a dentine adhesive system is used. Numerous cementation systems are available (e.g. Calibra®, Nexus™, Variolink®). The resin composite luting cement is placed thinly on the fitting surface of the veneer and the veneer carefully positioned. Excess luting cement should be removed with a brush or microbrush before curing. Adjustments are made with a flame-shaped diamond or multi-blade tungsten carbide bur before polishing. The patient should be instructed in the use of floss.

Porcelain slips These are veneered corners or edges used to restore # incisors or close spaces by building out the tooth mesially or distally. Now rarely used as direct placement of resin composite is preferred.

Anterior crowns

▶ Defer preparation of any crowns until the patient can attain good OH. Not only will this help to ↑ their motivation, but also healthy gingivae are necessary for correct placement of preparation margins and accurate impressions.

A thorough examination should be carried out to assess appropriateness of crown placement. Disease such as periodontal disease and caries should be controlled prior to placement of definitive restorations such as crowns.

Preliminary Rx
- Check vitality; if non-vital, institute RCT first.
- Take a periapical radiograph to check for apical pathology, health of supporting tissues, and anatomy of pulp and bone levels.
- Get study models. A trial preparation and diagnostic wax-up on a duplicate model can be helpful (especially for the less confident operator). This helps to anticipate any complications.
- Record the shade, so that it can be checked at subsequent visits.
- Examine the occlusion.

All-ceramic crowns are becoming more popular than porcelain fused to metal but there is little evidence as to which material to use in which situation.

Porcelain fused to metal (PFM) crown ↑ strength, but ↑ labial reduction (NB: some ceramic crowns can be more destructive than PFMs). ↑ aesthetics compared with all-ceramic and proven clinical track record. Preparation requires 0.5mm reduction of lingual surface with chamfered margin and labial reduction of 1.2–1.5mm, with shoulder. Transition from shoulder to chamfer is on proximal surface. The junction between porcelain and metal must not be in an area of contact with the opposing teeth. Ideally, all occlusal surfaces in contact with opposing teeth should be finished in metal.

Porcelain jacket crown (PJC) This was previously the first choice for aesthetics in cases where occlusal loading was not a problem. Now being superseded by newer ceramic systems.

Dentine bonded crowns These are full coverage ceramic restorations which are bonded to the underlying dentine. The bond is formed between a dentine bonding agent, composite resin luting material, and a ceramic fitting surface which has been made micromechanically retentive by etching. The labial preparation is minimal, but incisal reduction is the same as for other porcelain crowns. They are useful for tooth wear cases or where preparation taper is large or crown height poor. Chair-side fitting is more time-consuming than for conventional crowns.

All-ceramic crown Where there is a large restoration in place or there is a pre-existing crown it may not be possible to use a dentine-bonded crown. In this case, an all-ceramic crown provides better aesthetics and ↑ strength compared with PJC (e.g. E-max, In-Ceram®, Empress II®, Procera®, Lava™).

Which system to use depends on clinical situation. Glass-based, etchable ceramics provide superior aesthetics but won't mask out an underlying dark substrate (e.g. IPS Empress®, IPS e.max®). IPS e.max® crowns are made from a single block of lithium disilicate ceramic, a material known for its translucency, toughness, and durability. They must be bonded with resin cement to achieve clinically acceptable strength. Crystalline alumina- or zirconia-based ceramics are relatively opaque so can mask underlying darker substrate and have high strength (e.g. Procera®, Lava™, In-Ceram®, Zircon). They are not etchable and can be cemented with RMGIC or resin cement.

Principles
- Sufficient tooth reduction to permit adequate thickness of crown for strength and aesthetics.
- Reduction should follow tooth contours. NB: two-plane reduction on labial face of incisor teeth.
- Chamfer preparation: 1.0mm labial (just into gingival crevice) and palatal (supragingival).
- 6° taper of opposing walls for retention.

Preparation
- Check shade in natural and artificial light with dental nurse and patient.
- *Interproximal*. Use a long, tapered chamfer bur. Walls should have 6° taper and converge lingually.
- *Labial*. With the same bur, first place three depth grooves and remove intervening tooth tissue. Extend a maximum of 0.5mm subgingivally.
- *Lingual*. If possible carry out under direct vision. Continue interproximal shoulder round to form cingulum wall, supragingivally. Remainder of palatal surface should be prepared with a flame-shaped bur to give 0.8–1.0mm clearance from opposing teeth.
- *Incisal*. A reduction of 1.5–2mm is required.
- *Finishing*. Finishing burs should be used to round off line angles.
- *Fabricate temporary crown* (➲ Temporary crowns, p. 270) next, as if time runs out impressions can be deferred, but a temporary crown cannot.
- *Impressions*. (➲ Impression techniques, p. 668). Record preparation in elastomeric material. Opposing arch can be recorded in alginate (cheaper), inter-occlusal record, and facebow if required. Fit temporary crown and arrange next appointment. Optical impressions are becoming used as an alternative.
- *Fitting crown*. Isolate with rubber dam. Remove temporary crown and cement. Check marginal fit and contact points. Cement with resin cement or RMGIC. Check occlusion. If any adjustments are required, polish with porcelain polishing wheels. Make sure the patient is happy before you cement the crown.

Confirm preparation requirements for each material as this can vary. If using a digital, in-house system, temporary crowns may not be necessary, and impressions may be digital. This can reduce the number of appointments required and save time for both the clinician and patient.

Common problems with anterior crowns

- *Preparation likely to expose pulp.* Consider veneer as an interim measure.
- *Completed crown does not seat.* Check: (i) no temporary cement left on preparation; (ii) approximal contacts with floss, and if too tight, adjust; (iii) ? distorted impression—check no undercuts on preparation and repeat impressions; (iv) die over-trimmed leading to over-extension of margin—cut-back crown margin.
- *Core material showing through crown.* Need to ↓ preparation so that sufficient bulk of enamel and dentine porcelain can be built up over core, and remake.
- *Colour not right.* If technician is handy, can see if surface stains will give sufficient improvement. If not, re-choose shade and remake.

Removing old crowns

- Protect airway.
- A crown-removing instrument can be used to try and remove a crown without destroying it.
- If a crown is to be replaced: cut a longitudinal groove in labial, occlusal, and palatal surfaces of crown, without damaging preparation. Insert an excavator or flat plastic and twist.

Anterior post and core crowns

In root-filled anterior teeth it may be necessary to insert a post and core prior to the placement of a crown if there is insufficient remaining coronal tooth tissue to support a core. Post and cores provide support and retention for a crown but they do *not* reinforce teeth. They transfer forces to the root of the tooth. A ferrule effect will protect the root from this to an extent. The placement of a post makes further orthograde endodontics difficult, so it is important to check first that the root-filling and apical condition are satisfactory. If in doubt, repeat RCT.

Preliminary preparation

The first step is to prepare the crown of the tooth to receive the appropriate coronal restoration. The appropriate reductions and margin preparations are carried out with the intention of retaining as much coronal dentine as possible. Grossly weakened tooth substance is removed, but the root face should *not* be flattened off. The retention of a core of tooth substance is important as it effectively ↑ the length of the subsequent post; obviously in some cases this will not be possible, e.g. if the tooth has fractured at gingival level. The coronal GP is removed with a heated instrument or Gates–Glidden bur, taking care not to disturb the apical seal. The root canal is then prepared according to the particular technique being used. As a general guide the post should be at least equal to the anticipated crown height, but a minimum of 5mm of well-condensed GP should be left. A periodontal probe or silicone stop is helpful to check prepared canal length.

Types of post and core system

Many different types of post system are available and they can be classified in numerous ways as follows:

Prefabricated or custom-made Prefabricated metal posts obviously have the advantage of being cheap and quick, however they lack versatility and many of the systems require all coronal dentine to be removed. Custom-made techniques are preferred for metal as they are more versatile, but they are also more expensive and require an additional laboratory stage. Prefabricated non-metal posts (ceramic or carbon fibre reinforced) are becoming more popular (e.g. LightPosts™, ParaPost® FiberWhite, and RelyX™ FiberPost). They are more flexible than metal posts and therefore less likely to cause root fracture. Failure with fibre posts is most commonly due to decementation or 2° caries rather than fracture so failure can be more retrievable.

Parallel-sided or tapered Parallel-sided posts are generally preferred to tapered as they provide greater retention and do not generate as much stress within the root canal. Tapered posts, however, are less likely to perforate in the apical region and are better for small tapered roots, e.g. lateral incisors.

Threaded, smooth, or serrated Threaded posts provide ↑ retention than smooth-sided; however, they will ↑ stress within the root canal and are therefore C/I. Serrated posts do not concentrate stress but simply ↑ the surface area for retention. Other design features include antirotational components and cementation vents.

Indirect custom-made posts

These are usually cast metal. First of all the root canal is prepared using parallel-sided twist drills, and an antirotation groove is placed in the coronal dentine. The post and core can then be constructed in one of two ways:

- From a pattern which is fabricated in the mouth using either inlay wax or a burn-out resin (e.g. DuraLay®) which is then sent to the laboratory for casting.
- From an impression taken using a matched plastic impression post placed in the prepared post hole. When using this technique it is generally inadvisable to have the post and subsequent crown constructed on the same impression. A good coronal seal must be maintained between visits, although this is difficult and so is a disadvantage compared to direct posts.

Direct prefabricated posts

Non-metal posts Fibre posts must be bonded to the root canal space which means remnants of GP/sealer must be removed from the walls of the post space. Rinse with alcohol if eugenol-based sealer has been used. The curing light may not be able to transmit light to all surfaces. Chemical- or dual-cure composites may be used. There are many different systems available. The advantage is they may be placed immediately after endodontic Rx is completed when individual root canal anatomy and orientation is clearly understood and the risk of microleakage is reduced. Rx time is also reduced. Once the post is cemented, the remainder of the core can be built up with the same composite or with a light-cured composite.

Metal posts These are available in various different forms:
- *Parallel, serrated*—e.g. ParaPost®.
- *Parallel, threaded*—e.g. Radix®, Kurer™.
- *Tapered, threaded*—e.g. Dentatus™ screw. These are the poorest design in terms of stress production. If they are used in small tapered roots they should be cemented 'passively'.

Some of these systems have a prefabricated core on the post while with others it must be built up around the neck using resin composite. For the majority of crowns, choice is one of personal preference. However, no one system will be versatile enough to cover every eventuality, so it is wise to be familiar with more than one method.

Anterior post and core crowns—practical tips

Some problems and possible solutions

- *Subgingival tooth loss*. Either extrude tooth orthodontically or use cast post and core method, extending post into defect in the form of a diaphragm.
- *Extensive tooth loss and calcified canal* (e.g. dentinogenesis imperfecta, severe tooth wear). Use adhesive system to retain resin composite core for porcelain bonded crown or consider crown-lengthening surgery.
- *Perforation of root by post*. If the post can be removed it may be possible to seal the perforation from an orthograde approach with the use of magnification, illumination, and MTA. If successful, re-prepare post hole to correct alignment. Alternatively, a surgical approach is needed to cut back excess post and seal perforation with MTA. Perforations of the coronal third have a poorer prognosis.
- *Loss of post*. Check: (i) ? length adequate. If not, remake with ↑ length. (ii) ? Loose fit or too much taper. Can try sandblasting post and re-cementing with adhesive cement, e.g. Panavia™ 21. Alternatively, correct and remake. (iii) ? Perforation. Take radiographs in parallax to check, and see previous bullet point. (iv) ? Root #. Extract.
- *Apical pathology*. If post and core, crown, and endodontics are satisfactory, periradicular surgery may be considered. If not, remove and carry out revision endodontic therapy and place new post and crown.

Causes of failure in post and core crowns

A survey of failed posts showed that most failed within 1yr, but that a post crown that has survived satisfactorily for 3yrs has a good chance of lasting for 10yrs. Common causes of failure were caries, root #, and mechanical failure of the post.[21]

Removing old posts and cores

Unretentive posts may be removed by grasping with Spencer–Wells forceps and twisting. Post removers are available (but C/I for threaded posts) that work by drawing out post using root face as anchorage, e.g. the Eggler post remover. Some proprietary kits, e.g. Masseran, can be used to cut a channel around the post to facilitate removal. In some cases an ultrasonic scaler tip can be used to vibrate the post loose, but copious water irrigation is needed as heat generation can be a problem.

21   R. Lewis & B. G. Smith 1988 *Br Dent J* 165 95.

Posterior crowns

Where there is significant tooth tissue loss (e.g. endodontically treated teeth, caries, tooth wear, or #), indirect restorations may be considered, e.g. inlay/onlay (⊃ Indirect resin composite or porcelain inlays/onlays, p. 246) or crowns. The decision to place a crown depends on an assessment of the amount of tissue removal required to provide a retentive restoration and the likelihood of pulpal involvement. Posterior crowns may be used as bridge abutments. Prior to preparation, replace any doubtful restorations, check vitality, and take a pre-operative radiograph.

The types of posterior crowns available are as follows:

Full veneer gold or non-precious metal crown
The least destructive but not as aesthetic as tooth-coloured restorations. The benefits vs risks of aesthetic restorations versus metallic need to be discussed with patients. More destructive preparations associated with tooth-coloured restorations ↑ the chance of pulpal problems. Fracture of porcelain from PFM crowns can be a problem.

Principles
- Remove enough tooth substance to allow adequate thickness of gold, i.e. 1.5mm on functional cusp, 1mm elsewhere, following original tooth contours.
- Wide bevel on the functional cusp (normally buccal—lowers, palatal—upper) for structural durability.
- Convergence of opposing walls <10°.
- Height of axial walls as great as possible (without compromising occlusal reduction).
- Chamfer finishing line.
- Where possible, margins should be supragingival and on a sound tooth substance.

Preparation
Occlusal
Using a short diamond fissure bur reduce the cusp height, maintaining the original anatomy.

Bucco-lingual
With a torpedo-shaped bur eliminate undercuts, retaining 5° taper in cervical two-thirds, but usually remaining one-third will converge occlusally.

Approximal
Using a fine tapered diamond bur within the confines of the tooth, eliminate undercuts at an angle of 5°.

Finishing
Round axial line angles and cusps. Check no undercuts and smooth preparation with fine diamonds.

See impressions, ⊃ Impression techniques, p. 668, and temporary coverage, ⊃ Temporary restorations, p. 270.

Porcelain fused to metal crown

Used where a combination of strength and aesthetics is needed. Preparation is similar to the full veneer gold crown except that where porcelain coverage is required, more tooth substance must be removed. The amount of porcelain coverage must be decided before the preparation is commenced, and the patient consulted at this stage to make sure that they are happy.

Occlusal reduction If acceptable to the patient, it is better to provide an all-metal occlusal surface, as less tooth substance needs to be removed. If not and an all-porcelain occlusal surface is required, 2mm will need to be removed from the supporting cusps and 1.5mm from the non-supporting cusps, which will compromise retention in teeth with short clinical crowns and vitality.[22] Porcelain occlusal surfaces can also introduce occlusal interferences and wear of the opposing teeth if unglazed.

Buccal reduction 1.2–1.5mm should be removed to provide enough room for the metal and porcelain.

Margins If it is acceptable to the patient, it is better to produce a metal to tooth margin, which will necessitate a narrow collar of metal around the gingival margin. In this case, the finishing line prepared should be a deep chamfer or a bevelled shoulder. If the patient insists on a porcelain to tooth margin then a 1.2–1.5mm shoulder must be produced. Where no porcelain coverage is needed, a chamfer finishing line is produced, as for the full veneer gold crown.

All ceramic crowns

These new systems (e.g. In-Ceram®, Empress I and II®, Procera®, Techceram) are built on high-strength alumina cores and may be used for posterior crowns. Zirconia all-ceramic restorations have high strength and are relatively opaque compared to glass-based etchable ceramics, and therefore can mask underlying darker substrates.

Single-rooted posterior teeth can be treated as anterior teeth (⊕ Anterior post and core crowns, p. 264). In multirooted teeth there is divergence of the root canals. Preformed posts can be cemented into one or more canals. Amalgam may also be packed into the coronal aspect of the root canals (Amalcore or Nayyar technique) and an amalgam core built up, which is the preferred technique. RMGIC or resin composite may also be used. These materials have the advantage that the preparation can be completed at the same visit. A dentine adhesive system should be used with resin composite to enhance retention.

A gold shell or porcelain-bonded crown can be used for the final restoration.

---

22 W. P. Saunders & E. M. Saunders 1988 *Br Dent J* **185** 137.

Temporary restorations

Indications
- Protection of pulp and palliation of pulpal pain.
- Restoration of function.
- Stabilization of active caries prior to permanent restoration.
- Aesthetics.
- Maintenance of position of prepared and adjacent teeth.
- To prevent over-eruption of opposing teeth.
- To prevent gingival overgrowth.

Temporary dressings
Choice of material depends upon the main purpose of the dressing, i.e. therapeutic or structural, but the dressing must also be capable of promoting a good seal and being readily removed. For palliation of pulpal pain ZOE is indicated, along with medicaments such as Odontopaste® (contains 5% clindamycin hydrochloride and 1% triamcinolone acetonide). For caries control, a calcium hydroxide liner and traditional GIC or RMGIC. If the remaining tooth tissue requires support, this can be gained using an orthodontic band. The interim seal during RCT is very important, a relatively strong material which prevents microleakage (e.g. GIC) should be used.

Temporary crowns
Three main types:

Preformed
- Polycarbonate crown (e.g. Directa™), which is trimmed to correct shape and customized by lining with a bis-acryl material (e.g. Protemp™). NB: roughen the inside of the crown to facilitate retention.
- SS crowns.

Laboratory custom-made Advisable if preparing multiple crowns or if temporary crown needs to last for several months while other aspects of Rx are completed. Preferred method for temporary bridges.

Chair-side This is a versatile technique. Crowns are custom-made using an alginate impression or putty index of the tooth taken prior to preparation as a mould. When the preparation is completed, any undercuts should be blocked out with carding wax to prevent the temporary crown material locking in the mouth. The material for the crown is then syringed into the impression/index of the prepared tooth/teeth and re-seated in the mouth. When the initial set has been reached the impression is removed and the temporary left to finish curing before being polished. Suitable materials are Protemp™ (a bis-acryl resin) and Trim™ (poly-*n*-butyl methacrylate). Care must be taken when using the latter due to high exotherm on curing. An alternative technique is to make the putty index of a diagnostic wax-up. This approach is useful for multiple crowns or where changes are being made to shape of teeth/occlusion/aesthetics. Applicable to both anterior and posterior crowns.

If preparing several adjacent teeth, consider linking temporary crowns to aid retention.

Temporary post and core crowns Some systems (e.g. ParaPost®) come complete with temporary posts, otherwise they can be made at the chair-side with a suitably sized piece of wire. The length of the post should be adjusted so that it protrudes 2–3mm out of the canal without interfering with the occlusion. A one-piece temporary post and crown is made either by the chair-side method (◑ Temporary crowns, p. 270) or with a polycarbonate crown-former and acrylic.

Temporary bridges The best type is made in the laboratory in acrylic and re-lined at the chair side. Alternatively, make a chair-side bridge using the diagnostic waxing.

Veneers Temporary coverage is usually not necessary, but if the patient complains of sensitivity tack a temporary composite veneer to the prepared surface by etching a spot of enamel.

Temporary inlays A light-cured temporary material (e.g. Fermit™, Clip™) is useful.

Temporary cements The preferred material is TempBond® or similar. Fears about eugenol-containing cements and subsequent use of resin composite materials are unfounded as the etching stage removes residual eugenol from the dentinal tubules.

Restorative dentistry 3: replacing teeth

Relevant pages in other chapters Occlusionl, ➔ p. 234;
acrylic and other denture materials, ➔ Denture materials—
acrylic resins, p. 680; casting alloys, ➔ p. 670; impression materials ➔ p. 666.

Further reading D. W. Bartlett 2004 *Clinical Problem Solving
in Prosthodontics*, Churchill Livingstone. D. Ricketts & D. W.
Bartlett 2011 *Advanced Operative Dentistry: A Practical Approach*,
Churchill Livingstone. G. A. Zarb et al. 2013 *Prosthodontic
Treatment for Edentulous Patients: Complete Dentures and Implant-
supported Prostheses*, Elsevier.

Treatment planning for patients with missing teeth

Solutions for missing teeth will vary depending on the number, their location and function, and the patient's wishes. A minimally invasive approach is preferable where possible. Twenty-one or more is considered the minimum number of teeth consistent with a functioning dentition but this may vary depending on the patient's age, pattern of tooth loss, and incisal relationship. Replacement of missing teeth, therefore, isn't always necessary. The Adult Dental Health Survey in 2009 showed that 86% of dentate adults had 21 or more natural teeth but this proportion ↓ significantly as age ↑.[1] In 2009, 6% of adults aged 16yrs or over were edentulous compared with 37% in 1968. These edentulous patients are also in the older age groups.

For those with insufficient teeth for satisfactory function and aesthetics, fixed or removable prosthodontic solutions will be needed. The use of bonding techniques and implants can help minimize unnecessary destruction of valuable tooth tissue.

Indications for the replacement of missing teeth

- ↑ masticatory efficiency.
- Improve speech.
- Preserve or improve health of the oral cavity by preventing unwanted tooth movements (vertical/rotational/tipping/drifting).[2]
- Improve distribution of occlusal loads.
- Space maintenance.
- Restore aesthetics.
- Prepare patient for complete dentures.

Treatment planning for the replacement of missing teeth

History Active listening in order to clarify the patient's aims and expected outcomes is essential.

It is important to enquire about previous denture history (just because a patient is not wearing a denture does not mean that they have not had one) and assess the reasons for failure or success.

PMH Medical factors can impact upon availability for Rx and ability to cope with dentures. Some drugs may ↓ salivary flow.

Social history Other considerations may affect Rx, e.g. transport arrangements.

Clinical examination EO and IO examinations, including a thorough assessment of any pathology, remaining teeth, existing restorations, periodontium, and edentulous areas (ridge form and extent, compressibility of mucosa). Assess tongue size, tonicity of the lips, and the volume and viscosity of saliva. An evaluation of any current dentures: what to copy and what to correct. Some patients present with a collection of unsuccessful dentures!

---

1 Health and Social Care Information Centre (ℬ http://www.hscic.gov.uk).

2 H. L. Craddock et al. 2007 *J Prosthodont* 16 485.

Special investigations Radiographs/sensibility testing (especially of potential bridge abutments). Mounted study models and wax-up in partly dentate cases.

Diagnoses These are then listed and will allow appropriate Rx planning after considering the Rx options. If pre-existing denture problems are diagnosed, some could be addressed via modifications to the existing dentures prior to embarking on the construction of replacement prostheses.

Options for the replacement of missing teeth

No replacement First consider whether benefits of replacing missing teeth (improved mastication, speech, occlusal stability, and aesthetics) outweigh disadvantages (↑ oral stagnation, tooth preparation, cost). If not, then replacement is C/I. An occlusion with the second premolar to the second premolar present in each jaw (shortened dental arch) is usually functionally adequate.

Bridges (➜ Bridges, p. 278.) These have the advantage that they are fixed. Resin-bonded cantilever design is minimally invasive. Conventional bridges can have good appearance, but are destructive of tooth tissue, moderately expensive, and require lengthy clinical time.

Implant-supported prostheses These can be fixed or removable and have the advantage of avoiding preparation of natural teeth but involve surgical procedures and are expensive. They help maintain supporting bone and have a high level of predictability if carefully planned and carried out.

Removable partial dentures (➜ Removable partial dentures—principles, p. 292.) These can be minimally invasive as only minor (or no) tooth preparation is required but ↑ plaque accumulation/changes in composition. Damage to soft tissues and remaining teeth is exacerbated by poor denture design and/or lack of patient care. Can be a good option when there are multiple edentulous areas or as a training/interim appliance prior to F/F. Can be used to replace missing soft tissue and aesthetics can be very good but patients often dislike removable prostheses.

Complete immediate dentures These are indicated for patients who have already mastered wearing a partial denture and whose remaining teeth have a poor prognosis.

Complete dentures These require patient compliance as well as good clinical and technical management for success. They can replace hard and soft tissue, but patients tend to dislike them and successful denture control can be difficult for patients to master.

In the older, partially dentate patient it is important to assess whether the patient is likely to retain some functional teeth for the remainder of their lifespan. If this is improbable, some advocate providing F/F dentures while the patient is still young enough to adapt.

Orthodontic space closure This is an option that is seldom used but may be appropriate, particularly in the imbricated dentition.

Treatment planning If replacement is indicated: consider fixed or removable prosthesis. A number of factors affect this decision (Table 7.1).

These factors need to be favourable if expensive and complex bridgework is required. Removable prostheses are indicated if general or local factors are less than ideal. Always consider implants or shortened dental arch therapy.

Treatment options These must be clearly explained to the patient with the advantages and disadvantages of each. This is essential in the management of expectations and to allow informed consent.

Initial treatment
- Relief of pain and any emergency Rx including temporary modification of existing dentures, if indicated.
- Unless immediate dentures are planned, extract any teeth with hopeless prognosis. Consider extraction of teeth with poor prognosis.
- OHI and periodontal Rx.
- Preliminary design of partial denture.
- Carry out restorations required.
- Modify design if necessary and commence prosthetic Rx (◆ Removable partial dentures—clinical stages, p. 300).
- Removal of pathological abnormalities (e.g. retained roots), and pre-prosthetic surgery, if required.
- Carry out definitive prosthetic Rx.

Table 7.1 Fixed or removable prosthesis?

General	Local
Patient's motivation/condition	OH and periodontal health
Age	Number of missing teeth
Health	Position of missing teeth
Occupation	Occlusion
Cost	Condition of potential abutments
	Length of span
	Degree of resorption

Bridges

Definitions

Bridge (fixed partial denture) A prosthetic appliance that is definitively attached to remaining teeth and replaces a missing tooth or teeth.

Abutment A tooth which provides attachment and support for a bridge.

Retainer The part of the fixed prosthesis that is cemented or bonded to an abutment tooth in order to provide retention. In the case of an implant, this may be screw or cement retained.

Pontic The artificial tooth that is suspended from the abutments.

Connector The component that joins the pontic to the retainer. May be rigid or non-rigid.

Saddle The area of edentulous ridge over which the pontic will lie.

Units Number of units = number of pontics + number of retainers.

Retention Prevents removal of the restoration along the path of insertion or vertical direction of the preparation.

Support The ability of the abutment teeth to bear the occlusal load on the restoration.

Resistance The features of tooth preparation that enhance the stability of a restoration and resists dislodgement along an axis other than the path of placement.

Types of bridge

Fixed–fixed The pontic is anchored to the retainers with rigid connectors at either end of the edentulous span. Both abutments provide retention and support. Both preparations must have at least one common path of insertion to allow the prosthesis to be fully seated.

Fixed–movable The pontic is anchored rigidly to the major retainer at one end of the span and via a movable joint to the minor retainer at the other end (Fig. 7.1). The major abutment provides retention and support while the minor abutment provides support only. This design allows some independent movement of the minor abutment and has the advantage that the preparations need not be parallel.

Direct–cantilever Pontic is anchored at one end of the edentulous span only.

Spring cantilever A tooth-retained, mucosal-supported bridge. The retainer and pontic are remote from each other and connected by a metal bar which runs along the palate. Usually an upper incisor is replaced from the premolars or a molar. It is useful where there is an anterior diastema or if the posterior teeth are heavily restored; however, they are often poorly tolerated. These are rarely used now.

Minimal or no preparation resin-bonded bridges Retained by resin composite (➔ Resin-bonded bridges, p. 288). May be adhered by glass ionomer adhesives when considered for temporary purposes.

Compound/hybrid Combination of more than one of the types listed.

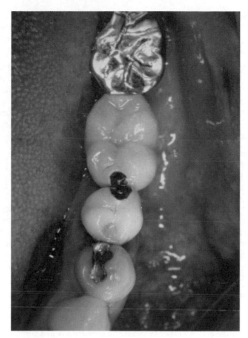

Fig. 7.1 Fixed movable bridge replacing the lower left first permanent molar.

Removable Can be used to describe screw-retained implant bridges and removable partial dentures. Can be removed by dentist for maintenance.

Types of retainers
- Full coverage crown.
- Three-quarter crown.
- Onlay.
- Inlay.

All of these restorations have been used as retainers in conventional bridgework. They are listed in order from most retentive to least retentive. Wherever possible, one of the first two should be used, as the failure rate of the last three is much higher. Post crowns should be avoided if possible, and onlays or inlays should only ever be used as minor retainers in fixed–movable bridges. It is ideal to aim for equal retention on abutments unless deliberately trying to 'build in' a failure point.

Selection of abutment teeth

General factors must be taken into account, e.g. caries status and existing restorations. Also, two other considerations specifically relate to bridgework—*retention* and *support*.

Assessment of retention Retention offered by a potential abutment tooth depends on clinical crown height and the available surface area. It is important to assess the amount of enamel present for retention for resin-bonded bridges. Obviously, larger teeth offer more retention and should be chosen in preference to smaller ones. The teeth of both arches are listed in Table 7.2 in order of the amount of retention offered (if a full coverage restoration is used).

Assessment of support Three factors are important:
1. *Crown–root ratio*. Ideally should be 2:3 but 1:1 is acceptable. As bone is lost, the lever effect on the supporting tissues is ↑.
2. *Root configuration*. Widely splayed roots provide more support than fused ones.
3. *Periodontal surface area*. Ante's law, 'the combined periodontal area of the abutment teeth must be at least as great as that of the teeth being replaced', has no scientific basis and no longer has a place in contemporary bridgework design. It does not take into account that we are dealing with a biological system—as the load is ↑ on the abutment teeth, a biofeedback mechanism operates to cause a reduction in this load.

The teeth of both arches are listed in Table 7.3 in order of the support offered, assuming that the periodontal tissues are intact.

Taper and parallelism
- For most designs, abutments should be prepared with a common path of insertion.
- Opposing walls of abutments should have a 6° taper or a total degree of convergence of 12°.
- Checking parallelism: direct vision, with one eye; survey mirror with parallel lines inscribed.
- Management of tilted abutments (➲ Tilted abutments, p. 282).

Types of pontic

Modified ridge lap This type of pontic should make (minimal) contact with the buccal aspect of the ridge. Gives good aesthetics and is the most popular type.

Bullet Makes point contact with the tip of the ridge. Can be used for posterior bridgework.

Ovate Aims to address the issue of emergence profile in the maxillary anterior region. Has greater mucosal contact and applies light pressure to the underlying mucosa. Needs a smooth, convex surface to allow flossing. The patient must have excellent OH. The 'modified ovate pontic' lies slightly more labial to the ovate pontic, so tends to be used more in aesthetic areas.

Table 7.2 Assessment of retention

	Greatest	→	→	→	→	→	Poorest
Maxilla	6	7	4	5	3	1	2
Mandible	6	7	5	4	3	2	1

Table 7.3 Assessment of support

	Greatest	→	→	→	→	→	Poorest
Maxilla	6	7	3	4	5	1	2
Mandible	6	7	3	5	4	2	1

Hygienic Does not contact saddle, therefore supposedly easy to clean but can still be challenging and may lead to food packing if insufficient clearance. Unaesthetic, therefore limited to molar replacement.

Saddle (ridge lap) Extends over ridge buccally and lingually, therefore difficult to clean. Should not be used.

Bridges—design

Designing bridges

- Assess prognosis of all teeth in vicinity to ↓ risk of another tooth requiring extraction in the near future.
- Assess possible abutment teeth (check restorations, endodontic status, periodontal condition, mobility, and take periapical radiographs).
- Select design of retainers, e.g. full or partial crown. Full coverage is preferred.
- Consider pontics and connectors.
- With this information compile a list of possible bridge designs.
- Consideration of the advantages and disadvantages of each design combined with a diagnostic wax-up should help to narrow down the choice. Where possible, try the least destructive alternative first.

Specific design problems

Periodontally involved abutments First control periodontal disease. Then consider whether a bridge is indicated. A fixed–fixed type of design is preferable to splint teeth together. Consider fibre-reinforced resin composite fixed partial dentures for this specific indication.

Pier abutments This is the central abutment in a complex bridge that supports pontics on either side, which are in turn anchored to the terminal abutments. In this situation, the pier abutment can act as a fulcrum and when one part of the bridge is loaded the retainer at the other end experiences an unseating force which can lead to cementation failure. To overcome this a stress-breaking element must be introduced, e.g. fixed–movable joint, or avoid pier abutments by simplifying the design.

Tilted abutments Occurs most commonly following loss of a molar. There are several approaches if bridgework is planned:
- Orthodontic Rx to upright abutments.
- Two-part bridge, e.g. fixed–movable.
- Telescopic crowns—placement of individual gold shell crowns on abutments, over which the telescopic sleeves of the bridge fit.
- Precision attachments—a precision screw and screw tube can be incorporated into a two-part bridge. After cementation the screw is inserted, which effectively converts the bridge to a fixed–fixed design.

Canines The canine is often the keystone of the arch, and a very difficult tooth to replace. The adjacent teeth are poor in terms of the amount of retention and support that they offer and the canine is often subject to enormous stresses in lateral excursion (in a canine-guided occlusion). If a canine is to be replaced with a bridge, the occlusal scheme should be designed to provide group function in lateral excursion—never canine guidance.

Bridges—practical stages

As always, a thorough history and examination are required (➲ Treatment planning for patients with missing teeth, p. 274). It is essential to clarify the patient's attitude to and expectation of Rx. They must be assessed for active disease due to poor OH or diet and for pre-existing TMD. The response to initial Rx to stabilize active disease should be monitored before embarking on definitive Rx. If bridgework is planned, the following stages are carried out:

- *Diagnostic mounting*—take accurate impressions of both arches, a facebow record, and have the models mounted on a semi-adjustable articulator. The mounting can be carried out either in ICP (best fit) or in RCP, for which a precentric record will be necessary. If a reorganized approach to reconstruction is being considered, or if the clinical examination has revealed significant occlusal interferences, an RCP mounting should be performed. Carefully examine the occlusion and consider what occlusal consequences the proposed restoration will have.

- *Diagnostic waxing*—in effect, this is a mock-up of the final restoration on the mounted models. Wax can be added to the teeth to simulate the effect that the restoration will have on the final occlusion and aesthetic result. In the anterior part of the mouth a denture tooth can be used. In addition to assessing aesthetics and occlusion, the diagnostic wax-up can serve as a template from which the temporary bridge can be constructed. An impression is taken of the wax-up in a silicone putty and saved for later. At this stage, the design of the prosthesis must be finalized.

- *Preparations*—before the preparations are carried out, any suspect restorations in the abutment teeth are replaced. Preparations are carried out in accordance with basic principles (see Chapter 6) and care is taken to ensure that a single path of insertion is established. When checking for parallelism, one eye should be kept closed and the use of a large mouth mirror is very helpful. Custom-made paralleling devices can be used but they are very cumbersome.

- *Temporary bridge*—this is normally constructed using the matrix which has been formed from the diagnostic wax-up; in this way the temporary bridge should reproduce the aesthetics and occlusion of the final bridge (if the wax-up was done properly!). The matrix is filled with one of the proprietary temporary crown and bridge resins (e.g. Protemp®) and seated over the preparations. After it has set it is removed, trimmed, polished, and cemented with a temporary cement (e.g. TempBond®). Or a laboratory-made temporary bridge may be used. The pontic should be contoured so that it is hygienic (e.g. to a modified ridge lap design).

- *Impressions*—an impression is taken using an elastomeric material. Ideally, all of the preparations should be captured on one impression, but this can be very difficult if multiple preparations are involved. If difficulties are encountered in this respect, they can often be overcome by using the transfer coping technique. In this technique, acrylic (DuraLay®) copings are made on dies of the preparations for which a successful impression has been achieved. These are then taken to the mouth and seated on the appropriate tooth, and the impression repeated to capture the other preparations. On removal, the coping will be removed in the impression and the dies can be reseated in the copings and a new model poured around them. CAD/CAM digital techniques can also be used.

- *Occlusal registration*—under most circumstances the models will be mounted in ICP in the position of best fit, and therefore an occlusal registration will not be necessary. Where numerous preparations have been carried out and it is difficult to locate this position, or where there is a lack of AP stability in the models, some form of inter-occlusal record will be necessary. A popular technique involves the use of transfer copings, and is described in the section on occlusion (◆ Occlusal records, p. 237).

- *Metal work try-in*—if a porcelain fused to metal bridge is being constructed, it is advisable to try-in the metal work before the porcelain is added, particularly for larger span bridges. At this stage the fit of the framework can be evaluated and the occlusion adjusted. On occasions it will be found that one retainer seats fully while the other does not. This can occur if there has been some minor movement of the abutments since the impression was taken. If this is the case the bridge should be sectioned, and hopefully both retainers will then seat. The two parts are then secured in their new position with acrylic resin (DuraLay®) and sent back to the laboratory for soldering.

- *Trial cementation*—the finished bridge is tried in and any necessary adjustments made. The bridge should then be temporarily cemented (with modified TempBond®) for a period of a week or so. The advantage of a trial cementation period is that if any further adjustments are necessary they can be carried out outside the mouth and the restoration repolished and reglazed. The patient is instructed in how to clean the bridge (use of Super Floss® or an interdental brush).

- *Permanent cementation*—after the period of trial cementation, the bridge is re-evaluated and the patient asked if they are happy with it. If all is well the bridge is removed and cemented with a permanent cement (usually traditional or RMGIC).

- *Follow-up*—arrangements are made to recall the patient to check that the bridge is still functioning satisfactorily.

Bridge failures

Patients should be warned about these prior to Rx.

Most common reasons for failure

- Loss of retention.
- Mechanical failure, e.g. # of casting.
- Problems with abutment teeth, e.g. 2° caries, periodontal disease, loss of vitality.

Management of failures Depending upon type and extent of problem:

- Keep under review.
- Adjust or repair *in situ*.
- Replace.

Replacement Before replacement of a bridge is embarked upon, a careful analysis of the reasons for failure is necessary. Minor problems in an otherwise satisfactory bridge should be repaired if at all possible. Fractured porcelain can be repaired with one of the specialized repair kits available (e.g. CoJet™). 2° caries or marginal deficiencies, if small, can be restored with traditional GIC. Failure may be due to loss of vitality. This is not necessarily an indication for removal of the bridge because RCT can often be carried out through the retainer of the abutment.

Removing old bridges   To remove intact, try a sharp tap at the cervical margin with a chisel or preferably a slide hammer. Orthodontic band-removing pliers can also be used but these require a small hole to be cut in the occlusal surface. If only one retainer is loose, support the bridge in position while trying to remove it so that it does not bind.

Retainers can be cut through, but this will destroy the bridge.

Resin-bonded bridges

This technique involves bonding a cast metal framework, carrying the pontic tooth, to abutment teeth using an adhesive resin. This type of bridge is almost exclusively used for cantilever adhesive bridgework, i.e. one abutment and one pontic (Fig. 7.2). Fixed–fixed designs have been problematic, with one retainer debonding being a common clinical finding. The resin bonds to the abutment tooth using the acid-etch technique and to the metal framework by either mechanical or chemical means. Fibre-reinforced bridges are also available.

Classification
Position
- Anterior.
- Posterior.

Retention
- Macromechanical:
  - Perforated (Rochette).
  - Mesh (Klett-O-Bond®).
  - Particular (Crystalbond™).
- Micromechanical:
  - Electrolytically etched (Maryland).
  - Chemically etched.
- Chemical:
  - Sandblasted.
  - Tin-plated.

Chemical retention to a sandblasted metal surface is now used virtually exclusively. A dual-affinity cement (e.g. Panavia™ 21) is used, which chemically bonds to both enamel and non-precious alloys.

Advantages
- Less expensive than conventional bridge or cobalt chromium partial denture or implant in the shorter term.
- Minimal or no tooth preparation required.
- No LA required as preparation is in enamel.
- Potential for rebond if debond occurs.

Disadvantages
- Tendency to debond especially if planning and preparation and placement technique is poor.
- Metal may show through abutments.
- Creation of a natural emergence profile can be challenging especially in very resorbed ridges. Use of an ovate pontic can be helpful.

Indications
- Short span-single tooth edentulous space.
- Sound abutment teeth (or only minimal restoration) and sufficient crown height to ensure sufficient surface area for acid etch bonding.
- Favourable occlusion.

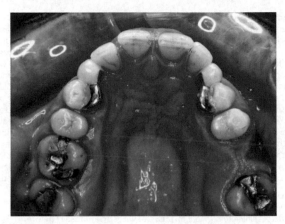

Fig. 7.2 Adhesive cantilever bridgework replacing missing upper canines.

Treatment planning This is as for conventional bridgework. If orthodontic Rx is needed to localize space or upright adjacent teeth, it is advisable to retain with a removable retainer for at least 3 months prior to bridge placement.

Design The design is usually cantilever. If a fixed–fixed design is used and there is a debond of one retainer, caries can develop quickly and undetected under this retainer. Fixed–fixed design may be used if periodontal splinting is required or retention required following orthodontics.

Tooth preparation There is debate as to what is the 'ideal' preparation and some advocate no preparation. The need for preparation will be defined by the individual clinical situation.

Guidelines for preparation
- Give a single path of insertion. Provide near-parallel guiding planes eliminating undercuts, which allow coverage of maximal surface area for bonding.
- Provide space in occlusion to accommodate bridge. Need at least 0.7mm for wings.
- ↑ retention, e.g. using a wrap-around design (covering >180° of tooth circumference) to resist lateral displacement and reduce stress on the cement bond.
- Mesial and distal grooves enhance resistance form.
- To prevent gingival displacement a minimal chamfer is recommended.
- Provide axial loading of the abutments—prepare cingulum or occlusal rests.
- A connector height of at least 2mm is required.

NB: tooth preparation should usually be confined to enamel, and the framework should be designed with maximal coverage (to ↑ surface area available for bonding).

Technique
Chemical method using Panavia™ 21 Following tooth preparation an elastomeric impression of the abutment teeth is taken plus an alginate impression
of the opposing arch. At the try-in stage the bridge should be assessed
for fit, aesthetics, etc., and then the fitting surface thoroughly cleaned with
alcohol (assessment of occlusion may not be possible until after cementation). Contamination of the fitting surface with saliva must be avoided
and cementation is best done under a rubber dam. Following etching and
washing of the abutment(s), and placement of a dentine adhesive system,
the wings of the bridge are coated with Panavia™ 21 and the bridge seated
into place and held firmly until set. Use of acetate strips and Super Floss®
at this stage will clear most of the excess cement and prevent it adhering
to the adjacent teeth. The cement must then be covered with a substance
known as OxyGuard®, which prevents O_2 inhibition of the surface layer.
After 3min the rubber dam is removed and any excess cement removed.

Problems
- *Dentine exposed during preparation.* Use a dentine adhesive system.
- *Metal shining through abutments.* Cut wings away incisally before
  cementation or use a more opaque cement. May have to consider
  conventional bridge or placing veneer on labial surface.
- *Debonds.* If one flange only, can usually detach other by a sharp tap
  with a chisel or by using ultrasonic scaler tips. If a persistent problem,
  consider conventional bridge. The trend is for these bridges to be used
  for cantilevered bridgework and it is not usual for fixed–fixed adhesive
  bridgework to be prescribed due to problems with unilateral debonding.
- *Caries occurring under debonded wings.* Remove bridge and repair.

Further reading
D. S. Thomas, et al. 2017 Article I. A systemic review of the survival
and complication rates of resin-bonded fixed dental prostheses after
a mean observation period of at least 5 years. *Clin Oral Implants
Res* **28** 11.

Removable partial dentures—principles

Definitions

Saddle That part of a denture which rests on and covers the edentulous areas and carries the artificial teeth and gumwork.

Connector (major and minor) Joins together component parts of a denture.

Support Resistance to vertical forces directed towards mucosa.

Retainers Components which resist displacement of denture.

Indirect retention Resistance to rotation about fulcrum axis by acting on the opposite side to the displacing force. Retention of the denture may be possible through other means as opposed to clasping, such as guide planes.

Fulcrum axis Axis around which a tooth- and mucosa-borne denture tends to rock when saddles are loaded.

Bracing Resistance to lateral movement.

Reciprocation The mechanism by which lateral forces generated by a retentive clasp passing over a height of contour are counterbalanced by a reciprocal clasp passing along a reciprocal guiding plane.[3]

Guide planes Two or more parallel surfaces on abutment teeth used to limit the path of insertion, and improve retention and stability.

Survey line This indicates the maximum bulbosity of a tooth in the plane of the path of withdrawal.

Free-end saddle Edentulous area posterior to the natural teeth.

Stress-breaker A device allowing movement between the saddle and the retaining unit of partial denture.

Gum-stripper A tissue-borne partial denture which can 'sink'.

Swinglock denture Has a labial retaining bar or flange which is hinged at one side of the mouth and locks at the other.[4]

Sectional denture Made in two or more sections which are then fixed together with screws or other devices.

Classification

Kennedy Describes the pattern of tooth loss (Fig. 7.3):
I.   Bilateral free-end saddles.
II. Unilateral free-end saddle.
III. Unilateral bounded saddle.
IV. Single, anterior bilateral bounded saddle. Must cross the midline.

Any additional saddles are referred to as modifications (except Class IV), e.g. Class I modification 1 has bilateral free-end saddles and an anterior saddle.

---

3 🔗 https://www.academyofprosthodontics.org/_Library/ap_articles_download/GPT9.pdf.

4 M. Chan et al. 1998 *Dent Update* 25 80.

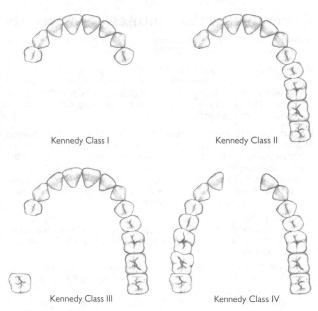

Fig. 7.3 Kennedy classification.

Craddock Describes the denture type:
- Tooth-borne.
- Mucosa-borne.
- Mucosa- and tooth-borne.

Acrylic versus metal dentures

Approximately 75% of the dentures provided in the UK have an acrylic connector and base. Although metal bases are generally preferred because the greater strength of metal permits a more hygienic design, an acrylic base is indicated for:
- Temporary replacement, e.g. following trauma or in children.
- Where there is inadequate support from the remaining teeth for a tooth-borne denture.
- When additions to the denture are likely in the near future.

However, where financial constraints C/I a metal base, attention to the following may avoid the production of a gum-stripper:
- Wide mucosal coverage to provide maximum support.
- Keep base clear of the gingival margins wherever possible.
- No interdental extensions of acrylic.
- Point contact and wide embrasures between natural and artificial teeth.
- Labial flanges for extra retention and bracing.
- Additional support from wrought SS rests.

Removable partial dentures—components

Saddles These can be made entirely of acrylic or have a sub-framework of metal overlaid by acrylic.

Rests These are an extension of the denture onto a tooth to provide support &/or prevent over-eruption. Occlusal rests are used on posterior teeth (usually over either the mesial or distal marginal ridge and fossa) and cingulum rests on anterior teeth. Rests may be wrought or cast; the latter is preferred for strength and fit.

Clasps These provide direct retention by engaging the undercut portion of a tooth (Fig. 7.4 and Fig. 7.5). The action of a clasp must be resisted either by a non-retentive clasp arm above the maximum bulbosity of the tooth or by a reciprocal connector. Clasps can be classified by their position (occlusally approaching or gingivally approaching) or by their construction and material. A minimum length of 14mm is generally advocated for cobalt–chrome clasps to prevent rapid distortion.

Cast Cast (cobalt–chrome) clasps are stiff, easily distorted, and liable to #. However, provided they are limited to undercuts of 0.25mm, the advantage of being able to cast them as an integral part of a denture framework offsets these drawbacks.

Wrought Wrought clasps are usually attached by insertion into the acrylic of a saddle. SS is the most commonly used alloy, but gold clasps are more flexible and easily adjusted (and distorted).

The stiffer the wire, the smaller the undercut that can be engaged. This can be offset by reducing the diameter of the wire to ↑ flexibility (but ↑ the likelihood of #) or by ↑ the length of the clasp arm (e.g. gingivally approaching clasp). Cast cobalt–chrome can be too stiff for occlusally approaching clasps on premolar teeth. The actual design used depends upon:

- Depth of undercut: 0.25mm—cast cobalt–chrome; 0.5mm—SS wire; <0.75mm—wrought gold.
- Position of undercut on tooth and relative to saddle, e.g.:
  - High survey line: gingivally approaching clasp or modify tooth shape by grinding.
  - Diagonal survey line, (i) sloping down from saddle: gingivally or occlusally approaching (ring or recurved) clasp; (ii) sloping up from saddle: gingivally or occlusally (circumferential) approaching clasp.
  - Medium survey line: as for previous bullet point.
  - Low survey line: modify tooth shape, e.g. with resin composite.
- Position of tooth. Gingivally approaching clasps are less conspicuous and are therefore preferred for anterior teeth.
- Occlusion: adequate inter-occlusal space should be present or created for a clasp arm to cross a contact point between two natural teeth, to prevent occlusal disruption.
- Shape of sulcus: fraenal attachments and alveolar undercuts may prevent use of gingivally approaching clasps.
- Periodontal health: reduced periodontal support requires more flexible clasps to avoid overload.
- Material of denture base. Cast clasp arms are easily cast as part of the framework but for acrylic dentures wrought clasps are more usual.

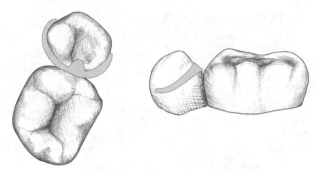

Fig. 7.4 Occlusally approaching three-arm clasp. One arm is the bracing reciprocal arm. One arm is the retentive component. One arm is the occlusal rest.

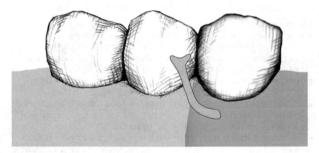

Fig. 7.5 Gingivally approaching T clasp.

Table 7.4 P/− connectors

	Patient tolerance	Indirect retention	Support	Comments
Ant. bar	−	+	−	Useful for Kennedy IV
Mid. bar	+	−	++	C/I torus
Post. bar	++	+	−	Need muco-compression
Ring	−	++	+	
Plate	+	++	++	Less hygienic
Horseshoe	+	+	++	Useful for multiple saddles

Connectors In addition to joining parts of the denture together, the connector can also contribute to support and retention (Table 7.4).

−/P connectors
- Lingual bar should only be used if there is >7mm between floor of mouth and gingival margin to give 3mm clearance from gingivae. Does not contribute to indirect retention. Usually cast. C/I if incisors are retroclined. If insufficient space can use sublingual bar.
- Sublingual bar lies horizontally in anterior lingual sulcus, but opinions differ as to patient tolerance. More rigid than lingual bar.
- Lingual plate is well tolerated and provides good support, bracing, and indirect retention if used in conjunction with rests but covers gingival margins. Can be made of cast metal or acrylic.
- Continuous clasp is really a bar which runs along the cingulum of the lower anterior teeth and is usually used in conjunction with a lingual bar. Poorly tolerated.
- Dental bar is similar to continuous clasp, but of ↑ cross-sectional area and without lingual bar. Useful for teeth with long clinical crowns. Provides support and indirect retention. May not be well tolerated.
- Buccal/labial bar is indicated when the lower incisors are retroclined.

Fig. 7.4 and Fig. 7.5 show the two most commonly used types of clasp.

Removable partial dentures—design

P/P design is carried out after assessment of the patient and with reference to any previous dentures. A set of accurately articulated study models is essential.

Surveying

Objectives:
- Establish path of insertion.
- Define those undercuts which may be used to retain the denture.
- Define those undercuts which require blocking out prior to finish.

If the path of insertion is at 90° to the occlusal plane, insertion of the denture will be straightforward; however, where the teeth are tilted or few undercuts exist, an angled path of insertion may be advantageous. Whether this provides more resistance to displacement during function is controversial.

A survey line can then be marked on the teeth to indicate their maximum bulbosity in the plane of the path of withdrawal. This is done using a dental surveyor.

Design

- *Outline saddles*. Usually straightforward. If less than half a tooth width or if in doubt of the need to replace a missing tooth, omit.
- *Plan support*. Support can be tooth only, mucosa only, or both. Tooth-borne support (occlusal and cingulum rests) should be used wherever possible, as teeth are better able to withstand occlusal loading and support will not be compromised following resorption. Tooth and mucosa support are inevitable with large or free-end saddles and where plate designs are used. Tissue-only support should be utilized when no suitable teeth are available, and is less damaging in the upper than the lower arch, because of the palatal vault.
- Need to assess the role of the denture, length of the saddles, the amount of support required (? denture opposed by natural or artificial teeth), and the potential of remaining teeth to provide support (root area in bone), before a final decision is made.
- *Obtain retention*. Retention can be:
  - Direct. E.g. clasps, guide planes, soft tissue undercuts, or precision attachments. Of these, clasps are the most commonly used. The best arrangement is to use three clasps as far away from each other as possible. Guide planes help to establish a precise path of insertion and withdrawal. Need be only 2–3mm in length, reducing reliance on clasps. Composite resin can be added to abutment teeth to maximize undercuts.
  - Indirect. This is derived by placing components so as to resist 'rocking' of the denture around direct retainers, e.g. by the position of clasps and rests and the type of connector. Particularly important with free-end and large anterior saddles.
- *Assess bracing required*. Bracing is provided by the connector, maximum saddle extension, and the reciprocal arms of clasps. Elimination of occlusal interferences ↓ need for bracing.
- *Choose connector*. After consideration of earlier listed points. Is there space in the occlusion to accommodate the chosen connector? Where possible, the connector should be cut away from the gingival margins.
- *Reassess*. ? As simple as possible. ? Aesthetic.

- *Instructions to technician.* Should include written details and diagram. Where some confusion may arise over the precise position of a component, it may be helpful to mark this directly on the cast. CAD programs are now available for design, communication, and production of prostheses.

Some design problems

The lower bilateral free-end saddle (Class I) This presents a particular problem because of a lack of tooth support and retention distally, small saddle area compared to force applied, and distal leverage on abutment tooth in function (which ↑ with resorption). Possible solutions include:

- Maximize indirect retention by placing rests and clasps on mesial aspect of the abutment tooth and using lingual plate design.
- Using a muco-compressive impression of saddle area to ↓ displacement in function—the altered cast technique.
- Use fewer, smaller teeth and maximize base extension.
- RPI system for distal abutment teeth—mesial *Rest*, distal guiding *Plate*, and mid-buccal *I* bar. During function the saddle moves tissue-ward and rotates around the mesial rest. The plate and I bar are constructed in such a way as to disengage from the tooth and avoid potentially harmful loading.
- Stress-breaker design (advantages more theoretical than practical).
- Use precision attachments (beware of overloading abutments).

Class IV Can sometimes avoid unsightly clasps anteriorly by the use of:
- A flange engaging a labial alveolar undercut.
- Avoiding distal facing clasps. A mesial-facing clasp will engage more as the anterior saddle tries to drop/rotate out.
- A rotational path of insertion[5] utilizing rigid minor connectors that are rotated into proximal undercuts anteriorly.
- Interproximal undercuts, which may allow minimal display of clasps—'hidden clasps' (Fig. 7.6).
- An acrylic spoon denture held in place by the tongue.

Multiple bounded saddles A horseshoe design, which utilizes guide planes for retention, may be indicated.

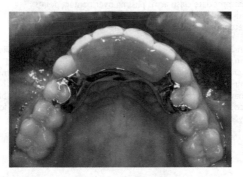

Fig. 7.6 Sectional partial denture (Implant bar retained).

5 T. W. Chow et al. 1988 *Br Dent J* **164** 180.

Removable partial dentures—clinical stages

- *Assessment and treatment plan.* ➲ Treatment planning for patients with missing teeth, p. 274.
- *Take first impressions.* These are usually taken using alginate in a stock tray. For free-end saddles modify the tray first with compound or silicone putty.
- *Record occlusion.* If ICP is obvious, the occlusion can be recorded conventionally (➲ Occlusal examination, p. 236) at the same visit as first impressions. If ICP is not obvious, wax record blocks will be required and a separate visit. Where there are no teeth in occlusal contact, the steps involved are the same as for recording the occlusion for F/F (➲ Complete dentures—recording the occlusion, p. 308). If there is an occlusal stop, but insufficient standing teeth to produce a stable relationship of the casts, the procedure is as follows:
  - Determine the occlusal vertical dimension (OVD) and mark the position of two index teeth with pencil.
  - Define the occlusal plane using the record block on which this is easiest, e.g. tooth to tooth in a bounded saddle, tooth to retromolar pad in a free-end saddle.
  - Check the record blocks in the mouth, using the mark on the index teeth as a guide, and adjust blocks if necessary.
  - Record occlusion with bite-recording paste.
  - Check the relationship of the index teeth on the articulated casts corresponds to that in the mouth.
- *Mounted casts are surveyed and denture designed* (➲ Occlusal considerations for restorative procedures, p. 236).
- *Tooth preparation* may be required to:
  - Accommodate rest seats. Rests need to be >1mm for strength, therefore if insufficient room in occlusion to accommodate this bulk, tooth reduction is required.
  - Establish guide planes.
  - Accommodate clasp arms passing over contact points.
  - Modify unfavourable survey line, e.g. ↓ bulbosity.
  - ↑ retention, e.g. by the addition of resin composite to create undercuts.
  - Consider crowning teeth with a poor long-term prognosis prior to denture construction.
- *Record second impressions* using a special tray. Alginate is the most commonly used material, but elastomers are preferable. It is helpful to have a wax try-in before the framework is made. This enables you to confirm the tooth position so that the retentive elements for the acrylic are placed appropriately.

- *Try-in of framework:*
  - Check extension, adaptation, and position of clasp, and rests. If casting does not fit, use of correcting fluid may reveal which areas to relieve.
  - Check upper and lower separately for OVD and occlusion, and then together.
  - Major faults: repeat second impressions.
  - Minor faults: adjust at finish.
  - Re-record occlusion, if required.
  - Select tooth mould and shade.
  - Altered cast technique, if required.
- *Try-in of waxed denture on framework:*
  - Check position of denture teeth.
  - Check flange extensions/thickness.
  - Check OVD and occlusion.
  - Check aesthetics with patient and only proceed when patient is satisfied.
  - Prescribe post-dam relief areas and management of undercuts.
- *Finish.* Once any fitting surface roughness is eliminated, the dentures are tried in separately, adjusting undercuts and contacts as required. The extension, occlusion, and articulation are then adjusted if necessary. Give the patient written and verbal instructions, and a further appointment.

Rebasing P/P Acrylic mucosa-borne dentures can be rebased at the chair-side with self-cure materials, but difficulty may be experienced in removing the denture in the presence of undercuts, and the materials are generally inferior to the original denture base. Alternatively, P/P can be rebased in the laboratory by means of a technique similar to that used for F/F (● Rebasing, p. 314). Alternatively, make a new denture. For cast metal dentures an impression can be recorded of the saddle area using an elastomer or ZOE, while holding the denture by the framework. In all cases care must be taken to avoid the introduction of occlusal errors, e.g. ↑ OVD.

Immediate complete dentures

When the remaining teeth have a poor prognosis, the transition from the partly dentate to edentulous state must be managed carefully. Patients must be warned about the effects of resorption and the need for early rebasing/replacement. Rx planning must be thorough.

Rx alternatives for partial denture wearer
- A gradual transition towards being edentulous via additions to a transitional P/P can ↑ the chances of successful adaptation to F/F especially for the older patient.
- Immediate complete denture. This has the advantage that the form and position of the natural teeth can be copied and is said to promote better healing and reduce resorption, but frequent adjustments and early replacement are necessary.
- Overdenture (◑ Overdentures, p. 324); may retain alveolar bone.

Rx alternatives for patients with no previous denture experience
- Provide a partial denture and allow the patient to adapt before progressing to an immediate complete denture—the best solution.
- Extract the majority of posterior teeth leaving sufficient only to maintain OVD and occlusal relationship, and then make immediate complete dentures when resorption has slowed.
- Extraction of the remaining teeth and provision of a denture after healing has occurred (post-immediate denture). Avoid if possible as considerable guesswork is involved in the subsequent denture and the chances of the patient coping successfully are ↓.

Types of immediate complete denture
- *Flanged*. Either full or part (extended 1mm beyond maximum bulbosity of ridge).
- *Open face*. No flange, artificial teeth sit over (or just into) the socket of the natural predecessor.

Flanged dentures are preferable as they afford better retention and make subsequent rebasing easier. However, where a deep labial undercut exists into which it would be impossible to extend a flange, the choice is either surgical reduction or an open-face denture. Most patients choose the latter.

Clinical procedures
- *1° impressions* (as for P/P, ◑ Removable partial dentures—clinical stages, p. 300).
- *2° impressions* in alginate or silicone.
- *Recording occlusion*. Where there are sufficient posterior teeth remaining, a hand articulation should suffice, and this can be taken at the same visit as impressions are recorded. Otherwise, record blocks will be required.
- *Try-in*. This will be limited to those teeth that are already missing. Check fit, extension, and stability, etc. In addition, need to prescribe:
  - Type of flange required.
  - Any proposed changes in position of anterior artificial teeth compared to natural teeth.

- *Extraction* of remaining teeth as atraumatically as possible.
- *Finish.* Repeated removal and insertion of the denture should be avoided, therefore adjustments should be limited to making the patient comfortable. They should be instructed not to remove the denture before the review appointment in 24h.
- *Review.* The fitting and occlusal surfaces are adjusted as required. If dentures are unretentive they will require temporary reline (➔ Denture problems and complaints, p. 318).
- *Recall.* Regular inspection of immediate dentures is important as rapid bone resorption means that they will require rebasing early. However, this should be deferred, if feasible, for at least 3 months after the extractions. A possible regimen is 1 week, 1 month, 3 months, 6 months, and then yearly.

Laboratory procedures These are similar to F/F except that the plaster teeth are removed and the cast trimmed to mimic the changes that will occur in the hard and soft tissues following extraction, before final processing.

Surgical procedures See ➔ The extraction of teeth, p. 383 and ➔ Minor pre-prosthetic surgery, p. 426.

Problems
- *Denture unretentive.* Use a temporary reline material (replaced regularly) to tide patient over initial 3 months and then reline with heat-cure acrylic.
- *Gross occlusal error.* Adjust occlusal surface of one denture until even contact attained. This denture can then be replaced after initial resorption has occurred.

Complete dentures—principles

Retention The resistance of a denture to displacement. It is dependent upon (i) peripheral seal, (ii) contact area between denture and tissues, (iii) close fit, and (iv) viscosity/volume of saliva. Neuromuscular control has more to do with stability than retention.

Stability The ability of a denture to resist displacing forces during function. Influenced by forces acting on polished and occlusal surfaces, as well as the form of the supporting tissues.

Neutral zone The area where the muscular displacing forces are in balance.

Ways to optimize retention and stability
- Maximum extension of denture base (as far as the surrounding musculature will allow). The upper denture should extend distally over the tuberosities and onto the compressible tissue just anterior to the vibrating line on the palate. The lower denture should extend the full depth and width of the lingual pouch, and halfway across the retromolar pad. NB: over-extension will result in a denture that is easily displaced in function.
- As close an adaptation of denture base to mucosa as possible, to maximize the surface tension effects of saliva.
- Placement of the teeth in the neutral zone. More important in −/F. The better retention of F/− often allows some latitude in this respect.
- Correct shape of the polished surfaces so that muscle action tends to re-seat the denture.
- A good border seal. This is achieved by ensuring that the flanges fill the entire sulcus width and by placing a post-dam on compressible tissue.
- Balanced occlusion free from interfering contacts.

Common denture faults
- Lack of freeway space (FWS).
- Failure to reproduce closely enough the features of previous successful dentures.
- Occlusal errors.
- Incorrect adaptation and extension.

Complete dentures—impressions

▶ Tissues must be healthy before final impressions are recorded. If necessary, use tissue conditioner in present F/F (➓ Tissue conditioners, p. 314).

Classically, two sets of impressions are recorded of the edentulous mouth. The purpose of the first is to record sufficient information for a special tray to be made in which to record the second or master impression.

Preliminary impressions

These are recorded using an (edentulous) stock tray and alginate, elastomer (both preferable for undercut or flabby ridges), or impression compound. A line should be marked on the impression to indicate to the technician the desired extension of the special tray. In the upper, the posterior limit should be the hamular notches and the vibrating line, and in the lower the retromolar pads.

Special trays These can be made in self-cure or light-cure acrylic. The space left for the impression depends upon the material to be used: ZOE = 0.5mm; elastomer = 0.5–1.5mm (depending on viscosity); alginate = 3mm. For trays with >1mm space use greenstick stops clinically to aid positioning.

Master impressions

These aim to record the maximum denture-bearing area, and to develop an effective border seal, the functional width and depth of the sulcus. The special tray should be modified by reducing any over-extension and the peripheries adapted by the addition of greenstick tracing compound. Non-perforated trays ensure that a peripheral seal with the upper tray can be demonstrated before taking the impression. However, a perforated tray reduces the compression of tissue leading to a more mucostatic impression. Gently manipulate the patient's soft tissues and ask them to slightly protrude their tongue to imitate functional movements.

Muco-compressive versus muco-static A muco-compressive impression technique is sometimes advocated to give a wider distribution of loading during function and to compensate for the differing compressibility of the denture-bearing area, thus preventing # due to flexion. ZOE or composition is used. However, dentures made by this method are less well retained at rest, which is the greater proportion of time. Alginate is said to be more muco-static. Tissue adaptation following a period of use probably reduces the clinical difference between the two techniques.

Special techniques

Neutral zone impression technique This is used for recording the neutral zone in patients with limited natural retention for −/F.
- Record second impressions and occlusion.
- A fully extended acrylic baseplate is made on the lower cast, with wire loops added which do not extend above the occlusal plane.
- The upper trial denture or record block is inserted.
- Tissue conditioner is placed on the baseplate and around loops, and inserted.
- Ask patient to swallow, purse lips and say 'Ooh' and 'Eee'.
- The impression is removed and trimmed down until it can be fitted onto the articulator to replace the lower occlusal rim.

- A mould of the impression is made into which wax is poured.
- The wax is cut away so that each denture tooth can be positioned within the zone recorded to make the trial denture. The polished surfaces should replicate the impression.

Flabby (displaceable) ridge Classically occurs under a F/− opposed by nat- ural lower teeth. If mild, then an impression recorded with alginate or elastomer in a tray perforated over the flabby area may suffice. For more severe cases a two-stage technique is required, using a special tray with a window cut out over the flabby tissue. First, an impression is recorded in the tray with ZOE and the paste trimmed away from the flabby area. This is then re-seated and low-viscosity elastomer or impression plaster placed into the window to complete the impression. NB: combination type cases should have the dentures constructed on a semi-adjustable articulator to minimize occlusal displacing forces.

Functional impression Tissue conditioner is placed inside the patient's existing denture. After several days of wear a functional impression is produced.

Common impression problems and faults

- A feather edge indicates under-extension. This can be corrected by the addition of greenstick to the tray and repeating.
- Tray border shows through impression material. Reduce tray in the area of over-extension and repeat the impression.
- Air blows. If small, can be filled in with a little soft wax. If large, retake the impression, or if using silicones or ZOE the impression may be added to.
- Tray not centred. Often partially due to using too much material so that it is difficult to see what is where. Remember to line up the tray handle with the patient's nose (except for ex-boxers).
- Retching. A calm and confident manner is necessary for successful impressions. Gain the patient's confidence by attempting the lower first and use a fast-setting, viscous material. Distraction techniques may help, e.g. wriggling the toes on the left foot and the fingers of the right hand at the same time (the patient, not the operator).
- Patient with dry mouth: ZOE is C/I; use elastomer instead.
- Areas where tray shows through in otherwise good impression. Can be overcome by prescribing a tin-foil relief when dentures are being processed.

Complete dentures—recording the occlusion

When recording the occlusion with wax rims mounted on rigid acrylic or shellac bases, the aim is to provide the technician with information for constructing trial dentures.

As head posture can affect FWS, position the patient so that the Frankfort plane is horizontal. A wax trimmer and a heat source are required to adjust the rims.

- Check fit of bases. If poor, can either repeat second impressions, or take a ZOE or low-viscosity elastomer impression with the base and proceed.
- Adjust upper rim to give adequate lip support.
- Trim occlusal plane of upper rim.
  - *Position of the occlusal plane.* This should be placed so that ~1–2mm (↓ with age) of tooth are visible below the patient's upper lip at rest. The occlusal plane should lie midway between the ridges parallel to the inter-pupillary and the ala-tragal lines. At rest, the tongue should rise just above the lower occlusal plane posteriorly. Centre lines, canine lines, and smile line should be marked.
- Trim lower record block to obtain correct lip support and bucco-lingual position of posterior teeth.
- Adjust lower rim so that it meets upper evenly in RCP, with 2–4mm of FWS:
  - *Vertical dimension.* The FWS is the space between the occlusal surfaces of the teeth when the mandible is in the rest position. In the majority of patients it is 2–4mm. The OVD for an edentulous patient can therefore be determined by measuring their resting face height and subtracting a FWS. Resting face height is assessed using:
    - A Willis gauge, to measure the distance between the base of nose and the underside of the chin. Is only accurate to ±1mm.
    - Spring dividers, to measure the distance between a dot placed on both the chin and the tip of the patient's nose. This method is less popular with patients and is C/I for those with a beard.
    - The patient's appearance and speech.
- Mark the centre lines.
- Locate rims in RCP, e.g. with bite-recording paste:
  - *Horizontal jaw relationship.* Record the more reproducible RCP. In the natural dentition, ICP is ~1mm forward of RCP; some prosthetists advise adjusting the finished dentures to allow the patient to slide comfortably between the two positions.
- Prescribe mould and shade of artificial teeth for try-in.
- Consider using a facebow registration to mount the maxillary cast on the articulator.

Position of the anterior and posterior teeth

Ideally, the artificial teeth should lie in the space occupied by the natural denti-tion. The extent to which it is possible to compensate for a Class II or III mal-occlusion depends upon the retention afforded by the ridges. In the natural dentition the upper incisors lie ~10mm anterior to the posterior border of the incisive papilla. With resorption this comes to lie on the ridge crest, there-fore the artificial teeth should be placed labial and buccal to the ridge, to give adequate lip support and a nasolabial angle of ~90°.

Posterior teeth should be narrow to ↑ masticatory efficiency. Low-cusped teeth are preferred, but cuspless teeth are useful for patients with poor natural retention or a 'wandering' ICP. When considering the colour, mould, and arrangement of the anterior teeth, the patient's age, facial ap-pearance, and most importantly their opinion, must be considered. If you disagree about the suitability of their choice, document it.

Type of articulator to be used for setting up the teeth

Most textbooks advocate semi-adjustable or average value articulators for F/F dentures. However, most dentures are made on simple hinge articula-tors to the satisfaction of the majority of patients, probably because they are able to adapt to the occlusion that results. An average value type is the preferred method. It will give some degree of balanced articulation which can then be refined in the mouth and will help avoid the introduction of occlusal interferences.

Common pitfalls

- Inaccuracies caused by poorly fitting bases.
- Rims contacting prematurely posteriorly and flipping-up anteriorly, or vice versa.
- Failure to provide adequate FWS. This is less likely to occur if the rest position is recorded with only one denture or rim in position.
- Attempting to correct too much when replacing old worn dentures and exceeding the adaptive capacity of the patient.

Complete dentures—trial insertion

Trial dentures are constructed by setting-up the prescribed teeth in wax on acrylic or shellac bases. Both the dentist and patient must be satisfied before the dentures are processed in acrylic.

Clinical procedures

Check the trial dentures

- On and off the articulator. Comparison with the patient's existing dentures is helpful to see if the features to be copied or modified have been successfully incorporated.
- Singly in the mouth. To check extension, stability, and the position of the teeth relative to the soft tissues.
- Together in mouth. Examine vertical dimension, occlusion, aesthetics, and phonetics ('S' sound will be affected by ↑ or ↓ FWS).

Seek the patient's opinion Some advocate getting patients to sign an acceptance slip before going to finish.

Prepare post-dam This should be placed just anterior to the vibrating line on the palate, which can be assessed by asking patient to say 'Aah'. The degree of compressibility of the tissues is assessed and the depth of the post-dam cut accordingly (usually ~1mm). The post-dam is recorded by marking the master impression with indelible pen and prepared on the upper cast with a wax knife in the shape of a Cupid's bow.

Complete prescription to the technician This should include:

- Any changes in posterior tooth position or anterior tooth arrangement.
- For fibrous undercuts >4mm and bony undercuts >2mm, decide whether they are to be plastered out or the flange thickened for adjustment at finish.
- Tin-foiling for relief of hard or nodular areas, if required.
- Gingival colour and contour.
- Denture base material. This is usually heat-cure acrylic; however, metal bases are indicated for patients with a history of fractured dentures.
- Identification marker, which is preferably legible.

Common problems and possible solutions

- Over-extension of flanges. Reduce.
- Under-extension of flanges. Try a temporary wax addition to flange first, to check effect of extending it. If this is satisfactory a new impression is required.
- Teeth outside neutral zone. Remove offending teeth and replace with wax which can be trimmed until correct.
- Incorrect OVD. If too small, can ↑ by adding wax to the occlusal surfaces of teeth, but if too large, will need to replace lower teeth with wax and re-record OVD.
- Occlusal discrepancy or anterior open bite or posterior open bite. Replace lower posterior teeth with wax and re-record OVD.

- Too little of upper anterior teeth visible. Reset anterior teeth to correct position and ask the laboratory to adjust occlusal plane accordingly.
- Too much of upper anterior teeth showing. The effect of reducing the length of the incisors can be judged by colouring the incisal region with a black wax pencil and then indicating desired change in position to lab.
- Inadequate lip support. An ↑ in support can be assessed by adding wax to the labial aspect of the upper try-in.

A new try-in will be required if large errors are being corrected or if any doubt still exists about the occlusion.

Complete dentures—fitting

Some adjustment of completed dentures is inevitable following processing. On average, a 0.5mm ↑ in height occurs and a slight shift in tooth contact posteriorly. The main steps are:

Adjustment of fitting surface First, smooth any roughness and if necessary gradually reduce the bulk of the flanges in areas of undercut until the denture can be easily inserted without compromising retention.

Check occlusion The vertical dimension of the dentures is maintained by contact between the upper palatal and lower buccal cusps, therefore adjustment of these should be avoided if possible.
- Get patient to occlude and check contact with articulating paper. If contact uneven, or heavy contacts seen, adjust the fossae.
- For cusped teeth only, place articulating paper between occlusal surfaces and ask patient to make small lateral movements and adjust buccal upper and lower lingual ('BULL' rule) cusps only to remove any interferences.
- Remove any interferences to protrusive movements.
- Balancing contacts are desirable, but not essential unless they can be established easily by minor adjustments to working side contacts. Some authorities suggest providing even occlusal contact only at the time of fitting, allowing the patient to adapt to their new dentures before trying to achieve balanced articulation.

Advice to the patient Verbal and written instructions should be given.
- Most patients take some time to adapt to their new dentures. During this time a softer diet is advisable.
- If pain is experienced, the patient should try to continue wearing their dentures and return for adjustment as soon as possible so that affected areas can easily be seen. If this is not possible, they should stop wearing the dentures until 24h prior to the next visit.
- Although patients should be encouraged not to wear their dentures at night, adaptation may be speeded up if they are worn full-time for the first 1–2 weeks.
- When the dentures are not being worn they should be stored in water to prevent them drying out and warping. Plastic denture boxes are cheap, and safer than a glass of water at the bedside.
- Cleaning (⊃ Cleaning dentures, p. 316).

Review The patient should be seen 1–2 weeks after fitting to ease the dentures and adjust the occlusion. Localization of the cause of any irritation due to a flaw on the fitting surface can be helped by:
- Pressure relief cream which is painted onto the fitting surface of the denture.
- Indelible pencil, or denture fixative powder mixed with zinc oxide, which is applied carefully to the area thought to be responsible and the denture inserted. On removal, the mark will have been transferred to the adjacent mucosa and should correspond with the damaged area.
- If there is no obvious cause relating to the fitting surface remember that occlusal faults can cause displacement and mucosal trauma, and an excessive OVD is a common cause of generalized soreness under −/F (➋ Denture problems and complaints, p. 318).

Stress the importance of regular review to all patients with dentures.

Denture maintenance

▶ Review patients with F/F annually. Regular maintenance will help prevent damage due to ill-fitting dentures and will ↑ the likelihood of early detection of oral pathology.

Problems caused by lack of aftercare of F/F

As a result of resorption all dentures become progressively ill-fitting, → loss of retention and stability. Movement of dentures in function may result in:
- Resorption.
- Predisposition to candidal infection.
- Denture irritation hyperplasia (◆ Problems in denture wearers, p. 426).
- Inflammatory papillary hyperplasia of the palate.

All of these are exacerbated by wear of the occlusal surfaces.

Rebasing

The terms 'rebasing' and 'relining' are commonly used interchangeably. Strictly speaking, relining is replacement of the fitting surface (e.g. with a temporary material) and rebasing is replacement of most or all of the denture base.

Rebasing is indicated where the only feature of F/F that requires improvement is the fitting surface; otherwise consider replacement F/F using the copy method. For rebasing, the material of choice is heat-cure acrylic (◆ Denture materials—rebasing, p. 682), but this necessitates the patient being without their dentures while the addition is being made. Self-cure acrylic applied at the chair-side appears attractive, but its properties are inferior. For a heat-cure rebase, a wash impression (ZOE or low-viscosity elastomer) must be recorded inside the denture.

Technique To avoid an ↑ in OVD, record the impression for one denture at a time.
- Check occlusion and adjust if required. Note OVD.
- Remove undercuts from fitting surface.
- Correct extension and place post-dam in greenstick.
- Apply impression material and insert in mouth. Get patient to close into contact with opposing denture. Check OVD and occlusion.
- Remove and examine impression; if unsatisfactory (or if in doubt) repeat.

An alternative method for inflamed tissues is to record a functional impression (◆ Functional impression, p. 307) over several days with a tissue conditioner (e.g. Visco-gel®), in which case the resulting impression needs to be cast immediately.

Tissue conditioners (e.g. Coe-Comfort™, Visco-gel set®)

These are r0esilient materials which give a more even distribution of loading and thus promote tissue recovery. They are particularly useful where ill-fitting dentures have caused trauma, as it is important to allow the tissues to recover before impressions for replacement dentures or a rebase are taken.

Technique Relieve any areas of pressure on the fitting surface and re-duce any over-extension. A minimum thickness of 2mm is required and the material should not be left for >1 week. Repeated applications may be necessary.

Tissue conditioners can also be used after pre-prosthetic surgery. They become less soft with time therefore they should be replaced at least weekly.

For patients who have very atrophic ridges and who struggle with denture wearing, a definitive soft lining aimed at distributing stresses more evenly to the denture bearing area may be helpful, e.g. GC reline™ or Permasoft®. GC reline™ may also be used to engage bony undercuts.

Soft linings These are indicated for:
- Older patients with a thin atrophic mucosa. Usually for −/F.
- Following prosthetic surgery.
- To utilize soft tissue undercuts for ↑ retention, e.g. following hemimaxillectomy, clefts.

It is wise to make a new denture first in acrylic and adjust the occlusion, before placing soft lining. A minimum thickness of 2mm is required, which may significantly weaken a lower denture necessitating placement of a metal strengthener on the lingual aspect. No material is ideal and soft linings are best avoided (➲ Soft liners, p. 682).

Cleaning dentures

When new dentures are fitted, the importance of regular, thorough cleaning, especially of fitting surfaces, with soap, water, and a brush to prevent the build-up of plaque, stain, and calculus should be emphasized. Unfortunately, few patients are sufficiently diligent, due in part to being conditioned by advertising, to expect to use a denture cleaner.

Advise patients to clean their dentures over a basin of water to act as a safety net (Table 7.5).

Practical tips Hypochlorite solutions are effective for acrylic dentures when used overnight, but if used with hot water are liable to cause bleaching, therefore warn patient.[6] The peroxide cleaners are popular but are ineffective if used for only 15–30min as the manufacturers advise. See Table 7.6.

Table 7.5 Cleaning dentures—formulations

Formulation	Active ingredients	Problems
Powder	Abrasives, e.g. calcium carbonate	Abrasion
Paste	Abrasives + eugenol	Abrasion + crazing
(Dentu-creme®)	Abrasive + phenol oil	Abrasion + sensitivity
Hypochlorite (Dentural®)	Sodium hypochlorite	Can corrode metal
Effervescent (Steradent®)	Dissolves to give alkaline peroxide solution	Doubts about effectiveness
Dilute acids (Denclen®)	3–5% hydrochloric acid or 5–10% phosphoric acid	Can corrode metal
Enzymatic	Proteolytic enzymes	Not widely available

Table 7.6 Cleaning dentures—peroxide cleaners

	Avoid	Use
Visco-gel®	Acids, alkaline peroxide	Hypochlorite
Molloplast®	Acids, alkaline peroxide	Hypochlorite
Coe-Comfort™	Hypochlorite, alkaline peroxide	Soap + water
Metal denture	Hypochlorite	Alkaline peroxide
Any denture	Household bleach	

6 C. A. Crawford et al. 1986 *J Dent* **14** 258.

Denture problems and complaints

The most common complaints are of pain and/or looseness, which can be due to denture errors or patient factors. The latter should be foreseen and the patient warned in advance of the limitations of dentures. Unless the cause is immediately obvious, e.g. a flaw on the fitting surface, a systematic examination of the fitting and the polished and occlusal surfaces (including the jaw relationship) should be carried out.

Pain This can be due to a variety of causes, including roughness of the fitting surface, errors in the occlusion, lack of FWS, a bruxing habit, a retained root, or other pathology. Forward or lateral displacement of a denture due to a premature contact can lead to inflammation of the ridge on the lingual or lateral aspect, respectively. With continued resorption, bony ridges become prominent and the mental foramina is exposed, which can lead to localized areas of specific pain.

Pain from an individual tooth on P/P
- Excessive load and/or traumatic occlusion.
- Leverage due to unstable denture.
- Clasp arm too tight.

Looseness This more commonly affects the lower than the upper denture (Table 7.7).

Burning mouth This can be due to (i) local causes, e.g. ↑ OVD or sensitivity to acrylic monomer, or be unrelated to the denture (e.g. irritant mouth washes, candidiasis); or (ii) systemic causes, e.g. the menopause, deficiency states, cancerophobia, or xerostomia.

Cheek biting Check first that teeth are in the neutral zone. If satisfactory, ↓ buccal 'overjet', i.e. reduce buccal surface of lower molars (provided there is a normal bucco-lingual relationship).

Speech See Table 7.8.

Retching
- Map out extent of sensitive area on palate using a ball-ended instrument and firm pressure, and check extension of denture.
- Palateless dentures may be a solution, but their retention is poor.
- Training dentures. These can take the form of a simple palate to which teeth are added incrementally, starting with the incisors.
- Hypnosis.
- Implants (➔ Introduction to implantology, p. 361) and a fixed prosthesis.

Table 7.7 Denture faults—looseness

Denture faults	Patient factors
Incorrect peripheral extension	Inadequate volume of saliva
Teeth not in neutral zone	Poor ridge form
Unbalanced articulation	↓ adaptive skills, e.g. elderly patient
Polished surfaces unsatisfactory	

Table 7.8 Denture faults—speech

Patient's complaint	Possible cause
Difficulty with f, v	Incisors too far palatally
Difficulty with d, s, t	Alteration of palatal contour
	Incorrect overjet and overbite
An s becomes th	Incisors too far palatally
	Palate too thick
Whistling	Palate vault too high behind incisors
Clicking teeth	OVD
	Inadequate FWS
	Lack of retention

The grossly resorbed lower ridge Resorption is progressive with time, which is a good argument for avoiding rendering young patients edentulous. The mandible resorbs more quickly than the maxilla, which exacerbates the problem of retention for −/F. Management is dependent upon the severity of the problem and the patient's biological age.
- Minimizing destabilizing forces upon the lower denture, e.g.
  - Maximum extension of denture base.
  - ↓ number and width of teeth.
  - ↑ FWS.
  - Lowering occlusal plane.
- Neutral zone impression technique (Ɔ Special techniques, p. 306).
- Surgery (Ɔ Problems in denture wearers, p. 426).
- Implants (Ɔ Introduction to implantology, p. 361).

Recurrent fracture Apart from carelessness, this is usually caused by occlusal faults or fatigue of the acrylic due to continual stressing by small forces. Flexing of the denture can occur with flabby ridges, palatal tori, and following resorption. Notching of a denture, e.g. relief for a prominent fraenum, can also predispose to #. Rx depends upon the aetiology, but in some cases provision of a metal plate or a cast-metal strengthener may be necessary.

Candida and dentures

Candida is a common oral commensal. It becomes pathogenic if the environment favours its proliferation (e.g. dentures, ↑ carbohydrate intake, antibiotic alteration of the bacterial flora) or the host's defences are compromised (➲ Oral candidosis (candidiasis), p. 438).

Denture stomatitis

Also known as denture sore mouth, a misnomer because the condition is usually symptomless. Classically, seen as redness of the palate under a F/ − denture, with petechial and whitish areas. 90% of cases due to *Candida albicans*, 9% to other *Candida* spp., and <1% to other organisms, e.g. *Klebsiella* spp.

Incidence A common condition, having been reported in 30–60% of patients wearing F/F. It affects F more commonly than M, in a ratio of 4:1, and usually affects the upper denture-bearing area only.

Aetiology This is still not completely understood.
- Infection with *Candida* spp.
- Poor denture hygiene.
- Night-time wear of dentures.
- Trauma is often cited as a contributing factor to denture stomatitis, *but*:
  - It occurs more commonly under F/− than −/F.
  - It can affect patients wearing F/− only.
  - It is also found under well-fitting orthodontic appliances.
- Systemic factors can predispose to *Candida* infection, e.g. iron and vitamin deficiency, steroids, drugs which cause xerostomia, and endocrine abnormalities.
- A high sugar intake provides substrate for *Candida* to multiply.

Management
- Patients should be encouraged to remove their dentures at night.
- They should cleanse denture thoroughly, e.g. brushing fitting surface and soaking in hypochlorite cleanser.
- New dentures may be required if these measures fail despite good compliance. The denture can act as a reservoir for *Candida*.
- Reduce sugar intake.
- Miconazole gel can be added to the fitting surface of the denture before insertion.
- If suspect systemic factors exacerbating condition, refer to GMP.
- Coexisting papillary hyperplasia of palate may need surgical reduction.
- Systemic fluconazole may be used in some cases.

Angular cheilitis See ➲ Chronic candidosis, p. 438.

Denture copying

Successful function with complete dentures depends to a marked degree upon the patient's ability to control them. This ability is learnt during a period of denture use. When replacement dentures become necessary, it is helpful if the new appliances require as little adaptation as possible to the existing skills. This is generally considered to be particularly important for the older patient. Not only may skills have been developed over a long period, but also the ability to relearn may be diminished. So-called denture copying techniques provide a more reliable method for provision of replacements.

Treatment planning Before undertaking Rx it is essential to decide which features of the previous dentures are satisfactory, and which require modification, and by how much. Consider:

- Fitting surface—if this is the only feature that requires improvement, then rebasing is a possibility.
- Polished surface shapes.
- Occlusal surface; jaw relationship; OVD. The effect of an ↑ in OVD can be assessed by self-cure addition to the existing dentures (occlusal pivots), but remember that this irreversibly alters them.
- Anterior tooth size, arrangement, and relation to lips.
- Posterior tooth mould and arch width (relation to tongue and cheeks).

Copying complete dentures A number of techniques have been described. They vary in the materials used, and these in turn affect the acceptability of laboratory work, and the clinical freedom to incorporate 'corrections'. In general, copies of the old appliances are used as substitutes for record blocks, and as special trays. A typical method is as follows[7]:

Step 1. Clinic
- Correct under-extension with greenstick tracing compound.
- Record impressions with silicone putty of polished surface and teeth, using large disposable tray. Complete mould with second mix of putty to record fit surface (use a separating medium—white soft paraffin or, better, emulsion hand cream).
- Open mould, clean dentures, and return to patient.
- Send putty moulds to laboratory.

Step 2. Laboratory
- Fabricate self-cure acrylic baseplates on the silicone model of the fit surface.
- Pour wax into remaining space.
- After cooling remove completed copy, cut off sprues, and polish.

Step 3. Clinic
- Employ the copies ('replica record blocks') to record required changes in denture shapes (➋ Treatment planning, p. 322), by adding or removing wax. Record working impressions in low-viscosity silicone *with adhesive* to aid retention on base.
- Record jaw relationship with 'bite recording paste'.
- Select shade/moulds for new teeth.

7 R. Yemm 1991 *Int Dent J* **41** 233.

Step 4. Laboratory
- Cast impressions and articulate.
- Set-up, cutting away modified replica rims to substitute new teeth (rather like setting up an immediate denture).
- Wax-up, including borders defined by working impressions.

Step 5. Clinic
- Try-in stage.

Step 6. Laboratory
- Finishing stages as normal.

Step 7. Clinic
- Normal insertion stage (and subsequent review).

Other methods use alternative materials (e.g. alginate for impressions of existing dentures, wax, and shellac to form the copy dentures). Choice will depend on acceptability to both clinic and laboratory. In no instance, however, is an all-wax copy regarded as being acceptable, since rigidity is inadequate for use as an impression tray.

Copying partial dentures for immediate dentures In patients with successful P/P, for whom extraction of the remaining teeth is planned, the transition to complete dentures can be facilitated by using a copy technique.[8]

Clinic 1 Correct under-extended flanges with greenstick and then take impressions of the dentures with putty in stock trays (see F/F technique, ➲ Copying complete dentures, p. 322). Record an alginate impression of the opposing arch, if no denture is planned for that arch.

Laboratory 1 Wax/shellac or acrylic replica of partial denture is constructed.

Clinic 2 Use the replica denture to develop the prescription and then record a wash impression inside the base with a light-bodied silicone. Record the occlusion using bite registration paste. Finally, take an overall impression in a stock tray with the modified replica denture *in situ*.

Laboratory 2 The impression is cast and used as a base for articulating the wax replica with the cast of the opposing arch. The teeth prescribed are then set up, and the wash impression retained in the replica, for the try-in.
  Try-in and finish as for complete immediate dentures (➲ Immediate complete dentures, p. 302).

8 J. R. Drummond et al. 1983 *Br Dent J* **155** 297.

Overdentures

An overdenture (OD) derives support from one or more abutment teeth or implants by completely enclosing them beneath its fitting surface. It can be a partial or complete denture.

Advantages
- Alveolar bone preservation around the retained tooth.
- Improved retention, stability, and support.
- Preservation of proprioception via PDL.
- Better crown-to-root ratio, which ↓ damaging lateral forces.
- ↑ masticatory force.
- Additional retention possible using attachments.
- Aids transition from P/P to F/F.
- Psychological benefits of maintaining natural teeth.

Disadvantages
- RCT probably required.
- To avoid excessive bulk in region of retained tooth (which may compromise aesthetics), denture base may need to be thinned, which ↑ likelihood of #.
- ↑ maintenance for both patient and dentist.
- Roots may be prone to caries.

Indications
- Motivated patient with good OH.
- Because of ↓ retention and stability of −/F and ↑ rate of mandibular resorption, ODs are particularly useful for −/F or free-end saddle.
- CLP.
- Hypodontia.
- Severe tooth wear.

Choosing abutment teeth
- Ideally: bilateral, symmetrical, with a minimum of one tooth space between them.
- Order of preference: canines, molars, premolars, incisors.
- Healthy attached gingiva, adequate periodontal support (more than half root in bone), and no or limited mobility.
- Is RCT required and if so is it feasible?

Preparation of abutment teeth
Alternatives include:
- If pulps have laid down lots of 2° dentine (e.g. severe tooth wear), can just cut down crowns and place dentine bonding agent.
- Preparation of crown for thimble/telescopic gold coping.
- RCT, tooth cut to dome shape, and access cavity restored with amalgam or an adhesive restoration.
- RCT and gold coping over root face.
- RCT and precision attachment.

Precision attachments These are useful for ↑ retention of dentures or bridges, especially in cases with tissue loss (e.g. trauma or CLP), but they ↑ loading on abutment teeth, and are expensive and difficult to rebase and repair.[9,10] Usually of two parts, which are matched to fit together. One part is attached to the abutment tooth and the other to the denture. A variety of attachments are available, including stud/anchor (e.g. Rotherman eccentric clip), bar (e.g. Dolder), and magnets.

Since precision attachments require the highest technical skill and are highly dependent on patient and professional maintenance, it is wise to first use a basic OD and then reassess the need for additional retention. Hybrid dentures are partial dentures that utilize precision attachments (either intra- or extracoronal) on the abutment teeth for retention. Implants which are inserted in edentulous areas can be used with precision attachments to ↑ retention.

Clinical procedures
- Assessment (clinical examination, study models, X-rays, etc.).
- RCT if required.

If abutment preparation is limited to crown reduction:
- The steps involved are as for immediate dentures, with the abutment teeth reduced less on cast than is planned clinically. At the visit during which the final dentures are to be fitted, the abutment teeth are prepared and the dentures relined with self-cure acrylic to improve their adaptation.

If precision attachments or copings to be used:
- The teeth are prepared and an impression of the abutments, including post holes, taken. In the laboratory, dies are prepared and transfer copings (usually metal) made. The transfer copings are tried on the abutments, and if satisfactory an overall impression is recorded to accurately locate the copings to the remainder of the denture-bearing area. Alternatively, a two-stage technique using a special tray with windows cut out over abutments can be used.
- Regular review (6-monthly) and maintenance is necessary for success.

Problems
The most important are:
- Caries of abutment teeth, therefore need good oral and denture hygiene and topical fluoride, e.g. toothpaste, applied to the fitting surface of the denture. Patients should be encouraged to remove their denture at night.
- Periodontal breakdown.

Restoration of the edentulous mandible
There is good evidence that a patient's satisfaction and quality of life is significantly ↑ with implant-supported ODs than with conventional full dentures. The York Consensus Statement on implant-supported ODs states that 'a large body of evidence supports the proposal that a two-implant-supported mandibular overdenture should be the minimum offered to edentulous patients as a first choice of treatment'.[11]

9 H. W. Preiskel 1984 *Precision Attachments in Prosthodontics*, Quintessence.

10 H. W. Preiskel & A. Preiskel 2009 *Dent Update* **36** 221.

11 British Society for the Study of Prosthetic Dentistry 2009 *Eur J Prosthodont Rest Dent* **17** 164.

Dentistry and the older patient

From a chronological, social, and healthcare planning perspective, being elderly means being >65yrs old. This is entirely different from biological age. Two factors are mainly responsible for the ↑ relevance of dentistry for the elderly: an ↑ in the proportion of the elderly in the population and the improvements in dental health that have resulted in more people keeping their natural teeth for longer. The proportion of edentulous adults in the UK fell from 37% in 1968 to 6% in 2009.[12]

Challenges
- Age changes, both physiological and pathological.
- Disease and drug therapy (see Chapter 13).
- Delivery of care.

Restorative problems
- Reduced adaptive capacity; therefore if teeth are unlikely to last a lifetime, the transition to at least partial dentures should be made while the patient is able to learn the new skills necessary.
- Age changes in the denture-bearing areas, including bone resorption and mucosal atrophy. This leads to reduced masticatory forces and reduced masticatory efficiency.
- Root caries, which can occur following exposure of root surfaces by gingival recession, in association with changes in diet, ↓ self-care, and ↓ salivary flow. Details of management are given in ➲ Root caries, p. 25. Prevention of root caries in susceptible patients is possible using a topical fluoride mouthrinse, high fluoride toothpaste, or fluoride-containing artificial saliva, e.g. Luborant® or Saliva Orthana®.
- Tooth wear (➲ Tooth wear/tooth surface loss, p. 252) is especially prevalent when partial tooth loss has occurred.
- Pulpal changes, including sclerosis (➲ Sclerosed canals, p. 354) and ↓ repair capacity.
- Reduced manual dexterity, making OH procedures difficult. Epidemiological studies of the periodontal needs of the elderly population are still sparse and some trends may be masked by a high rate of edentulousness. The available evidence suggests that, although older patients develop plaque more quickly, the need for periodontal Rx ↑ up to middle age, and thereafter the majority can be maintained by regular non-surgical management.

12 Health and Social Care Information Centre 2009 *Adult Dental Health Survey: Oral Health in the United Kingdom* (♫ http://www.hscic.gov.uk).

Age changes

Age changes are defined as an alteration in the form or function of a tissue or organ as a result of biological activity associated with a minor disturbance of normal cellular turnover.

In general ↓ microcirculation, ↓ cellular reproduction, ↓ tissue repair, ↓ metabolic rate, and ↑ fibrosis. Degeneration of elastic and nervous tissue. These result in reduced function of most body systems.

Oral

Oral soft tissues A ↓ in the thickness of the epithelium, mucosa, and submucosa is seen. Taste bud function ↓. With age, an ↑ occurs in the number and size of Fordyce's spots (sebaceous glands), lingual varices, and foliate papillae. Recent evidence suggests that stimulated salivary flow rate does not fall purely as a result of age. However, medications, head and neck radiotherapy, or systemic disease can affect salivary output.

Dental hard tissues Enamel becomes less permeable with age. Clinically, older teeth appear more brittle, but there is no significant difference between the elastic modulus of dentine in old or young teeth. The rate of 2° dentine formation reduces with age, but still continues. Occlusion of the dentine tubules with calcified material spreads crownwards with age.

Tooth wear is an age-related phenomenon and can be regarded as physiological in many cases. However, excessive and pathological wear can be caused by parafunction, abrasion, erosion (dietary, gastric, or environmental), or a combination of these factors (◑ Tooth wear/tooth surface loss, p. 252).

Dental pulp ↑ fibrosis and ↓ vascularity mean that the defensive capacities of the pulp ↓ with ↑ age, therefore pulp capping is less likely to succeed. Also ↑ 2° dentine and ↑ pulp calcification.

Periodontium ↑ fibrosis, ↓ cellularity, ↓ vascularity, and ↓ cell turnover are found with ↑ age. Gingival recession has been previously thought to be an age change but is now known to be a part of periodontitis.

Systemic

Immune system A ↓ in cell-mediated response and ↓ in number of circulating lymphocytes leads to an ↑ incidence of autoimmune disease as well as a ↓ in the older patient's defence against infection. Also an ↑ in neoplasia is seen. Steroid Rx for autoimmune disease may complicate dental Rx.

Nervous system Ageing involves both a physiological decline in function and dysfunction associated with age-related disease (e.g. strokes, parkinsonism, trigeminal neuralgia). A ↓ in acuity compounds the problem.

Cardiovascular Hypertension and ischaemic heart disease worsen with age. Anaemia is more common in the elderly. In general, the greatest problems arise when a GA is required.

Pulmonary system Lung capacity ↓ with age and chronic obstructive airways disease ↑ in prevalence.

Endocrine system Diabetes is more common.

Muscles ↓ bulk, slower contractions, and less precision of control occur. This is highly relevant to dentures and function.

Nutrition Poverty, impaired mobility, ↓ taste acuity, and ↓ masticatory function can result in nutritional deficiencies in the elderly. These can manifest as changes in the oral mucosa.

Mucosal disease, which is more common with ↑ age
- Oral cancer (**⊃** Oral cancer, p. 452).
- Lichen planus (**⊃** Lichen planus, p. 468).
- Herpes zoster is more common with ↑ age due to a ↓ in T-cell function. Neuralgia occurs more frequently after an attack in the elderly.
- Benign mucous membrane pemphigoid (**⊃** Mucous membrane pemphigoid, p. 444).
- Pemphigus (**⊃** Pemphigus, p. 442).
- Candidal infection is seen more frequently in the older age groups due to an ↑ proportion of denture wearers and ↑ immune deficiencies.

This list is obviously not exhaustive.

Dental care for the elderly

General management problems

Medical and drug history (see Chapter 13.) It is wise to check any complicated medical problems with the patient's GMP or physician. Unfortunately,
many doctors are only familiar with the dental Rx they have personally received, therefore give details of what is proposed.

Communication Communication with the elderly may sometimes require
patience and understanding. Older patients may try to cover up deafness,
poor eyesight, and lack of comprehension, so it is better to err on the side
of over-stressing an important point or instruction, but avoid sounding pat-
ronizing. Active listening and questioning to check understanding is helpful.
It is often helpful to enlist the assistance of a relative or friend of the older
patient (with the patient's consent).

Oral hygiene OH may be compromised by arthritis &/or a stroke. Advise
an electric toothbrush or modifying the handle of an ordinary toothbrush
to make it easier to grip, e.g. with an adhesive bandage or bicycle handlebar
grips. Alternatively, self-cure acrylic can be used to make a custom grip for
a toothbrush.

Delivery of care

Dental practice Consideration should be given to:

- Access for a wheelchair or Zimmer frame. Dental practices are required
  to provide reasonable adjustments to ensure Rx is accessible (Equality
  Act 2010).
- Timing of appointments; e.g. for a diabetic patient these need to be
  arranged around meals and drug regimens, and early morning visits are
  probably C/I for arthritic patients as it may take them a couple of hours
  to 'get going'.
- Positioning of the patient. Some elderly patients are unhappy to be
  recumbent in the dental chair. In addition, this position is C/I for those
  with cardiovascular or pulmonary disease. Adjust dental chair gradually
  as rapid movement from a flat to upright position can result in postural
  hypotension.

Domiciliary care An estimated 12–14% of the elderly population is bed-
ridden or housebound to such a degree that they cannot visit their GMP or
GDP. Domiciliary care aims to provide care for those patients.[13] There is an
↑ demand for domiciliary oral healthcare and guidelines for delivering these
services have been published.[14]

13 D. Lewis & J. Fiske 2011 *Dent Update* **38** 231.

14 British Society for Disability and Oral Health 2009 *Guidelines for the Delivery of a Domiciliary Oral
    Healthcare Service* (🖰 http://www.bsdh.org.uk).

Key points
- Can Rx be carried out successfully?
- Consider maintenance required by any proposed Rx. Elaborate procedures which fail may leave the patient worse off.
- The objective is to maintain optimum oral function. Sometimes retention of a few teeth can be disadvantageous.
- Medical crises (e.g. a period in hospital) can result in a very rapid change in a previously stable oral state (e.g. rapid caries attack, loss of denture-wearing skill through lack of use).
- Avoid sudden changes in occlusion. The shape/form of dentures should not be changed anteriorly. During restorative work refrain from introducing significant occlusal change. If necessary to extract teeth, do so a few at a time, with additions to existing dentures.

Some clinical techniques of particular value in elderly patients
- Adhesive restorations, e.g. GI for root caries.
- Acid-etch bridgework is less destructive to abutments and is therefore more fail-safe.
- Gradual tooth loss, with additions to existing P/P, is less demanding of a ↓ adaptive capacity.
- Replacement dentures should be made with careful regard to existing appliances. Use of copying techniques again ↓ amount of adaptation required.
- If recording the occlusion proves difficult, use cuspless teeth or lingualized occlusion.
- Mark dentures with the patient's name.
- Bleaching and bonding and minimally invasive dentistry should be considered.

Chapter 8

Restorative dentistry 4: endodontics

Principal sources and further reading J. L. Gutmann et al. 2010 *Problem Solving in Endodontics* (5e), Mosby; S. Patel & J. Barnes 2019 *The Principles of Endodontics* (3e), OUP; J. M. Whitworth 2002 *Rational Root Canal Treatment in Practice*, Quintessence.

Preserving pulp vitality

Endodontics is the study of the prevention and management of problems affecting the dentine, pulp, and periapical tissues.

A healthy pulp is essential for:
- Completion of root formation in immature teeth (1° dentine).
- Continued lifelong tooth development (2° dentine).
- Protecting against infection when there is loss of enamel/dentine integrity as a result of caries/trauma/tooth surface loss (reactionary and reparative 3° dentine).
- Maintaining sensory/nociceptive function.
- Maintaining elasticity of dentine.

Infection of the pulp can result in irreversible pulpitis and, if left untreated, periapical periodontitis. The overall aim of endodontic Rx is to prevent or treat periapical periodontitis by controlling infection. This is achieved by disinfecting infected teeth and sealing well thereafter. The scope of endodontics is wider, therefore, than just non-surgical and surgical root Rx but also covers therapies which preserve pulp tissue that has been affected by caries, trauma, and tooth surface loss.

Pulp-preserving therapies

These include biological caries removal, pulp protection (capping), and pulpotomy.

Principles An improved understanding of the carious process and the development of adhesive materials which can provide a seal have changed the approach to cavity preparation. Fundamentally, a vital dental pulp and the surrounding dentine (pulp–dentine complex) is a dynamic connective tissue with inherent repair properties. As such, some caries-affected dentine can be left in the depths of a cavity once caries-infected dentine has been removed (see Chapter 6). This removal of the bacteria and their toxins which act as a noxious stimulus and subsequent sealing allows the pulp–dentine complex to deposit dentine at the advancing front of the lesion and reactionary or reparative (3° dentine) at the pulp/dentine interface. If caries is very close to the pulp or the pulp is exposed then indirect or direct pulp protection can be considered, respectively. Pulpotomy removes part or all of an inflamed coronal pulp to leave healthy, uninflamed radicular pulp within the root canal. Haemostasis must be achieved after pulpotomy (if not, then pulpectomy is required). Indirect pulp protection is achieved by a layer of one of multiple materials, Biodentine™, calcium hydroxide, or resin-modified calcium silicate (TheraCal LC™). Direct pulp protection is via calcium silicate cement (e.g. ProRoot® MTA, Biodentine™) the aim being to prevent bacterial ingress following restoration and to stimulate dentine bridge formation.

Prerequisites for pulp-preserving therapies These include no symptoms of irreversible pulpitis, a positive response to pulp testing, and no radiographic evidence of periapical periodontitis. The procedure is carried out under rubber dam isolation and a well-sealed adhesive restoration must be placed.

Follow-up Follow-up is required within 6–12 months of these procedures to check for signs/symptoms and to carry out sensibility testing and radiographic examination. If symptoms of irreversible pulpitis or signs of periapical periodontitis occur then conventional RCT is required. At present, there is not enough evidence to consider pulpotomy for the final Rx of permanent teeth but it has much potential and requires further study.[1]

In the future, regeneration of pulp and dentine via stem cell therapy, tissue engineering, or revascularization may be an alternative to RCT in selected cases. These procedures are collectively referred to as regenerative endodontic procedures.

1 S. Simon et al. 2013 *Int Endod J* **46** 79.

The root canal system

The root canal system is complex and can only be viewed in two dimensions with plain-film radiography (Table 8.1). The apical foramina are usually sited 0.5–0.7mm away from the anatomical and radiographic apex. The apical constriction usually occurs 0.5–0.7mm short of the foramina. These distances ↑ with age due to deposition of 2° cementum. Root filling to the constriction provides a natural stop to instrumentation, thus the working length should be established 1–2mm from the radiographic apex. Electronic apex locators are frequently used to assess the approximate position of the apical constriction and should be used in conjunction with radiographs to optimize the working length.

Table 8.1 The root canal system

Average working lengths (in mm)

	1	2	3	4/5	6	7
Maxilla	21	20	25	19	19	18.5
Mandible	19	19.5	24	20	19.5	18.5

Most canals are flattened mesio-distally, but become more rounded in the apical third. Lateral canals are branches of the main canal and occur in 17–30% of teeth

NB	
Maxillary	
4	74% have >1 canal with >1 foramen
5	75% have 1 canal with 1 foramen
6,7	Assume these teeth have 4 canals (2 MB; 1 P; 1 DB) until second MB canal cannot be found
Mandibular	
1,2	>40% have 2 canals, but separate foramina are seen in only 1%
4,5	May have 2 canals, but these usually rejoin to give 1 foramen
6,7	Generally have 3 canals (MB; ML; D), but one-third have 4 canals (2 in D root)

Root canal treatment—rationale

Conventional RCT is aimed at the Rx and prevention of apical periodontitis. It involves the cleaning and shaping of the root canal system to remove bacteria and pulpal remnants, followed by obturation of the resultant space to prevent reinfection.[2]

Indications
- Pulp irreversibly damaged or necrotic &/or evidence of apical periodontitis.
- Elective devitalization prior to further restorative Rx, e.g. overdenture.

Contraindications
- Non-functional or non-restorable teeth.
- Insufficient periodontal support.

Aims of RCT Aims of RCT are the elimination of microorganisms and remaining pulp tissue by chemomechanical debridement of the root canal system followed by the obturation of the root canal system to create an apical and coronal seal, preventing reinfection.

Shaping aims The aims of shaping are to remove pulpal debris and microbes and produce the ideal shape and space for effective penetration of irrigant and the resistance form to allow filling of the space with root filling material.

Shaping objectives

Shape The prepared canal should be a continuously tapering cone from crown to apex and should maintain the original anatomy. The apical constriction and original canal length should be maintained as far as possible.

Length The termination point of the preparation has been controversial. In teeth with vital inflamed pulp, bacteria are not present in the apical region of the canal and several authors recommend terminating instrumentation 2–3mm short of the radiographic apex in order to leave a clinically normal apical pulp stump.[3] In teeth with necrotic infected pulp, bacteria may penetrate to the most apical part of the root canal. Therefore, the length of instrumentation should be the entire root canal.

Apical width The apical width is gauged with hand files once the working length is reached.

Cleaning aims The aims of cleaning are to remove bacteria and organic debris from the root canal by chemomechanical preparation. Mechanical preparation alone does not reduce bacterial biofilm sufficiently. A classic study showed that only 50% of teeth treated with hand files and saline were free from cultivable bacteria.[4] Therefore, antibacterial irrigation is also required to reach those parts of the root canal system inaccessiblnse to mechanical instrumentation.

2 European Society of Endodontology 2006 *Int Endod J* 39 921.

3 M. K. Wu et al. 2000 *Oral Surg Oral Med Oral Pathol Oral Radiol Endod* 89 99.

4 Bystrom & Sundqvist 1981 *Scand J Dent Res* 89 321.

Cleaning objectives Cleaning objectives are to flush out debris and eliminate microorganisms, lubricate root canal instruments, dissolve organic debris, and remove smear layer. Frequent exchange of fluid and flooding of the root canal system is important as it ↓ torsional forces on the root canal files and aids disinfection. The irrigant solution should have broad antimicrobial spectrum, be active against endodontic pathogen biofilms, and dissolve pulp remnants and the smear layer created by instrumentation, with no irritant effect on the periradicular tissues. Solution can be delivered gently with a syringe and activated within the canal with ultrasonic or sonic systems. Sodium hypochlorite is the gold standard. It is an effective irrigant as it is both bactericidal and dissolves organic debris. There is some controversy over the appropriate concentration. The higher-concentration solutions have been shown to dissolve tissue at a quicker rate. Sodium hypochlorite is available in many different concentrations and it is often used at 2.5%. It should not be extruded beyond the apex as it can cause inflammation and tissue necrosis. The use of a side vented needle 2–3mm short of working length reduces the risk of sodium hypochlorite extrusion.

Instrumentation of the root canal wall produces a smear layer. EDTA is a calcium ion chelating agent which dissolves the inorganic component of the smear layer which sodium hypochlorite cannot do, as it only dissolves the organic tissue. EDTA solution can be used after instrumentation is complete followed by a final rinse of sodium hypochlorite.

Paste or gel type chelators can be useful for negotiating canal blockages but are not recommended for use with rotary instruments as they can ↑ torque for some instruments.

Aims of obturation
- Incarceration of residual bacteria.
- Apical seal: prevent reinfection of bacteria and ingress of inflammatory exudate into the root canal system.
- Coronal seal: prevent bacteria and tissue fluid from entering the root canal system.

Root canal treatment—instruments

It is helpful to make up RCT kits with commonly used instruments, e.g. front surface mirror, double-ended endodontic explorer, endo-locking tweezers, long-shanked excavator, flat plastic, root canal spreaders and condensers, and a metal ruler. The whole kit can then be sterilized.

Files

Stainless steel files See Table 21.1.

K-type files (K-File™, K-Flex™, K-Flexofile™)
Usually used in a watch-winding action[5] or with balanced force which involves using blunt-tipped (non-cutting) files and rotating clockwise to bind the flutes into the dentine and then rotating anticlockwise while applying an apically directed force to remove dentine. It requires practice to master but is very useful when preparing the apical part of severely curved canals.

Hedström file
Made by machining a continuous groove into a metal blank. More aggressive than K-type files. Use with push–pull filing motion. Must never be used with a rotary motion as this can ↑ torsional forces and ↑ chances of fracture. Liable to #.

Nickel titanium (NiTi) files NiTi files are popular as they are much more flexible, even with ↑ diameters. Benefits also include ↓ preparation time, ↓ files required to complete preparation, and ↓ operator and patient fatigue. Unlike conventional hand files which have a constant taper of 0.02 (2%), they have a range of tapers (0.05–0.12) and often have matched GP cones. There are a number of different systems (e.g. ProTaper® (Table 21.2), K3, TF, RaCe). Any chosen technique must be carefully learned and practised. NiTi files are vulnerable to fracture due to cyclic fatigue and torsional stress. They should be used with care in very (especially coronally) curved canals. They are designed to be used following the production of a negotiable glide path that has been created by small hand files. Initial hand preparation to at least a size no. 10 ISO instrument and production of a glide path is always required. More recently, NiTi glide path files have been produced to improve the transition between the size 10 K-File™ and the NiTi motorized file. Frequent irrigation is important and recapitulation with a small hand file between each rotary file helps maintain a glide path and avoid blockages with dentine mud/debris. A light touch and slow speed is essential. NiTi files for use in a motor with reciprocating (clockwise/anticlockwise) motion are now commonplace (e.g. WaveOne™, Reciproc®). The main advantage of these is that the reciprocating action reduces torsional forces on the file and therefore a single NiTi file is used in the majority of cases. A crown-down preparation strategy should still be used with adequate coronal flaring and irrigation before progressing the file further into the canal.

NiTi hand files can be used where a motor is not available or where greater manual control is required. Greater taper (GT®) files are one of

---

5 E. M. Saunders & W. P. Saunders 1997 *Dent Update* **24** 241.

these file types in which the flutes are machined in reverse and as such are used with a reverse balanced force method. Hand ProTaper® files have a variable taper over the length of the instrument (like the Eiffel tower!). Used with balanced force technique and same sequence as for the rotary ProTaper® series.

Ultrasonic instrumentation These can be used for shaping but are less effective than other methods. Useful for activating irrigant during canal cleaning, for assisting with loosening of posts/crowns prior to removal, removing # instruments, identifying canal orifices, and for apical surgery.

Spiral root fillers These may be used to deposit paste materials within the canal, but are liable to #, therefore the novice should use them by hand. Alternatively, coat a file with the paste and spin it by hand in an anticlockwise direction to deposit the paste in the canal.

Gates–Glidden burs These are bud-shaped with a blunt end and are used, at slow speed, for preparing the coronal two-thirds of the canal. An 'orifice opener' works in the same fashion and is generally considered less aggressive and less prone to endodontic misadventure.

Silicone stops These are used to indicate the working length. Some have a notch or mark to indicate the direction of a curvature. This is especially useful when using pre-curved SS files to establish a guide path or negotiate ledges and blockages.

Finger spreaders These are used to condense the cones of GP during canal obturation with the cold lateral condensation techniques. May be sized to match the GP accessory cones.

Other equipment This includes sterile cotton-wool pledgets and paper points for drying canals, and a syringe and side-vented endodontic needle (gauge 27 or 30) for irrigating them. Machtou pluggers are additional endodontic pluggers available in a range of sizes used to condense GP following warm obturation techniques.

There are concerns about the ability to effectively decontaminate files after contact with pulpal tissue. It is unclear whether vCJD prions could be transmitted in this way. No evidence has yet linked vCJD transmission with endodontic Rx but the single use of endodontic files was advised by the Chief Dental Officer in the United Kingdom due to the theoretical risk of transmission.

Root canal treatment—materials

Irrigants These are required to flush out debris and lubricate instruments. Dilute sodium hypochlorite is generally considered to be the best irrigant as it is bactericidal and dissolves organic debris. The normal concentration is 2.5% available chlorine. Chelating agents which soften dentine by their demineralizing action are particularly helpful when trying to negotiate sclerosed or blocked canals (e.g. EDTA paste, File-Eze®, RC Prep™). Organic acid (e.g. citric acid) can also remove inorganic material. The overall effect is optimized by agitating and alternating the irrigants.

Canal medication Non-setting calcium hydroxide paste (Hypocal™, Ultracal®) is used as an inter-appointment medicament. It can be very effective in treating an infected canal where there is a persistent inflammatory exudate from the periapical tissues.

Antibiotic/steroid paste (Odontopaste®) This is useful if anaesthesia of a hyperaemic pulp is not successful. Dressing with zinc oxide-based Odontopaste® ↓ inflammation and may allow pulp extirpation under LA during the next visit. It contains calcium hydroxide, the broad-spectrum antibiotic clindamycin hydrochloride, as well as a steroid-based anti-inflammatory agent, triamcinolone acetonide.

Iodine-containing pastes (Vitapex®, Calcipast-I®se) These are useful in retreatment cases as certain organisms are resistant to calcium hydroxide.

Filling material GP, an isomer of latex extracted from tropical trees, comes the nearest to meeting the requirements of an ideal filling material. It is supplied in cones which come in two main forms: *master cones*, sized to match the master apical file, and *accessory cones*, sized to match the finger spreaders. Some systems advise that only one cone is required (single-cone obturation techniques); however, this does create a relatively high proportion of sealer in the obturation and not all canals will be a uniform cone shape.

Sealers A wide variety is available. Calcium hydroxide materials (e.g. Sealapex™) and the eugenol-based sealers (e.g. Tubliseal™) are popular. Other sealers based on resin (AH Plus®) and GI (Ketac™ Endo) are available. Calcium silicate sealers are also used (BioRoot™ RCS, TotalFill®) and have shown good biocompatibility.

Calcium hydroxide This is useful in endodontics due to its antibacterial properties and which then allows the body to form a calcific barrier also known as a dentine bridge. The former is thought to be due to a high pH and also to the absorption of carbon dioxide, upon which the metabolic activities of many root canal pathogens depend. It is also proteolytic. Non-setting calcium hydroxide is used as an inter-visit medicament in two-stage RCT. In setting form, it was previously used for apexification and Rx of perforations but is now largely superseded by MTA. It is effectively placed with a Lentulo spiral filler or a cannula-based system. The spiral filler has a reduced risk of extrusion.

Mineral trioxide aggregate MTA is a calcium silicate cement, originally developed as a root-end filling material. It is biocompatible and can set in the presence of moisture. It is the material of choice in apexification procedures and can be used as a pulp-capping agent. It creates a physical barrier and releases calcium hydroxide when it is setting. It can be difficult to handle and can cause grey discoloration when used as a root canal filling (RCF) material or pulp-capping agent, this is thought to be due to the presence of bismuth oxide. Other biocompatible products have been developed (ProRoot MTA®, MTA Angelus®, Biodentine®).

Root canal preparation—1

Preparation for treatment

Magnification and illumination Magnification and illumination with loupes or an operating microscope are of great benefit.

Pre-operative radiograph A pre-operative radiograph must show the full length of the root(s) and 2–3mm of the periapical region.

Local anaesthesia LA should be given if required.

Preparation of tooth Before starting RCT all caries must be removed from the tooth and an interim restoration placed to allow placement of a rubber dam, prevent ingress of bacteria from the mouth, and provide a stable reference point for measurement of working length. This may mean removal of existing full coverage restorations (with the patient's consent) in order to ensure the tooth is free from caries or fracture. It will also establish whether the tooth can be predictably restored. If not, then there is no point in carrying out RCT.

Isolation A rubber dam is mandatory to prevent inhalation or ingestion of small root canal instruments, maintain an aseptic environment, and protect the patient from toxic materials. The seal may be optimized with use of OraSeal®/OpalDam®.

Access The aim is total removal of the pulp chamber roof. This allows unimpeded, smooth-walled access with instruments to the coronal third of root canals. Careful removal of dentine needs to be balanced with conservation of as much sound tooth tissue as possible. The shape of the access cavity depends on the anatomy of the tooth (Fig. 8.1). Initial access is made at a point where the pulp chamber roof and floor are furthest apart (usually the pulp horns). This can be done using tungsten carbide burs or diamond burs. Diamond burs are used to cut through ceramic and newer generations of diamond burs can be used to cut through ceramic and reduce the possibility of fracturing of the ceramic crown. Following initial penetration, a non-end-cutting bur can be used for removal of the rest of the pulp chamber roof without damaging the floor. When completed the access cavity should have a smooth funnel shape. Proprietary access cavity burs are available.

Identification of root canal orifices This is achieved by careful examination of the pulp chamber floor with an endodontic explorer. Magnification and additional illumination are helpful. Knowledge of tooth morphology is essential. Developmental lines on the dark pulp chamber floor can form useful landmarks. If a single canal is located towards one side of the root there may be a second, hidden canal on the other side. 3° dentine can narrow orifices. Tends to be white in colour. Gates–Glidden burs, NiTi orifice shapers, and non-end-cutting burs can be used carefully to create straight line access. Ultrasonic endodontic tips can assist with the removal of 3° dentine and the identification of canal orifices.

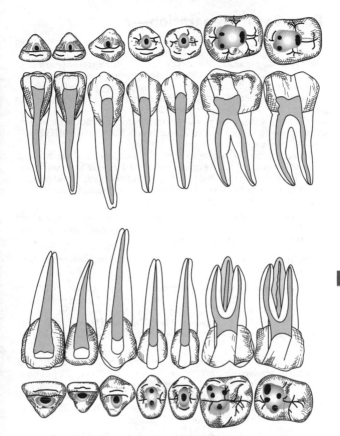

Fig. 8.1 Access cavity preparations.

Root canal preparation—2

Current thinking favours the development of shape in a crown-down manner. Many single-file systems are in use now and the techniques recommended by each manufacturer vary. When using a progressive sequence of files, preparation of the coronal part of the canal is done first with larger instruments. Then the root canal is prepared with progressively smaller instruments. This principle is adhered to whether hand or rotary techniques are used. The advantages of this are that it:[6]

- Effectively ↓ the curvature in the coronal part of the root canal, allowing straighter access for files to the apical region. Therefore ↓ the likelihood of apical transportation (zipping).
- Allows improved access for the flow of irrigant solution within the canal.
- ↓ the likelihood of apical extrusion of infected material as most of the canal debris is removed before apical instrumentation takes place. Important because the majority of bacteria in an infected root canal are located in the coronal region.

Whether using hand or rotary instruments, adequate access is required and the choice of technique, instrument, and final preparation size have to be decided for each root canal system (Fig. 8.2).

Sequence of canal preparation Next, the root canal orifices are identified and the canals prepared as follows:

Initial negotiation Coronal two-thirds of canal is negotiated with an ISO size 10 or 15 file in a watch-winding movement and then flooded with sodium hypochlorite. EDTA lubricant is also helpful. In very fine canals, one may need to start with an ISO size 6 or 8 first. Files should be worked gently to the coronal two-thirds with sequentially larger files up to ISO size 20. This creates a 'glide path'.

Coronal % flaring After creating a glide path, the coronal two-thirds is flared. This can be achieved using proprietary 'orifice shaper' files or a combination of SS hand files or NiTi hand or rotary files or Gates–Glidden drills. Files with sequentially ↓ taper or diameter are used in a crown-down approach. Copious irrigation is needed throughout and frequent recapitulation with an ISO size 10 or 15 hand file to prevent blockage.

Apical negotiation Next, the remaining one-third of the canal can be negotiated up to ISO size 15 to develop a glide path to allow the entire length of the canal to be prepared.

Working length determination This is defined as the distance from a fixed reference position on the crown of the tooth to the apical constriction of the root canal.[7] The apical constriction is normally 0.5–2mm short of the radiographic apex of the tooth. There are two methods of establishing the working length: (i) a radiograph—a file fitted with a silicone stop and of sufficient size is inserted into the canal to the estimated working length prior to taking the radiograph, and (ii) an electronic apex locator—this works by

6 M. A. al Omari & P. M. Dummer 1995 J *Endod* **21** 154.

7 P. Carrotte 2004 *BDJ* **197** 603.

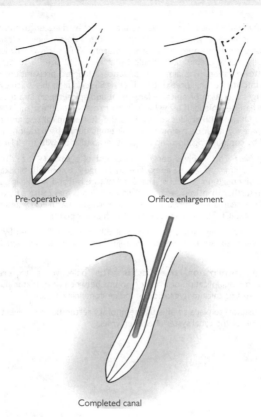

Pre-operative

Orifice enlargement

Completed canal

Fig. 8.2 Stages in preparation.

measuring electrical impedance with an electrode attached to a file in the root canal; when the file reaches the apical foramen the device emits an audible or visible signal. Working length is determined by subtracting 0.5mm from the length indicated by the device. This allows thorough cleaning, and preservation of the constriction facilitates a good apical seal while reducing extrusion of infected debris. Ideally, both methods of working length determination should be used in each case. It is advisable to prepare 1mm from the zero reading of an apex locator on lower 5s and 7s as the apices are potentially very close to the inferior dental nerve (IDN).

Apical third preparation Preparation to the correct working length and apical width is done next. The size of the apical width is determined by 'gauging' the root canal at the apex by passively inserting SS files to working length. Generally, apical preparation should be at least ISO size 25 to facilitate adequate irrigation. The aim is to produce a tapered preparation which blends into the coronal preparation. If using SS hand files, this is achieved in two stages (creation of apical enlargement and apical taper) in a modified double-flare technique. If using NiTi hand or rotary files, the manufacturers generally have finishing files to produce the desired apical size and taper. Canal patency must be maintained at all times during preparation. This is helped by copious irrigation and frequent recapitulation with small files.

Patency filing This involves passive placement of a small (< size 10) ISO file 0.5–1.0mm through the apex. The advantage is to prevent blockage at the apex by build-up of debris. The disadvantage is that if the file is pushed through further than 1mm, extruded infected debris may cause a flare-up.

Finally, smear layer removal is achieved by irrigating with EDTA and a final rinse of NaOCl. The root canal is dried with paper points.

Balanced force filing This is performed at 90° clockwise followed by 270° anticlockwise using a k-flexofile. Its benefit is to remove dentine equally on all walls.

Inter-appointment medication The objective is to prevent growth and multiplication of microorganisms between visits. Materials used are non-setting calcium hydroxide or iodine-containing pastes.

▶ It is essential to place an effective temporary restoration to prevent contamination of the canal system between visits.

Common errors in canal preparation

Incomplete debridement and missed anatomy For example, working length short and missed canals.

Lateral perforation This often occurs as a result of poor access or bur angulation.

Apical perforation and overpreparation This makes filling difficult.

Ledge formation This can be very difficult to bypass.

Apical transportation (zipping) A file will tend to straighten out when used in a curved canal and straightening can transport the apical part of the preparation away from the curvature. The use of flexible files reduces the likelihood of this happening.

Elbow formation When apical zipping happens, a narrowing often occurs coronal to this in the canal such that the canal is hourglass in shape. This narrowing is termed an elbow.

Strip perforation This is a perforation occurring in the inner or furcal wall of a curved root canal, usually towards the coronal end.

Anticurvature filing This was developed to minimize the possibility of creating a 'strip' perforation on the inner walls of curved root canals. It is used in conjunction with other techniques or preparation, and the essential principle is the direction of most force away from the curvature. Filing ratio is 3:1 outer wall:inner wall.

Establishing straight line access reduces the chances of errors occurring.

NiTi rotary instruments reduce creation of blocks, ledges, transportations, and perforations by remaining centred within the natural path of the canal. The newer generation of controlled memory wire M wire, gold wire, and blue wire nickel titanium reduces the transportation of the root canal during preparation.

Root canal obturation

Objectives To provide a 3-D hermetic seal to the root canal to:
- Prevent the ingress of bacteria or tissue fluids which might act as a culture medium for any bacteria that remain in the root canal system. Called a coronal seal.
- Incarcerate any microbes remaining in the root canal system.
- Prevent reinfection of the root canal system.
- Prevent diffusion of inflammatory exudate into the canal, called an apical seal.

Timing RCF should be done after completion of canal preparation, infection is considered to be eliminated, and the canal can be dried. There is no evidence that single- or multiple-visit RCT is more effective, in terms of radiological success. Single-visit RCT may result in a slightly ↑ frequency of swelling and ↑ need of analgesics.[8] The presence of pretreatment symptoms/swelling, complex anatomy, or patient management factors may influence the decision to carry out single- or multiple-visit RCT. If done over multiple visits, placement of inter-visit medicament (usually calcium hydroxide) is essential.

Materials[9]

Core materials
- GP: a form of latex derived from tropical trees.
- Resin-based core materials.

Both types are supplied as master/accessory points for placement with lateral condensation and as pellets for thermoplastic, vertical condensation techniques. The proposed advantage of adhesive (Resilon™) obturation systems is ↓ risk of root # by creating a 'monoblock' of dentine and obturation materials but clinical studies to back this up are lacking. It is very difficult to bond atubular root dentine.

Sealers These fill the space between the root canal wall and core material and between GP points and fill accessory and lateral canals.
   A wide variety is available:
- ZOE-based sealers (e.g. Tubliseal™).
- Calcium hydroxide-based materials (e.g. Sealapex™).
- Resin-based sealers (e.g. AH Plus®), RealSeal® for use with Resilon®.
- Silicone-based sealers (e.g. RoekoSeal®).
- Gutta flow is a material based on RoekoSeal® with powdered GP added.
- Bioceramic sealers (TotalFill® Endo sequence)
- Glass ionomer based (e.g. Ketac™ Endo).

Techniques Numerous techniques have been described; all of those mentioned here use GP. The aim is to fill the entire root canal from the orifice to the apical constriction with a dense RCF with no voids. There is no evidence that any technique is superior in terms of promoting healing. Cleaning and shaping of the root canal is the single most important factor in preventing and treating endodontic diseases.

8 L. Figini et al. 2007 *Cochrane Database Syst Rev* 2007 **4** CD005296.

9 J. Whitworth 2005 *Endod Topics* **12** 2.

Cold lateral compaction This is a commonly taught method of obturation and is the gold standard by which others are judged. The technique involves placement of a master point chosen to fit the apical section of the canal. Obturation of the remainder is achieved by compaction of smaller accessory points. The steps involved are as follows:

- Select a GP master point to correspond with the master apical file instrument. This should fit the apical region snugly at the working length so that on removal a degree of resistance or 'tug-back' is felt. The point should be notched at the correct working length to guide its placement to the apical constriction.
- Take a radiograph to confirm that the point is in the correct position.
- Coat walls of canal with sealer using a small file.
- Insert the master point, covered in cement.
- Condense the GP laterally for 20sec with a finger spreader set to within 1mm of working length to provide space into which an accessory point can be inserted. Repeat until the canal is full.
- Excess GP is cut off with a hot instrument at the base of the pulp chamber and the remainder packed vertically into the canal with a cold plugger to 1mm below the amelo-cemental junction.

Single-cone obturation techniques are very popular with matched GP points, corresponding to the file size/shape used.

Warm GP techniques
Warm lateral compaction
As for cold lateral compaction, but uses a warm spreader after the initial cold lateral condensation. Special heat carriers can be used with a flame or a special electronically heated device (Touch 'n Heat™).

Vertical compaction
The GP is warmed using a heated instrument and then packed vertically. A good apical stop is necessary to prevent apical extrusion of the filling, but with practice a very dense root filling can result. Time-consuming. The System B™ heat carrier has simplified this technique.

Thermoplasticized injectable GP (e.g. Obtura®, Ultrafil®, Calamus® Dual, BeeFill® 2in1, Elements™ Free)
These commercial machines extrude heated GP (70–160°C) into the canal. It is difficult to control the apical extent of the root filling, and some contraction of the GP occurs on cooling. Useful for irregular canal defects, e.g. following internal root resorption. Can be used for backfill in combination with System B™.

Coated carriers (e.g. Thermafil®, Gutta Core™, Gutta Fusion™, Soft Core™)
These are cores of metal or plastic-coated or a cross-linked GP carrier with surrounding GP. They are heated in an oven and then simply pushed into the root canal to the correct length after size verification and sealer placement. The core is then severed with a bur or in the case of GP carriers, a sharp spoon excavator. A dense filling results, but again apical control is difficult and extrusions are common. They are relatively expensive and the materials without the GP carriers can be difficult to remove.

Once the RCF is in place the tooth will need to be permanently restored, provided the follow-up radiograph is satisfactory. RCFs that appear inadequate radiographically may be reviewed regularly, or replaced, depending upon the clinical circumstances.

Coronal seal After completing obturation, a good coronal seal must be achieved by placement of an ideal restorative material on the pulp chamber floor and canal orifices and placement of a definitive restoration. This is now recognized as very important for success in endodontics. Too often good endodontic therapy is jeopardized by a poor restoration that does not provide a good coronal seal.[10]

10   H. A. Ray & M. Troupe *Int Endod J* **28** 12.

Some endodontic problems and their management

Acute periapical abscess Relief of symptoms requires drainage of the abscess and where possible this should be obtained through the tooth under a rubber dam. Open the pulp with a diamond bur in a turbine handpiece while supporting the tooth to ↓ vibration. Regional anaesthesia and occasionally sedation may be required. Once opened, the canal is irrigated with sodium hypochlorite and, if at all possible, resealed. It may be necessary to see the patient again in 24h, rather than leaving the tooth on open drainage. Relieve any traumatic occlusion.

If a fluctuant abscess is present this should be incised. If drainage can be obtained through the tooth and there is no evidence of a cellulitis, then antibiotics are not required (◐ Dento-facial infections, p. 408).

Pain following instrumentation This is usually due to instruments or irrigants, or to debris being forced into the apical tissues. Occasionally, an acute flare-up of a previously asymptomatic tooth occurs following initial instrumentation so pre-warn patients.

Sclerosed canals As the incidence of pulp necrosis following canal obliteration is only 13–16%, elective RCT is not warranted. However, where pulp death has occurred, finding the canal orifice may be difficult. If careful exploration with a small file is unsuccessful, investigation of the expected position of the canal entrance with a small round bur or ultrasonic tips, aided by magnification and illumination, may help. Once the canal is found, a no. 8 or 10 file should be used to try and negotiate it, using EDTA-containing File-Eze®, Glyde™, or RC Prep™ as a lubricant, and the canal prepared and filled conventionally. Success rates of 80% have been reported for canals that were hairline or undetectable on radiographs.[11] Occasionally, a total blockage of the canal is encountered, in which case the filling is placed to this level &/or periradicular surgery done.

Pulp stones Pulp stones in the pulp chamber can usually be flicked out. If they occur in the canal, use EDTA and a small file to dislodge them.

Fractured instruments The success of removal depends on root canal anatomy and type and design of the # instrument and location of the # portion. The fractured file may be bypassed. Sometimes it is possible to pull out the # portion with a pair of fine Steiglitz forceps. If not, insertion of a fine file beside the instrument or ultrasonic tips to create a staging platform used at a low power setting may dislodge it. Otherwise, a Masseran kit (◐ Removing old posts and cores, p. 266) may be required but these weaken the root dentine. Should the # piece be lodged in the apical portion of the canal it may be better to fill the canal coronal to it and keep it under observation, resorting to periradicular surgery as a last-ditch solution.

---

11 J. O. Andreasen et al. 2007 *Textbook and Color Atlas of Traumatic Injuries to the Teeth* (4e), Wiley-Blackwell.

Immature teeth with incomplete roots See ➲ RCT of teeth with immature apices, p. 112.

The length of the root can be obtained by using radiographs, an electronic apex locator, or making a hook from a K-type file. Preparation often involves activation of irrigants due to the width of the root canal. The apex is often filled with a bioceramic cement or MTA to aid in apexification and then the canal filled using warm GP. Revascularization is also a Rx modality for non-vital teeth with incomplete root formation.

Removing old root-fillings Single GP points can be removed with a Hedström file. Thermal softening using Gates–Glidden drills (coronally) or rotary NiTi files may help. There are specially designed retreatment NiTi files (e.g. ProTaper® Universal Retreatment files, Mtwo® retreatment files). Chemicals, e.g. chloroform, or oil of eucalyptus can be used but they can create a smear on the root canal walls which is difficult to remove. All methods leave some RCF on canal walls. This can be assessed with the operating microscope.

Perforations These can be iatrogenic or caused by resorption (➲ Resorption, p. 112). In the latter case, dressing with non-setting calcium hydroxide may help to arrest the resorption and promote formation of a calcific barrier. Increasingly, MTA is being used for the repair of perforations and in surgical endodontics as a retrograde filling material with excellent results.[12] Management of traumatic perforations depends upon their size and position:

• *Pulp chamber floor*—if small, can cover with MTA or a bioceramic material, but if large, hemisection or extraction may be necessary. MTA can also be used.
• *Lateral perforation*—if near the gingival margin, can be incorporated in the final restoration, e.g. a diaphragm post and core crown. If in the middle third, the remainder of the canal may be cleaned by passing instruments down the side of the wall opposite the perforation. Then the canal can be filled with GP, using a lateral compaction technique to occlude the perforation as well. Larger perforations may require a surgical approach and in multirooted teeth hemisection or extraction may be unavoidable.
• *Apical third*—it is usually worth trying a vertical compaction technique to attempt to fill both the perforation and the remainder of the canal. If this is unsuccessful, periradicular surgery will be required.

Ledge formation If this occurs, return to a small file curved at the apex to the working length and use this to try and file away the ledge, using EDTA or RC Prep™ as a lubricant.

Periodontal–endodontic lesions See ➲ Periodontitis associated with endodontic lesions, p. 201.

Partial (Cvek) pulpotomy See ➲ Injuries to permanent teeth—crown fractures, p. 104.

12 M. Torabinejad & N. Chivian 1999 J Endod 25 197.

Restoration of the root-treated tooth

Once RCT is completed, a definitive restoration will be required.

Aims
Coronal seal—the restoration acts as a first-line defence against infection by oral microbes so it should form a good coronal seal.

Protection of remaining tooth structure—root-treated teeth are substantially weakened by:
- Loss of tooth substance as a result of the original cavity/restoration and also by subsequent access cavity and root canal preparation.
- Dehydration.
- Loss of elasticity of dentine due to effect of irrigants and medicaments on collagen.

Therefore the restoration needs to protect the remaining tooth structure from #.

Restoration of form, function, and aesthetics.

Principles Cuspal coverage for root-treated molar teeth enhances survival. The success of this restoration will depend on how much sound coronal tooth substance remains and whether a 'ferrule effect' can be achieved, i.e. an extra-coronal restoration surrounds a 'collar' of dentine of at least 2mm height coronal to the preparation margins.

Timing of restoration Definitive restoration needs to be carried out as soon as possible. A provisional restoration is in place the higher the risk of coronal leakage and #.

If there is a delay in placement of the final restoration (e.g. awaiting resolution of sinus tract) then molar restorations should have cuspal coverage in the temporary restoration.

Restoration design This will depend on a number of factors including amount of coronal tooth substance remaining, position of tooth in arch, aesthetics, patient preferences, cost, occlusal load, and parafunction.

Use of adhesive materials where possible allows for preservation of tooth tissue. Where cuspal protection is needed, onlays or partial coverage crowns can provide the necessary occlusal form without excessive tooth tissue loss which would result from full crown preparation.

Anterior root-treated teeth do not require crowning unless there has been substantial loss of tooth structure.

Core build-up Usually done in composite or amalgam. GI has poor compressive strength. Where there is insufficient tooth structure remaining to support a core, a post and core will be required (see Chapter 6).

Treatment outcomes

Following RCT the ideal outcome is prevention or resolution of periapical periodontitis and absence of clinical signs and symptoms. In some cases, however, periapical periodontitis will persist, develop, or recur.

Previously, the terms 'success' and 'failure' were used. It may be more pragmatic to consider that the absence of clinical signs and symptoms and a ↓ in size of any apical area be deemed acceptable. Considering this as tooth *survival* (having an asymptomatic functional tooth) is more in line with the criteria used to judge the outcome of implant placement.[13,14]

Three main prognostic factors influence the outcome:

- *Pre-treatment status of the periapical tissues*—if there is no pre-treatment radiolucency, outcome is more favourable and can be up to 95%. If there is a lesion, outcome is more favourable for smaller (<5mm) lesions.
- *Quality and length of RCF*—outcome is more favourable if well compacted and reaches within 2mm of the radiographic apex.
- *Quality of coronal restoration*.

Outcomes

There are no standard terms for endodontic outcomes and this subject is hotly debated. They can be described as:

Favourable Symptom free, functional tooth, clinical healthy tissues, radiographic evidence of healthy periapical tissues or healing by scar tissue formation.

Uncertain Symptoms or symptom free. May be low-grade tenderness to palpation/percussion. Radiographically, periapical radiolucency persists within the 4yr assessment period.

Unfavourable Presence of symptoms, tooth not functional, clinical signs of infection, e.g. sinus tract/swelling. Radiographically, a new radiolucency or radiolucency has persisted or ↑ in size.

Assessment of outcome is by clinical history and examination to check for post-treatment signs and symptoms and radiographic assessment of outcome using the long-cone parallel technique and film holders.

Conventionally, 1yr is considered the time at which a decision on outcome can be made. If there are symptoms, the patient may be reviewed sooner. If the outcome is uncertain, follow-up for a total of 4yrs is needed.

The radiology report should include an assessment of:

- Quality of RCF (length and compaction), presence/absence of radiolucency, size of any radiolucency compared with pre-treatment status, quality of coronal restoration, presence of caries, and periodontal status.
- CBCT may be indicated where there are symptoms but conventional radiography shows no radiolucency or where missed canal anatomy may be suspected.

---

13 Y.-L. Ng et al. 2011 *Int Endo* J **44** 583.

14 Y.-L. Ng et al. 2011 *Int Endo* J **44** 610.

Retreatment

Endodontic causes of unfavourable outcome are mainly due to reinfection or persistent infection due to missed or inadequately treated canals. Retreatment involves removal of the original RCF (see ➔ Removing old root-fillings, p. 355). Microflora in endodontically treated teeth with persistent infection differs from that of untreated, infected teeth; *Enterococcus faecalis* and *Candida albicans* are found more frequently in retreatment cases.

Where the root canal is not accessible for retreatment (e.g. post crown), surgical endodontics may be required.

Chapter 9

Restorative dentistry 5: dental implants

Principal sources and further reading Association of Dental Implantology 2012 *A Dentist's Guide to Implantology* ($\mathcal{R}$ http://www.adi.org.uk). J. Malet et al. 2018 *Implant Dentistry at a Glance* (2e), Wiley Blackwell. G. A. Zarb et al. 2012 *Prosthodontic Treatment for Edentulous Patients: Complete Dentures and Implant-supported Prostheses* (13e), Elsevier.

Introduction to implantology

Single or multiple dental implants have become a well-accepted method of replacement of missing teeth and their supporting structures. They have the advantage of replacing teeth often using available bone without preparing healthy remaining teeth. Single tooth implants are an alternative to conventional tooth-supported bridgework for this reason (Fig. 9.1). Implantology in restorative dentistry is based on the principle of osseointegration, i.e. a direct functional and structural connection between a load-carrying titanium implant with bone, with no intervening connective tissue. Successful long-term osseointegration depends on meticulous planning, careful surgery and restoration, as well as a favourable host response. There is little point in a successfully integrated implant in the wrong place! However, while an attractive option to many patients, not all teeth need replacing and case selection is important to ensure appropriate treatment provision.

Implants tend to be used in one of three ways:
- For fixed restorations which are either:
  - Screw-retained.
  - Cement-retained.
- To retain a removable prosthesis.
- For orthodontic anchorage purposes.

Why replace missing teeth? For adequate functioning and aesthetics, it has been proposed that a minimum of 20 teeth are required. The shortened dental arch (SDA) concept[1] is advocated by many dentists due to its practicality and cost-effectiveness. This is defined as reduced dentition with missing posterior teeth and remaining intact anterior teeth, i.e. premolar to premolar in both arches. However, the number of teeth required to have a good quality of life can vary between patients due to their personal beliefs, values, and preferences. It should also be noted that the SDA concept is not a well-accepted concept in many countries of the world.

Teeth are required for mastication, to facilitate breakdown of food in the mouth allowing for adequate nutrition to be achieved through a balanced diet. Teeth also contribute to self-esteem, phonation, and aesthetics. What is acceptable to one patient may not be acceptable to another and therefore an in-depth consultation involving discussion of the patient's expectations and motives for wanting implant treatment is paramount. In general, a high number of patients are willing to pay more for implants than conventional dentures and accept the difference in cost. Despite the initial costs of implant treatment being higher than that of tooth-supported or conventional removable prostheses, this may well be deemed worth it to patients in terms of the potential benefits.

---

1 A. F. Kayser 1981 *J Oral Rehabil* **8** 457.

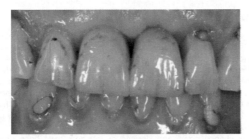

Fig. 9.1 Two cement-retained implants to replace both central incisors.
Courtesy of Dr Nilesh R. Parmar, Parmar Dental, UK.

History of dental implants

Numerous procedures for oral implants have been described, dating back hundreds of years; all had advocates but most failed. Genuine advances in the discipline came about, thanks to a major contribution by Brånemark, in the 1960s. The term 'osseointegration' was coined, meaning the direct functional and structural connection of the implant to bone. All current implants are based on this now well-accepted concept. Many materials and coatings for implants have been used in the past (e.g. ceramics and hydroxy-apatite) but success rates have been found to be greatest with titanium fixtures. As a result, almost all modern implants are titanium.

Various shapes, sizes, and designs of implants have been used over the years. Nowadays, virtually all designs are of a cylinder-shaped fixture (known as 'root-form' implants) with an external screw-thread to screw the implant into the bone. Internally, the implant has an internal screw thread and some form of internal shape coronally to prevent rotation of the abut-ment (i.e. an internal hex or star shape) (Fig. 9.2).

Modern implants usually have a roughened outer surface to ↑ the sur-face area for integration. The surface may be roughened by a subtractive technique such as being grit-blasted (e.g. with titanium dioxide) and/or acid-etched. Additive techniques can also be used such as coating with hy-droxyapatite or a fluoride-modified surface.

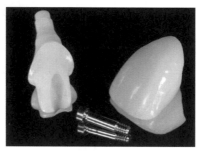

Fig. 9.2 Implant components. Left: zirconia abutment; centre: abutment screw; right: crown.

Courtesy of Dr Nilesh R. Parmar, Parmar Dental, UK.

Types and sizes of dental implants

Root-form implants There is a wide range of implant diameters and lengths available. Typically for root-form implants this would be a range of diameters from 3mm to 6mm and lengths from 5mm to 17mm. An average implant would be around 4mm in diameter and 10mm long. The exact size to be used in a given situation is determined from the planning process (⊖ Planning for dental implants, p. 366). Generally, wider diameter implants are used to replace wider teeth (e.g. molars) and narrower implants are used for smaller teeth (e.g. lower incisors). Larger implants have a greater surface area for integration but as implants ↑ in size, there becomes a greater risk of complications during surgery, such as insufficient bone volume surrounding the dental implant or damage to adjacent anatomy.

Other types of dental implant As well as conventional root-form implants, there are also:
- Mini-implants.
- Zygomatic implants.
- Orthodontic implants used for anchorage.

Mini-implants are those with a diameter of <3mm, these are not used to support a permanent fixed prosthesis. They can be used to support a removable overdenture or temporary prosthesis.

Zygomatic implants are placed into the zygomatic arch and are an alternative for patients who do not have enough bone in the maxilla for conventional root-form implants. This includes those patients with very resorbed ridges, after ablative cancer surgery, or severe traumatic defects.

Orthodontic mini-implants are used as a temporary anchorage device in fixed orthodontics.

Planning for dental implants

Assessment of suitability for implant placement This is achieved by taking a thorough history, clinical examination of hard and soft tissue availability, periodontal health, dentition, occlusion, available inter-dental and interocclusal space, and mouth opening ability. The volume, quality, and shape of bone are also important considerations when planning implant suitability and placement. Radiographic examination with plain films can look at the height of bone and adjacent anatomical structures (e.g. tooth roots, ID canal, maxillary antrum, and bony pathology). All prosthetic options (i.e. no treatment, removable partial denture, fixed bridge, or implant) should be considered and, if appropriate, included in the consent process.

Indications for implants
- Edentulous or partially edentulous mouths unable to retain dentures.
- Multiple missing teeth.
- Single tooth replacement (providing the space is >6.5mm).
- Maxillofacial or dental prostheses post cancer surgery or trauma.

Relative contraindications for implants
- Poor plaque control.
- Poor bone quality or soft tissue biotype.
- Smoking.
- Anticoagulation therapy.
- Active chemotherapy.
- Alcohol or drug abuse.
- Radiotherapy to the jaw bones (past or present).
- Diabetes (particularly if poorly controlled).
- Unfavourable smile line.
- Unrealistic patient expectations.
- Oral medicine conditions may compromise healing.
- Cardiac conditions considered high risk for infective endocarditis.
- Chronic kidney disease (healing impairment).
- Immunocompromised (transplant patients, AIDS/HIV).
- Medications predisposing to medication-associated osteonecrosis, such as denosumab or bisphosphonate use (past or present, risk IV > oral).
- Active periodontal disease or history of treated periodontitis (slightly more susceptible to peri-implantitis, implant failure, and peri-implant bone loss).

Planning of implant position This uses the 'top-down' or 'pros-thetically driven' approach. This means deciding on tooth position by first using wax-ups on mounted study models, or digitally.

The wax-up can be used to produce a radiographic stent which is used to help plan the appropriate size and position of the implant. Further radiographs may be indicated with the stent in position such as a CBCT scan. CT scanning has the advantage over plain film radiography of allowing a 3-D assessment of the bone volume. This radiographic stent can often also be converted into a surgical stent to help guide implant placement. Digital implant planning systems (e.g. SimPlant®) are now available. These allow for 3-D planning and the production of surgical guides. A disadvantage of

CBCT scanning is an additional patient dose of radiation. There is an ↑ drive towards lower dose systems which can also provide a limited field of view.

When planning implants, 1.5mm or more is left between the implant and adjacent teeth. So, for a single tooth implant the minimum space between adjacent teeth is 7mm for a 4mm diameter fixture; 3mm of space is usually required between adjacent implants. If there is insufficient bone available to allow correct implant positioning, then either bone augmentation is required or other prosthetic options need to be considered.

Bone augmentation Bone augmentation may be achieved by a variety of techniques such as guided bone regeneration (GBR), block bone grafting, ridge expansion, sinus elevation, or distraction osteogenesis. The materials used may be:
- Autogenous bone (the patient's own bone, e.g. mandible/iliac crest).
- Allografts (bone from another human, e.g. tissue banks).
- Xenografts (animal-derived bone, e.g. bovine, porcine, or equine origin).
- Alloplastic materials (inorganic or non-animal derived, e.g. hydroxyapatite, calcium sulfate).

Barrier membranes can be used with these materials to exclude soft tissue ingrowth and to support the graft material. Bone morphogenetic proteins may be used as bioactive mediators.[2] Plasma rich in growth factors (PRGF) produced by the patient's own blood may be applied directly to the implant surface—they are believed to accelerate bone regeneration, improving the osseointegration of titanium dental implants.

It may be feasible to simultaneously carry out bone augmentation at the time of implant placement if there is sufficient bone to allow 1° stability of the implant fixture and soft tissue closure. Alternatively, the bone may need to be augmented prior to implant placement and allowed to heal (for 3–6 months) before the implant can be placed, known as a two-stage approach. The later bone augmentation procedures are performed after tooth extraction, the more bone resorption will occur, therefore timing of such procedures should be planned carefully and implant assessment should take place before extraction of a tooth where possible.

2 M. Esposito et al. 2008 *Cochrane Database Syst Rev* 3 CD004152.

Risks of dental implants

There are risks associated with dental implants as with any surgical procedure—these should be discussed in detail with the patient. Risks include:

- Pain, swelling, and bruising.
- Bleeding.
- Failure to osseointegrate and lack of stability.
- Peri-implantitis and late failure.
- Bony necrosis in patients with a history of radiotherapy or bisphosphonate use.
- Nerve damage.
- Sinus problems (due to protrusion of implant into sinus).
- Accidental damage to adjacent teeth and structures.
- Very rarely, mandible fracture and necrosis of surrounding flap tissue.
- Infection (including peri-implantitis and peri-implant mucositis) (Fig. 9.3).
- Implant fracture.
- Gingival recession.
- Broken, loosened, worn, or discoloured prosthesis.
- Fracture of abutment screw or implant.

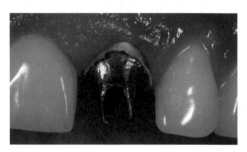

Fig. 9.3 Peri-implant disease due to cement left below the gingival margin.
Courtesy of Dr Nilesh R. Parmar, Parmar Dental, UK.

Implant placement

Timing of placement Following extraction of an existing tooth or root, implant placement may be immediate or following a period of healing. Timing of implant placement is often categorized as:[3]

- Immediate (placement just after tooth extraction).
- Immediate-delayed (inserted after weeks up to a couple of months to allow for soft tissue healing).
- Delayed (placed thereafter in partially or completely healed bone).

If implants are placed immediately, less overall surgical time may be required and post-extraction healing will occur at the same time as osseointegration. Bone volumes may also be partially maintained which can improve the aesthetic result. However, there can be challenges in achieving 1° stability of the implant and there may be residual dental infection associated with the extracted tooth, with a potential to cause a failure of osseointegration. Bone healing and remodelling are also unpredictable.

Delayed implant placement can mean the overall treatment time is longer but there is time for soft tissue healing and bone healing to occur. Not only does this allow for existing infection to clear, it also makes placement, surgical site closure, and achieving 1° stability of the implant more predictable. However, excessive healing time following extraction may lead to bone resorption and inadequate natural bone for implant placement.

Techniques for placement The patient must be both dentally and medically fit for surgery. Planning should have been completed. It is crucial that key anatomical structures are identified by the surgeon prior to and during implant placement to ensure injuries (e.g. laceration, section, or compression) are avoided where possible. Moderate- to high-risk structures include the inferior alveolar nerve, mental nerve, lingual nerve, and sublingual/submental arteries. The surgical procedure is highly equipment dependent and the surgeon needs to be trained in the particular technique and implant system to be used. Careful technique with constant irrigation is required to avoid overheating bone resulting in bone necrosis.

A gingival–mucosal flap is raised and a receiving channel is prepared in the bone, using drills matched to the implant size and type. The fixture, depending on the type of implant, is either pressed or screwed into place. When placing multiple implants, direction indicators/surgical guides are helpful for achieving parallelism. Intraoperative periapical radiographs can be used to further assess the position of the osteotomy site. This may be more relevant to smaller spaces where adjacent roots could potentially become damaged. In two-stage procedures, the implant has a 'cover screw' placed and is entirely covered by the flap at the end of the procedure. In a single-stage procedure, a 'healing abutment' is placed on the implant that extents transgingivally—the gingivae are sutured around this, meaning it is visible at the end of the placement appointment (Fig. 9.4).

In two-stage procedures, the implant head needs to be uncovered (or 'exposed') following a suitable period of integration, during which the cover screw is removed and the healing abutment placed.

3 M. Esposito et al. 2010 *Cochrane Database Syst Rev* 9 CD005968.

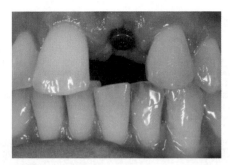

Fig. 9.4 A healing abutment in place.
Courtesy of Dr Nilesh R. Parmar, Parmar Dental, UK.

Healing Osseointegration is a time-dependent healing process. Following creation of an intraosseous channel and implant insertion, blood cells enter the space between the implant threads, sitting within a fibrin network that acts as a provisional matrix for erythrocytes, macrophages, and neutrophils. The fibrin clot is replaced by collagen-rich granulation tissue. The granulation tissue is invaded by osteoblasts, which start to deposit woven bone. Over the following weeks to months, lamellar bone and marrow replace the initial woven bone as the bone remodels.

Peri-implant mucosa—soft tissue healing surrounding the implant after placement establishes the peri-implant mucosa. The outermost surface of the peri-implant mucosa is pink, firm, and covered by keratinized epithelium. It is poor in fibroblasts, rich in collagen fibres, and has a limited blood supply, and thus has a lower potential for repair than gingival tissue.

Integration times Traditionally the time from placement to integration and loading has been accepted as 2–6 months. In certain circumstances, implants may be loaded earlier than this, even immediately.[4] However, there are few indications for this and if the implant is prematurely loaded or overloaded during the healing phase, there may be connective tissue encapsulation of the implant body, preventing osseointegration. The most predictable treatment plan and gold standard remains the conventional approach.

4 M. Esposito et al. 2007 *Cochrane Database Syst Rev* 2 CD003878.

Restoration of dental implants

Abutment connection Once integrated (and, if necessary, exposed), an abutment is connected to the implant (Fig. 9.5). This allows the prosthetic superstructure to be manufactured and connected via the abutment to the implant. Implant superstructures may be a single tooth crown, an implant-retained bridge, or implant-retained overdentures. There are multiple different abutment/implant connection types available, including internal hexagon design, external hexagon, conical connection, and Morse taper. Connections may have an anti-rotation device.

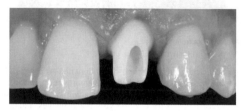

Fig. 9.5 Implant abutment in position prior to cementation of final restoration.
Courtesy of Dr Nilesh R. Parmar, Parmar Dental, UK.

Follow-up and maintenance

Follow-up and maintenance

If implants survive the first 2yrs, there is a 98% success rate with dramatic improvement in all functional parameters.[5] Success rates for the mandible are higher than those for the maxilla (due to bone quality). Implant-retained restorations need to be carefully maintained by the patient. The implant needs to be followed up long term clinically and radiographically by the clinician. Implant failure may be early or late. Early failure may be due to inadequate site preparation, overheating of bone, infection, premature loading, or lack of 1° stability. Late failure may be due to overloading or infection (peri-implantitis). Literature shows maintenance of restorations will be an ongoing problem for the implant patient (e.g. # screws, clips, porcelain, acrylic).

Implant success Success rates of dental implants are reported to be in excess of 90% after 10yrs. There are two ways an implant can be considered to fail: 1° failure, which is failure of osseointegration, and 2° failure, which is failure to maintain osseointegration. The implant can be considered to be successful if it is present and functioning (acceptable mastication, phonation, and pain-free) with a lack of mobility, associated radiolucency, and bone loss of <1.5mm. There should not be associated paraesthesia although this is a risk of treatment. The majority of implant failures are due to peri-implantitis. Aesthetic failure has been measured in the literature with the Pink Aesthetic Score (PES) and the White Aesthetic Score (WES).

Peri-implantitis Peri-implant mucositis is a condition of reversible inflammation of the soft tissue around an implant but which does not show any peri-implant bone loss (similar to gingivitis around teeth).

Peri-implantitis is a condition with destructive inflammation of the soft and hard tissues surrounding an osseointegrated implant (similar to periodontitis around teeth). Although implants have a 90%+ chance of 10yr survival, >40% of patients may experience peri-implantitis to some extent.[6]

Peri-implantitis and peri-implant bone loss is not well-understood but ↑ risk is associated with:

- Inadequate OH.
- Prosthesis designs that hinder OH.
- An excessive occlusal load on the implant.
- Poorly controlled diabetes.
- Existing periodontal disease (treated and untreated).
- Smoking.
- Thin bone coverage at the time of implant placement.
- Residual cement from a cemented implant restoration.
- Thin gingival biotype and tissue thickness.

Diagnosis involves radiographic examination to look for bone loss around the implant, assessment of the gingival tissue (colour and bleeding), evidence

5 R. Adell 1983 *J Prosthetic Dent* **49** 251.

6 H. Dreyer et al. 2018 *J Peridontal Res* **53** 657.

of suppuration, and ↑ probing depth of peri-implant pockets. Management can range from local debridement and improved OH to surgery with bone grafts and regenerative procedures.

Craniofacial implants (➲ p. 523.) Prosthetic eyes, ears, and noses can be securely fixed to the facial skeleton with implants using techniques similar to oral implants.

Oral surgery

Principal sources and further reading J. R. Hupp et al.
2008 *Contemporary Oral and Maxillofacial Surgery* (5e), Mosby.
D. A. Mitchell and A. N. Kanatas 2015 *An Introduction to Oral
and Maxillofacial Surgery* (2e), CRC Press. J. Pedlar & J. Frame
2007 *Oral and Maxillofacial Surgery: An Objective Based Textbook*
(2e), Churchill Livingstone. Additional background pathology: J. V. Soames & J. C. Southam 2018 *Oral Pathology* (5e),
OUP. Third molars: NICE 2000 *Guidance on the Extraction of
Wisdom Teeth* ℰ http://www.nice.org.uk/. Medication-related
osteonecrosis of the jaw (MRONJ)—full guidance available ℰ
http://www.sdcep.org.uk.

Principles of surgery of the mouth

The mouth is a remarkably forgiving environment in which to operate, because of its excellent blood supply and the properties of saliva. It is compromised less than could be expected by its teeming hordes of commensal organisms. This does not, however, constitute carte blanche for ignoring the basic principles of surgery, although these can and should be modified to suit the nature and the site of the surgery.

Asepsis and antisepsis See ➲ Asepsis and antisepsis, p. 380.

Analgesia Nowadays, all patients should expect and receive painless surgery, both peri-operatively and post-operatively. For analgesia and anaesthesia, see Chapter 15.

Anatomy and pathology These are the interdependent building blocks of surgery. Know the anatomy and you can understand the operation. Know the pathology and you know why you are doing it, what can be sacrificed, and what must be preserved.

Access For all minor and certain major oral surgical procedures, access is through the mouth via IO incisions. For EO surgery, see Chapter 12.

Incisions Incisions for dento-alveolar surgery are full thickness, i.e. mucoperiosteal flaps; for mucosal and periodontal surgery, split thickness flaps are raised (➲ Periodontal surgery—types of surgery, p. 212; ➲ Periodontal surgery—mucogingival surgery, p. 218). For mucoperiosteal flaps, although the base does *not have* to be longer than its length, this design improves the blood supply to the flap and should be used where this is a concern. Improved access via a large flap, allowing minimally traumatic surgery, virtually always outweighs the trauma of additional periosteal stripping.

Always plan the incision mindful of local structures. *One cut*, at right angles, through mucoperiosteum to bone, is the aim. Blade blunts on touching bone. Do not split interdental papillae. Try to cut in the depth of the gingival sulcus. Raise the flap cleanly, working subperiosteally with a blunt instrument, moving from easily elevated areas to the more difficult (➲ Forceps, elevators, and other instruments, p. 382).

Retraction Retraction of the raised flap should be gentle and precise. It is the assistant's duty to prevent trauma to the tissues by sharp edges, overheated drills, or bullish surgeons.

Bone removal Bone removal by drills must be accompanied by sterile irrigation to prevent heat necrosis of bone, damage to soft tissues, and clogging of the bur. When using chisels to remove bone, remember the natural lines of cleavage of the jaws and make stop cuts (chisel technique, ➲ Dento-alveolar surgery: third-molar technique, p. 400).

Removal Removal of the tooth/root is carried out using controlled force.

Debridement   Debridement is removal from the wound of debris generated by both the pathology and the operation. It is as important as any other part of the operation. Subperiosteal bone dust is a common cause of pain and delayed wound healing.

Haemostasis   Haemostasis and wound closure are covered in ➔ Suturing, p. 388.

Post-operative oedema   Post-operative oedema is, to some degree, inevitable; it is minimized by gentle efficient surgery, which is more important than such measures as ice packs and peri- or post-operative steroids, although these can help.

Asepsis and antisepsis

Asepsis Asepsis is the avoidance of pathogenic microorganisms. In practical terms, 'aseptic technique' is one which aims to exclude all microorganisms. Surgical technique is aseptic in the use of sterile instruments, clothing, and the 'no touch' technique.

Antisepsis Antisepsis is an agent or the application of an agent which inhibits the growth of microorganisms while in contact with them. Scrubbing up and preparation of operative sites are examples of antisepsis.

Disinfection *Disinfection* is the inhibition or destruction of pathogens, whereas *sterilization* is the destruction or removal of *all* forms of life. Prepackaged sterile supplies and the use of an autoclave (121°C for 15min or 134°C for 3min) for resterilizable equipment are the only really acceptable techniques in dentistry. Disinfection using glutaraldehyde or hypochlorite is second choice, for use where true sterilization is not feasible. There are strict restrictions on the use of glutaraldehyde which limit its usefulness outside hospitals. It is not possible to render the mouth aseptic and it is fruitless to try; there are, however, three basic techniques which are of value:

Avoid introducing infection This is achieved by *always* using *sterilized* instruments and wearing gloves.

Avoid being infected yourself by the operative site Wear gloves and face and eye protection.

Reduce the contaminating load to the site By pre-extraction cleaning of teeth, use of chlorhexidine mouthrinse, and prophylactic antimicrobials, when appropriate. There is a minimal evidence base, but it is common sense.

Cross-infection and its control Much attention has been focused on this problem in recent years, first with hepatitis B (Hep B) and its related agents, then with HIV, and now with prions. Although screening is possible in some instances, this is of little real value since the majority of individuals with communicable viral particles are *asymptomatic* and hence not identifiable. Therefore, safe practice mandates the use of sound cross-infection control as part of everyday practice on all patients.

Aerosols These are easily created and are a potential source of cross-infection. Minimize wherever possible by high-vacuum suction. Wear glasses and a mask if exposure to an aerosol cannot be avoided. Masks are routine in theatre, although of unproven value in preventing wound infection.

Cleaning and sterilizing Use disposable equipment when possible and never reuse. Clean instruments prior to sterilization. Use disposable or easily disinfected work surfaces. The cover of the printed version of this book can be wiped down with a variety of antiseptics!

Gloves Gloves should be worn routinely. Sterile gloves for surgery.

Immunization Immunization against Hep B is available. Get it and get all staff with clinical contact to do likewise.

Waste disposal It is everyone's responsibility to ensure sharps are carefully placed in rigid, well-marked containers and disposed of by an appropriate service. Dealing with potentially contaminated impressions and appliances, see ➲ Disinfection of impressions, p. 669. Treatment of the known high-risk patient, see ➲ Cross-infection prevention and control, p. 750.

Needlestick injuries If this happens to you, stop the procedure, ensure patient safety, rinse wound under running water, and record date and patient details. The patient needs to be informed and will require testing. In hospital, follow local policy; in practice, contact your local public health laboratory. DH guidance in the UK recommends universal source testing for Hep B, C, and HIV after an appropriate risk assessment. Highly active antiretroviral treatment (HAART) 'prophylaxis' post contamination with HIV has been shown to reduce the risk of seroconverting.

Forceps, elevators, and other instruments

Extraction forceps These come in numerous shapes and sizes. The choice of forceps is largely down to individual preference or, more frequently, availability. 'Universal' forceps are straight-bladed upper or lower forceps used to grip the roots of teeth to allow a controlled extracting force. 'Eagle beak' forceps are upper and lower molar forceps which engage the bifurcation of molar teeth allowing a buccally directed extraction force. 'Cowhorns' are designed to penetrate the molar bifurcation either to be used in a figure-of-eight loosening pattern or to split the roots. Most forceps come with a deciduous tooth equivalent.

Elevators These are used to dilate sockets to facilitate extraction or to remove dental hard tissue by themselves. These are the instruments which should *always* be used to remove impacted teeth. They should be used with gentle (finger pressure) forces. The commonly used patterns are Couplands no. 1, 2, and 3, Cryers right and left, and Warwick–James right, left, and straight.

Luxators These are sharp instruments with a less concave blade than the elevators. They are used to cut Sharpey's fibres within the periodontal ligament and loosen the teeth. Use with care.

Scalpel A Bard–Parker handle with a no. 15 blade is the usual choice.

Periosteal elevators A number are available; the Howarths, originally designed as a nasal rasparatory, is a favourite. McDonalds and 'no. 9' are others.

Retractors Tongue, cheek, and flap retractors are needed and are legion in number; Dyson's tongue retractor, Kilner's cheek retractor, Bowdler–Henry's rake retractor, and the Minnesota flap retractor are favourites. Lack's is an all-purpose retractor (really a bent bit of metal)!

Chisels versus burs Depends upon your training. Generally, burs (no. 8 round T-C for bone removal, medium taper fissure T-C for tooth division) are kinder on the conscious patient and the best bet for the inexperienced. Chisels are more appropriate in theatre and are particularly useful (3mm and 5mm TC tipped) for disto-angular third molars and upper third molars.

Curettes The Mitchell trimmer is probably the most valuable instrument in this category.

Needle holders and sutures These vary more than any of those previously mentioned, depending on your location. The usual suture size for IO work is 4/0; the material may be non-absorbable (silk) or absorbable (Dexon®, Vicryl®). It is difficult to justify the continued use of any non-absorbable IO suture for routine use.

Scissors Remember to keep dissecting scissors, e.g. McIndoe's, separate from suture-cutting scissors, and keep both sets sharp.

Dissecting forceps These are designed to hold soft tissue without damaging it; Gillies dissectors are popular. College tweezers are not dissecting forceps and are used to lift up sutures prior to removing them.

Aspirator This has a sterile/disposable suction tip small enough to get into the defect.

The extraction of teeth

The extraction of teeth must be viewed as a minor surgical procedure; therefore, the medical history will be pertinent, e.g. bleeding diathesis, etc. More common and specific considerations are the sex, age, and build of the patient. NICE guidelines currently state that patients at risk of bacterial endocarditis do *not* require antibiotic cover. Extractions in children are technically simple; it is the child who is most likely to be a problem, whereas stoical old men who may not bat an eye at the procedure often have teeth aptly described as 'glass in concrete'. Malpositioned teeth present problems of access and isolated teeth, especially upper second molars, tend to be ankylosed. Heavily restored and root-filled teeth can be very brittle. In all these cases a pre-extraction X-ray can help.

Extraction of teeth Extraction of teeth begins with *positioning*. After LA has taken, the patient is positioned supine at the height of the operator's elbow for upper teeth, sitting with the operator behind for (right-handed) dentists) lower extractions on the right and in front for lower extractions on the left. The position is reversed for left-handers, but unfortunately the world seems biased against this group, and many dental chair systems seem to preclude comfortable positioning for them.

Common technique The socket is dilated either using an elevator between the bone of the socket wall and the tooth or by driving the forceps blades into the socket. The blades of the forceps are applied to the buccal and palatal/lingual aspects of the tooth and pushed either along the root of the tooth or, in certain molar extractions, into the bifurcation. The tooth is then gripped in the forceps and, maintaining a consistent and quite substantial vertical force, the tooth is moved depending on its anatomy:
- 1, 2, 3 have conical roots—rotate then pull.
- 4, 5 have either two fine roots or a flattened root—move bucco-palatally until you feel them 'give', then pull down and buccally.
- 6, 7 have three large divergent roots—these are moved buccally while maintaining upward pressure, but frequently need a variety of rocking movements before they are sufficiently disengaged to complete extraction.
- $\overline{1}$, $\overline{2}$, $\overline{3}$ can usually be removed with a simple buccal movement, but sometimes need to be rocked or even rotated.
- $\overline{4}$, $\overline{5}$ are rotated and lifted out.
- $\overline{6}$, $\overline{7}$ are two-rooted and can usually be removed by a controlled buccal movement. Remember to support the patient's jaw.

Deciduous teeth These are extracted using the same principles, but while permanent molars can be removed using forceps which engage the bifurcation, these should not be used on deciduous teeth.

Third molars See ● Dento-alveolar surgery: removal of third molars, p. 396; ● Dento-alveolar surgery: coronectomy, p. 398; ● Dento-alveolar surgery: third-molar technique, p. 400.

Difficulties and complications of extracting teeth

Access Small mouths present an obvious, but usually manageable problem. Crowded or malpositioned teeth may need a trans-alveolar approach. Trismus, if due to infection, e.g. submasseteric abscess, should be managed in hospital where facilities for external drainage and airway protection are available.

Pain Has the LA worked? Try further LA as regional block, infiltration, or intraligamentary injection. Is it pain or pressure? If pressure, reassure and proceed. If pain and other signs of adequate LA are present, then acute infection is the most likely culprit. Can the extraction wait by using delaying tactics such as draining an abscess? The vast majority can and very few adult extractions really justify a GA.

Inability to move the tooth Don't worry; it happens to us all. Have you got an X-ray? If not, get one and look for: bulbous or diverging roots, very long roots, ankylosis, or sclerotic bone. Do not press on regardless; it will work sometimes but shows lack of consideration and will cost you in time and goodwill in the long run. Most 'solid' teeth have an easily identifiable cause, e.g. diverging roots, and raising a flap and using a trans-alveolar procedure (➔ Surgical methods, p. 392) will quickly and easily remedy this.

Breaking the tooth This is a common occurrence and may even assist extraction if, e.g. the roots of a molar are separated. More often, unfortunately, the crown #, leaving a portion of root(s) *in situ*. It is quite acceptable to leave small (<3mm) pieces of deeply buried apex, but provide antibiotics, tell the patient, and review. Larger pieces of root must be removed as they have a high incidence of infective sequelae (➔ Dento-facial infections, p. 408).

# of alveolar &/or basal bone Breaking the alveolar bone is relatively common. If # only involves the alveolus containing the extracted tooth, remove any pieces of bone not attached to periosteum and close the wound. Rarely, the alveolus carrying other teeth will be involved, in which case remove tooth by a trans-alveolar procedure and splint remaining teeth (➔ Splinting, p. 109). Basal bone # is rare; ensure analgesia (LA &/or systemic analgesics) and arrange reduction and fixation (➔ Open reduction and internal fixation (ORIF), p. 500).

Loss of the tooth Stop and look; in the mouth, is it under the mucoperiosteum or in a tissue space? These can usually be milked out. Look in the suction apparatus. Is it in the antrum (➔ The maxillary antrum, p. 422), through the lingual cortex, or even the ID canal? Has it been swallowed or inhaled? A CXR is mandatory if not found.

Oro-antral communication This is a complication that can occur during root removal, whereby a communication between the maxillary antrum and the oral cavity is created. If the root is removed, then the operator should close the communication with local full-depth mucoperiosteal flaps. If not able to carry out this procedure, a referral should be made to the local oral surgery department. The patient should be encouraged to avoid blowing their nose until resolved and a nasal decongestant prescribed (0.5% ephedrine nasal drops for 5 days).

Damage to other teeth/tissues and extraction of the wrong tooth Prevent this by confirming with the patient the teeth to be removed and making careful notes. One clever idea is to draw the teeth to be removed on the patient's cheek. Plan the operation; do not use inappropriate instruments or ones which you don't know how to use. If the wrong tooth is extracted, replant if feasible and proceed to remove the correct tooth. Tell the patient and make careful notes.

Dislocated jaw Reduce (➲ Dislocation, p. 504); bleeding (➲ Suturing, p. 388); pain, swelling, and trismus are common sequelae, and are discussed in ➲ Post-operatively, p. 400.

Medication-related osteonecrosis of the jaw (MRONJ) Several anti-resorptive and anti-angiogenic drugs that are prescribed in the UK have been associated with MRONJ but commonly it is due to bisphosphonates (➲ Bisphosphonates, p. 614). Risk assessment is required and the Rx needs to be tailored according to the risk. The principle is not to carry out any surgery which requires osteoclast activity for healing on someone taking these drugs. If this is inevitable, explain relative risks to patient and take recommended precautions (➲ Dento-alveolar surgery: bisphosphonates, denosumab, or anti-angiogenic medication, p. 390).

Post-operative bleeding

Bleeding disorders are covered in → Bleeding disorders, p. 530.
  Principles of management of post-operative bleeding:
• Support the patient. If hypotensive and tachycardic, establish IV access and replace lost blood volume.
• Diagnose each cause, nature, and site of blood loss.
• Control the bleeding point.

Classically, post-operative bleeding is described as immediate (1°), reactionary, and 2°.

Immediate When true haemostasis has not been achieved at completion of surgery.

Reactionary Occurs within 48h of surgery and is due to both general and local rises in BP opening up small divided vessels which were not bleeding at completion of surgery.

Secondary Occurs ~7 days post-operatively and is usually due to infection destroying the clot or ulcerating local vessels. In practice, bleeding following removal of teeth is common and usually simple to diagnose. The patients are seldom shocked or hypotensive but are often very anxious and nauseated by the taste, smell, and sight of blood, and by blood in the stomach, which is irritant. Bleeding usually comes from one or all of three sources: (i) gingival capillaries; (ii) vessels in the bone of the socket; and (iii) a large vessel under a flap or in bone, such as the inferior alveolar artery. The first two are by far the more common.

Management
Reassure the patient they won't bleed to death. Remove accompanying entourage and get the patient to an area with reasonable facilities. Take a drug history (anticoagulants?). *Wear gloves and apron*: patients often vomit. (If patient has to wait to be seen they should bite firmly on a clean handkerchief or gauze, rolled to fit the area the bleeding seems to be coming from.) In good light, with suction, clean the patient's face and mouth, remove any lumps of clot, and identify the source of bleeding. Is it from under a flap? If from a socket, squeeze the gingivae to the outer walls of the socket between finger and thumb; if bleeding stops it is from a gingival vessel. In these cases, LA and suturing are needed. If bleeding continues it is from vessels in bone, which need some form of pack.

Technique
Give LA if needed, and have assistance with suction. If a flap is involved, remove old sutures, evacuate clot, identify bleeding point, and place a tight suture around it. Bleeding should be much ↓; if not, repeat until it is, then close wound and have the patient bite on a swab for at least 15min. If it is a gingival bleed, a tight interrupted or mattress suture will compress the capillaries, again followed by a swab to bite on. If bleeding is from the depths of the socket, the clot may need to be removed and replaced by a pack or supported by a resorbable mesh (oxidized cellulose) &/or agents such as tranexamic acid, adrenaline, or epsilon

aminocaproic acid soaked into the mesh. If removing clot and packing the socket, remember this will delay healing and predispose to infection, so use bismuth iodoform paraffin paste (BIPP) or Whitehead's varnish packs. If all else fails, use all the earlier mentioned measures plus a pressure pack, analgesia, an antiemetic, and a night in a hospital bed. Patients requiring this degree of Rx should be investigated haematologically and for liver disease.

Suturing

Every dentist should master the basic skills of suturing.

Materials Most sutures are suture material fused to a needle, although threaded reusable needles are used in some countries. Needles may be round-bodied, cutting, or reverse cutting, and straight, curved, or J-shaped. Almost all IO work is done with a 16–22mm curved cutting or reverse cutting needle held in a needle holder. Suture material may be resorbable (Dexon®, Vicryl®, or Monocryl®) or non-resorbable (silk, nylon, Prolene™, or Novafil®). Monofilament suture (e.g. nylon) causes less tissue response than braided (e.g. silk).

Skin Skin is best closed with nylon, Prolene™, or Novafil®. *Mucosa* and *deep tissues* are best closed with an absorbable. *Vessels* are tied off using resorbables, except major veins and arteries, which are transfixed and tied with silk. Black silk suture (BSS) can be used for skin but must be removed *early*. Suture strength is described as 0 (thickest) to 4/0 (commonest in IO use) to 11/0 (thinnest for microvascular work).

Types of stitch These are shown in Fig. 10.1.

Suture technique Closure of a wound or incision should, whenever possible, be without tension, by closing deep layers and over supporting tissue. Hold the needle in the needle holder about two-thirds of the way from its tip. Suture from free to fixed tissue taking a bite of 2–3mm on both sides. Leave the sutured wound edges slightly everted in apposition. Except when swaging tissue to bone, e.g. when arresting haemorrhage or when tying vessels, do not overtighten the suture as wound margins become swollen, and you need to allow for this.

Knot tying The two most useful are the square (reef) knot and the surgeon's knot (Fig. 10.1).

Instrument tying Instrument tying is easy to learn from a book but needs considerable practice to perfect. The knot is started by passing the suture once (square knot) or twice (surgeon's knot) around the tip of the needle holders; the knot is tightened and then locked by passing the suture around the needle holder in the opposite direction once. It is possible to control the suture tension by completing the knot in three loops instead of two.

Hand tying Hand tying is invaluable for those wishing to develop surgical expertise or be involved in major maxillofacial surgery. It takes a substantial amount of time and practice and is impossible to learn from a book. Get a sympathetic senior to demonstrate.

Suture removal Suture removal is not someone else's job to be casually forgotten about. Do the stitches need to be removed? In inaccessible sites, difficult patients, or areas in which scar quality is less important, a resorbable suture should be used. An alternative is tissue glue, e.g. Dermabond®, Indermil®. Facial skin sutures should be removed at 4–6 days. When removing sutures use sharp scissors (avoid 'stitch cutters' if you can), lifting up and cutting a bit of suture that has been in the tissue, thus avoiding dragging bacteria through the incision on removal.

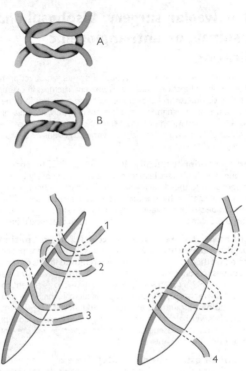

Fig. 10.1 (A) Reef knot. (B) Surgeon's knot.
1 Simple interrupted suture.
2 Horizontal mattress suture.
3 Vertical mattress suture.
4 Continuous subcuticular suture.

Dento-alveolar surgery: bisphosphonates, denosumab, or anti-angiogenic medication

Bisphosphonates constitute a wide group of agents which act primarily by inhibiting osteoclast function which helps prevent fractures in osteoporosis, stabilizes Paget's disease, relieves bone pain and fractures in bone metastases in a range of malignancies, and can treat hypercalcaemia of carcinomatosis. Unfortunately, one of their side effects is necrosis of jaw bone, usually (although not always) associated with extractions or dento-alveolar surgery (Fig. 10.2).

If asked to render 'dentally fit' If you are asked to render 'dentally fit' someone who is to start bisphosphonates, it is probably best to adopt a similar approach to those having head and neck radiotherapy—try to ensure they never need to have a tooth removed in the future. Obviously a balance has to be struck between inappropriately rendering everyone edentulous and the optimistic watch-and-wait approach that would be usual.

If you have to remove a tooth in a patient on bisphosphonates There will be many instances where patients have been started on these drugs and need teeth removed. If this can be avoided by endodontics, coronectomy, etc. then do it. If not, warn the patient of risks (range from <1% for low-risk drug in osteoporosis patient to 30% in a myeloma survivor at 10yrs). Use prophylactic chlorhexidine and broad-spectrum antibiotic, atraumatic extraction, and alveolar septoplasty to ensure all bone lies well below the gingival margin and close mucosa primarily. This is on the basis that vascularized mucosal coverage will prevent super-infection of bone that will not remodel.

Treatment of established MRONJ There are no agreed effective Rxs to date. Tactics that work for osteoradionecrosis do not seem to help. Limited sequestrectomy coupled with some form of coverage of the exposed bone seems to help and a variety of supplemental drug Rxs are being used but there is no established evidence base for this. Refer to your local oral and maxillofacial surgery department.

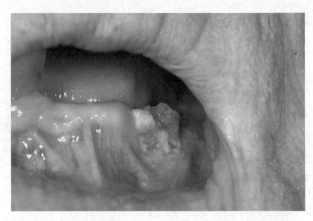

Fig. 10.2 Clinical example of bisphosphonate-related osteonecrosis of the jaw (BRONJ).

Dento-alveolar surgery: removal of roots

Does the root need to be removed? If large, being extracted for pulpal or apical pathology, is symptomatic, is an impediment to denture construction, or is in a patient in whom risk of minor local infection is not tolerable (e.g. immunocompromised), then the answer is yes.

Non-surgical methods The use of root forceps or elevators may allow simple removal of roots close to the alveolar margin. When using root forceps ensure the root can be seen to be engaged by the blades. Elevators can be used to direct a root along its path of withdrawal providing (i) one exists, and (ii) an elevator can be introduced between bone and root. Do not waste time persisting with non-surgical methods if your initial attempt is unsuccessful.

Surgical methods Plan your operation. Do you know why the root cannot be delivered, exactly where it is, and about any adjacent structures? If not, get an X-ray.
- The flap: if edentulous, incise along the crest of the ridge; if dentate, in the gingival margin. Flaps may be envelope, two-sided (Fig. 10.3), or three-sided. Relieving incisions make reflection of the flap easier but must be avoided in the region of the mental nerve ($\overline{45}$) and are better avoided around the buccal branch of the facial artery (mesial root $\overline{7}$). Include an interdental papilla at either side of the flap and start vertical cuts two-thirds of the way distal to the included papilla. Big flaps heal as well as small ones; the important consideration is access.
- Identify obstructions to the path of withdrawal of the root; these are either removed or the root is sectioned to create another path of withdrawal, depending on which approach is the least traumatic.
- Remove the minimum amount of buccal bone compatible with exposing the maximum diameter of the root and a point of application for an elevator (no. 8 round T-C surgical bur).
- Elevate by placing an elevator between bone and tooth (remember to apply to the convex surface of curved roots) and direct the root along its natural path of withdrawal.
- Finally, debride and close the wound.

Special cases
- Small apical fragments: use an apicectomy approach.
- Multirooted teeth: always divide the roots, as this makes life much easier.
- Cannot find the root: re-X-ray and look in the soft tissues. The root may have been displaced into another cavity or even be in the aspirator; look carefully but remember discretion is the better part of valour. Tell the patient.
- Patient refuses operation: it's their body—record your advice and their decision.

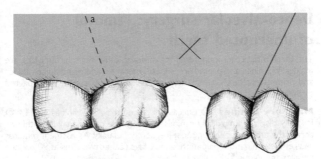

Fig. 10.3 Outline of two-sided flap in heavy shade.
X   Retained root or similar.
a   Line of additional incision to convert to three-sided flap.

Dento-alveolar surgery: removal of unerupted teeth

The teeth most commonly requiring removal, other than third molars, are maxillary canines and premolars, supernumeraries, and mandibular canines and premolars. Rarely, permanent or deciduous molars may be impacted or infraoccluded.

Maxillary canines (➲ Buccally displaced maxillary canines, p. 143; ➲ Palatally displaced maxillary canines, p. 144.) The canine may lie within or across the arch, buccally, or, most frequently, palatally. Assessment requires a careful examination, palpation, and X-rays (either two films at 90° or the parallax technique ➲ Parallax technique, p. 19; ➲ Assessment, p. 144).

Techniques Buccal impactions are approached via a buccal flap, palatal via a palatal flap, and cross- or within-arch impactions need a combination of the two. Buccal flaps are as previously described (➲ Surgical methods, p. 392). Palatal flaps involve the reflection of the full thickness of the mucoperiosteum of the anterior hard palate, the incision running in the gingival crevice from 6| to |6 for bilateral canines or to the contralateral canine region for single impactions. The neurovascular bundle emerging from the incisive foramen is often sacrificed, with no noticeable morbidity (if it bleeds, use bone wax). *Never* incise the palate at 90° to the gingival crevice and *always* use an envelope flap, otherwise you will section the palatine artery. Remove bone over the bulge of the crown of the tooth until the maximum bulbosity of the crown and the incisal tip are exposed. If the root curvature and path of withdrawal are favourable, the entire tooth can be elevated out. If not, section at the cervical margin with a tapered fissure bur and winkle the pieces out separately. Debride the socket and close with vertical mattress sutures to minimize haematoma formation.

Mandibular canines Most lie buccally, and can be elevated or removed with root forceps. Unerupted, deeply impacted buccal or lingual canines rarely need to be removed. If necessary, a degloving incision provides good access.

Maxillary premolars Most lie palatally. If partially erupted and conically rooted, they are simply elevated. Otherwise, a similar approach to that used for palatal canines is used. Premolars within the arch are approached buccally, sectioned, and removed piecemeal.

Mandibular premolars These are often angled lingually. The 'broken instrument' technique can be invaluable. Otherwise, an extended buccal flap is raised to visualize and protect the mental nerve, buccal bone is removed, and the tooth sectioned at its cervical margin. The crown is then displaced downwards into the space created and the root elevated upwards.

Submerged deciduous molars If they must be removed, they are approached buccally and sectioned vertically, then elevated along the individual roots path of withdrawal.

Supernumeraries (⊙ Hyperdontia, p. 68.) These are removed using the approach used for the tooth they impede or replace. This can be a surprisingly difficult operation, usually because of difficulty in finding and identifying the supernumerary.

Piezosurgery® This is a technique that uses a cutting tip vibrating between 60 and 200mm/sec. Benefits of avoiding trauma to soft tissues such as nerves and vessels are claimed, as the device selectively cuts hard tissues. This may be of use in situations where structures such as the mental nerve or antral lining are in close proximity and is particularly useful in implantology during bone augmentation or sinus lift procedures. Outside these indications, it has yet to become a popular alternative to the conventional rotary drill.

Dento-alveolar surgery: removal of third molars

Not all wisdom teeth need to be removed.[1] Most clinicians will follow the NICE guidance although currently the guidelines are under review. Those which have space to erupt into functional occlusion should be left to do so, and those which are deeply impacted and asymptomatic are best left alone. Decisions about surgery vary widely.[2] In the UK the absolute number removed has not changed despite guidelines but the age at which they are removed has become older.[3]

Aetiology As the last tooth to erupt, the third molar is most liable to be prevented from doing so in a crowded mouth. *Causes:* a soft Western diet doesn't create space by contact point abrasion, inherited tooth–jaw size incompatibility, and possibly an evolutionary tendency towards ↓ jaw size.

Symptoms Pain, swelling, pericoronitis (❷ Dento-facial infections, p. 408), and sometimes a foul taste. Mostly due to localized infection, less commonly due to caries or resorption of the second molar or cyst associated with the third molar. Third molars covered by bone are very unlikely to become infected, whereas those where the crown has breached mucosa will almost inevitably do so. Infections in older, less vascular bone are more difficult to treat.

Indications for removal Recurrent pericoronitis, unrestorable caries in 7 or 8, external or internal resorption, cystic change, or periodontal disease distally in 7. The prevention of LLS crowding on its own is *not* an indication, nor is vague TMJ pain.

Timing Symptoms are most common in the late teens and twenties; bone is soft, spongy, and elastic in this age group, so this is the usual and most favourable time to operate. Prophylactic removal of symptomless third molars is currently hard to justify.[4]

Choice of anaesthetic Bilateral impacted third molars are more kindly treated under GA, as are those where surgery may be technically more difficult, e.g. disto-angular 8s. LA &/or sedation is appropriate for most unilateral impactions not presenting particular difficulty. Consider the medical history.

Assessment Look first: unerupted or partially erupted? Take a pre-operative X-ray (DPT is ideal; see Fig. 10.4).

Assess angulation (vertical, mesio-angular, disto-angular, horizontal, or transverse); depth of impaction from the alveolar crest to the maximum diameter of the crown; degree of impaction (and against what); root shape; bone density; the relationship to the ID canal; and the presence of any other pathology or complicating factors.

1 NICE 2000 *Guidance on the Extraction of Wisdom Teeth* (⅍ https://www.nice.org.uk/guidance/ta1).

2 D. M. Hyam 2018 *Aust Dent J* 63 s19.

3 L. McArdle & T. Renton 2012 *Br Dent J* 213 E8.

4 T. G. Mettes et al. 2012 *Cochrane Database Syst Rev* 6 CD003879.

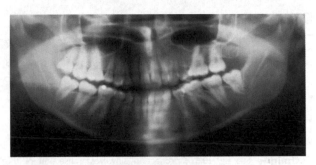

Fig. 10.4 A DPT example of simple, vertically impacted, conically rooted third molars suitable for removal in the ambulatory setting.

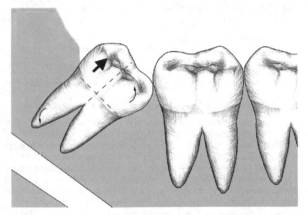

Fig. 10.5 A schematic showing planning for third molar removal. Bold arrow—natural path of withdrawal, this causes impaction against second molar. Dashed lines are the lines of tooth sectioning. Top curved arrow—rotational movement to disimpact. Lower curved arrow—compensatory rotational movement which puts nerve at risk if tooth is not sectioned vertically.

Plan the path of withdrawal (Fig. 10.5). What impedes it? How much bone needs to be removed to provide a point of application for an elevator? How much to clear the path of withdrawal? Can this be done less traumatically by sectioning the tooth? In what direction?

Warn the patient about pain, trismus, swelling, and the possibility of damage to the ID and lingual nerves.

Dento-alveolar surgery: coronectomy

This is used as an alternative to the complete removal in selective cases only.[5] It involves removal of the crown of a lower 8, with deliberate retention of the roots. This may be indicated if the roots of the lower 8 are radiographically assessed as being closely involved with the ID canal. Radiographic signs of ↑ risk of nerve damage include:

- Proximity to nerve canal.
- Narrowing or diversion of canal.
- Darkening of root/interrupting white lines of canal.
- Interruption of lamina dura.
- Juxta-apical area.

Technique See Fig. 10.6. Coronectomy involves transection of the tooth 3–4mm below the ADJ. The pulp is left untreated. The root is further reduced with a rose head bur to 3–4mm below the level of the alveolar crest. This may not be possible if there are defects in the lingual plate, due to risk of damage to the lingual nerve. Irrigate the socket with saline and close with a single suture.

Exclusion criteria

- Predisposition to local infection/medically compromised.
- Mobile teeth.
- Non-vital lower third molar.
- Horizontal or disto-angular impaction where sectioning crown puts nerve at risk.
- If root becomes mobile during sectioning, it must be removed.

Coronectomy compares favourably to surgical removal of lower wisdom teeth in terms of altered sensation: reported rates for conventional surgical removal are 8% temporary, and 3.6% permanent (personal rates vary). There is a similar incidence of dry socket (10–12%). Long-term data on late infection and cyst development are not yet available. If the coronectomy fails and the root is mobilized, there appears to be a reduced risk of nerve damage, although this probably reflects the fact that the nerve was not involved in the root in the first place. Post-coronectomy migration of the root may occur, necessitating a second procedure. The root is likely to erupt away from the nerve thereby reducing the risk of damage. Failure of coronectomy may occur, particularly in women with conical roots that narrow into the ID canal.

5 T. Renton et al. 2005 *Br J Oral Maxillofac Surg* **43** 7.

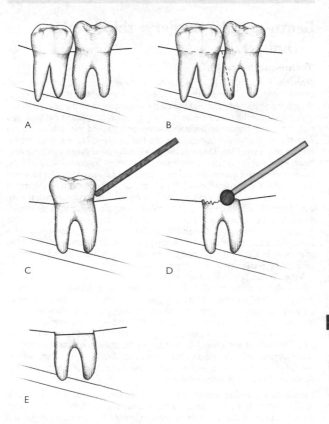

Fig. 10.6 A step-by-step illustration of coronectomy.
A   Vertical impaction with high likelihood of nerve involvement.
B   Gingival incision.
C   Crown is sectioned through ADJ.
D   Remaining root is reduced 3–4 mm below the alveolar crest.
E   The residual roots (now lying below the surrounding bone) are then covered with the mucosal flap.

Dento-alveolar surgery: third-molar technique

Technique See Fig. 10.7.

Mandible A buccal flap is incised along the external oblique ridge (lies well lateral to the arch) over the crest of the ridge if unerupted, or in the gingival margin if partially erupted. Extend to the distal aspect of the second molar and down into the buccal sulcus. Cut on to bone to create a full-thickness flap. If a mesio-angular or horizontal impaction, extend the incision around $\overline{7}$ to the mesial border, but beware the buccal branch of the facial artery. Reflect and retract flap. There is now good evidence to suggest that manipulation from the lingual aspect results in unnecessary lingual nerve morbidity. Bone and tooth removal should be from a buccal approach. An attached mucosa disto-lingual flap for visibility which does not encroach on the lingual nerve is reasonable. Wide exposure and subperiosteal protection of the lingual nerve should be undertaken by those using the lingual split technique. Remove bone to provide a point of application for an elevator and clear obstruction to the path of withdrawal. This can be done with chisels or a bur. With a bur this is done by creating a disto-buccal gutter, exposing the maximum bulbosity of the tooth. If needed, the bur can then be used to section the $\overline{8}$ to provide an unimpeded path of withdrawal.

With chisels, place mesial and distal stop cuts around the tooth and split off a collar of buccal and distal bone to expose the bulbosity of the crown. This can then be extended into a lingual split, taking off a piece of lingual plate and allowing the tooth to be elevated lingually. Whichever technique is used, it is important to remember that if it has been done properly, a minimum of directed force via an elevator will deliver the tooth or fragment out along its path of withdrawal. If this cannot be done, look carefully for another obstruction. Once the tooth is removed, debride the socket, remove the follicle, and close the wound with loose sutures to allow for swelling. Achieve haemostasis with pressure.

Maxilla A flap similar to that in the mandible can be used for inaccessible wisdom teeth but many can be approached using a 'slash' incision (from disto-palatally on the tuberosity to disto-buccally at the second molar and into the buccal sulcus). Reflect and retract the flap. Bone removal can usually be effected with a hand-held chisel. The much softer bone rarely causes any problem with elevation, but care has to be taken to prevent displacement into the pterygoid space. The 'slash' incision often needs no closure, whereas a conventional incision will need repositioning with sutures.

Post-operatively Pain can be quite severe and responds best to NSAIDs. Peri-operative LA works well and leaves patients pain-free but numb for the duration. Trismus is due to pain and muscle spasm and can be ↓ by adequate analgesia (⊃ Acute and post-operative pain, p. 584). It has obvious but often forgotten connotations for meals post-operatively. Swelling can also be ↓ by high-dose peri-operative steroids. There is no evidence that ice-packs help, although they are often used. Haemorrhage can usually be controlled by biting on pressure packs. Rarely, it may be necessary to re-explore the wound. Antibiotic prophylaxis is probably beneficial.[6]

6 J. M. V. Martin et al. *BDJ* **198** 327.

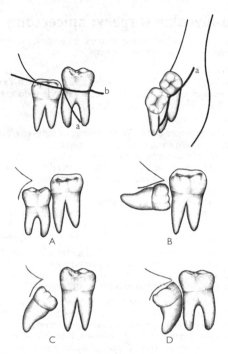

Fig. 10.7 A step-by-step illustration of the third molar technique.
a   Outline of incision for raising a third-molar buccal flap.
b   Modification to create an envelope flap.
A   Vertically impacted third molar.
B   Horizontally impacted third molar.
C   Mesio-angular impaction of a third molar.
D   Disto-angular impaction of a third molar.

Dento-alveolar surgery: apicectomy

There are three surgical aids to endodontics: apicectomy, root hemisection, and removal of extruded endodontic paste.

Apicectomy

See Fig. 10.8 and Fig. 10.9. This is by far the commonest Rx. It is a *second-line* Rx after failure of, or as a supplement to, orthograde endodontics (which has an 86–96% success rate in expert hands).[7]

Indications
- Impossible to prepare and fill apical one-third of tooth (e.g. pulpal calcification, curved apex, open apex).
- Irretrievable broken instrument in canal.
- Post crown on tooth with apical pathology (only if post crown has sealed the coronal root and crown margin adequately).
- Root perforation.
- Fractured and infected apical one-third.
- Persistent infection due to apical cyst or other lesion requiring biopsy, and repeat root canal therapy has been performed and is adequate or 'pull through' technique is planned. A coronal seal must be achievable.

Assessment IO X-ray, best possible root filling *in situ*, free from acute infection, and crown sealed with good quality restoration.

Remember—non-surgical Rx: 72% success; apicectomy and retrograde root filling: 60%, apicectomy no retrograde root filling: 51%.

Technique This operation is best performed under LA. Ensure an area of two tooth widths either side of the tooth being treated is anaesthetized, and give palatal infiltration. In the mandible, give a block plus infiltration to aid haemostasis. If associated with infection, prophylactic antibiotics, e.g. amoxicillin 1g 1h pre- and 6h post-operatively, or metronidazole 400mg 1h pre- and 6h post-operatively can help.

Flaps Flaps may be two- or three-sided, semilunar or sublabial; the latter two avoid post-operative recession but give inferior access. Semilunar flaps are prone to breakdown. Reflect and retract well above the apex (there is often a bulge or perforation of the cortical plate to aid location of the apex). A bony window is created to visualize the apex, which is often found sitting in a mass of granulation tissue. Excise the apical 1–2mm and curette out the cystic and granulation tissue. Pack the cavity with bone wax or adrenaline-soaked ribbon gauze, identify the canal and prepare it with a no. 1/2-round bur or ultrasonics (depending on availability). Seal with super ethoxy benzoic acid (EBA), Intermediate Restorative Material® (IRM®), or MTA and debride. Close, using interrupted or vertical mattress sutures.

Operating microscopes These have become popular with those specializing in surgical endodontics (who would claim this to be the 'gold standard'). It can minimize loss of tooth and allow visualization of accessory canals and precise preparation (with the right instruments) and seal of the apical canal. Cost and availability remains a significant issue.

7 N. Chandler 2002 *J R Coll Surg Edin* **47** 600.

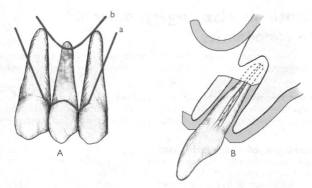

Fig. 10.8 Apicectomy technique. A, An approach to apicectomy. a, Outline of incision for three-sided flap, good access, best flap for the novice. b, Outline of semilunar flap incision. B, An approach to apicectomy, a window is created in the buccal cortex to expose the apex, which is resected, leaving a smooth raw bony cavity.

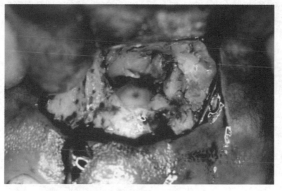

Fig. 10.9 Clinical view of the apical preparation.

Special points in apicectomy   Warn patients about post-operative swelling. Lower incisors present an access problem eased but not erased by a degloving incision and experience. Think twice about the mental nerve in lower premolar apicectomies. Think hard about alternatives to apicectomy of 6. Don't think at all about 7, 8. Remember the buccal and palatal roots in 4̲; section the buccal root low to see the palatal. Apicectomy of 6̲ is fine provided the palatal root can be treated by an orthograde approach, is hemisected, or you are happy to deal with breaching the antrum.

Dento-alveolar surgery: other aids to endodontics

Root perforations are approached as for apicectomy; however, multirooted tooth perforations, un-rootfillable roots, or untreatable periodontal pockets may be dealt with by the following:

Root hemisection   This simply involves raising a flap around the tooth, identifying and horizontally sectioning the root, and atraumatically elevating it out. The wound is closed and a cleanable undersurface sealed with super EBA, IRM®, or MTA left.

Removal of extruded paste   Usually, all that is required is an apicectomy approach. However, careless use of 'paste only' techniques can result in paste in the floor of the nose, the antrum, or the ID canal. The nasal floor can be approached sublabially or intranasally, the antrum by standard methods (⊃ The maxillary antrum, p. 422), and the ID canal by sagittally splitting the buccal cortex of the mandible.

Prognosis   Single-rooted tooth apicectomies should succeed 58–96% of the time. The range is due to an ill-defined definition of 'success' and operator technique. Multirooted teeth, revision apicectomy, and perforation repair have a much lower success rate.

Dento-alveolar surgery: helping the orthodontist

Many minor oral surgical procedures, e.g. extraction of 4s or removal of 8s, are carried out at the instigation of an orthodontist. This topic concerns itself with the specific procedures of fraenectomy, pericision, tooth exposure, and tooth repositioning (see Fig. 10.10 and Fig. 10.11).

Fraenectomy This is of value in closing a median diastema only if gentle traction on the upper lip and fraenum produces blanching in a palatal insertion around the incisive papilla. It follows that the excision of the fraenum must include those fibrous insertions, which leaves a raw area of alveolus after excision—this can be dressed with Surgicel®, BIPP, or a periodontal pack. It is a different operation from pre-prosthetic fraenectomy and is performed for a different reason.

Pericision This technique means simply incising supra-alveolar periodontal fibres to prevent relapse when de-rotating teeth.

Tooth exposure Orthodontic traction is the Rx of choice for malpositioned, unerupted canines and incisors if the apices are in a good position for eruption. The essential aspect of the operation is to remove any sacrificable impediments to tooth movement. Bonding an eyelet and gold chain or other bracket technique has a lower incidence of reoperation; this is fiddly and requires use of composite in a hard-to-dry field.

Technique Palatal teeth are exposed by a palatal flap. Remove bone carefully with chisels; expose the greatest diameter of the crown and the tip. (Moving the tooth is counter-productive, therefore don't do it.) Excise palatal mucoperiosteum generously, it grows back; bond a bracket if you're going to do. The wound may be packed firmly with, e.g. Whitehead's varnish and ribbon gauze, and secure, or use an acrylic dressing plate with periodontal paste dressing, or cauterize and leave open. Close the remainder of the flap with vertical mattress sutures. Buccally located teeth are approached by a buccal flap, in order to preserve attached gingiva, and bonding should be done at operation. The flap can be repositioned coronally with the elastics or chain tunnelling subgingivally. Teeth within the arch are approached buccally removing crestal bone as needed.

Tooth repositioning (transplantation) Although there are claims of success rates as high as 93%, few people match this and most would transplant only when exposure and orthodontic movement were rejected. The most commonly transplanted tooth is the maxillary canine. It is essential to measure the available space and compare this with the erupted contralateral tooth or a good X-ray estimation, as it is not acceptable to grind down healthy teeth at operation to accommodate the retrieved tooth. If the tooth appears to be too big for the available space, then orthodontic Rx is required to create space. As this is often the reason the patient rejected exposure, an impasse is sometimes reached.

Technique The tooth is exposed by buccal or palatal flap, and once it is certain that it can be removed atraumatically, the deciduous tooth, if present,

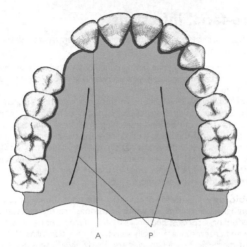

Fig. 10.10 A, Outline (heavy red line) of the incision for a palatal flap raised to expose a buried right maxillary canine. P, Position of the palatine arteries. Do not attempt a palatal 'relieving' incision; exposure is achieved by the length of the envelope flap.

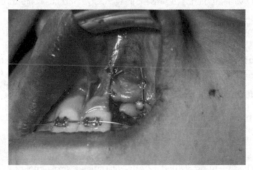

Fig. 10.11 An apically repositioned flap allows access to the buccal surface without loss of attached gingivae.

is extracted and a new socket surgically prepared with a bur. The tooth is reimplanted without force, the flaps sutured, and a close-fitting but *not* cemented splint placed. Functional splinting is continued for 7–10 days and the tooth root-filled as soon as possible after surgery. Regular follow-up is essential to allow early detection of root resorption which is common.

Dento-facial infections

▶ Infection associated with teeth is rarely, if ever, treated *definitively* by antibiotics and analgesics.

Ask about the airway. Anyone having difficulty swallowing their own saliva should be admitted immediately as the airway is at risk. People can die from these infections.

The vast majority of infections in this area requiring surgical Rx are bacterial, usually arising from necrotic pulps, periodontal pockets, or pericoronitis. They can be life-threatening if allowed to progress, e.g. to the fascial spaces of the neck, mediastinum, or the cavernous sinus, or as a focus for infective endocarditis (➔ Dental implications, p. 533). There has been a substantial ↑ in the number of hospital admissions for severe cervicofacial infection of dental origin in the UK over the last decade.[8] This ↑ is greater in lower socio-economic groups.[9]

Microbiology Culture of dento-facial infections usually produces several commensal organisms, of which anaerobes are the most important. The predominant species, *Bacteroides* species (anaerobe) and streptococci (aerobe and anaerobe), are usually sensitive to the penicillins. Resistance is reported rarely. *Bacteroides* species are nearly always sensitive to metronidazole. Remember the aerobic pathogens in established infection (don't just rely on metronidazole), and *Haemophilus* and *Staphylococcus aureus* near the antrum (➔ The maxillary antrum, p. 422); *Streptococcus milleri* is a particularly virulent pathogen present in aggressive potentially life-threatening infections.

Diagnosis This is usually simple and clinical based on pain, swelling, temperature, and discharge.

Apical abscess Teeth with an apical abscess are TTP and non-vital. They may be discoloured or crowned and have a history of trauma or RCT. Pain and TTP are often diminished when the intrabony pus tracks through the soft tissues and discharges, usually in the buccal sulcus (exceptions are 2̲, and palatal roots of maxillary molars which discharge palatally, and 1̅2̅ which often discharge on the chin). May be associated periostitis with severe thickening.

Rx Drainage of pus either via the root canal, by incision of any fluctuant abscess, or by extraction under LA or GA. Palatal or buccal abscesses can be drained quite simply under LA by infiltrating a small amount of LA *between* the abscess cavity and the overlying mucosa, then incising the abscess. Explore using blunt closed forceps and keep patent either by excising an ellipse of tissue or inserting and suturing a small rubber drain; this is particularly important in the palate. Cover the procedure with 'best guess' antibiotics such as amoxicillin 500mg tds PO for 5–7 days, or metronidazole 400mg tds PO for 5–7 days, or both. For severe infections, in-patient management with EO drainage may be needed.

8 S. Thomas et al. 2008 *BMJ* **336** 1219.

9 D. Moles 2008 *BMJ* **336** 1323.

Periodontal abscesses These arise in a pre-existing periodontal pocket (➔ Periodontal abscess, p. 200). Initial Rx involves incision and drainage, followed by elimination of the pocket, unless extraction is considered the only option.

Pericoronitis Pericoronitis is inflammation and infection of a gum flap (operculum) overlying a partially erupted tooth, usually an $\overline{8}$ often traumatized by an overerupted $\underline{8}$. Rx: involves removal of the opposing $\underline{8}$, irrigation under the operculum with saline or chlorhexidine, and antibiotics (as for abscess) if necessary. Nearly all third molars associated with pericoronitis need removal.

Dry socket Dry socket is osteitis of a socket following tooth removal. It is commonest in the mandible after removal of molars, especially $\overline{8}$. Predisposing factors are smoking, surgical trauma, LA, history, bone disease, oral contraceptives, or immunodeficiency.

Diagnosis Pain onset after (usually 2–4 days) extraction, similar in nature but worse than the preceding toothache. The socket looks inflamed and exposed bone is usually visible. Rx is to gently clean the socket by irrigation and dress the exposed bone with Alvogyl®, BIPP, or ZOE packs (provide remarkable analgesia but are a horror to remove). Topical metronidazole is an alternative.[10] Chlorhexidine &/or hot salt mouthwashes may help. NSAIDs are the systemic analgesic of choice (➔ Analgesics in general dental practice, p. 598; ➔ Analgesics in hospital practice, p. 600). Prophylactic anaerobicidals such as metronidazole reduce the incidence of this condition.[11]

Actinomycosis (➔ *Actinomyces israelii*, p. 183.) Persistent low-grade infection, multiple sinuses. Rx: drainage and up to 6 weeks amoxicillin 500mg tds. Doxycycline 100mg od is an alternative.

Staphylococcal lymphadenitis This is especially seen in children; small occult skin or mucosal breach allows ingress. May mimic a 'slapped face' due to exotoxin. Drain and give flucloxacillin 125–500mg qds (depending on age ➔ Prescribing for children, p. 596).

Atypical mycobacteria Lymphadenitis with no obvious cause. Cold nodes, non-febrile patient. Drain or excise. Culture for up to 12 weeks. Do *not* start antituberculous therapy as many atypical mycobacteria are resistant and side effects are common and significant. Clarithromycin is the most useful 'conventional' antibiotic. Excision of nodes is definitive Rx.

Ludwig's angina This is a combination of abscess and cellulitis affecting both submandibular and sublingual spaces bilaterally. The floor of the mouth is raised and the tongue pushed up and back. The floor of mouth, tongue, and soft tissues of the neck are board hard. The patient is systemically unwell and often cannot swallow their own saliva. The airway is seriously at risk and this is an urgent case for admission.

10 J. Kaur et al. 2017 *J Clin Exp Dent* **9** e284–e288.

11 G. Lodgi et al. 2012 *Cochrane Database Syst Rev* **14** CD003811.

Necrotizing fasciitis This is a rare but life-threatening infection often with a highly virulent streptococci. Treatment involves wide local excision of necrotic tissue combined with resuscitation and IV antibiotics. Often fatal if untreated.

Abscess An abscess is a collection of pus (white cells, inflammatory exudates, tissue fluid, and bacteria), it is relatively isolated from the circulation (and hence antibiotics). Treatment is drainage which continues until all pus is gone.

Cellulitis This is intra- and intercellular oedema generated by inflammatory exudates. The overlying surface is red and hot and it allows the rapid migration of bacteria to surrounding areas (Fig. 10.12). It has a good blood supply and high-dose antibiotics are the Rx of choice.

Head and neck infections These are usually a combination of both.

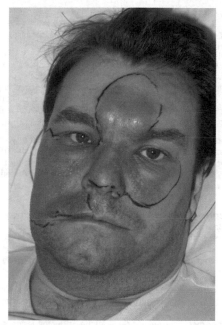

Fig. 10.12 A clinical example of spreading facial cellulitis—the blue markings allow the assessment of the impact of treatment.

Biopsy

A biopsy is a sample of tissue taken from a patient for histopathological examination.

Types of biopsy Biopsies may be incisional or excisional. Examples of incisional biopsies are fine-needle aspirate (really cytology), punch biopsy, trephines, and 'true-cut' needle biopsy. The commonest technique by far, however, is to excise an ellipse of tissue that includes a portion of the lesion and surrounding normal tissue. Excisional biopsy provides after the fact information on the excised sample (reserve for very small lesions).

What should be biopsied? Nearly everything that is worth excising is worth histological review, and so all excised specimens should be examined histopathologically. Any soft tissue lesion not amenable to accurate clinical Δ (by a reasonably trained eye) should be biopsied. All red lesions of oral mucosa and most white patches should be biopsied. If you think 'Should I biopsy this?' then do it; you will always get some unpleasant surprises.

Special considerations Frozen sections are biopsy specimens taken during major surgery, either when the extent of the procedure will depend on the histological Δ of the lesion or to verify clearance of excision. It is essential to contact the pathology lab before the patient goes to theatre to warn them. Advance warning is also necessary for certain special tests, e.g. immunohistochemistry.

How it is done Tell the patient you need a piece of tissue to help make the Δ. LA or GA. For simple incisional biopsy, stabilize the tissue to be sampled. Transfixing with a 3/0 BSS helps avoid crush artefact, and orientates the specimen. Cut an ellipse of tissue, including lesion and normal surrounding tissue, lift up and dissect out, then close primarily with sutures.

Biopsy and oral cancer Incisional biopsy carries a (theoretical) risk of shedding malignant cells into the circulation. The alternative is to subject a patient to mutilating surgery before definitive Δ. If you suspect an oral malignancy, refer *before* biopsy because most consultants have a preferred approach. This also allows integrated Δ and counselling.

Specimens Specimens are best laid out on paper if small or pinned out on a cork board if large. This allows orientation and $\downarrow$ shrinkage artefact, which can be considerable. Usual preservative is 10% formalin; ask if you are not sure, as some specimens are needed fresh. Consider a specimen for culture as well (e.g. lymph node biopsy). Make a diagram of the specimen on the pathology form to accompany the clinical details. A photograph of the operative site can help.

▶ Tell the pathologist what you are thinking!

Non-tumour soft tissue lumps in the mouth

Abscess (→ Apical abscess, p. 408.) This consists of a generalized gingival swelling and gingivitis (→ Gingivitis, p. 192).

Brown 'tumour' This is not a tumour but a giant cell lesion sometimes found in soft tissue but more commonly within bone (→ Brown 'tumour', p. 416). It occurs $2°$ to hyperparathyroidism, although this is usually suggested after enucleation on finding giant cells in a fibrous stroma histologically. Check bone biochemistry (Ca^{2+}, PO_4^{3-} ↓, alkaline phosphatase ↑, PTH ↑). If hyperparathyroidism is confirmed and treated, these lesions regress.

Dermoid cyst This is a developmental cyst most commonly found at the lateral canthus of the eye where it may extend intracranially, but next most often found in the midline of the neck above the mylohyoid, where it causes elevation of the tongue. Rx: complete but conservative excision.

Congenital epulis By definition, this is present at birth; it usually presents as a pedunculated nodule. Histology reveals large granular cells. Rx: complete but conservative excision.

Peripheral giant cell granuloma (Giant cell epulis.) This is a deep red gingival swelling, probably caused by chronic irritation. Histology reveals a vascular lesion with multinuclear giant cells. Rx: excision with stripping of periosteum and curettage of underlying bone.

Pregnancy epulis An ↑ inflammatory response to plaque during pregnancy causes a lesion indistinguishable from a pyogenic granuloma. Onset usually in third month. Rx: none (other than OHI) if possible, as it regresses after delivery. If very troublesome, simple excision is performed; but it may recur.

Pyogenic granuloma A red fleshy swelling, often nodular, occurring as a response to recurrent trauma and non-specific infection. Histology shows proliferation of vascular connective tissue, therefore it bleeds easily. Rx: excision, debride area, and good OH.

Fibroepithelial polyp This is an over-vigorous response to low-grade recurrent trauma. May be sessile or pedunculated and ranges from small lumps to lesions covering the entire palate. Excise with base. Histology shows dense collagenous fibrous tissue lined by keratinized stratified squamous epithelium.

Irritation (denture) hyperplasia This is a very common hyperplastic response to repeated trauma, e.g. following denture-induced ulceration. Classically, seen as rolls of tissue in the sulcus related to a denture flange. Histology is similar to a fibroepithelial polyp. Rx: complete excision with temporary removal of dentures allows healing. Consider simple pre-prosthetic measures and replace F/F.

Mucoceles These are usually mucous extravasation cysts, where saliva leaks from a traumatized duct and pools, creating a compressed connective tissue capsule. Rarely, they are mucous retention cysts. They mostly affect the lower lip—similar swellings in the upper lip are often minor salivary gland tumours (➜ Salivary gland tumours, p. 513). Rx: excision with associated damaged glands and duct.

Ranula These are mucoceles of the floor of the mouth, arising from the sublingual gland. They tend to recur if marsupialized. A plunging ranula crosses deep to the mylohyoid and appears as a neck and floor of mouth swelling. Rx: excision of cyst and associated sublingual gland; the submandibular gland may have to be excised if the duct is damaged.

Granulomata Lumps characterized by the histological finding of granulomata may be caused by Crohn's disease (➜ Crohn's disease, p. 470) or its localized variant orofacial granulomatosis, sarcoidosis (➜ Sarcoidosis, p. 455), or implanted foreign bodies such as amalgam.

Haemangioma This is a developmental lesion of blood vessels. Present at birth, they can grow with the child, remain static, or regress. Blanch on pressure. *Do not* biopsy. 80% spontaneously regress; Rx for those that don't: laser or cryotherapy, can be excised if very small.

Lymphangioma This is a rarer developmental lesion, this time of lymphatics. Can be microcystic or macrocystic. May present as an enlarged tongue, cheek, or lip (usually microcystic) or neck swellings (usually macrocystic). Rx: microcystic difficult as no clear plane of excision although some can be beneficially excised. Macrocystic lymphangiomas do have definable planes in most cases and can be excised with little damage to the surrounding structures. Sclerosant picibanil is often used in the larger cyst cavities, despite these being easiest to remove.

Vascular malformations These are developmental lesions of blood vessels which *do not* regress but grow with the patient. Characterized by rate of blood flow in lesion. Rx: interventional radiology and surgery.

Warts/squamous papillomata The main aetiological factor is HPV. True warts are rare in the mouth and usually transmitted from skin warts. Found in those with a STD or AIDS, but most have no such link.

Papillomata are common in the mouth; they appear as multiple papillated pink or white asymptomatic lumps. Rx: excision biopsy (if on a stalk—ligate or diathermy base as they contain a prominent vessel).

Non-tumour hard tissue lumps

Cysts (◆ Cysts of the jaws, p. 418); benign tumours (◆ Benign tumours of the mouth, p. 420); malignant tumours (◆ Oral cancer, p. 452).

Tori These are bony exostoses found in both jaws. *Torus palatinus* is found in the centre of the hard palate; *torus mandibularis* on the lingual premolar/molar region of the mandible. Rx: reassurance that these developmental anomalies cause no harm (they are *not* part of the Gardener syndrome, ◆ Gardener syndrome, p. 783). Rarely, excision for denture construction is indicated.

Giant cell granuloma (◆ Peripheral giant cell granuloma, p. 414.) This can present as an intrabony swelling or symptomless radiolucency. Carefully enucleate.

Brown 'tumour' (◆ Brown 'tumour', p. 414.) Again, this imitates the giant cell granuloma; the difference is in bone biochemistry.

Paget's disease of bone This is relatively common over the age of 55yrs and affects the skull, pelvis, and long bones, as well as the jaws. Although aetiology is uncertain, both the measles and respiratory syncytial viruses have been implicated. The maxilla is more frequently affected than the mandible. Hypercementosis of roots makes extractions difficult in this group. There is a replacement of normal bone remodelling by a chaotic alternation of resorption and deposition, with resorption dominating in the early stages. Bone pain and cranial neuropathies can occur. X-rays show a 'cotton wool' appearance. Biochemistry shows an ↑ in alkaline phosphatase and urinary hydroxyproline. Avoid GA; use prophylactic antibiotics and plan extractions surgically. Bisphosphonates (◆ Bisphosphonates, p. 614) and calcitonin are used in Rx.

Fibrous dysplasia In this disorder, areas of bone are replaced by fibrous tissue. Onset is in childhood; lesions ossify and stabilize with age. Jaw involvement usually presents as a painless, hard swelling. Characteristic X-ray appearance is of 'ground-glass' bone. Histology shows fibrous replacement of bone with osseous trabeculae which look like irregular 'Chinese characters'. Rx: skeletal resculpting after stabilization of growth &/or orthognathic surgery/orthodontics.

Cherubism Cherubism is hereditary, and presents at 2–4yrs. It is a bilateral variant of fibrous dysplasia. In addition to the histological pattern for fibrous dysplasia there are also multinucleated giant cells. The natural history is not well understood—it may burn out or regress. Skeletal resculpting after cessation may be necessary.

Cysts of the jaws

Cysts are abnormal epithelium-lined cavities which often contain fluid but only contain pus if they become infected. Jaw cysts predominantly arise from odontogenic epithelium and grow by a means not fully understood but involving epithelial proliferation, bone resorption by prostaglandins, and variations in intracystic osmotic pressure.

Diagnosis

Many are detected as asymptomatic radiolucencies on X-ray; others present as painless swellings, almost always of the buccal cortex. Infected cysts present with pain, swelling, and discharge. Vitality test associated teeth. Take a DPT and a periapical film when possible to screen for size and coexisting pathology. Transillumination rarely helps, but aspiration is sometimes useful and can help distinguish some lesions. Rarely, cysts may present with a pathological #, especially of the mandible.

Treatment

- Enucleation with 1° closure is commonest and generally the Rx of choice. It consists of removing the cyst lining from the bony walls of the cavity and repositioning the access flap. Any relevant dental pathology is treated at the same time, e.g. by apicectomy.
- Enucleation with packing and delayed closure is used when badly infected cysts, particularly very large ones, are unsuitable for 1° closure. Pack with Whitehead's varnish or BIPP.
- Enucleation with 1° bone grafting. Rarely useful.
- Marsupialization. This is the opening of the cyst to allow continuity with the oral mucosa; healing is slower than with enucleation and a cavity persists for some time. It is useful to allow tooth eruption through the cyst or where enucleation is C/I.

▶ Always submit cyst lining for histopathology.

Types of cysts Many classifications exist, few are helpful.

Inflammatory dental cysts These are very common, and may also be called radicular cysts. Described as apical or lateral depending on position in relation to tooth root, or residual if left behind after tooth extraction. Necrotic pulp is the stimulus, and the epithelium comes from cell rests of Malassez. Rx: enucleation plus endodontics or extraction.

Eruption cysts See ➋ Eruption cyst, p. 66.

Dentigerous cysts These form around the crown of an unerupted permanent tooth and arise from reduced enamel epithelium. May delay eruption. Rx: marsupialization or enucleation, depending on position and desired fate of the tooth.

Keratocysts Keratocystic odontogenic tumour (KCOT) is an odontogenic cyst that can be rapidly growing. In 2005 the WHO reclassified the lesions as KCOT due to their propensity to reoccur and invade local tissues. This term was not used commonly and in 2017 the name reverted to odontogenic keratocyst. They are lined by parakeratinized epithelium derived from the remnants of the dental lamina and are thought to replace a missing tooth. They have a fluid filling with a protein content <4g/dL. Aspiration of samples for biochemistry and cytology for parakeratinized squames can be helpful. It is important to identify these cysts, as outpouching walls and 'daughter' or 'satellite' cysts make them more liable to recur. Their multiloculated appearance on X-ray may confuse them with an ameloblastoma (➲ Ameloblastoma, p. 420). Rx: careful enucleation, &/or cryotherapy &/or Carnoy's solution, or aggressive curettage of the cavity. Rarely, excision is needed if recurrent.

Calcifying epithelial odontogenic cysts These are rare and distinguished by areas of calcification and 'ghost cells' on histology. Rx: enucleate.

Solitary bone cysts These are usually an incidental finding on X-ray and devoid of a lining, but may contain straw-coloured fluid. They probably arise following breakdown of an intraosseous haematoma, and are distinguished by a scalloped upper border on X-ray where the cyst pushes into cancellous bone between teeth but spares the lamina dura. Opening the cyst, gentle curettage, and closure heals these 'cysts'; associated teeth need no Rx.

Aneurysmal bone cysts These are expansile lesions full of vascular spongy bone. They present as a symptomless swelling, unless traumatized, when bleeding causes pain and rapid expansion. Small ones can be carefully enucleated, but larger aneurysmal bone cysts need excision and possible reconstruction since they will recur if incompletely excised.

Fissural cysts These are not associated with dental epithelium but arise from embryonic junctional epithelium. They are rare and include incisive canal cysts, incisive papilla cysts, and nasolabial cysts. Rx: enucleation.

Benign tumours of the mouth

Non-odontogenic tumours

Epithelial

Squamous cell papilloma (❸ Warts/squamous papillomata, p. 415). Resembles a white or pink cauliflower and is caused by papilloma virus. Usually presents on the palate. Does not undergo malignant change. Excise.

Connective tissue

- *Fibroma*. Very rare. Benign fibrous tumour, usually pink and pedunculated. Excise with a narrow margin.
- *Lipoma*. Soft, smooth, slow growing yellowish lump composed of fat cells. Enucleate or excise with narrow margin.
- *Osteoma*. Smooth, hard, benign neoplasm of bone. Usually unilateral and covered by normal oral mucosa. Not situated in the classical position of tori (❸ Tori, p. 416). Gardener syndrome (❸ Gardener syndrome, p. 783).
- *Neurofibroma*. Rare tumour of the fibroblasts of a peripheral nerve. Usually affects the tongue; may be part of von Recklinghausen disease (❸ von Recklinghausen neurofibromatosis/syndrome, p. 788). Can undergo sarcomatous change. Excise with a small margin.
- *Neurolemmoma* (schwannoma). Tumour composed of Schwann cells (cells of the axonal sheath). Rx: excision; nerve fibres can sometimes be preserved due to eccentric tumour growth.
- *Granular cell myoblastoma*. Rare tumour of histiocyte origin, usually arising as a nodule on the tongue. Excise with a margin.
- *Ossifying fibroma*. May be neoplasm or developmental anomaly. It is a well-demarcated fibro-osseous lesion of the jaws. Presents as a painless slow-growing swelling, expanding both buccal and lingual cortices. X-ray shows a radiolucent area, circumscribed by a radio-opaque margin. Histology is similar to fibrous dysplasia. Enucleation or conservative excision is curative. A faster-growing but equally benign version occurs in children.

Odontogenic tumours

Many of these are fascinating (to some) rarities. Only the more important are discussed.

Ameloblastoma One of the commoner odontogenic tumours. Commonest in men and Africans, and in the posterior mandible. There are three basic types: unicystic, polycystic, and peripheral. The unicystic type is the least aggressive; the polycystic and peripheral types show a tendency to invade surrounding tissue, whereas the unicystic expands it. Metastases are very rare. Histologically, two types are seen: plexiform and follicular. Rx: unicystic can be enucleated provided a rim of enclosing bone is removed as well; the other types require excision with a margin.

Adenoameloblastoma This tends to occur in the anterior maxilla in females. Rx: conservative excision, as recurrence is not a problem.

Calcifying epithelial odontogenic tumour (Pindborg tumour) Characteristically, this is radiolucent on X-ray with scattered radio-opacities. Needs excision with a margin.

Myxoma This occurs in both hard and soft tissues. Those arising in the jaws are tumours of odontogenic mesenchyme. This is a tumour of young adults arising within bone and can invade the surrounding tissue extensively. Characteristically, has a 'soap bubble' appearance on X-ray. Histology reveals spindle cells in a mucoid stroma. These tumours need excision with a margin of surrounding normal bone.

Ameloblastic fibroma Rare; affects young adults and appears as a unilocular radiolucency on X-ray, causing painless expansion of the jaws. Enucleation is usually curative.

Odontomes These are not true neoplasms, but malformations of dental hard tissues. Classically, they are classified as *compound* when they are multiple small 'teeth' in a fibrous sac, and *complex* when they are a congealed irregular mass of dental hard tissue. These are best regarded and treated as unerupted, malpositioned, or impacted teeth, and removed using standard dento-alveolar techniques when required (➲ Dento-alveolar surgery: removal of unerupted teeth, p. 394).

Disturbances in tooth formation can lead to isolated abnormalities of enamel, dentine, and cementum. Cementomas are worthy of mention because they create extreme difficulty in tooth removal. For dens in dente, see ➲ Dens in dente, p. 74.

The maxillary antrum

These are the largest of the four paired paranasal air sinuses, lying in each half of the maxilla between the alveolus inferiorly, nasal cavity medially, and orbits superiorly.

Antral pathology Often mimics symptoms attributable to maxillary teeth. Δ is by exclusion of dental pathology, nasal discharge or stuffiness, tenderness over the cheeks, and pain worse on moving the head. Occipito-mental X-rays (15° and 30°) may reveal antral opacity, fluid level, or # (◐ Nasal and malar fractures, p. 498). To define fluid level, repeat film with head tilted. Other X-rays: DPT for cysts and roots and CT scans for tumours, pansinusitis, and blow-out #.

Extractions and the antrum The proximity of maxillary cheek teeth to the antral floor makes it easy for roots and even teeth to be displaced into the antrum. It also predisposes to # of the alveolar process during 6, 7, 8 extraction. Displaced roots can be retrieved either by an extended trans-alveolar approach similar to that for removing roots (useful when the roots are lying under the antral lining) or via a *Caldwell–Luc* approach.

Maxillary sinusitis

Acute sinusitis This usually follows a viral upper respiratory tract infection which has ↓ cilia activity, and is due to bacterial superinfection (usually mixed; anaerobes, *Haemophilus*, staphylococci, and streptococci). Less commonly, due to foreign body (e.g. roots, water). Poor drainage via the ostium exacerbates the situation. Δ as earlier described and confirmed by proof puncture if necessary. Rx: erythromycin 500mg PO qds or doxycycline 100mg PO od. Decongestants, e.g. oxymetazoline or xylometazoline spray.

Chronic sinusitis Chronic sinusitis may then develop, particularly if a foreign body or poor drainage is present. Mucosal lining hypertrophies and may form polyps. A post-nasal discharge (drip) is often present. Rx: aimed at re-ventilation of the sinus. Foreign bodies, if present, should be removed via an incision in the canine fossa (above the premolars) and creation of a bony window into the antrum (Caldwell–Luc approach). Ventilation is provided either by intra nasal antrostomy or (ideally) by endoscopic enlargement of the ostium &/ or drainage of anterior ethmoids, depending on cause (functional endoscopic sinus surgery—FESS ◐ Functional endoscopic sinus surgery (FESS), p. 429).

Oro-antral fistula This is the creation of a pathological epithelium-lined tract between the mouth and maxillary sinus. This most often occurs following the extraction of isolated molar teeth when the fistula tends to persist. Post-extraction reflux of fluids into the nose or minor nosebleeds are diagnostic pointers. Confirm by getting the patient to attempt to blow out against a closed nose; air bubbles through the fistula. Occasionally, antral mucosa prolapses through the socket. Rx: many small fistulae are asymptomatic and close spontaneously. Closure if Δ is made at the time of extraction: close the socket by suture or buccal advancement flap (Fig. 10.13), give antibiotics and decongestants as for maxillary sinusitis, and advise not to blow the nose. Closure if Δ is made >2 days after extraction: place on antibiotics, etc., for 2 weeks and review after 6 weeks. Many will have closed. If not, repair by:

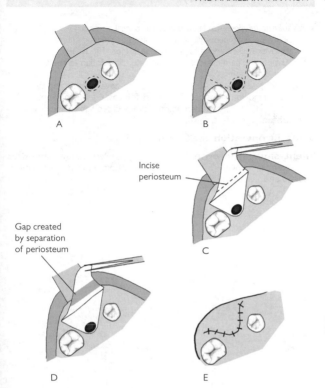

Fig. 10.13 The buccal advancement flap (after Rehrmann).
A   Excise the fistulous tract; easiest with a no. 11 blade.
B   Outline (dashed) of incision for a full thickness mucoperiosteal buccal flap.
C   Reflect full thickness mucoperiosteal flap and incise the periosteal layer only. This makes it possible to mobilize the flap.
D   'Stretch' the flap to assess the degree of elasticity once the restraining effect of the periosteum is lost.
E   The flap is advanced across the fistula and sutured to palatal mucosa over bone.

- *Buccal advancement flap*—excise fistula to prepare a line of closure over bone and raise a broad-based buccal flap. Incise periosteum to allow mucosa to stretch over the socket and close, over bone, with vertical mattress sutures. Use antibiotics, etc., remove sutures at 10 days. Disadvantages: thin tissue may break down; reduces sulcus depth.

- *Palatal rotation flap*—excise fistula as for buccal advancement flap. Dissect a palatal mucoperiosteal flap based on palatine artery, rotate over socket, and suture in similar fashion (Fig. 10.14). Disadvantages: bare bone left to granulate; difficult flap to rotate without distortion.
- *Buccal fat pad flap*—if after raising the buccal advancement flap the periosteal incision is opened with artery forceps, the buccal fat pad is exposed. This can be easily mobilized as a pedicled flap to suture into and obtund the defect.

Sinus lift operation See ⊃ Sinus lift, p. 506.

Silent sinus syndrome This is a rarity in which the maxillary sinus spontaneously involutes probably due to ventilatory abnormalities and can result in enophthalmos.

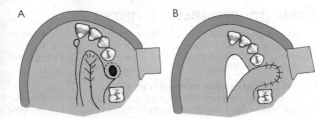

Fig. 10.14 The palatal rotation flap (after Ashley).
A   Excise fistula; outline palatal flap based on greater palatine artery.
B   Mobilize and rotate palatal flap, suturing its leading edge to buccal mucosa over bone. Leave donor site to granulate under surgical dressing or pack.

Minor pre-prosthetic surgery

When teeth are extracted, alveolar bone resorbs, therefore you should aim to preserve alveolar bone whenever possible, either by not extracting teeth (overdentures, ⊃ Overdentures, p. 324) or by using a minimally traumatic technique.

At time of extraction of remaining teeth

Extract carefully, compress the sockets, remove only small unattached pieces of bone, cover any exposed areas of bone with gingival flaps, and surgically remove roots *only* when necessary (infected, loose, > one-third root length). Consider interseptal alveolotomy if ridge is prominent and heavily undercut (e.g. Class II). This consists of creating a labial osteomucosal flap by dividing the septa and extending bone cut at the 3 region through the buccal plate and collapsing-in the bone flap. Prominent fraena should simply be excised. Attempts at ↓ the rate of ridge resorption have been made by leaving roots under mucosal flaps and by implanting hydroxyapatite or Biocoral® cones into extraction sockets.

Problems in denture wearers

▶ Only use surgery fresh I when denture faults and psychogenic disorders have been excluded. Screen jaws with DPT.

Retained roots and bone sequestra These are removed using a standard trans-alveolar technique, except in the maxilla where buried canines may be removed using an osteoplastic flap (where bone is raised on a mucoperiosteal hinge).

Small bony irregularities These can be smoothed with a bur but consider ridge augmentation if extensive.

Fibrous (flabby) ridges ↓ by raising a flap of attached gingiva to repair the defect, excise remaining soft tissue ridge, and repair with flap raised first. Fibrous tuberosities can be dealt with similarly.

Fibrous bands and irritation hyperplasia See Fig. 10.15. These should be excised. Results are improved if palatal mucosal grafts are used to repair the defects and minimize scarring.

Tori These can be reduced with a bur under a local flap or resected with a combination of bur and chisel.

Muscle attachments Muscle attachments to the mylohyoid ridge or genial tubercles can be displaced by resecting the bone from the mandible with a chisel and dissecting away the muscles. Genioglossus and geniohyoid muscles should be reattached to the labial sulcus.

Ridge augmentation (⊃ Major pre-prosthetic surgery, p. 506.) The use of subperiosteally injected porous hydroxyapatite as an out-patient procedure under LA is useful in a very limited number of cases, mainly due to ridge type. In this technique, a subperiosteal tunnel is raised along the crest of the ridge and filled with hydroxyapatite/saline sludge. It is very dependent on the shape of the ridge, and works best with concave ridges as opposed to the more often seen feather-edge ridge. *Problems*: migration of particles after periosteal elevation.

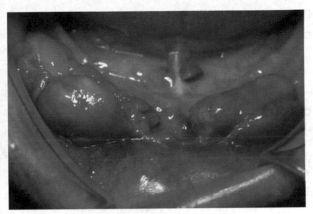

Fig. 10.15 A clinical example of irritation hyperplasia caused by an ill-fitting lower denture.

Sulcus deepening (➔ Epithelial inlay (vestibuloplasty), p. 506.) When adequate vertical and horizontal basal bone exists but there is a shortage of ridge &/or attached gingiva, these procedures can help. Depends on: (I) dissecting away non-attached mucosa to leave a raw 'new' sulcus; (ii) lining this new sulcus with skin or mucosa; (iii) *securing the new depth with a 'stent'*—a denture or baseplate lined with tissue conditioner or impression compound, which is held in place by nylon sutures for 10–14 days, then replaced immediately by a new denture with a soft lining extended to the new sulcus and worn continually for the first 3 months.

Lasers

Definition 'Laser' is an acronym for 'light amplification by the stimulated emission of radiation'. Light consists of packets of photons transmitted in electromagnetic waves (visible light 400–700nm). Laser energy is produced by light stimulation of active media to generate collimated light energy at a specific frequency. The active media determines the characteristics of the laser.

Clinical lasers These consist of two main groups, hard and soft lasers.

Hard lasers Hard lasers work principally by thermal effect, although certain benefits such as ↓ scarring and pain are thought to be due to the photochemical effects of the laser beam.

Carbon dioxide laser This is a hard laser in common use in the hospital service. Its main role is as a cutting beam which seals small vessels as it cuts. It is also used to evaporate benign white patches of oral mucosa. It is used as continuous wave or pulsed beam at 10–20 watts of energy.

KTP laser This is similar to the carbon dioxide laser, giving initially painless wounds. These become painful after 48–72h, however.

Argon laser This produces a light beam which is selectively absorbed by haemoglobin and melanin, therefore it is particularly useful for pigmented and vascular lesions.

Neodymium–yttrium aluminium garnet (Nd–YAG) laser This was originally marketed as a hard laser with a relatively low power output; it is now available as a soft dental laser.

Tuneable dye laser This is an expensive variable frequency laser.

Soft lasers These are thought to work by stabilizing cell membranes by a non-thermal photochemical process, ↑ cellular metabolism by a minor thermal change, and possibly by inducing endorphin release.

Helium–neon This forms the red aiming beam on hard lasers, classroom pointers, and the 'Terminator's' weaponry. Part of the soft laser group, it has no cutting effect but seems to act photochemically on cells. A similar non-thermal red light laser at highly specific frequency is used to active photosensitive chemicals as part of photodynamic therapy (PDT).

Neodymium–YAG A system using this active media is now marketed for use in dentistry and is purported to ↑ cell turnover, ↑ inflammatory response, inhibit oedema, ↑ rate of cell regeneration, e.g. peripheral neurones, and ↑ wound scarring. All this without any recognized side effects. Many of these claims have yet to be widely validated.

Summary Lasers are available for a range of uses in dentistry; they are expensive and require special safety precautions. Some benefits can be achieved in other ways and some have yet to be proven. They are a tool, not a magic wand.

Minimally invasive surgery

While some specialties such as orthopaedics and gynaecology have been using endoscopic technology for many years, a recent surge in fibre-optic technology coupled with the 'discovery' of the laparoscope by general surgeons made minimally invasive (minimal access) surgery one of the hot topics of the late 1990s.

One of the spin-offs of the sudden uncontrolled ↑ in the number of laparoscopic operations was bad publicity about some of the adverse outcomes following this type of surgery, and questions about surgeons' training. One very positive result of this has been the development of surgical skills laboratories, structured courses, and a real interest in training and education.

In the field of oral and maxillofacial surgery, minimally invasive surgery has yet to make a significant impact. Current examples include the following:

Temporomandibular joint arthroscopy This uses specialized small rigid endoscopes with a fibre-optic light source which can be placed in the TMJ space (usually upper joint space) through a tiny incision in the preauricular skin. The joint is distended by a throughflow of sterile irrigant which exits via a needle placed about 1cm anterior to the arthroscope. Reasonable visualization is possible but significant surgery is fairly limited.

Functional endoscopic sinus surgery (FESS) Rigid endoscopes with angled viewing ports allow visualization and a certain amount of surgery of the paranasal sinuses. Biopsy and sampling of a wide range of paranasal tissues is possible and specific surgical expansion of the ostium may prove to be the Ideal Rx for resistant chronic sinusitis. This technique has been rapidly developed by many ENT enthusiasts; however, its evidence base is still being established.

Endoscopically assisted internal fixation Internal fixation of facial # is now widely accepted and standard practice; however, some areas, particularly of the mandible, are very difficult to access safely. Condylar neck # and some angle # may be more easily treated using a modified trocar system and an endoscope with light source.

Endoscopically assisted face and brow lifting Aesthetic facial surgery by its very nature requires distant and minimalist scars. Endoscopic brow lifting from the anterior scalp is reasonably straightforward and has become standard. Endoscopic facelifting makes a tedious operation more so.

NB: while flexible fibre-optic scopes play quite an extensive role in examination of the upper aerodigestive tract, the extent to which significant head and neck surgery can be performed is currently limited.

Oral medicine

Principal sources and further reading Much of the skill of oral medicine lies in the clinical recognition of lesions, therefore a colour atlas of oral mucosal disease is invaluable, e.g. B. Neville et al. 2018 *Colour Atlas of Oral and Maxillofacial Diseases*, Elsevier. Other useful sources of information are A. Field & L. Longman 2003 *Tyldesley's Oral Medicine* (5e), OUP; C. Scully 2013 *Oral & Maxillofacial Medicine—The Basis of Diagnosis and Treatment* (3e), Churchill Livingstone. Related subjects are covered in R. Cawson & E. Odell 2017 *Cawson's Essentials of Oral Pathology & Oral Medicine* (9e), Elsevier; M. Robinson et al. 2018 *Soames' & Southam's Oral Pathology* (5e), OUP; M. Vahedifar 2018 *Temporomandibular Joint Clinical Considerations for Practice*, Lulu Publishing Company.

Bacterial infections of the mouth

Caries (◆ Dental caries, p. 24); periodontal disease (see Chapter 5); dento-facial infections (◆ Dento-facial infections, p. 408). This topic refers primarily to mucosal infections.

Scarlet fever Scarlet fever, an infectious disease of 4–8yr-olds, may be due to a delayed-type hypersensitivity to streptococcal erythrogenic toxin. Symptoms include sore throat, general malaise, fever, and characteristic red rash. The oral mucosa is reddened and the tongue undergoes pathognomonic changes; the dorsum develops a white coating through which white oedematous fungiform papillae project—the 'strawberry tongue' of scarlet fever. Later the white coating is shed and the dorsum becomes smooth and red with enlarged fungiform papillae—'raspberry tongue'. Rx is directed towards the systemic condition with penicillin. The oral manifestations resolve within 14 days.

Tuberculosis (TB) TB is a re-emerging infectious disease caused by *Mycobacterium tuberculosis*. It is commonly seen in immunocompromised patients, including elderly persons. TB is rare in Western countries; however, it is being reported more frequently in recent years. This has been attributed to ↑ migration and spread of HIV. Although one-third of the global population is affected by TB, oral involvement is rare. When it does occur it is usually due to open pulmonary infection or coexisting HIV. The oral lesion presents as a deep, painful ulcer with raised borders, gradually ↑ in size. Any part of the oral mucosa may be involved, although the posterior aspect of the dorsum of the tongue is the commonest site. PCR may facilitate definitive Δ, especially in cases with an unusual presentation. Histopathology shows necrotizing granuloma with Langhans giant cells and epithelioid cells and a Ziehl–Nielsen stain reveals mycobacteria. Previous infection can sometimes be seen on facial views as radio-opacities due to calcifications within lymph nodes. Refer to a chest physician for management as combination chemotherapy is required. Often in children a lymph node excision may be required.

Syphilis Syphilis is a sexually transmitted disease cause by *Treponema pallidum*.
- *1° lesion*. A chancre (a firm, painless ulcerated nodule) develops at the site of inoculation. Genitalia and anus are the most common sites, however it can present on the lips or tongue. This lesion is highly infectious and *T. pallidum* can easily be isolated. There is usually marked cervical lymphadenopathy which resolves spontaneously in 1–2 months.
- *2° lesion*. Develops 2–4 months after the 1° with a cutaneous rash, condylomata, and systemic features such as malaise, fever, headache, and weight loss. The oral lesions include sensitive sloughy mucous patches known as snail-track ulcers (serpiginous ulceration). These are also highly contagious and *T. pallidum* can be easily isolated. Syphilis serology is positive at this stage. The ulcers generally clear up by 12 weeks, although there may be recurrences up to 1yr.

- *3° lesion*. Develops several years later in 30% of patients and is marked by gumma formation. This is a necrotic granulomatous reaction usually affecting the palate or tongue, which enlarges and ulcerates and may lead to perforation of the palate. Lesions are non-infectious. Tertiary syphilis is a multisystem disorder causing CNS involvement and vasculitis.

Congenital syphilis Due to *T. pallidum* crossing the placental barrier leading to the classical appearance of saddle nose, frontal bossing, sensori-neural deafness, Hutchinson incisors (peg-shaped with notch), and mulberry (Moon) molars.

Gonorrhoea Gonorrhoea is 15 times more common than syphilis. It results from oro-genital contact with an infected partner and presents as a non-specific stomatitis or pharyngitis with frequent persisting superficial ulcers and purulent gingivitis caused by *Neisseria gonorrhoeae*. Swabs may reveal Gram −ve intracellular diplococci. Rx is with high-dose penicillin; sexually transmitted infections should be referred to a genitourinary medicine specialist.

Viral infections of the mouth

Human papilloma virus (HPV) HPV is now established as the principal cause of an ↑ in incidence of a subset of head and neck squamous cell cancers. HPV has been associated with squamous cell papilloma (◑ Warts/squamous papillomata, p. 415), condyloma acuminatum (multiple white/pink nodules), focal epithelial hyperplasia (multiple painless papules), and verruca vulgaris (white exophytic lumps). HPV type 16 is a cause of oropharyngeal cancer and oral cavity cancer. In general oropharyngeal cancer incidence rates were higher and ↑ more sharply in men. Rx: topical solutions for the benign growths. For cancer, surgery or chemoradiotherapy are the Rxs of choice. ◑ Oral cancer, p. 452.

Herpes simplex virus (HSV) (Human herpesvirus type 1 and 2.) Most common viral infection affecting the mouth. Although oral infection with HSV types 1 and 2 has been described, type 1 remains the dominant pathogen (type 2 usually causes genital infection). Antibodies indicating past infection are present in >60% of adult population.

Primary HSV This varies widely in severity (↑ with age); it is often subclinical, and asymptomatic in 80%. In infancy it is often mistakenly attributed to 'teething'. It presents with a single episode of widespread stomatitis and unstable mucosa with vesicles which break down to form shallow painful ulcers, enlarged, tender cervical lymph nodes, halitosis, coated tongue, fever, and a general malaise for 10–14 days. Although generally self-limiting, rare complications include herpetic encephalitis and meningitis. Δ: based on the clinical features and history, although the virus can be grown in cell culture. Microscopically ballooning degeneration of epithelial cells with intranuclear viral inclusions, 'Lipshutz bodies', are seen. A fourfold ↑ in convalescent-phase antibodies is also diagnostic, *but* give the Δ only retrospectively. Rx: bed rest, topical and systemic analgesia, a soft or liquid diet with extra fluid intake, and prevention of 2° infection (chlorhexidine mouthwash) is usually adequate in healthy patients. Severely ill or immunocompromised patients should receive systemic aciclovir.

Recurrent HSV infections These are seen in up to 30% of patients affecting the mucocutaneous junction of the lips (herpes labialis, cold sore) and result from reactivation of the 1° infection which is believed to lie dormant in the dorsal root, and autonomic or cranial nerve ganglia (trigeminal or geniculate). Precipitating factors include trauma, e.g. during removal of 8 and immunosuppression and, less commonly, exposure to sunlight, stress, and febrile illness. Usually recurs on area of distribution supplied by one branch of the trigeminal nerve. Prodromal phase (burning/tingling) over 24h is followed by vesiculation and pain. Lesions may respond to 1% penciclovir or aciclovir 5% cream if used in the prodromal stage. Should consider systemic aciclovir (◑ Aciclovir, p. 612) in the immunosuppressed or frequent recurrences.

Varicella zoster (Human herpesvirus 3.) This is a neurogenic DNA virus which causes chickenpox as a 1° infection (varicella) and shingles as a reactivation (zoster).

Chickenpox Classically, an itchy, vesicular, cutaneous, centripetal rash affects children with a peak age of 5–9yrs, rarely affecting the oral mucosa. Patients are contagious from 1–2 days before the rash, until all lesions crusted.

Shingles Shingles is commoner in the immunocompromised, alcoholics, and elderly people. It is confined to the distribution of a nerve, the virus staying either in the dorsal root ganglion of a peripheral nerve or the trigeminal ganglion. It always presents as a unilateral lesion, never crossing the midline. Facial or oral lesions may arise in the area supplied by the branches of the trigeminal nerve. Δ: pre-eruption pain, followed by development of painful vesicles on skin or oral mucosa, which rupture to give ulcers or crusting skin wounds, in the distribution outlined previously. These usually clear in 2–4 weeks, with scarring and pigmentations and is often followed by severe post-herpetic neuralgia (up to 15%) which may continue for years. Rx: symptomatic relief for chickenpox. There is some evidence to suggest that aggressive early Rx of shingles with aciclovir (within 3 days of first vesicle) ↓ the incidence and severity of post-herpetic neuralgia in immunocompromised patients. Urgent referral to an ophthalmologist is required if the eye is involved as there is a risk of corneal ulceration and visual loss.

Herpangina Herpangina is caused by Coxsackie A virus, is confined to children, and presents with widespread small ulcers on the oral mucosa with fever and general upset. Clinically it resembles herpetic stomatitis, but is site pathognomonic, affecting uvula, palate, and fauces with no *gingivitis*. May be preceded by sore throat and conjunctivitis. Can also be mistaken as 'teething'. Self-limiting in 10–14 days. Spread by faeco-oral route.

Hand, foot, and mouth disease This is caused by Coxsackie virus (usually A16, but less commonly types 5 and 10) and is similar to herpangina but the lesions are present throughout the oral cavity. A papular, vesicular rash appears on the hands and feet in conjunction with nasal congestion and oral mucosal vesicles. These break down, leaving painful superficial ulcers, particularly on the palate. The gingivae are rarely involved. It is self-limiting in 10–14 days. Rx: as for herpetic stomatitis.

Measles The prodromal phase of measles may be marked by small white spots with an erythematous margin on the buccal mucosa, known as Koplik spots. A few days later the maculo-papular rash of measles appears, usually behind the ears, then spreading to the face and trunk. Complications include pneumonia and encephalitis which may lead to neurological deficits in 40% and has a 15% mortality.

Glandular fever (infectious mononucleosis) This is seen mostly in children and young adults and is spread by infected saliva. It varies widely in severity and presents with sore throat, generalized lymphadenopathy, fever, headaches, general malaise, and often a maculo-papular rash. There may be hepatosplenomegaly. Oral manifestations may mimic 1° herpetic gingivostomatitis, with widespread oral ulceration, and in addition petechial haemorrhages, especially at the junction of hard and soft palate (pathognomonic), and bruising may be present. The cause is usually Epstein–Barr virus (EBV) and, less commonly, cytomegalovirus (CMV). Toxoplasmosis can give a similar picture. Δ: initially monospot test, Paul–Bunnell test to exclude EBV, and acute and convalescent titres for CMV and toxoplasmosis. Be aware that early HIV infection can mimic this condition. Rx: symptomatic as for 1° herpes, except toxoplasmosis, which may respond to sulfa drugs; seek expert advice. NB: ampicillin should not be given to patients with a sore throat who may have glandular fever as it inevitably produces an unwanted response, ranging from a rash to anaphylaxis.

Opportunistic infection on the tongue mucosa by EBV is thought to be the pathological mechanism behind 'hairy leucoplakia', which is found in transplant and HIV-positive patients.

Reiter syndrome (reactive arthritis) The causative agent is unknown but it appears to be a post-infective response (after 2–3 weeks). Consists of urethritis, arthritis, conjunctivitis, &/or oral ulcers or erosions. Predominantly affects young males and is associated with human leucocyte antigen (HLA) B27 in 80% of patients—leucocytosis and ↑ ESR are common.

Oral candidosis (candidiasis)

Although >100 *Candida* species can be isolated only a handful are clinically important. *C. albicans* and *C. dubliniensis* are by far the most important. It is found in the mouths of >40% of the symptom-free population. Overt infection occurs when there are local or systemic predisposing factors, therefore the prime tenet of management is to look for and treat these factors. The ↑ risk is seen in denture wearers, immunocompromised (including diabetics, steroid users, and HIV-infected patients), smokers, and those with xerostomia, malignancy (radiotherapy/chemotherapy), malnutrition, and those taking broad-spectrum antibiotics.

Acute candidosis

Pseudomembranous candidosis (thrush) This affects 5% of newborn infants and 10% of elderly debilitated individuals. Δ: appears as creamy, lightly adherent plaques on an erythematous oral mucosa, usually on the cheek, palate, or oropharynx. Occasionally symptomless, but more commonly cause discomfort on eating and also may cause a burning sensation and bad taste. These plaques can be gently stripped off, leaving a raw under-surface and, with Gram staining, show candidal hyphae. In infancy, widespread oral candidosis can be associated with a livid facial rash and an associated nappy rash. Colonization of a breastfeeding mother's nipples can lead to mutual recolonization. Rx: a variety of topical formulations such as nystatin and miconazole are available, but provide only limited benefit. Fluconazole and itraconazole are very effective. Chlorhexidine mouthwash is an effective adjunct to Rx. *C. glabrata*, *C. tropicalis*, and *C. knusel* are fluconazole resistant, therefore, *Candida* subtyping should be performed for resistant cases. Most antifungals especially the azole group, interact with a number of drugs including warfarin and statins.

Erythematous candidosis This is an opportunistic infection following the use of broad-spectrum antibiotics, sometimes inhaled steroids, and in patients with HIV as well as those with xerostomia. It is painful and exacerbated by hot or spicy foods. The oral mucosa has a red, shiny, atrophic appearance and there may be coexisting areas of thrush. Rx: eliminate cause (if due to inhaled steroids rinse mouth with water after inhaling and/or use a spacer device), otherwise as for thrush.

Chronic candidosis

Chronic atrophic candidosis (denture stomatitis) (◐ Denture stomatitis, p. 320.) Reported prevalence of denture stomatitis: 10–75%.

Angular cheilitis A combined staphylococcal, β-haemolytic streptococci, and candidal infection, involving the tissues at the angle of the mouth (Fig. 11.1). Aetiology is multifactorial with local and systemic precipitating factors, e.g. trauma, inadequate vertical dimension of denture, iron deficiency, and vitamin B_{12} deficiency anaemia. Therefore, FBC and haematinics should be investigated. Clinically, red, cracked, macerated skin at angles of the mouth, often with a gold crust. Rx: miconazole cream, which is active against all three infecting organisms. Rx needs to be prolonged, up to 10 days after resolution of clinical lesion, and carried out in conjunction with elimination of any underlying factors. Mupirocin cream applied to the anterior nares helps eradicate sources of *Staphylococcus aureus*.

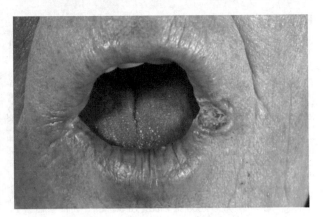

Fig. 11.1 Clinical example of severe angular cheilitis associated with chronic oral candidosis.

Median rhomboid glossitis This is a form of chronic atrophic candidosis affecting the dorsum of the tongue. It is seen in patients using inhaled steroids and smokers. Some patients have lesions in the centre of the dorsum of tongue and palate (kissing lesions). Rx only if symptomatic as discomfort can be improved with topical antifungals, but the appearance cannot. Exclude haematinic deficiency and diabetes.

Chronic hyperplastic candidosis (candidal leucoplakia) This is more commonly seen in middle-aged men who are heavy smokers. It typically presents as a white patch on the oral commissural buccal mucosa bilaterally or dorsum of tongue. Although there is an ↑ risk of malignant change, the initial approach *after ensuring the diagnosis microbiologically and histopathologically* is to eradicate the candidal infection. Candidal hyphae can be seen in the superficial layers of the epidermis, one reason why eradication is so difficult. Rx: systemic antifungals such as fluconazole and itraconazole are indicated. Often associated with iron, folate, and vitamin B_{12} deficiency, and smoking, which should be corrected. Most lesions will resolve after such Rx; if not, reassess degree of dysplasia and surgical excision may be indicated. Patients should be encouraged to stop smoking.

Chronic mucocutaneous candidosis A rare syndrome complex with several subgroups, including *candidal endocrinopathy*, where skin and mouth lesions occur in conjunction with endocrine abnormalities; *granulomatous skin candidosis*, a *late-onset predominantly male-affecting group*; and an *AIDS-associated group*. Rx: difficult, high-dose fluconazole 100mg od or 200mg od for 3 weeks (➌ Fluconazole, p. 612). Voriconazole has recently been introduced as a Rx.

Histoplasmosis This and other rare fungal infections have occasional oral manifestations.

Recurrent aphthous stomatitis (ulcers)

Recurrent aphthous stomatitis (RAS) is the term given to a fairly well-defined group of conditions characterized by recurrent oral ulceration. There are three subgroups:

Minor aphthous ulcers A very common condition (~25% of population) affecting ~80% of RAS patients. Start at childhood or adolescence. Usually appear as a group of 1–6 ulcers at a time, of variable size (usually 2–5mm diameter) (Fig. 11.2). Mainly occur on non-keratinized mucosa and heal within 1–2 weeks without scarring. Usually recur at an interval of 1–4 months. Prodromal discomfort may precede painful ulcers. Exacerbated by stress, local trauma, menstruation (fall in progesterone level), sodium lauryl sulfate (in some toothpastes), drugs (NSAIDs, alendronic acid, and nicorandil), smoking, allergy to some foods, and may be an oral 'marker' of iron, vitamin B_{12}, or folate deficiencies. In some cases, they are a manifestation of Crohn's disease, ulcerative colitis, or gluten enteropathy. Aetiology, although not fully understood, is almost certainly a T-cell-mediated immunological reaction in patients with a genetic predisposition (HLA A1, A11, B12, and DR2). There is a familial history in 45% of cases. Rx: prevent superinfection with chlorhexidine mouthwash and relieve pain (simple analgesics, benzydamine mouthrinse). Topical tetracycline and steroid preparations are sometimes useful (➔ Hydrocortisone 1% and oxytetracycline 3%, p. 602). It is important to look for and treat any underlying deficiency or coexisting pathology (FBC, haematinics, vitamin B_{12} and red cell folate, serum antiendomysium, and transglutaminase assay).

Major aphthous ulcers Seen in 10% of RAS patients. A more severe and more frequent variant with fewer, but larger ulcers >10mm which may last 5–10 weeks and most commonly affect keratinized mucosa. Associated with tissue destruction and scarring, and any site in the mouth and oropharynx may be affected. There is an even higher association between major aphthae and gastrointestinal and haematological disorders. They are also seen in AIDS. Seldom a cyclical pattern. Rx: as for minor aphthae, plus topical or systemic steroids (➔ Anti-inflammatory drugs, p. 602).

Herpetiform ulcers Least common. So named due to their resemblance to 1° herpetic stomatitis; however, they are not related to viral infection. Commoner in older females. Manifest as a crop of small but painful ulcers (up to 100) which usually last 1–2 weeks, the commonest site being the floor of mouth, lateral margins, and tip of tongue, occurring on both keratinized and non-keratinized surfaces. Rarely, they merge to form a large ulcer which heals with scarring. There are frequent recurrences (may be almost continuous for 2–3yrs). Rx: as for minor aphthous ulceration.

Behçet's disease A severe relapsing and remitting systemic vasculitis, characteristically affecting venules. All organs of the body can be affected. It has a worldwide distribution but is most prevalent in the Far East, along the Silk Route, and in the Middle East. In the UK a prevalence of 0.064 in 10,000 has been reported from Yorkshire. It is a disease of young adults, more common and more severe in males. It is associated with HLA subtype.

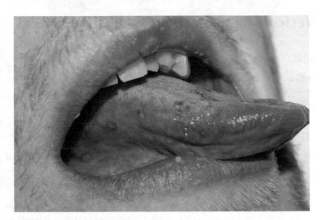

Fig. 11.2 Classically, aphthous ulceration affects the non-keratinized mucosa although it is not an exclusive finding.

Δ: clinical and based on the presence of recurrent oral ulcers and two of the following: recurrent genital ulceration, eye lesions (uveitis), or skin lesions (erythema nodosum, folliculitis). Oral signs are frequently the first manifestation of autoimmune diseases. Dentists can play an important role in the detection of autoimmune pathologies. Skin hyper-reactivity is common and the patient may have raised ESR and IgA. In order to diagnose the Behçet syndrome, according to the International Study Group (ISG) criteria at least two of the main features (oral, genital, or ocular lesions) must be present when another clinical explanation is excluded. Managed in consultation with rheumatologist. Rx: ophthalmic referral if eye involved. Monoclonal anti-TNF is helpful in severe mouth ulcers. The Rx of Behçet syndrome is based on the use of local and systemic cortisones often in addition to immuno-suppressant drugs. Behçet syndrome could be fatal in the case of vascular involvement with aneurysm rupture and thrombosis.

Oral ulcers   See ➔ An approach to oral ulcers, p. 482.

Vesiculo-bullous lesions—intraepithelial

Vesicle A vesicle is a small blister, a few millimetres in diameter.

Bulla A bulla is a larger blister (0.5cm or more).

Intraepithelial bullae Intraepithelial bullae are caused by loss of attachment between individual cells (acantholysis).

Subepithelial bullae Subepithelial bullae separate the epithelium from the underlying corium.

Ulcer An ulcer is a breach in the mucous membrane.

Immunopathology Immunofluorescence is a prime diagnostic test. Direct immunofluorescence is performed on a fresh biopsy specimen. Indirect is performed on a serum sample.

Erosions Erosions are shallower than ulcers. Because the vesiculo-bullous lesions constitute a defined group with examples from several different pathological processes, they are a favourite examinations topic. One method of classifying this group is into intraepithelial and subepithelial, according to where the blisters form.

Pemphigus Pemphigus is a chronic skin disease which can be rapidly fatal if not treated (mortality 10%). Affected patients have immunoglobulin G (IgG) autoantibodies against desmosomal components like desmoglein-1 and desmoglein-3. Oral mucosa is affected in 95% of patients with pemphigus vulgaris (most common type) and may be the initial presentation of pemphigus in 50%. Autoimmune in aetiology, there are circulating autoantibodies to epithelial desmosome tonofilament. Acantholysis and intercellular IgG &/or C3 are typical and cause separation of epithelium above the basal cell layer, and oedema into this potential space produces a superficial, easily burst, fluid-filled bulla. Rupture leaves a large superficial, easily infected ulcer. The first identifiable lesions are quite often found in the mouth, especially on the palate, although these are usually seen as ulcers because the bullae break down rapidly. It is mainly a disease of middle age (F > M), with ↑ incidence in Jews and Arabs. Rarely, it may be drug induced or paraneoplastic. The pemphigus can be easily confused with other disorders that present lesions like aphthae, lichen planus, candidiasis, and pemphigoid. Δ: stroking the mucosa produces a bulla (Nikolsky sign), but this is inducing pathology for the sake of Δ. Other methods are by histology and direct or indirect immunofluorescent techniques (biopsy samples need to be fresh). Rx: systemic steroids &/or azathioprine, dapsone, mycophenolate mofetil, or gold; also cyclophosphamide, especially in refractory and severe cases. Newer therapies include biologic agents (rituximab) and calcineurin inhibitors appear promising. The titration of circulating antibodies is carried out to evaluate the progress of the disease.

Benign familial chronic pemphigus (Hailey–Hailey disease) This differs from other pemphigus by having a strong family history, with onset of the disease in young adults.

Viral infections See ➲ Viral infections of the mouth, p. 434.

Epidermolysis bullosa (Simplex is most common form.) Other variants are subepithelial. A group of uncommon bullous conditions that are inherited with an autosomal dominant or recessive pattern. Skin blisters due to mild trauma, leading to scarring and disfigurement. Great care should be taken to prevent IO lesions during dental Rx. Simplex type is due to mutations in the *K5* or *K14* gene, leading to disruption of basal cells and formation of bullae. No cure and Rx is symptomatic and preventive.

Vesiculo-bullous lesions—subepithelial

Angina bullosa haemorrhagica An acute, localized oral blood blister of unknown aetiology, although trauma may cause break in epithelium–connective tissue junction leading to bleeding from superficial capillaries and formation of bulla. Invariably develops during eating and can be alarming to the patient. Most common in elderly. Steroid inhalers may predispose. Soft palate, cheeks, and tongue most common sites. Δ: exclude other bullous conditions. Rx: puncture &/or reassure (must differentiate from pemphigus/pemphigoid).

Mucous membrane pemphigoid Commonest in females >60yrs. Presents as mucous membrane bullae which rupture and heal with scar formation. Rare to see skin bullae. Conjunctiva may be affected and if scarring occurs can lead to loss of vision, therefore regard oral signs as a warning to prevent ocular damage. The natural history is of a long-lasting disease which persists with alternating periods of activity and inactivity and may be quiescent for several years. The bullae are blood-filled and tense and may be found in conjunction with desquamative gingivitis. Δ: again histology and direct or indirect immunofluorescence are used, the antibodies (mainly IgG and C3) being found at the level of the basement membrane. The mucous membrane pemphigoid is a chronic disease that requires a continuous Rx strategy although the prognosis is benign. Rx: topical steroids, systemic steroids with or without azathioprine, methotrexate, or dapsone. Refer to ophthalmology.

Bullous pemphigoid This affects the >60yrs age group. Subepithelial bullae form which are firm and less likely to break down than those in pemphigus; it is due to autoantibodies (IgG) to the epithelial basement membrane. The oral mucosa is only affected in ~20% of patients. May be an external 'marker' of internal malignancy or a drug-related immune response.

Dermatitis herpetiformis This is a rare chronic condition of unknown aetiology, but often associated with gluten sensitivity with autoantibodies against reticulin, gliadin, endomysium, and transglutaminase. Oral lesions are seen in 70% of patients with a skin lesion. Commoner in middle-aged men; it affects both skin and mucous membranes; bullae in the mouth break down to leave large erosions. Rx: dapsone may be used both diagnostically and therapeutically. A gluten-free diet helps.

Lichen planus This affects both skin and mucous membranes. Bullous lichen planus is a rare variant in which subepithelial bullae form and break down, leaving large erosions. See also ➲ Lichen planus, p. 468.

Epidermolysis bullosa This is a rare skin disease which exists in numerous different forms. The dystrophic autosomal recessive form is most likely to present with oral manifestations and appears shortly after birth. Associated with bullae formation after minor trauma to skin or mucosa; these break down leaving painful erosions. Dentine may be affected leading to hypoplasia and high susceptibility to caries. Healing is with scarring, resulting in difficulty in eating, speaking, and swallowing as scar tissue limits movement. Skin involvement can lead to destruction of extremities and may be overtaken by carcinomatous change. Prognosis varies widely depending on type. Phenytoin and steroids may help some varieties.

Erythema multiforme This is an immunologically mediated hypersensitivity reaction affecting skin and mucous membrane, usually in young adult males. Trigger agents can be identified in half of the cases and these include drugs (carbamazepine, penicillins, NSAIDs), infection (HSV, mycoplasma pneumonia), pregnancy, malignancy, sunlight, and chemicals such as perfumes and food additives. Δ: from clinical features which include 'target lesions', concentric rings of erythema on the palms, legs, face, or neck. Oral lesions seen in 70% in which the oral mucosa is covered in bullae which break down, the lips and gingivae becoming crusted with painful erosions. There is usually a fever. It is a self-limiting condition in 3–4 weeks but can recur once or twice a year. The symptoms range from mild to life-threatening conditions. Stevens–Johnson syndrome and toxic epidermal necrolysis (TEN) represent the severest forms of the spectrum.

Management Withdraw or treat trigger factor if identified. Hospitalization may be required in severe forms for supportive therapy with IV rehydration. Biopsy; virological studies to exclude herpes; aciclovir may be needed if it is related to herpes. Improve OH with 0.2% chlorhexidine mouthwash. Severe form: Rx with steroids and azathioprine. Minor form: Rx with topical steroids.

Linear IgA disease This is rare and identified pathologically. May be variant of dermatitis herpetiformis. Produces non-specific oral ulceration and rarely bullae. Systemic steroids or mycophenolate mofetil for Rx.

White patches

Numerous conditions manifest as white patches of the oral mucosa; some of these are transient, such as thrush (➲ Oral candidosis (candidiasis), p. 438) or chemical burns (e.g. aspirin). May be localized (due to trauma or neoplasia) or widespread (hereditary or systemic).

White spongy naevus This is a rare, benign autosomal dominant condition affecting keratin. It appears as asymptomatic diffuse, soft, uneven thickening of the superficial layer of the epithelium, which characteristically has no definite boundary and may affect any part of the mouth. Histology shows hyperplastic epithelium with gross intraepithelial oedema. Usually noticed in second decade of life, although developmental in origin. Rx: reassurance.

Frictional keratosis This is a white patch due to hyperplastic hyperkeratotic epithelium induced by local trauma, e.g. sharp tooth, denture, or cheek biting. It is managed by removal of the source of the friction, which will generally allow complete resolution of the lesion. If this doesn't happen, biopsy is indicated. Can be seen as self-mutilation in psychiatric disorders or learning disability.

Smokers' keratosis Characteristically a white patch affecting buccal mucosa, tongue, or palate. Due to a combination of low-grade burn and the chemical irritants of smoke, and seen particularly in pipe smokers. There is little evidence that these patches are premalignant and they resolve on stopping smoking.

Stomatitis nicotina Affects palate; numerous red papules on a white/grey base. The papules have a dark 'head' which is the opening of a distended minor salivary gland. May indicate a risk of dysplasia or neoplasm at high-risk sites such as floor of mouth, retro-molar region, or lateral tongue.

'Syphilitic leucoplakia' A white patch on the dorsum of the tongue is one of the classical appearances of tertiary syphilis (➲ Syphilis, p. 432). Active disease must be treated; however, this will not resolve the area of leucoplakia, which has a propensity to undergo malignant change. Δ is usually suggested by histology, serology, or dark-field microscopy of smears.

Chronic hyperplastic candidosis/candidal leucoplakia See ➲ Chronic hyperplastic candidosis (candidal leucoplakia), p. 439.

Lichen planus See Fig. 11.3; see also ➲ Erosive lichen planus, p. 451.

Lupus erythematosus See ➲ Systemic lupus erythematosus (SLE), p. 469.

Leucoplakia See ➲ Leucoplakia, p. 450.

Hairy leucoplakia See ➲ Hairy leucoplakia, p. 478.

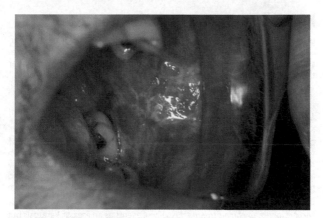

Fig. 11.3 The typical appearance of reticular pattern oral lichen planus, a condition with no premalignant potential (this is found in the erosive variant, ➔ Erosive lichen planus, p. 451).

Panoral leucoplakia This is where the entire oral mucosa appears to be undergoing hyperplastic field change. Risk of malignant change.

Oral carcinoma Occasionally, oral cancer may appear as a white patch, as distinct from a leucoplakia becoming malignant.

Skin grafts These may appear as a white patch in the mouth—and are a trap for the unwary in exams.

Renal failure Can produce soft, oval, white patches which resolve on Rx of renal failure.

Darier's disease A rare skin condition whose oral lesions (present in ~50%) are coalescing white papules on gingivae and palate. It is clinically manifested with hyperkeratotic papules affecting seborrheic areas on the head, neck, and thorax with less frequent involvement of the mouth.

Pachyonychia congenita A rare genetic condition affecting nails, skin, and sweat glands. Oval, benign, white patches on tongue are common.

Proliferative verrucous leucoplakia This is a hard-to-define white patch which appears to have a high incidence of long-term malignant transformation. Clinicians often wrongly diagnose such lesions as oral leucoplakia and treat simply. Lesions nearly always recur and turn malignant. Clinicians should treat these lesions aggressively because they can progress to SCC or verrucous carcinoma. F > M.

Pigmented lesions of the mouth

In many respects, the pulling together of pigmented lesions of the oral mucosa is artificial, as they are not related by pathology or Rx. Pigmented lesions are, however, a popular exam question and with this in mind we offer the following well-recognized conditions.

Δ is aided by whether the pigmentation is localized, or generalized throughout the mouth.

Localized

Foreign body Amalgam tattoo is the commonest, a localized dense blue/black area of mucosal pigmentation. May result from implantation at time of restoration or from broken filling. Radio-opaque. May be palpable but often not. Amalgam tends to become granular and fragmented and if removal is planned, cut out as full-thickness wedge. If asymptomatic, diagnose and reassure. 'Road rash' from grit after road traffic accident or graphite from pencils can cause similar lesions.

Local response to chronic trauma Usually presents as an area of keratosis but sometimes can appear pigmented.

Ephelis A freckle of the oral mucosa. Harmless.

Pigmented naevi Rare and benign. Analogous to a mole. Mostly harmless. Most commonly seen on vermilion border of lips and palate. If <1cm, they do not change in size or colour.

Peutz–Jeghers syndrome (➲ Peutz–Jeghers syndrome, p. 786.) Multiple small perioral naevi.

Kaposi's sarcoma (➲ Kaposi's sarcoma (KS), p. 478.) A HHV-8-related radiosensitive vascular tumour associated with AIDS.

Malignant melanoma Potentially lethal, relatively rare IO malignancy. Very dark, irregular outline, enlarges rapidly; poor prognosis. Rare variant is non-pigmented.

Generalized

Racial pigmentation Racial pigmentation of the oral mucosa varies with skin type and is obviously not pathological.

Foodstuffs A variety can cause superficial mucosal discoloration. Tobacco is the major offender, and paan in South Asian cultures.

Drugs Antimalarials, phenothiazines, cisplatin, zidovudine, busulfan, and oral contraceptives can all cause mucosal pigmentation. Commonest offender is chlorhexidine mouthwash, especially if 'blended' with tea and tobacco.

Heavy metal salts Now rare; classically deposited along the gingival margin in lead or mercury poisoning.

Endocrine associated Addison's disease, ACTH-secreting tumours, adenomatous pituitary dysfunction (Nelson syndrome), ACTH Rx. Δ: low BP, low sodium, cortisol levels, and response to ACTH stimulation (Synacthen® test).

Haemochromatosis Haemosiderin deposits cause hyperpigmentation. Rare.

Black hairy tongue Caused by overgrowth of pigment-producing micro-organisms combined with benign overgrowth of the filiform papillae of the dorsum of the tongue and a lack of normal desquamation. Rx: reassurance, improve OH, tongue scrape or tongue shave depending on patient need/severity.

Premalignant lesions

There exists a group of conditions which have an ↑ risk of malignant transformation of the oropharyngeal mucosa. Although a great deal of attention has been paid to these premalignant conditions, it should be remembered that only a small number of oral cancers are preceded by them, and also that the designation 'premalignant' does not necessarily imply certain malignant transformation. Indeed, the majority of patients with so-called premalignant lesions will not go on to develop oral cancer. The ↑ risk of progression to carcinoma necessitates accurate Δ, Rx if indicated, and long-term follow-up in an attempt to pre-empt life-threatening disease.

Leucoplakia 'White patch or plaque which cannot be characterized clinically or pathologically as any other disease' (WHO). 3% of the white population is affected.

The histopathology of these lesions varies widely from the essentially benign to carcinoma *in situ*. They are usually characterized by a thick surface layer of keratin with thickening of the prickle cell layer of the epithelium, acanthosis, and infiltration of the corium by plasma cells; however, the most important variable is cellular atypia among the epithelial cells. Pointers to look for are nuclear hyperchromatism, an ↑ nuclear/cytoplasmic ratio, cellular and nuclear pleomorphism, ↑ &/or atypical mitoses, individual cell keratinization, and focal disturbance in cell arrangement and adhesion. The degree of dysplasia is one of the most important factors to be considered in the management of a leucoplakia; however, there is a significant inter- and intra-observer variability among pathologists on its diagnosis. Furthermore there is no guarantee that the biopsy specimen is representative of the whole lesion. The second major consideration is the site, e.g. floor of mouth and ventral surface of tongue are more likely to undergo malignant change than most. Third, relation to cause, e.g. buccal leucoplakia, the preferred site for a paan quid is at high risk of malignant change if the habit is not discontinued.

One meta-analysis[1] revealed that the overall malignant transformation rate of leucoplakia was 12.1% and there was a significant difference between mild/moderate and severe dysplasia (10.3% vs 24.1%). In certain sites, e.g. floor of mouth, >25% may progress and certain variants, e.g. 'candidal leucoplakia', have a claimed 10–40% incidence of malignant change. Δ and Rx: specialist referral is indicated—biopsy (possibly guided by toluidine blue to select most appropriate area) and Rx as appropriate. Malignant transformation is more common among non-smokers (idiopathic leucoplakia).

Erythroleucoplakia (speckled leucoplakia) This is basically leucoplakia with areas of erythroplakia. Exhibits an ↑ risk of malignant transformation.

Erythroplakia This is any lesion that presents as bright red velvety plaques, which cannot be characterized clinically or pathologically as any other recognizable condition (WHO). Most of these lesions are carcinoma *in situ* or frank carcinoma and are found at high-risk sites (at least 85%).

1 H. M. Mehanna et al. 2009 *Head Neck* **31** 1600.

Erosive lichen planus This is a comparatively rare variant of lichen planus, which some authorities believe to be premalignant (<1%). The common forms of lichen planus have no proven premalignant potential.

Submucous fibrosis This is a condition found particularly in those of South Asian origin. It is characterized by chronic and progressive scarring of oral connective tissue due to hyperplasia of fibroblasts induced by chewing betel nuts (without tobacco). The addition of tobacco to areca nut and slake lime appears to ↑ the risk of developing SCC. The mucosa is pale, with constraining fibrous bands, and fibrosis of the submucosa occurs, making the lips and cheeks immobile and resulting in trismus. The histology may reveal epithelial atrophy and cellular atypia. Pathogenesis is unclear; ↑ levels of copper due to areca nut chewing leading to cross-linking of collagen by upregulation of lysyl oxidase and thus ↑ fibrosis and DNA damage.

Malignant transformation is seen in 10% in 10–15yrs. Rx: stop habit, intralesional steroids/exercise, surgery with flap reconstruction.

Dyskeratosis congenita A rare autosomal dominant condition of pigmented skin, nail dystrophy, and leucoplakia evident in childhood. White plaques have premalignant potential (● Dyskeratosis congenita, p. 468).

Patterson–Brown–Kelly syndrome (Plummer–Vinson syndrome) See ● Patterson–Brown–Kelly syndrome (Plummer–Vinson syndrome), p. 786.

Management of premalignant lesions Record site, preferably photographically. Consider site, histology, age, and health of the patient, in conjunction with aetiological factors, before deciding on long-term observation or active intervention. Completely stop patient from smoking. Observation may consist of clinical examination with repeated biopsy if change is seen. Guided biopsy with toluidine blue may ↑ diagnostic accuracy. Rx options: laser excision, cryotherapy, surgical excision, or medical therapy with vitamin A, retinoids, beta-carotene, or lycopene[2] after removal of any identifiable aetiological factors. Follow-up at 3-monthly intervals.

---

2 G. Lodi et al. 2008 Interventions for treating oral leukoplakia. *Cochrane Database Syst Rev* **4** CD001829.

Oral cancer

Cancer of the mouth (Fig. 11.4) accounts for ~2% of all malignant tumours in northern Europe and the US, but ~30–40% in the Indian subcontinent. >90% of these are SCCs. Globally it is the sixth commonest cause of cancer-related death. >2000 new cases of oral cancer are registered per year in the UK and each year half that number die from or with the disease. Oral cancer is preventable in 75% of cases. Overall mortality rate is just over 50% despite Rx. Recent survival data suggests that the UK has the best survival figures for diagnosed oral cancer at all stages.

Site The floor of the mouth is the commonest single site, accounting for >75% of carcinomas seen in European or American practice. The other high-risk sites are the retromolar region and lateral tongue. M > F, although this difference is less than it has been in the past, partly due to changes in smoking habits. Most common in sixth and seventh decades, however there appears to be an increasing incidence in younger patients and those who do not use tobacco.

Aetiology The main aetiological factor in cancer of the lip is exposure to sunlight, as with skin cancer. It is estimated that the risk of developing lip cancer doubles every 250 miles nearer the equator. Excessive alcohol and tobacco use are the important factors in the aetiology of cancer of the mouth showing a 'synergistic effect'. Perhaps the most clear-cut aetiological factor is the chewing of tobacco and paan. HPV type 16 and 18 infection is now recognized as an independent risk factor for oropharyngeal SCC. Immunosuppression, e.g. in renal transplant patients or patients with HIV, ↑ the risk of this and other tumours.

Clinical appearance Oral cancer is most often seen as a painless ulcer, although it may present as a swelling or as an area of leucoplakia, erythroleucoplakia, or erythroplakia. Patients may present with a history of a neck lump as a result of metastatic spread to cervical lymph nodes. Malignancy should be suspected if any of these lesions persists for >3 weeks. Pain is usually a *late* feature. Referred otalgia is a common manifestation of pain from the tongue or oropharyngeal cancer. The ulcer is described as firm with raised edges, with an indurated, inflamed, granular base and is fixed to surrounding tissues.

Survival This is dependent on site and stage,[3] (prognosis for stage I is >85% and for stage IV is 10% over 5yrs), and co-morbidity. The presence or absence of extracapsular spread of tumour in metastatic cervical nodes is the most important single prognostic factor. Nodal involvement ↓ cure rates by 50%.

Histopathology Mostly SCC. Characteristically shows invasion of deep tissues with cellular pleomorphism and ↑ nuclear staining. The presence of a lymphocytic response may have prognostic value, as does the manner of invasion (pushing or spreading). Can spread via local infiltration or lymphatic system (cervical nodes), and late spread via bloodstream.

3　⅋ https://www.cancerresearchuk.org/about-cancer/mouth-cancer/stages-types-grades/TNM.

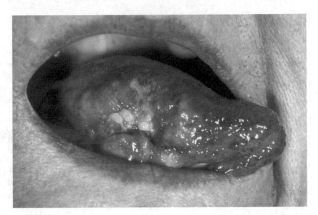

Fig. 11.4 A typical location for an oral cancer which presents as a slow growing, painless, non-healing ulcer or granular lesion; refer immediately for investigation and management through your local urgent cancer referral service.

Verrucous carcinoma A distinctive exophytic, wart-like lesion which grows slowly, spreading laterally rather than deeply, is locally invasive, and is regarded as a lower-grade SCC, characterized by folded hyperplastic epithelium and a lower degree of cellular atypia. Surgical excision &/or radiotherapy is the Rx. Historically, inadequate radiotherapy has been reported to induce more aggressive behaviour.

Other tumours Malignant connective tissue tumours (sarcomas) are rare in the mouth, but fibrosarcoma and rhabdomyosarcoma are seen in children. The malignant tumours of the facial bones include osteosarcoma, multiple myeloma, and 2° metastatic disease. Osteosarcoma of the jaws has a slightly better prognosis than when found in long bones.

Also see ➔ Salivary gland tumours, p. 508; ➔ Facial skin cancer, p. 516.

Management of oral malignancy See ➔ Oral cancer, p. 518.

Abnormalities of the lips and tongue

Although many diseases of the oral mucosa will involve the lips and tongue, there are a number of conditions specific to these structures, due in part to their highly specialized nature. The tongue is a peculiar muscular organ covered with specialized sensory epithelium and the lips form the interface between skin and mucosa.

The tongue

Ankyloglossia (tongue tie) The commonest of the developmental variations of the tongue and may be associated with microglossia. Rx: frenectomy. The current evidence suggests significant improvement in breastfeeding following division of tongue tie.

Macroglossia Congenital: Down syndrome, Hurler syndrome, Beckwith–Wiedemann syndrome. Benign tumours (e.g. lymphangioma), or acquired; acromegaly, amyloidosis ➜ Amyloidosis, p. 529. Surgical reduction of the tongue may be indicated.

Fissured tongue Deep fissuring of the tongue is not pathological in itself (affects 3% of tongues) but may harbour pathogenic microorganisms. Commoner in Down syndrome patients than average population. Melkerson–Rosenthal syndrome is a deeply fissured tongue in association with recurrent facial nerve palsy and swelling. Sjögren syndrome can have a tongue with a lobulated appearance. Rx: reassurance for most, referral for Melkerson–Rosenthal syndrome.

Hairy tongue This is a peculiar condition of unknown aetiology probably due to elongation of the filiform papillae, which may or may not be accompanied by abnormal pigmentation. More common in smokers and people with poor OH and hyposalivation. Sometimes responds to podophyllin paint, a thorough scrape, eating pineapple chunks, sucking a peach/plum stone, or surgical shave.

Median rhomboid glossitis See ➜ Median rhomboid glossitis, p. 439.

Geographic tongue (benign migratory glossitis, erythema migrans) This is a peculiar inflammatory condition of unknown aetiology. Seen in 1–2% of adults. Involves the rapid appearance and disappearance of atrophic areas with a white demarcated border on the dorsum and lateral surface of the tongue, giving it the appearance of moving around the tongue surface. It is due to temporary loss of the filiform papillae. Pain is usually 2° to other stimuli, e.g. acidic foods (e.g. tomatoes or fruits) or cheese. Familial pattern is common. 4% have psoriasis and histology is similar. Rx: reassurance.

Depapillation of the tongue Also appears in a number of haematological and deficiency states and in severe cases may also appear lobulated.

Sore tongue (glossodynia) May occur in the presence or absence of clinical changes; however, it should be remembered that even the presence of glossitis may not explain the symptoms of a sore or burning tongue. Main causes of glossitis are iron deficiency anaemia, pernicious anaemia, candidosis, vitamin B group deficiencies, and lichen planus. Sore, but clinically normal tongue is a common problem and often psychogenic in origin; however, the first line of Rx is to exclude any possible organic cause, e.g. haematological deficiency states and unwanted reactions to self-administered or professionally administered medicines or mouthwashes.

The lips

Granulomatous cheilitis (Orofacial granulomatosis.) This is characterized by diffuse swelling of the lips, cheeks, or face and is histologically similar to Crohn's disease (non-caseating granuloma being found on biopsy). It may be the initial manifestation of Crohn's disease or related to sarcoidosis or completely isolated. It may be an allergic reaction to benzoates (toothpaste ingredient) or tomatoes. A patch test for allergens may be indicated. Intralesional steroids, e.g. triamcinolone into affected lip, anti-TNF therapies, or clofazimine 100–200mg daily for 3–6 months may help.

Persistent median fissure This may be found as a developmental abnormality but is usually secondarily infected, which is extremely difficult to eradicate. May be associated with granulomatous cheilitis. Rx: excision ± intralesional steroid.

Sarcoidosis A chronic multisystem granulomatous condition of young adults (more common in black people). Lip swelling, and gingival and palatal nodules occur. Heerfordt syndrome, ⊃ Heerfordt syndrome (uveoparotid fever), p. 784. Biopsy reveals non-caseating granuloma with inclusion bodies in 20–50%). CXR: hilar lymphadenopathy. Serum adenosine deaminase, angiotensin converting enzyme, and calcium level is ↑. Ask an ophthalmologist to exclude uveal tract involvement. Mortality rate for disseminated systemic disease is 10–20%. Rx: steroids, intralesional or systemic.

Actinic cheilitis Sun damage to the lower lip causes excessive keratin production and ↑ mitotic activity in the basal layer. Premalignant. Advise sun blocks and regular follow-up.

Exfoliative cheilitis This is similar to actinic cheilitis but of unknown aetiology.

Dry sore lips Except when accompanied by frank cheilitis, this is usually entirely innocent and can be treated symptomatically. Common causes are lip licking, and exposure to wind or sunlight. It is also a manifestation of viral illness. Rx: lip salves.

Peutz–Jeghers syndrome See ⊃ Peutz–Jeghers syndrome, p. 786.

Herpes labialis See ⊃ Recurrent HSV infections, p. 434.

Mucocele See ⊃ Mucoceles, p. 415.

Allergic angio-oedema Severe type I allergic response affecting lips, neck, and floor of mouth. Usually an identifiable cause. Rx: mild—antihistamine PO; severe—as anaphylaxis, ⊃ Anaphylactic shock and other drug reactions, p. 564.

Hereditary angio-oedema Defect of C1-esterase inhibitor. Lip, neck, floor of mouth swelling, and swelling of feet and buttocks. Precipitated by trauma. Diagnosis from family history, bloods: low C4, normal C3, and absence of C1 esterase inhibitor activity. Rx: acute attacks—fresh frozen plasma (contains C1-esterase inhibitor) or partially purified (seek advice in your locality). Prophylaxis: long term, tranexamic acid; short term, danazol.

Kawasaki disease This systemic vasculitis affecting children <5yrs causes death in the UK in <4% (US and Japan ~0.1%).[4] It can be treated if Δ. The criteria include red, dry cracked lips, strawberry tongue, and erythematous oropharyngeal mucosa, bilateral conjunctivitis, cervical lymphadenopathy, generalized rash, desquamation of hands and feet, and fever. If suspected, refer to a paediatrician.

4 N. Curtis 1997 *BMJ* **315** 322.

Salivary gland disease—1

The salivary glands consist of the major glands, the paired sublingual, submandibular, and parotid glands, and the minor salivary glands present throughout the oral mucosa, but which are particularly dense in the posterior palate and lips.

Xerostomia Dry mouth can be both a sign and a symptom. Note that some patients complain of a dry mouth when, in fact, they have an abundance of saliva. True xerostomia predisposes the mouth, pharynx, and salivary glands to infection (candidosis, ascending sialadenitis) and caries. Common causes include irradiation of the head and neck, drugs (e.g. anticholinergics and sympathomimetics), anxiety states, and salivary gland diseases (aplasia of salivary glands, Sjögren syndrome, sarcoidosis). Rx is aimed at the underlying cause. Symptomatic relief with frequent sips of water, ice chips, or artificial saliva helps. Optimal OH is essential. Pilocarpine systemically ↑ salivary flow at the expense of unwanted effects.

Sialorrhoea/ptyalism Rare. Not necessarily due to excessive saliva production, but more commonly due to a lack of coordinated swallowing mechanism resulting in pooling of saliva in the oral cavity and spillage. It is due to inflammatory conditions in the mouth or neurological conditions such as cerebral palsy and Parkinson's disease. Management includes review of posture and positioning, speech therapy, anticholinergics, and rarely posterior repositioning of submandibular ducts. Botulinum toxin injected into the relevant glands is also found to be extremely effective as a short-term (3–6 months) measure.

Sialadenitis Inflammation of, usually, the major salivary glands. *Acute bacterial sialadenitis* presents as a painful swelling, usually with a purulent discharge from the duct of the gland involved. It may also develop as an exacerbation of *chronic bacterial sialadenitis*, which often exists as a complication of duct obstruction. Ascending infection of the parotid glands occurs in dehydrated elderly patients. Both acute and chronic conditions are almost always unilateral and common infecting organisms are oral streptococci, oral anaerobes, and *Staphylococcus aureus*. Rx: rehydration and exclusion or removal of an obstructing calculus. Plain radiographs may reveal calculus, but 50% are radiolucent (➲ Salivary duct calculi, p. 514). Culture of pus from the duct and aggressive antibiotic therapy (co-amoxiclav or amoxicillin and metronidazole). Stimulation of salivary flow by chewing or massage helps chronic recurring sialadenitis. Rarely, loculated pus collection within the gland necessitates incision and drainage; USS can localize collection. Once the acute symptoms have resolved, sialography is indicated to define duct structure and may prove therapeutic. Other Rxs include irrigation with antibiotics &/or steroids via sialendoscopy. Recurrent chronic sialadenitis is an indication for removal of the gland (➲ Recurrent sialadenitis, p. 514). *Viral sialadenitis*, commonly mumps, is an acute, infectious paramyxoviral disease which primarily affects the parotid (10% submandibular gland). It is transmitted by direct contact with droplets of saliva and usually affects children and young adults with sudden onset of fever, pain, and parotid swelling. Classically, one gland is affected first, although bilateral swelling is the norm. In adults, the disease is more severe, with multisystem problems such as epididymo-orchitis, oophoritis/mastitis, pancreatitis, thyroiditis, and meningoencephalitis. Protection is conferred by the measles, mumps, and rubella (MMR) vaccine, however the incidence in the UK has ↑ following reduced vaccine intake 2° to fraudulent but highly publicized 'research'. Rx: supportive, isolate patient for 7–10 days.

Rarely, sialadenitis can occur as a manifestation of allergy to various drugs, foodstuffs, or metals.

Sialolithiasis See ⊃ Surgery of the salivary glands, p. 514.

Recurrent parotitis of childhood Unknown aetiology; congenital malformation of portions of ducts and infections ascending from mouth following dehydration. Ages 5–9yrs; recurrent unilateral parotitis with malaise. Eased by antibiotics. Resolves by puberty. EBV implicated in aetiology, possibly by structural damage to ducts. Rx: antibiotics, duct irrigation, sialogram (if tolerated).

Salivary duct and salivary gland fistulae Communications between the duct or gland and the oral mucosa or skin may occur post-traumatically or post-operatively. Although most stop spontaneously after 10 days, duct repair or gland excision may be needed. Propantheline 15mg tds before food can ↓ salivary flow and dry up small fistulae as can botulinum intraglandular injection.

Mucocele, ranula See ⊃ Mucoceles, p. 415.

Salivary gland disease—2

Sialosis This is a non-inflammatory, non-neoplastic swelling of the major salivary glands, usually the parotids and usually bilateral. Of unknown aetiology, although linked with endocrine abnormalities, nutritional deficiencies, and alcohol abuse. Sialography is essentially normal. Histology is of serous acinar cell hypertrophy. Rx: aimed at any aetiological factors. Δ: exclusion of underlying organic disease by history, haematology, and biochemistry.

Sjögren syndrome (secondary Sjögren syndrome) About 90% of patients with Sjögren syndrome are female. It comprises the triad of xerostomia, keratoconjunctivitis sicca, and a connective tissue disorder, usually rheumatoid arthritis. When the connective tissue component is absent the condition is called *primary Sjögren syndrome (sicca syndrome)*. This is an autoimmune disease affecting salivary and lacrimal glands and causing a reduction of the secretion activity. The aetiology is probably autoimmune and there is a 5% risk of malignant lymphomatous transformation of the affected gland. Δ: antinuclear antibodies (70% +ve), SSA (70% +ve), SSB (40% +ve). Rheumatoid factor (70% +ve), ESR (↑), immunoglobulins (↑), labial gland biopsy may show lymphocytic infiltrate. Saliva flowmetry, sialography, Schirmer test, and slit lamp exam can be performed. Diagnosis is made on the basis of four positive findings out of the six categories which include ocular symptoms, oral symptoms, ocular signs, histopathological features, salivary gland involvement, and autoantibodies. Management is symptomatic Rx which may include synthetic saliva (➜ Artificial saliva, p. 618), synthetic tears, meticulous OH, Rx of candida, and patient awareness of the risk of lymphomatous change. See also ➜ Sjögren syndrome (secondary Sjögren syndrome), p. 787, and the British Sjögren Syndrome Society website (℻ http://www.bssa.uk.net). In major cases, corticosteroid and immunosuppressive drugs may be needed.

Salivary gland tumours About 80% are benign; 80% occur in the parotid and 80% of these are in the superficial lobe. The majority are *pleomorphic salivary adenomas* (PSAs) which have a mixed cellular appearance on histopathology. Although benign, the cells lie within the capsule of the tumour and satellite cells may lie outside the capsule, creating a tremendous propensity for recurrence if simply enucleated. A tumour in the parotid should therefore be removed by parotidectomy or at minimum formal extracapsular dissection, taking a safe margin of normal tissue if possible (➜ Parotidectomy, p. 514). *Lymphangiomas* and *haemangiomas* are the commonest tumours found in salivary glands in children. *Adenolymphoma (Warthin's tumour)* is found almost exclusively in the parotid, and adenoid cystic carcinoma is more commonly found in the minor than the major salivary glands. Tumours of the submandibular, sublingual, and minor salivary glands are more likely to be malignant than those found in the parotid. Pointers to malignant change in salivary gland tumours are fixation to surrounding tissues, nerve involvement (particularly the facial nerve in parotid tumours), pain, rapid growth, size >4cm, and lymphadenopathy. For management, see ➜ Surgery of the salivary glands, p. 514.

Other salivary tumours These include mucoepidermoid carcinoma and acinic cell carcinoma, both of which can behave indolently or aggressively. Monomorphic adenomas are benign, with many histological varieties.

Miscellaneous Lymphoepithelial lesion (Mikulicz disease) is essentially an aggressive form of Sjögren syndrome without the eye or connective tissue component. NB: Mikulicz syndrome is salivary enlargement of known cause.

Frey syndrome See ➲ Frey syndrome, p. 783.

Drug-induced lesions of the mouth

One way of thinking of these reactions is to divide them into local and systemic effects.

Local reactions

Chemical burns Chemical burns, e.g. from an aspirin tablet being held against the oral mucosa beside a painful tooth, are still seen in some patients. The burns are superficial necrosis of the epithelium and can appear as a transient white patch. Rx: re-education and removal of the irritant. The mucosa will spontaneously heal. Iatrogenic causes include trichloroacetic acid, sodium hypochlorite, and phenol. Also caused by accidental ingestion of corrosives (e.g. paraquat).

Interference with commensal flora Prolonged or repeated use of antibiotics, particularly topical antibiotics, can lead to the overgrowth of resistant organisms, especially *Candida*. Corticosteroids can cause a similar problem by immunosuppression.

Oral dysaesthesia A sore but normal-appearing tongue can be caused by certain drugs (e.g. captopril).

Systemic effects

Depressed marrow function There are a wide range of drugs which will depress any or all of the cell lines of the haemopoietic systems and these in turn can affect the oral mucosa, e.g. phenytoin. Long-term use can result in folate deficiency and macrocytic anaemia which can produce severe aphthous stomatitis. Chloramphenicol and certain analgesics can induce agranulocytosis, leading to severe oral ulceration. Chloramphenicol can also induce aplastic anaemia, which affects haemostasis, although spontaneous oral purpura and haemorrhage are a rare presentation.

Immunosuppression Steroids and other immunosuppressants (azathioprine) predispose to viral and fungal infection.

Lichenoid eruption Classically associated with the use of gold in the Rx of rheumatoid arthritis (➋ Rheumatoid arthritis, p. 544). NSAIDs, oral hypoglycaemics, and beta blockers are commoner offenders.

Erythema multiforme (Stevens–Johnson syndrome) See ➋ Stevens–Johnson syndrome, p. 787.

Exfoliative stomatitis This is simply an oral manifestation of the very dangerous drug reaction known as exfoliative dermatitis, in which the skin and other membranes are shed. Again, gold has been implicated.

Gingival hyperplasia Common in patients on phenytoin, ciclosporin, nifedipine, and certain other calcium channel blockers; less commonly the oral contraceptive pill can have this effect. It is characterized by progressive fibrous hyperplasia and, while improved by OHI, will occur even in the presence of meticulous OH. Rx: ask if drug can be safely changed and improve oral hygiene. Gingival surgery may be needed.

Oral pigmentation Black lines in the gingival sulcus are described as being a sign of heavy metal poisoning. Chlorhexidine causes a black or brown discoloration of the dorsum of the tongue, and some antibiotics can also do this. Tetracycline discoloration of teeth is well known.

Xerostomia See ➔ Xerostomia, p. 458.

Allergic reactions Penicillin is a common offender.

There are a host of conditions affecting the oral mucosa which may be ascribed to the use of drugs. Recognition by history and patch testing of these is, of course, important, providing the drug can be withdrawn, but one has to pay attention to the reason the drug was given in the first place, and it may be that minor oral symptoms have to be tolerated when the drug is essential for the overall well-being of the patient.

Facial pain

Pain is an unpleasant sensory and emotional experience caused by actual or potential tissue damage, or described in terms of such damage. It is a complex and multifaceted symptom and several other sections of this book are relevant. The commonest source of pain in the region of the jaws and face is the tooth pulp. Pain not directly related to the teeth and jaws is dealt with here.

Trigeminal neuralgia This is the most common neurological cause of facial pain, it is an excruciating condition affecting mainly the >50s, F > M. It presents as a paroxysmal shooting 'electric shock' type of pain of rapid onset and short duration (few seconds to less than 2min), affecting one side of the face in the distribution of the trigeminal nerve. It is often stimulated by touching a trigger point in the distribution of the trigeminal nerve. Patients may refuse to shave or wash the area which stimulates the pain although, strangely, they are rarely woken by it. In the early stages of the disease there may be a period of prodromal pain not conforming to the classical description and it may be difficult to arrive at a Δ; patients often have multiple extractions in an attempt to relieve the symptoms. It is thought to be a sensory form of epilepsy, although some cases are due to vascular pressure or nerve demyelination intracranially. Δ is by the history, and carbamazepine is useful both therapeutically and diagnostically, with an 80% response rate. Injection of LA can break pain cycles and be useful diagnostically. Other useful drugs are gabapentin and pregabalin. Surgical management includes peripheral Rxs such as cryotherapy, chemical destruction of nerve (alcohol/phenol), or radiofrequency ablation and central neurosurgical procedures such as microvascular decompression, glycerol or radiofrequency rhizotomy, or gamma knife radiosurgery.

Glossopharyngeal neuralgia This is a similar condition to trigeminal neuralgia but much less common. It affects the glossopharyngeal nerve, causing an intense paroxysmal shooting pain on swallowing. There may be referred otalgia. Topical LA to the ipsilateral tonsillar/pharyngeal region immediately relieves symptoms which may help with the diagnosis. Again, carbamazepine is the drug of choice.

▶ Patients under the age of 50yrs presenting with symptoms of cranial nerve neuralgia require full neurological examination and a MRI scan, as these may be the presenting symptoms of an intracranial neoplasm, skull base metastases, HIV, syphilis, or multiple sclerosis. Bilateral neuralgic symptoms indicate demyelination until proven otherwise.

Temporal arteritis (cranial arteritis) This is a condition affecting older age groups (average age of onset 70yrs) and related to polymyalgia rheumatica. The pain is localized to the temporal and frontal regions and usually described as a severe ache, although it can be paroxysmal. The affected area is tender to touch. Jaw claudication is seen in 20%. Major risk is involvement of retinal arteries, with sudden deterioration and loss of vision; underlying pathology is inflammatory arteritis. Biopsy shows the arterial elastic tissue to be fragmented with giant cells. Δ: pulseless temporal arteries, classical distribution of pain, and raised ESR (60–100). Temporal artery biopsy helpful only if positive (as negative result does not exclude the diagnosis due to the possibility of skip lesions). Rx: aim is to relieve pain and prevent blindness with the use of systemic prednisolone.

Migraine See ➔ Headache, p. 546.

Periodic migrainous neuralgia (cluster headache) This has a similar aetiology to migraine but with a different clinical presentation: periodic attacks of severe, unilateral pain, boring or burning in character, lasting 30–60min, located around the eye; commonly associated with autonomic symptoms such as watering of eye on affected side, congestion of conjunctiva, and nasal discharge. Attacks often occur at a particular time of night (early morning 'alarm clock wakening'), and tend to be closely concentrated over a period of time, followed by a longer period of remission. Most sufferers describe alcohol intolerance. Rx: O_2 inhalation (effectiveness in acute attack is diagnostic), NSAIDs, ergotamine or sumatriptan, intranasal lidocaine. Pizotifen is used prophylactically.

Pain associated with herpes zoster See ➔ Varicella zoster, p. 434.

Glaucoma Glaucoma gives rise to severe unilateral pain centred above the eye, with a tense, stony hard globe due to raised intraocular pressure. Acute and chronic forms are recognized. The acute form presents with pain and responds to acetazolamide. Will need ophthalmological referral.

Myocardial infarction and angina This may on occasion radiate to the jaws.

Multiple sclerosis This may mimic trigeminal neuralgia or cause altered facial sensation. Differs from trigeminal neuralgia in that different neurological signs and symptoms in time and place are evident from the history. Eye pain (retrobulbar neuritis) is associated. Δ: depends upon finding multiple focal neurological lesions, disseminated in time and place. MRI reveals features of demyelination of neural tissue.

Atypical facial pain Diagnosis is of exclusion. Constitutes a large proportion of patients presenting with facial pain. Mostly middle aged women (70%). Classically, their symptoms are unrelated to anatomical distribution of nerves or any known pathological process, and these patients have often been through a number of specialist disciplines in an attempt to establish a Δ. This Δ tends to be used as a catch-all for a large group of patients, with the connecting supposition that the pain is of psychogenic origin. There may be a florid psychiatric history or undiagnosed depression (50% are depressed or hypochondriacal). Pointers to a psychogenic aetiology include imprecise localization, crosses midline, often bilateral pain, frequently moves to another site or 'all over the place'. Bizarre or grossly exaggerated descriptions of pain. Pain is described as deep, constant ache or burning and there are no relieving or exacerbating factors. Sleeping and eating are not obviously disturbed, despite continuous unbearable pain. Most analgesics are said to be unhelpful, although many will not have tried adequate analgesia. No objective signs are demonstrable and all investigations are essentially normal. After exclusion of any possible organic cause, tricyclic antidepressants, gabapentin, or pregabalin can help. The specialist pain team with access to psychological input may be of help.

Oral dysaesthesia Oral dysaesthesia or burning mouth syndrome is an unpleasant abnormal sensation affecting the oral mucosa in the absence of clinically evident disease. Five times more common in women aged 40–50yrs than other groups. Related to atypical facial pain. Patients may complain of altered or bad taste. A burning sensation usually crosses the midline. Δ: by exclusion of haematological, metabolic, nutritional, microbiological, allergic, and prosthetic causes. With experience the patient type often becomes obvious. Rx: reassurance, patients are often cancerophobic. 50% achieve remission in 6–7yrs. A recent Cochrane review[5] has identified alpha-lipoic acid, clonazepam, and cognitive behavioural therapy to reduce symptoms in limited randomized studies. Tricyclic antidepressants are frequently prescribed by clinicians.

Bell's palsy Caused by inflammation of cranial nerve VII in the stylomastoid canal. Although the main symptom is facial paralysis, pain in or around the ear, often radiating to the jaw, precedes or develops at the same time in ~50% of cases. Rx: steroids improve chance for full recovery if Rx early (within 3 days of onset). If no Rx, 20% of patients will not completely recover. Protect cornea with eye pad. Combining aciclovir with steroid or aciclovir alone does not appear to improve recovery over steroid alone.[6]

Ramsay Hunt syndrome (➔ Ramsay Hunt syndrome, p. 786.) Pain is associated with herpes zoster virus in the facial nerve. Systemic aciclovir and steroids improve recovery.

5 R. McMillan et al. 2016 *Database Syst Rev* **11** CD002779.

6 D. Gilden 2007 *N Eng J Med* **357** 1653.

Oral manifestations of skin disease

Lichen planus This is a chronic inflammatory disease of adults involving skin and mucous membranes. It affects up to 2% of the general population; 50% of patients with skin lesions have oral lesions, whereas 25% have oral lesions alone. The oral lesions persist longer than the skin lesions. It affects females more commonly than males at the ratio of 3:2. It is an autoimmune condition mediated by a T-lymphocyte attack on stratified squamous epithelia which leads to hyperkeratosis and the typical histological appearance. Lichenoid reactions are an unwanted reaction to some systemic drugs and may also be related to amalgam restorations. Usually the oral lesions are bilateral and posterior in the buccal mucosa; it is not seen on the palate but can, however, affect the tongue, lips, gingivae, and floor of mouth. The most common oral lesion is a lacy reticular pattern of hyperkeratotic epithelia seen bilaterally on the buccal mucosa. Five other types described are papular, plaque-like, erosive, atrophic, and bullous pattern. Desquamative gingivitis is a common variant affecting the gingivae. The skin lesions affect the flexor surfaces of the arms, and wrists and legs, and are particularly common on the shin as purple papules with fine white lines (Wickham striae) overlying them. Histology shows hyperparakeratosis, elongated rete ridges with a saw-tooth appearance, with dense sub- and intra-epithelial lymphocyte infiltrate and degeneration of basal keratinocytes. Lichen planus can last for months or years. It is essentially benign; however, some controversy exists about the risk of malignant transformation in erosive forms of lichen planus.

Rx: biopsy may be indicated to exclude dysplasia or malignancy; if there are lichenoid eruptions, the implicated drugs should be identified and avoided if possible. Reassurance for asymptomatic reticular lesions. If painful or if ulceration is present, topical steroids such as betamethasone (at least 1mg rinsed for 3min tds–qds), prednisolone mouthwash or topical dexamethasone are usually helpful. In severe cases, oral steroids, azathioprine, topical tacrolimus, or tretinoin gel may be used in 3° care setting. Erosive type lichen planus should be followed up 6-monthly to exclude the transformation to malignancy. Clinical photographs and repeat biopsy may be indicated.

Dyskeratosis congenita A rare autosomal dominant condition, characterized by oral leucoplakia, dystrophic changes of the nails, and hyperpigmentation of the skin; the oral lesion is prone to malignant change (➔ Leucoplakia, p. 450).

Vesiculo-bullous lesions See ➔ Vesiculo-bullous lesions—intraepithelial, p. 442.

Oral manifestations of connective tissue disease

Ehlers–Danlos syndrome A rare inherited connective tissue disease characterized by hyperextensible skin, hypermobile joints, and fragile vessels due to mutations in collagen. This results in very easy bruising and bleeding of skin as well as oral mucosa. Oral features include severe early-onset periodontal disease, small teeth with short roots, pulp stones, and occasional hypermobility of the TMJ. Bleeding during surgery, weak scars, sutures 'pulling through', and difficulty with root canal Rx are the main practical points. Some types of Ehlers–Danlos syndrome can lead to an ↑ susceptibility to infective endocarditis and significant heart damage due to mitral valve prolapse, and some types are prone to cerebrovascular accident due to weakness of intracranial blood vessels. Rx: aimed at the symptoms.

Rheumatoid arthritis (➔ Rheumatoid arthritis, p. 544). Main associations are Sjögren syndrome (15%) and rheumatoid of the TMJ (10% cases), which may cause pain, swelling, and limitation of movement. Rarely, pannus formation within the joint may occur. Rx: as for systemic rheumatoid arthritis, which may include methotrexate or TNFα.

Systemic lupus erythematosus (SLE) SLE is a systemic multisystem disease of uncertain aetiology, although viruses, hormonal changes, and drug therapy have all been implicated. The association with the presence of antinuclear factor is more common in females. Gives rise to skin lesions, classical malar 'butterfly' rash, and oral mucosal lesions in 30%, which include ulceration and purpuras. Antinuclear antibodies are present. The so-called LE cells can be detected in the blood stream. The demonstration of intact adjacent tissues towards given lesions through histological and immunohistochemical confirmation is still the standard criterion for a definitive diagnosis. F > M. Arthritis and anaemia frequent, but all major organ systems may be affected.

Chronic discoid lupus erythematosus (DLE) The lesions of this condition are limited to skin and mucosa. May present as disc-like white plaques in the mouth and can progress to SLE, although is more likely to remain as a chronic and recurring disorder. Oral lesions are present in 30%. Lip lesions in women may be premalignant. Butterfly rash may be present. DLE can be distinguished from SLE by the presence of specific double-stranded DNA antinuclear antibody in serum. Rx: SLE—systemic steroids; DLE—topical steroids, refractory lesions may respond to dapsone or thalidomide.

Systemic sclerosis A chronic disease characterized by diffuse sclerosis of connective tissues. F > M (30–50yrs). It has an insidious onset and is often associated with Raynaud's phenomenon (painful, reversible digital ischaemia on exposure to cold). Classically, the face has a waxy mask-like appearance ('Mona Lisa face'). Eating becomes difficult due to immobility of underlying tissues, and dysphagia occurs due to oesophageal involvement. Autoantibodies are present. Circulating levels of E-selectin and thrombomodulin are useful markers in monitoring disease activity. Rx: a combination of cyclophosphamide and steroids may help in early disease; penicillamine has always been used but has numerous unwanted effects. The 5yr survival is 70%.

Polyarteritis nodosa Characterized by inflammation and necrosis of small and medium-sized arteries; necrosis at any site may occur and is seen as ulceration in the mouth. Up to 60% of patients die in the first year; Rx with systemic steroids ↑ the 5yr survival to 40%.

Dermatomyositis Inflammatory condition of skin and muscles; 15% are associated with internal malignancy. May occasionally present with mouth ulcers and soreness of tongue, palate, or gingiva.

Reiter syndrome See ➔ Reiter syndrome, p. 786.

Oral manifestations of gastrointestinal disease

Patterson–Brown–Kelly syndrome See ⊃ Patterson–Brown–Kelly syndrome (Plummer–Vinson syndrome), p. 786.

Coeliac disease (gluten-sensitive enteropathy) This common form of intestinal malabsorption may present with oral ulceration as the only symptom in adults. Although children also present with ulceration, they are more likely to show weight loss, weakness, fatty diarrhoea, and failure to thrive. Other findings are glossitis, stomatitis, and angular cheilitis. Up to 5% may have RAS without anaemia. Rx: haematological and gastrointestinal investigations are required, blood picture, and haematinic assay. ↑ malabsorption. Antibodies to gluten, reticulin, endomysium (anti-endomysial antibodies are a marker for coeliac disease); small bowel biopsy required for definitive Δ. Vitamin B₁₂, folate, iron ↓ should be corrected. Rx: gluten-free diet.

Ulcerative colitis Rarely, pyostomatitis vegetans, a papilliferous, necrotic mucosal lesion can occur; more commonly, ulcers indistinguishable from aphthae are seen. Gastrointestinal symptoms predominate. Arthritis, uveitis, and erythema nodosum also occur. Topical steroids and systemic sulfasalazine are used in Rx. Most of these patients are managed by gastrointestinal specialists.

Crohn's disease Chronic granulomatous disease of unknown aetiology affecting any part of the gut from mouth to anus. Primarily affects the terminal third of the ileum, although ~1% of cases will present with oral ulceration predating any other symptoms. These tend to affect the gingiva, buccal mucosa, and lips with purplish-red non-haemorrhagic swellings, linear long-standing ulcers and cobblestoning of buccal mucosa with mucosal tags and folds (Fig. 11.5). Orofacial granulomatosis is probably a variant. Painful oral lesions seem to respond well to topical steroids or simple excision but Rx is aimed at the systemic disease.

Orofacial granulomatosis This is clinically and histologically identical to oral manifestations of Crohn's disease. Δ of exclusion (Crohn's, sarcoid). Probable aetiology is as a hypersensitivity response to certain foods, additives such as benzoates, etc. Δ is biopsy to demonstrate granulomata histologically and exclusion of systemic disease ⊃ Gastrointestinal disease, p. 534. Rx: specific to the local problem; e.g. lips (granulomatous cheilitis) intralesional steroid. Most beneficial Rx is to identify and avoid the irritant factors. Patients who have generalized Crohn's or very severe orofacial granulomatosis may benefit from systemic Rx with sulfasalazine or infliximab.

Gardener syndrome See ⊃ Gardener syndrome, p. 783.

Peutz–Jeghers syndrome See ⊃ Peutz–Jeghers syndrome, p. 786.

Cirrhosis glossitis This occurs in ~50% of patients. Sialosis is another association.

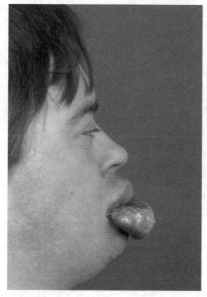

Fig. 11.5 An extreme case of lip swelling secondary to severe orofacial granulomatosis associated with Crohn's disease.

Oral manifestations of haematological disease

Anaemia The nutritional deficiencies associated with anaemia, iron, vitamin B_{12}, and folate, are all associated with *recurrent oral ulceration* (➔ Recurrent aphthous stomatitis (ulcers), p. 440) and specific deficiencies may be present, even in the absence of a frank anaemia. *Atrophic glossitis* was formerly the commonest oral symptom of anaemia but is less often seen now. Red lines or patches on a sore, but normal-looking tongue may indicate vitamin B_{12} deficiency. *Candidosis* (➔ Oral candidosis (candidiasis), p. 438) may be precipitated or exacerbated by anaemia, particularly iron deficiency, and *angular cheilitis* is a well-recognized association. The sore, clinically normal tongue (*burning tongue*) is sometimes a manifestation or even precursor of anaemia.

Patterson–Brown–Kelly syndrome See ➔ Patterson–Brown–Kelly syndrome (Plummer–Vinson syndrome), p. 786.

Leukaemia This and other haematological malignancies are associated with a ↓ in resistance to infection leading to candidosis or herpetic infections. Other oral problems include bleeding and petechial haemorrhage (even with minimal trauma), gingival swelling, ulceration, and mucosal pallor. Prevention of superinfection with chlorhexidine mouthwashes and aggressive appropriate Rx of infections which arise are of real help. Management of the bleeding is aimed at the underlying disorder; local techniques include improving OH, avoiding extractions, and using local haemostatic methods (➔ Post-operative bleeding, p. 386). Spontaneous gingival bleeding may be controlled by using impressions as a made-to-measure pressure dressing.

Cyclical neutropenia This condition may manifest as oral ulceration, acute exacerbations of periodontal disease, or NUG. As the name suggests, it recurs in 3–4-week cycles.

Myeloma This malignant neoplasm of plasma cells may occasionally cause macroglossia due to amyloid deposition. Classically, multiple osteolytic punched-out lesions in skull and jaws associated with pain, paraesthesia, and pathological fracture are seen. Bisphosphonates form part of these patients' Rx and 10yr survivors have a 30% risk of BRON (➔ Dento-alveolar surgery: bisphosphonates, denosumab, or anti-angiogenic medication, p. 390; ➔ Bisphosphonates, p. 614).

Purpura Purpura is due to platelet deficiency. Commonest as idiopathic thrombocytopenic purpura (ITP) in children. Palatal petechiae or bruising may be seen. Palatal petechiae are also seen in glandular fever, rubella, HIV, and recurrent vomiting.

Angina bullosa haemorrhagica Oral blood blisters; irritating but of no known significance (➔ Angina bullosa haemorrhagica, p. 444).

Oral manifestations of endocrine disease

Acromegaly Due to excess growth hormone production after the closure of epiphyseal plates. Oral signs include enlargement of the tongue and lips, spacing of the teeth, and an ↑ in jaw size, particularly the mandible resulting in a Class III malocclusion. Jaw pain is sometimes described, which can respond to Rx of the growth hormone-secreting pituitary tumour responsible for the disease. Rx: trans-sphenoidal hypophysectomy for pituitary adenoma.

Addison's disease (See ➋ Addison's disease, p. 540; ➋ Addison's disease, p. 590). (Adrenocortical hypofunction.) Classically, causes melanotic hyperpigmentation of the buccal mucosa. May also be part of the endocrine–candidosis syndrome.

Cushing syndrome A 'moon face' and oral candidosis are the common head and neck manifestations as a result of excess cortisol production (endogenous) or steroid medication (exogenous). Facial acne and skin atrophy is also seen. Note a need for steroid prophylaxis.

Hypothyroidism Congenital hypothyroidism is associated with enlargement of the tongue, with puffy enlarged lips and delayed tooth eruption. In adult hypothyroidism, puffiness of the face and lips also occurs, but there are no particular oral changes.

Hyperthyroidism Not associated with any particular oral changes. Ocular proptosis characteristic of Graves disease. Rx of hyperthyroidism with carbimazole is a rare cause of oral ulceration.

Hypoparathyroidism May be a component in the endocrine–candidosis syndrome; facial twitching and paraesthesia due to hypocalcaemia can be seen. Occasionally delayed eruption and enamel hyperplasia can be seen.

Hyperparathyroidism Rare. Caused by hyperplasia or adenoma of the parathyroids. ↑ parathormone causes ↑ plasma Ca^{2+} liberated from bone. Irreversible renal damage in absence of Rx so worth detecting (diagnosis confirmed by ↑ Ca^{2+}, ↑ PTH, ↓ alkaline phosphatase). Appears in the jaws as loss of lamina dura; a 'ground-glass' appearance of bone and cystic lesions (often looking multilocular), which contain dark-coloured tissue; 'brown tumour' histologically indistinguishable from a giant cell granuloma (➋ Giant cell granuloma, p. 416).

Diabetes No *specific* oral changes, although manifestations of ↓ resistance to infection can be seen if poorly controlled (e.g. severe periodontal disease). Xerostomia and thrush are prominent features of ketoacidosis. Sialosis is sometimes seen as a late feature of diabetes. Burning mouth may be a presenting feature, and oral or facial dysaesthesia may reflect the peripheral neuropathies seen in diabetics. There is a tendency to slower healing following surgery. Lichenoid reactions due to oral hypoglycaemic drugs may be seen.

Sex hormones There is a well-recognized ↑ in the severity and frequency of gingivitis at puberty and in pregnancy. Some females have recurrent aphthae clearly associated with their menstrual cycle, and several symptoms, usually burning tongue or mouth or general soreness of the tongue or mouth, have been described during the menopause. It should be remembered, however, that there are profound psychological changes at this time of life in many women, and these symptoms may be a manifestation of atypical facial pain rather than a direct hormonally mediated effect. Hormone replacement does not seem to help.

Oral manifestations of neurological disease

Examination of the cranial nerves, → Cranial nerves, p. 546; general concepts of neurological disease, → More neurological disorders, p. 548. Of the cranial nerves, the trigeminal and facial nerves contribute most to disorders affecting the mouth, face, and jaws.

Trigeminal nerve *Ophthalmic* lesions result in abnormal sensation in skin of the forehead, central nose, upper eyelid, and conjunctivae. Maxillary lesions affect skin of cheek, upper lip and side of nose, nasal mucosa, upper teeth and gingiva, and palatal and labial mucosa. The palatal reflex may be lost. Mandibular lesions affect skin of lower face, lower teeth, gingivae, tongue, and floor of mouth. Lesions of the motor root manifest in the muscles of mastication. Taste sensation is not lost in such lesions, although other sensations from the tongue are. Testing is performed by having the patient close their eyes and report on sensations experienced, in comparison to each other, while the areas of superficial distribution of the nerve are stimulated by light touch (cotton wool) and pin-prick (probe or blunt needle). The motor branch is tested by moving the jaws against resistance. A blink should be elicited by stimulating the cornea with a wisp of cotton wool (corneal reflex).

Facial nerve The facial nerve is motor to the muscles of facial expression and stapedius, secretomotor to the submandibular and sublingual salivary glands, and relays taste from the anterior two-thirds of the tongue via the chorda tympani. It is tested by having the patient raise their eyebrows, screw their eyes shut, whistle, smile, and show their teeth. Upper and lower motor neurone lesions can be distinguished because the forehead has a degree of bilateral innervation and is relatively spared in upper motor neurone lesions. Taste is tested using sour, salt, sweet, and bitter solutions. If taste is intact, flow from the submandibular duct can be assessed by gustatory stimulation. Test hearing to assess stapedius.

Neurological causes of facial and oral pain See → Facial pain, p. 464.

Neurological conditions causing altered sensation *Intracranial*: e.g. cerebrovascular accident, multiple sclerosis, polyarteritis, cerebral tumours, infection, trauma, sarcoidosis. *Extracranial*: nasopharyngeal or antral carcinoma, trauma, osteomyelitis, Paget's disease, viral or bacterial infection, leukaemic infiltrate. Psychogenic causes include hyperventilation syndrome and hysteria.

Neurological causes of facial paralysis Upper motor neurone or lower motor neurone; of the former, strokes are the commonest. Combination lesions can be caused by amyotrophic lateral sclerosis of the cord. Lower motor neurone paralysis can be caused by Bell's palsy (→ Bell's palsy, p. 466), trauma, infiltration by malignant tumours, Ramsay Hunt syndrome, or Guillain–Barré syndrome (post-viral polyneuritis, may even appear to be bilateral). Apparent paralysis may occur in myasthenia gravis where abnormally ↑ fatigue of striated muscle causes ptosis and diplopia. Therapeutic paralysis may be induced for facial spasm, using botulinum toxin injected locally. Horner syndrome results in ptosis, enophthalmos (sunken eye), miosis (constricted pupil), and anhidrosis of facial skin (↓ sweating) due to sympathetic impairment.

Neurological causes of abnormal muscle movement   Tetanus is an obvious cause. Muscular dystrophy may present with ptosis and facial paralysis. Hemifacial spasm and other tics may be caused by a tumour at the cerebello-pontine angle. Orofacial dyskinesia can be a manifestation of Parkinson's disease or an unwanted effect of major tranquillizers. Phenothiazines and metoclopramide are notorious for causing dystonic reactions in young women and children. Bizarre attacks of trismus due to masseteric spasm have been ascribed to metoclopramide.

Oral manifestations of HIV infection and AIDS

AIDS is the terminal stage of infection with the human immunodeficiency virus (HIV), which is recognized as undergoing a number of mutations. It is discussed in general terms in ➔ AIDS, p. 556. The underlying severe immunodeficiency leads to a number of oral manifestations (75% have orofacial disease) which, although not pathognomonic, should raise the possibility of HIV infection. They have been classified as follows:

Group I—strongly associated with HIV

Candidosis Seen in 70% of HIV patients as early manifestation (➔ Oral candidosis (candidiasis), p. 438). Erythematous (early), hyperplastic, pseudomembranous (late), and angular cheilitis in young people (most common oral feature of HIV). 50% of patients with HIV-associated thrush develop AIDS in 5yrs.

Hairy leucoplakia Bilateral, white, non-removable corrugated lesions of the tongue, unaffected by antifungals but usually resolve with aciclovir or valaciclovir (but return on discontinuation of Rx), and associated with EBV. It is a predictor of a bad prognosis and possible development of lymphoma.

HIV gingivitis Unusually severe gingivitis for relatively good OH. Often characterized by linear gingival erythema, an intense red band along the gingival margin.

Necrotizing ulcerative gingivitis (➔ NUG, p. 199.) Occurs in young, otherwise healthy mouths.

HIV periodontitis Severe localized destruction out of place with OH.

Kaposi's sarcoma (KS) Commonest malignancy among HIV patients. One or more erythematous/purplish macules or swelling, frequently on the palate. 50% occur intra- or peri-orally. It is pathognomonic if seen in a young male who is not receiving immunosuppression. Rx: radiotherapy, intralesional vincristine, or local excision.

Non-Hodgkin's lymphoma Also common. Burkitt's lymphoma is 1000 times more common than in HIV-negative persons in the West.

Group II—less strongly associated with HIV
Atypical oropharyngeal ulceration:
- ITP.
- *HIV-associated salivary gland disease*—lympho-epithelial cysts or focal lymphocytic sialadenitis (mainly parotid glands), more common in children.
- Wide range of common viral infections.

Group III—possible association with HIV
- Wide range of rare bacterial and fungal infections.
- Hyperpigmentation.
- Cat scratch disease.
- Neurological abnormalities.
- SCC oropharynx.
- *Persistent generalized lymphadenopathy*—otherwise inexplicable lymphadenopathy >1cm persisting for 3 months, at two or more extra-inguinal sites. Cervical nodes particularly commonly affected. May be prodromal or a manifestation of AIDS.

Rx Antiretroviral drugs prolong and improve quality of life in those with active AIDS. HAART has revolutionized the long- to medium-term prognosis, these are changing regularly and the combinations used are complex. Currently HIV positivity if treated with HAART is unlikely to manifest as AIDS and life expectancy approaches the age-matched norm. Facial manifestations of their use include a severe facial lipoatrophy. Early detection and Rx of opportunistic infections and neoplasms also has a major impact on quality of life.

Dental Rx for patients with AIDS This group present two risks with regard to dental Rx:
- Risk of transmission to personnel carrying out the Rx (risk from needlestick injury from an infected patient is 0.3–0.45%). Routine cross-infection control measures are necessary in all patients.
- As these patients are immunocompromised, any Rx with a known risk of infective complications, e.g. extractions, should be covered with antiseptic and antimicrobial prophylaxis, and any surgery should be as atraumatic as possible. There may also be a slight tendency to bleeding in these patients, and local haemostatic measures (➔ Post-operative bleeding, p. 386) may be needed.

Prophylaxis after contaminated needlestick injury Prophylaxis after contaminated needlestick injury, e.g. a hollow point needlestick injury from HIV-positive patient, should be given within 24h. HAART offers the best chance of preventing HIV seroconversion.[7]

7 CMO Expert Advisory Group on AIDS (✎ http://www.dh.gov.uk).

Cervicofacial lymphadenopathy

You cannot palpate a normal lymph node, therefore a palpable one must be abnormal (and is usually >1cm) (Fig. 11.6). The most important distinction to make is whether this is part of the node's physiological response to infection or whether it is undergoing some pathological change. The finding of an enlarged node or nodes in children is relatively common and can be reasonably managed by watchful waiting. Undiagnosed cervical lymphadenopathy in adults mandates establishing a definitive Δ.

History

Ask about pain or swelling in the mouth, throat, ears, face, or scalp. Was there any constitutional upset when the lump appeared? Has it been getting bigger progressively or has it fluctuated? Is it painful, and how long has it been present?

Examination

Fully expose the neck and palpate from behind, with the patient's head bent slightly forward to relax the neck. Examine systematically, feeling the submental, facial, submandibular, parotid, auricular, occipital, deep cervical chain, supraclavicular, and posterior triangle nodes. Differentiating between the submandibular salivary gland and node can be a problem, made simpler by palpating bimanually; the salivary gland can be felt moving between the external and internal fingers. Supraclavicular nodes are more liable to be due to an occult tumour in the lung or upper gastrointestinal tract, whereas posterior triangle nodes are more liable to be haematological or scalp skin in origin.

If a node is palpable, note its texture, size, and site, and whether it is tender to touch or fixed to surrounding tissues.

- Acutely infected nodes tend to be large, tender, soft, and freely mobile.
- Chronically infected nodes are soft to firm and less liable to be tender.
- Metastatic carcinoma in nodes tends to be hard and fixed.
- Lymphomatous nodes are described as rubbery and have a peculiar firm texture.

Extra-oral and intra-oral inspection Perform EO and IO inspection to identify 1° source for enlarged node. Examine axillary and inguinal nodes, liver, and spleen.

Investigations

Carry out a FBC to look for leucocytosis. Specific blood tests such as serology for EBV, CMV, cat scratch disease, and toxoplasmosis may be required according to the history. Once infection is excluded it is essential to exclude, as far as possible, an occult 1° malignancy of the head and neck; the best way to do this is by direct examination, flexible nasendoscopy, and CXR. If access for examination is limited, examination under anaesthesia (EUA) is indicated.

US-guided fine-needle aspiration cytology (FNAC) is probably the gold standard minimalist investigation. Although previously controversial, USS-guided core biopsy has an evidence base supporting it. MRI and CT scanning will confirm the presence, shape, size, and presence of necrosis within nodes and may reveal an occult tumour. MRI/CT cannot, however, confirm the pathological process within the node.

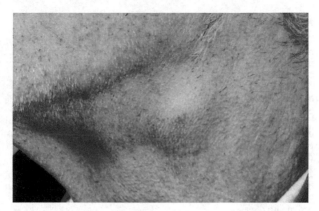

Fig. 11.6 A prominent palpable cervical lymph node arising at the junction of levels I and II in the neck; all such masses should be rapidly and fully investigated prior to any form of open biopsy. Biopsy is often requested by haematologists to diagnose lymphoma but carries the risk of decreasing the patient's prognosis if the diagnosis is squamous or salivary cancer of the head and neck.

If the Δ has still not been established it is reasonable to proceed to excision biopsy of the node, which should be cultured for mycobacteria as well as examined histologically. Find out how your pathology department likes the nodes sent; some want them fresh.

Common causes Dental abscesses, pericoronitis, tonsillitis, glandular fever, lymphoma, metastatic deposits, and leukaemia.

Rare causes Brucellosis, atypical mycobacteria (although commoner in children), TB, AIDS, toxoplasmosis, actinomycosis, sarcoidosis, cat scratch fever, syphilis, drugs (e.g. phenytoin), mucocutaneous lymph node syndrome (Kawasaki disease), and Crohn's disease. Other neck lumps, ◉ Neck lumps, p. 520.

An approach to oral ulcers

Oral ulceration is probably the commonest oral mucosal disease seen; it may also be the most serious. It is important, therefore, to have an approach to the management of oral ulcers firmly established in your mind.

Duration How long has the ulcer been present?

▶ If >3 weeks, referral for appropriate specialist investigation, including biopsy, is mandatory.

If of recent onset, ask whether it was preceded by blistering. Are the ulcers multiple? Is any other part of the body affected and have similar ulcers been experienced before? Then look at the site &/or distribution of the ulcer(s).

Blistering Blistering preceding the ulcer suggests a vesiculo-bullous condition (◐ Vesiculo-bullous lesions—intraepithelial, p. 442). Blistering with lesions elsewhere in the body suggests erythema multiforme or hand, foot, and mouth disease.

Distribution If limited to the gingivae, suggests NUG (◐ NUG, p. 199). Unilateral distribution suggests herpes (◐ Viral infections of the mouth, p. 434). Under a denture or other appliance suggests traumatic ulceration.

Recurrence Recurrence of the ulcers after apparent complete resolution is characteristic of RAS (◐ Recurrent aphthous stomatitis (ulcers), p. 440).

Pain Its presence or absence is not particularly useful diagnostically, although the character of the pain may be of value. Pain is often a late feature of oral carcinoma and the fact that an ulcer may be painless never excludes it from being a potential cancer.

For most ulcers of recent onset, and a few present for an indeterminate period, a trial of therapy is often a useful adjunct to Δ. This is especially useful in RAS, viral conditions (where Rx is essentially symptomatic), and lesions probably caused by local trauma (Rx being removal of the source of trauma and review after 1 week).

Ulcers which need early diagnosis These include:
- *Herpes zoster* as early aggressive Rx with aciclovir may reduce post-herpetic neuralgia.
- *Erythema multiforme* in order to avoid re-exposure to the antigen.
- *Erosive lichen planus* as this may benefit from systemic steroids or other specialist Rx and will require specialist long-term follow-up.
- *Traumatic ulcerative granuloma with stromal eosinophilia (TUGSE)* because it can be clinically indistinguishable from SCC but spontaneously resolves in most cases (after up to 6 weeks).
- *Oral SCC* for obvious reasons.

Temporomandibular pain—dysfunction/facial arthromyalgia

Fig. 11.7 is a practice-based protocol for a patient with TMJ symptoms.

What is it? The problem being addressed is pain in the preauricular area and muscles of mastication with trismus, with or without evidence of internal derangement of the meniscus. Conditions which can otherwise be classified as facial pain syndromes or other forms of joint disease are excluded and can be found in the relevant sections (❸ Facial pain, p. 464).

Prevalence Affects ~50% of the population at some time in their lives. F > M. Onset 20–30yrs of age.

Aetiology Idiopathic. Multiple theories put forward regarding occlusion, trauma, stress, habits, and joint hypermobility. To date, the concept of stress-induced parafunctional habits (bruxism, clenching) causing pain and spasm in the masticatory apparatus coupled with a ↓ pain threshold has seemed the most reasonable. This is compatible with the observed high association with depression, back pain, tension headache, migraine, irritable bowel syndrome, and fibromyalgia. It does not, however, explain the cause in those patients who can identify no different levels of stress in their lives nor does it help explain the high incidence of internal derangement of the meniscus.

Clinical features Pain, clicking, locking, crepitus, and trismus are the classical signs and symptoms. Some patients may be clinically depressed but most are not. Pain is elicited by palpation over the muscles of mastication &/or the preauricular region. Clicking commonly occurs at 2–3mm of tooth separation on opening and sometimes closing. This is due to the meniscus being displaced anteriorly on translation of the head of the condyle and then returning to its usual position (the click). A lock is when it does not return.

Management Success has been claimed for a wide range of Rxs, reflecting confusion over Δ and the multifactorial and self-limiting nature of the condition. Simple conservative Rx within the range of every dentist is successful in up to 80% of cases. In unsuccessful cases, a referral to an appropriate 2° setting specialist is recommended.

Reassurance and explanation Advice as to the nature of the problem and its benign and frequently self-limiting course is all that many patients require. Do not create a problem where there is none! This is also the time to take a gentle but thorough social and family history to identify clinically depressed patients or those with significant stress. An information leaflet is helpful.

Simple analgesia, rest, gentle heat, and remedial exercises Whether these are given by the dentist, physiotherapist (in the form of short-wave diathermy and US), or ancillary staff is unimportant, as the crucial part is the patient compliance at home.

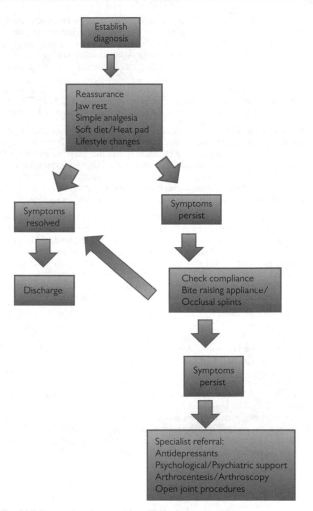

Fig. 11.7 Practice-based protocol for a 'TMJ' patient.

Splint therapy Upper/lower, hard/soft have all been used with varying success. The initial aim of a splint is to (i) show something is being done (placebo); (ii) ↓ bruxism and joint load; and (iii) ↑ the gap between condyle and fossa, whereby the disc may be freed. A simple, full-coverage upper or lower splint should be worn as often as possible, nights and evenings especially, and reassessed after 4–6 weeks.

These three simple measures should relieve symptoms in ~80% of patients and identify those needing referral to a specialist (Fig. 11.7). Do not persist with ineffective Rx if symptoms have not improved within 3 months.

Drug therapy There is a natural reluctance among many patients to take drugs, particularly those associated with psychiatry. There is also a misconceived reluctance among clinicians to use the tricyclics and related compounds. They are non-addictive and the commoner side effects of weight gain, constipation, and dry mouth can be overcome. Nortriptyline, dosulepin, and related compounds have been demonstrated to have analgesic and muscle relaxant effects independent of their antidepressant effect.

Occlusal adjustment There are a group of patients where a significant occlusal problem exists. In these cases, a hard diagnostic occlusal splint can be constructed for the mandible (Tanner) or for the maxilla (Michigan), and should be made to give multiple even contacts in centric relation and anterior guidance. The patient attempts to wear this full-time for up to 3 months. If pain is abolished while wearing the appliance, returns when it is removed, and is abolished on reinstitution, then occlusal adjustment by orthodontic, surgical, or restorative means is a reasonable option.

Surgery for internal derangement If pain can be abolished by other methods and the patient continues to be bothered by a painful click, particularly with recurrent locking, Rx aimed specifically at the meniscus is justified. The first line which may be useful diagnostically and improve pain due to capsulitis is arthrocentesis or arthroscopy. This includes irrigation of the upper joint space, through which lysis and lavage of adhesions and synovial inflammatory mediators, and injection of steroids and LA can be performed. These techniques have surprisingly high published success rates (>90%). The next line of surgical Rx includes open procedures such as meniscopexy, menisectomy, condylar shave, and eminectomy. However, the consensus dictates that the minimum of interference to the articulatory surfaces and the articular meniscus is carried out. Rarely, completely ruined joints will benefit from total joint replacement.

Maxillofacial surgery

Relevant pages in other chapters Oral cancer, ➲ p. 452; neck lumps, ➲ Cervicofacial lymphadenopathy, p. 480; TMJ, ➲ Temporomandibular pain—dysfunction/facial arthromyalgia, p. 484; salivary glands, ➲ Salivary gland disease—1, p. 458; clefts, ➲ Cleft lip and palate, p. 170; orthognathic surgery, ➲ Orthodontics and orthognathic surgery, p. 168; pre-prosthetic surgery, ➲ Minor pre-prosthetic surgery, p. 426; ➲ Introduction to implantology, p. 361.

Principal sources and further reading ACS 2018 *ATLS Core Course Manual*. R. Ferris & M. L. Gillison 2017 Nivolumab for squamous cell cancer of head and neck. *N Engl J Med* **376** 596. J. R. Hupp et al. 2018 *Contemporary Oral and Maxillofacial Surgery* (7e), Mosby. B. Jones 2008 *Facial Rejuvenation Surgery*, Mosby. C. Kerawala & C. Newlands 2014 *Oral and Maxillofacial Surgery* (Oxford Specialist Handbook) (2e), OUP. D. A. Mitchell and A. N. Kanatas 2015 *An Introduction to Oral and Maxillofacial Surgery* (2e), CRC Press. J. Shah 2003 *Oral Cancer*, Dunitz. J. Watkinson 2000 *Head & Neck Surgery*, Butterworth-Heinemann. K. Wolffe & F. Hölzle 2017 *Raising of Microvascular Flaps* (3e), Springer. Personal experience, 1988–2018.

In general, maxillofacial surgery is a postgraduate subject which has evolved from oral surgery, with foundations in medicine, dentistry, and surgery. It is included here as an introduction to students, an aide-memoire for junior hospital staff, and a guide for those who will be referring patients.

Advanced trauma life support (ATLS)

ATLS is a system providing one safe way of resuscitating a trauma victim. It was first conceived in Nebraska, subsequently developed by the ACS, and has now reached international acceptance. It is not the only approach but it is one which works. The principles of basic life support are included during trauma management and can be applied during emergencies in general dental practice.

Trauma deaths

These have a trimodal distribution. The first peak is within seconds to minutes of injury. The second is within the first hour, the 'golden hour', and is the area of main concern. The third is days to weeks later but may reflect management within the golden hour.

The core concept behind ATLS

The core concept is the *primary survey* with *simultaneous resuscitation*, followed by a *secondary survey* leading to definitive care.

Primary survey

This uses the mnemonic *ABCDE* on the basis of identifying and treating the most lethal injury first.

- *Airway with cervical spine control.* Establish a patent airway and protect the cervical spine from further injury. Chin lift, jaw thrust, oral airway, nasopharyngeal airway, intubation, surgical airway as needed, coupled with manual inline immobilization of cervical spine or rigid cervical collar, sandbags, and tape.
- *Breathing and ventilation.* Inspect, palpate, and auscultate the chest. Count respiratory rate. Give 100% O_2. Chest decompression by needle puncture in second intercostal space mid-clavicular line if indicated for tension pneumothorax. Chest drain fifth intercostal space anterior axillary line if needed.
- *Circulation with haemorrhage control.* Assess level of consciousness, skin colour, pulse and BP, manual pressure control of extreme haemorrhage. Establish two large venous cannulae; take blood for X-match and baseline studies. Give 2L of pre-warmed Hartmann's solution. Establish ECG, seek help for operative control of bleeding if needed. Establish urinary catheter unless urethral transection is suspected, and oro- or nasogastric tube. Tranexamic acid IV in first 3h.
- *Disability* (neuro-evaluation). Glasgow Coma Scale (GCS) score. Pupillary response to light, visual acuity. Prevent hypotension and hypoxia.
- *Exposure.* Remove all clothing to allow full assessment of injuries. Ensure monitoring: respiratory rate, BP, pulse, arterial blood gases, pulse oximetry, and ECG. Prevent hypothermia.

If all these can be established and monitored parameters are normalized, the patient's chances of living are optimized.

X-rays At this stage obtain a chest and pelvis film in the resuscitation room. Cervical spine film may help but the cervical spine should remain immobilized until fully assessed if the mechanism of injury suggests spinal trauma.

Reassess the ABCs

If all is stable, move to the *secondary survey*, which is a head-to-toe examination of the patient. It is at this stage *only* that specific non-immediately life-threatening conditions should be identified and dealt with in turn.

Maxillofacial injuries Other than those with a direct effect on the airway or cervical spine, or causing exsanguinating haemorrhage, maxillofacial injuries should not be dealt with until the *ABCs* have been completed and this question should be asked of all referring doctors prior to accepting responsibility for a patient. Intracranial, visceral, and major orthopaedic injuries with neurovascular compromise should be identified and managed first.

While ATLS is designed primarily for front-line physicians, dental graduates training in oral and maxillofacial surgery can complete the course, and it's strongly recommended to anyone who may undertake care of the trauma patient.

Primary management of maxillofacial trauma

The first consideration is whether the patient has suffered polytrauma, which may have multiple and life-threatening ramifications, or, as is more commonly the case, trauma confined to the face. In the former, the prime concern is keeping the patient alive, and the maxillofacial injuries can await Rx (⊃ Advanced trauma life support (ATLS), p. 488). Remember that isolated facial injuries rarely cause sufficient bleeding to induce hypovolaemic shock. Bleeding can cause pressure to the optic nerve and can cause blindness. Visual acuity must be checked.

Airway The brain can tolerate hypoxia for ~3min. Most conscious patients can maintain a patent airway if the oropharynx is cleared. Give all traumatized patients maximal O_2 initially. Oral airways are not tolerated unless the patient is unconscious. Nasopharyngeal airways are only of value if they can be inserted safely and kept patent. If the patient is unconscious and the airway is obstructed, they should be intubated. If this is not possible, an emergency airway can be maintained by cricothyroid puncture with a wide-bore cannula. Long-term security of the airway can be achieved by surgical cricothyroidotomy as an emergency, or tracheostomy as a planned operation. Conscious patients with severe isolated facial trauma maintain their airway by sitting leaning forward—let them.

Cervical spine injuries Until these are excluded, the patient should be immobilized; must balance with need to remove from spine boards as soon as possible (painful, prevent pressure sores). Use common sense to decide between immobilization and sitting/leaning forward.

Bleeding As for airway. Gunshot wounds and lacerated major vessels are exceptions which can cause extensive bleeding. Specific techniques to control naso- and oropharyngeal bleeding are bilateral rubber mouth props to immobilize the maxilla; bilateral balloon catheters passed into the postnasal space, inflated then pulled forward; and bilateral anterior nasal packs.

Scalp wounds Can exsanguinate children; control with pressure and heavy full-thickness sutures.

Head injuries The main cause of death and disability in patients with isolated maxillofacial trauma. Assessment, ⊃ Assessing head injury, p. 492.

Can they see? Orbital compartment syndrome (retrobulbar haemorrhage), ⊃ Retrobulbar haemorrhage, p. 496. Assess and document visual acuity, can they count fingers? Use a Snellen chart to formally document vision. If evidence of lost or decreasing visual acuity, request formal ophthalmological review.

Cerebrospinal fluid (CSF) leaks Facial and skull # can create dural tears, leading to CSF rhinorrhoea (from the nose) or otorrhoea (from the ear). Although controversial, prophylactic antibiotics are used by many. A combination penicillin in high dose is often used, despite the fact that conventional antibiotics do not cross the healthy blood–brain barrier in adequate levels, the rationale being that the blood–brain barrier is damaged in these cases. It was the concern that low levels of antibiotic in the CSF would only suppress *signs* of meningitis while selecting resistant organisms that prompted influential recommendations against prophylaxis.[1]

Tetanus immunity If in doubt, give tetanus toxoid.

Analgesia This may not be needed. Avoid opioids if possible as they interfere with neuro-observations by limiting pupillary response. If needed, use diclofenac 75mg IM bd or codeine phosphate 60mg IM 6-hourly.

Patients to admit Any question of danger to the airway, skull #, history of unconsciousness, retrograde amnesia, bleeding, middle-third #, mandibular # (except when very simple), malar # if +ve eye signs, children, and those with domestic or social problems. If in doubt *admit*. Place on, at least, initial hourly neurological observations (most will need 15min observations initially). IV access and antibiotic. If not admitting, give the patient a head-injury card.

If teeth have been lost, ensure they are not in the chest (CXR) or soft tissues.

X-rays See ➲ X-rays, p. 495; ➲ X-rays, p. 497.

1 Working Party of the British Society for Antimicrobial Chemotherapy 1992 *Lancet* **344** 1547.

Assessing head injury

▶ All patients with recent facial trauma warranting hospital admission need at least initial assessment for head injury.

Change in the level of consciousness is the earliest and most valuable sign of head injury.

A combination of the scales in Table 12.1 is generally used.

Pulse and BP ↓ pulse and ↑ BP is a late sign of ↑ intracranial pressure.

Pupils Measure size (1–8mm) and reaction to light in both pupils.

Respiration ↓ rate is a sign of raised intracranial pressure.

Limb movement

Indicate   normal

mild weakness

severe weakness

extension

no response

For arms and legs Record right and left separately if there is a difference.

CT scan The definitive investigation. However, patients must be stabilized first. Never transfer a patient before correcting hypoxia and hypovolaemia.

Using the GCS Severe head injury &/or deterioration = call for help.

One accepted method of categorizing head-injured patients by severity is by using the GCS score:
- Severe: <8.
- Moderate: 9–12.
- Minor: 13–15.

In addition A severe head injury is present if the following are seen:
- Unequal pupils (except traumatic mydriasis).
- Unequal limb movement (except orthopaedic injury).
- Open head injury (i.e. compound to brain).
- Deterioration in measured parameters.
- Depressed skull #.

Subtle signs of deterioration include:
- Severe &/or worsening headache.
- Early unilateral pupillary dilatation.
- Early unilateral limb weakness.

A GCS score of <6 in the absence of drugs has a dismal prognosis.

A change in GCS score of 2 or more is significant. Beware changes in monitoring staff!

Table 12.1 Glasgow Coma Scale (GCS) score

Eyes open			
• spontaneously	4		
• to speech	3		
• to pain	2		
• do not open	1		

Best verbal response		Best motor response	
• orientated	5	• obeys commands	6
• confused	4	• localizes pain	5
• inappropriate	3	• normal flexion	4
• incomprehensible	2	• abnormal flexion	3
• none	1	• extension	2
		• none	1

Reproduced from Teasdale, G., Jennet, B., Assessment of coma and impaired status. *The Lancet* (1974) **304**:7872, with permission from Elsevier.

Optimizing outcome You are preventing 2° brain injury:
- Oxygenate.
- Moderate hyperventilation to control partial pressure of carbon dioxide (PCO_2).
- Control haemorrhage and optimize fluid balance, use tranexamic acid.
- Contact neurosurgery and ask advice.
- Only use mannitol under expert advice.

Do not use steroids at all.[2]

2 ACS 2018 *ATLS Core Course Manual.*

Mandibular fractures

These are the commonest # of the facial skeleton (Fig. 12.1). Most are the result of fights and road traffic accidents (the former ubiquitous in Western countries whereas the latter are commoner in the Middle East; the role of alcohol, laws, and attitudes to driving are self-evident). Rarely, they may be comminuted with hard and soft tissue loss, e.g. gunshot wounds.

Classification The most useful is based on the site of injury: dento-alveolar, condyle, coronoid, ramus, angle, body, symphyseal, or parasymphyseal. Further subclassification into unilateral, bilateral, multiple, or comminuted aids Rx planning. In common with all # they can be grouped into simple (closed linear #), compound (open to mouth or skin), pathological (# through an area weakened by other pathology), or comminuted; again, this influences Rx.

Muscle pull Pull on # segments renders the # favourable or unfavourable depending on whether or not the # line resists displacement. This is of less importance than recognizing the # and its associated injuries.

Common # Condylar neck # are commonest and range from easiest to most difficult. Often found with a # of the angle or canine region of the opposite side of the jaw. Rarely, bilateral condylar # is found with a symphyseal #—'guardsman's #' from falling on the point of the chin. Angle # usually occurs through wisdom-tooth socket, and body # commonly through canine socket. Condylar neck fractures may be fixed several days later and usually within 2 weeks.

Diagnosis History of trauma. Ask if the patient can bite their teeth or dentures together in the manner which is normal to them. Inability to do this and a lingual mucosal haematoma is pathognomonic of a mandibular #. Look at the face; there is usually bruising and swelling over the # site and sometimes lacerations. If the # is displaced, there may be gagging on the posterior teeth and the mouth hangs open. The saliva is usually bloodstained. The patient may complain of paraesthesia in the distribution of the IDN. Gentle palpation over the mandible will reveal step deformities, bony crepitus, and tenderness. All have trismus to some degree, opening <40mm.

Examination of the mouth This may reveal broken teeth or dentures which should be removed. Suction the mouth to clean away blood clots prior to examining both the buccal and lingual sulcus. Look for step deformities in the occlusion, and examine the teeth. Palpate for steps in the lingual and buccal sulcus. If Δ is uncertain, it is sometimes worth trying to elicit abnormal mobility across the suspected # site, using gentle pressure. In cases where you are very unsure, place one hand over each angle of the mandible and exert gentle pressure; this will produce pain if there is a #, even if it is only a crack #. Never perform this if you have proved otherwise that there is a #.

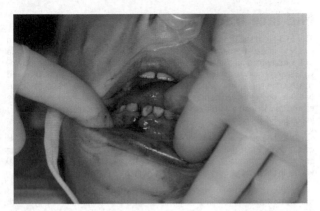

Fig. 12.1 Malocclusion and abnormal mobility are pathognomonic of a fractured mandible.

X-rays DPT and PA mandible are the essentials in order to diagnose and assess a mandibular fracture. Most patients in trauma centres will have additional assessment with a CT scan. CT scans are required to assess condylar fractures before fixation.

Preliminary Rx (⊙ Primary management of maxillofacial trauma, p. 490.) Most patients will be admitted to hospital, nursed sitting up and leaning forward as this is the most comfortable position. Keep nil by mouth and maintain hydration by IV crystalloid. Compound # need antibiotics. Assess need for analgesia; LA, temporary immobilization with circumdental wire (bridle wire), parenteral NSAIDs, or opioids may be needed.

Mid-face fractures

The mid-facial skeleton is a complex composite of fine fragile bones, which rarely # in isolation. It forms a detachable framework which protects the brain from trauma. Severe trauma can move the entire mid-face downwards and backwards along the base of the skull, lengthening the face and obstructing the airway (clot and swelling exacerbates this). Most *conscious* patients, however, can compensate for this. # of the cribriform plate of the ethmoids can lead to dural tears and CSF leak (➜ Cerebrospinal fluid (CSF) leaks, p. 490).

Orbit The globe and optic nerve are well protected by the bony buttress of the orbit. Most # lines pass around the optic foramen; however, swelling and roof # can cause proptosis. Late changes, particularly floor and medial wall # include tethering and enophthalmos.

Retrobulbar haemorrhage This is an arterial bleed behind the globe following trauma. It presents as a painful, proptosed eye with decreasing visual acuity, and is a surgical emergency. The clot must be decompressed and evacuated. Medical management with mannitol 20% 2g/kg, acetazolamide 500mg and prednisolone at least 1mg/kg all IV may help while theatre is being arranged. Evacuation is by lateral canthotomy. Involve ophthalmology.

Bleeding Severe bleeding is rare, but severe mid-facial trauma may lacerate the third part of the maxillary artery, resulting in profuse bleeding into the nasopharynx which requires anterior and posterior nasal packs and possibly direct (endoscopic) ligation.

Classification Mainly based on the experimental work of Rene Le Fort. Le Fort I # detaches the tooth-bearing portion of the jaw via a # line from the anterior margin of the anterior nasal aperture running laterally and back to the lower third of the pterygoid plate. Le Fort II detaches the true mid-face in a pyramidal shape (Fig. 12.2). Le Fort III detaches the entire facial skeleton from the cranial base (Fig. 12.2).

Diagnosis Le Fort I may occur singly or be associated with other facial #. The tooth-bearing portion of the upper jaw is mobile, unless impacted superiorly. There is bruising in the buccal sulcus bilaterally, disturbed occlusion, and posterior 'gagging' of the bite. Grasp the upper jaw between the thumb and forefinger anteriorly, place thumb and forefinger of the other hand over the supraorbital ridges, and attempt to mobilize the upper jaw to assess mobility. Spring the maxillary teeth to detect a palatal split. Percussion of the upper teeth may produce a 'cracked cup' sound. Le Fort II and III # produce similar clinical appearances; namely, gross oedema of soft tissues, bilateral black eyes (panda facies), subconjunctival haemorrhage, mobile mid-face, dish-face appearance, and extensive bruising of the soft palate. Look for a CSF leak and assess visual acuity. Le Fort II may also show infra-orbital nerve paraesthesia and step deformity in the orbital rim. Peculiar to Le Fort III # are tenderness and separation of the frontozygomatic suture, deformity of zygomatic arches bilaterally, and mobility of entire facial skeleton.

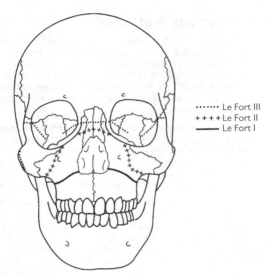

Fig. 12.2 Each line represents a different fracture line although these lines are in reality more often produced surgically, trauma being less predictable.

X-rays Occipito-mental 10° and 30°, submento-vertex, lateral skull, PA **skull** *only* if C-spine is confirmed to be intact. Otherwise secure C-spine and await CT scan as the definitive imaging technique.

Preliminary Rx See ⊃ Advanced trauma life support (ATLS), p. 488; ⊃ Primary management of maxillofacial trauma, p. 490; *definitive Rx*, ⊃ Treatment of facial fractures, p. 500.

Nasal and malar fractures

Malar (or zygoma) # A common and easily missed injury, usually the result of a blow with a blunt object (e.g. fist). The malar forms the cheekbone and resembles a four-pointed star on occipito-mental X-ray. The 'star' points to the maxilla (orbital margin and lateral wall of antrum), frontal bone, and temporal bone. # can involve the arch alone or the whole malar, which may or may not be displaced. The nature of the displacement is of value in planning the Rx.

Diagnosis Δ is from history, examination, and X-ray. Bruising around eye with subconjunctival haemorrhage (unilateral) (Fig. 12.3). Diplopia, a step deformity of the orbital rim, sometimes paraesthesia of the infra-orbital nerve, limitation of lateral excursion of the mandible on mouth opening, and unilateral epistaxis. There is often tenderness on palpation of the zygomatic buttress IO and usually some flattening of the cheek prominence.

Orbital floor # Main signs are those of the malar # (or middle third # if that is the presenting injury). Signs are enophthalmos and diplopia in upwards gaze (inferior rectus). Late enophthalmos caused by fibrosis of herniated periorbital fat. Also known as orbital blowout #; fat and muscle herniates through the thin orbital floor (a similar injury can occur to the medial wall). Classically, seen on X-ray as 'hanging drop sign' (radiolucent fat hanging into antrum) (Fig. 12.4). Confirm with coronal CT scan. Lateral wall &/or roof # are much less common.

White eye blowout Seen in children, often a trapdoor blowout # with no subconjunctival haemorrhage but severe pain and intractable vomiting. Repair resolves the condition. Rare but one of the few indications for emergency orbital surgery.

Nasal # Simple nasal trauma is seen by a number of different specialities and considered rather trivial. This is unfair to the patients, as long-term results of nasal # leave a lot to be desired. Nasal # are frequently associated with deviation or crumpling of the septum, obvious nasal deformity, epistaxis, and a degree of nasal obstruction. Rx: often consists of simply manipulating the nasal bones with the thumb and splinting. This leaves the septum untreated and contributes to poor long-term results, with many needing septorhinoplasty later.

Nasoethmoid # This consists of nasal bones, frontal process of maxilla, lacrimal bones, orbital plate of ethmoid, and displacement of the medial canthus of the eye. These # require accurate reduction, stabilization, and fixation of the medial canthus. Δ: bilateral black eyes, obvious nasal deformity (particularly depression of the nasal bridge), septal deviation, epistaxis, and obstruction. Look for CSF leak.

Septal haematoma A comparatively uncommon complication of nasal trauma which demands immediate evacuation as, if ignored, it can lead to septal necrosis.

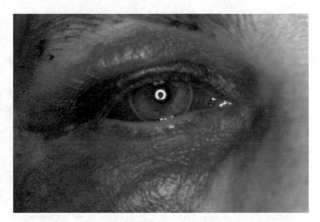

Fig. 12.3 The presence of subconjunctival haemorrhage (seen here medially and laterally) is usually indicative of underlying fracture.

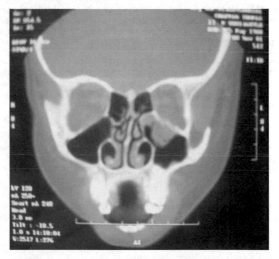

Fig. 12.4 A coronal CT scan demonstrating prolapse of the contents of the left orbit into the maxillary antrum—the 'hanging drop' of a blowout fracture.

Treatment of facial fractures

Essentially involves reduction, fixation, and immobilization of the # segments. In mandibular and maxillary #, this was traditionally achieved by IMF, i.e. immobilizing the jaws in occlusion. Nowadays, elastic traction is sometimes used to supplement internal fixation. Wisdom teeth and grossly broken down or periodontally infected teeth in the # line should be removed. Otherwise, provision of antibiotics and adequate reduction and immobilization with good follow-up (including endodontics as a 2° procedure) often allows preservation of teeth in the # line.

Open reduction and internal fixation (ORIF) ORIF of facial bone # has revolutionized Rx. # sites are exposed, usually via mucosal incisions, and reduced under direct vision; the teeth are placed in temporary IMF &/or a wire around the tooth on either side of the # (tension band or bridle wire) and small bone plates fixed by monocortical screws are placed to immobilize the reduction. IMF can then be released for recovery and elastics placed instead on the ward if needed. Resorbable plating systems are now on the market (polylactic and polyglycolic acid) but are yet to match titanium's reliability.

Edentulous mandible The absence of teeth in occlusion created problems when relying on IMF, and modified dentures called Gunning splints were used. This technique has been superseded by the use of bone plates in virtually all cases. Pencil-thin edentulous mandibles are best managed by thick (2.4mm) plates with bicortical screws inserted transcutaneously (either by trochar endoscopically or open operation).

Condylar # Management depends on age and type of injury. <12yrs: analgesia, soft diet, and intermaxillary elastic guidance (if needed) produces optimal results. >12yrs: pain-free, pre-injury occlusion should be established (by elastic traction if need be), and the patient reassessed at 7 days. If spontaneous pain-free occlusion not possible at this stage: ORIF.[3]

Mid-face # Use one of the following methods:
- Internal fixation—interosseous plating (by far the commonest), wiring, transfixation with Kirschner wires. Plating to recreate the pyriform and zygomatic buttress system is currently most widespread.
- External fixation—e.g. Levant frame, box frame, which fix the mid-face to the cranium.

Malar # These are elevated by a temporal approach (Gillies) or bone hook percutaneously and supplemented by internal fixation with a range of plating techniques through small eyelid incisions.

Nasal bones These are manipulated and splinted. Some benefit from mini-submucous resection of the septum.

---

3 Faculty of Dental Surgery 1997 *National Clinical Guidelines* (⅋ http://www.rcseng.ac.uk).

Nasoethmoidal # These are openly reduced and wired or microplated to reposition the medial canthi and restore anatomy often through a coronal flap incision.

Fractures in children These are considerably rarer. Plates and pins tend to be avoided because of risk to unerupted teeth. Patients <10yrs may require a form of Gunning splint which fits over the mixed dentition. # are usually firmly united within 3 weeks. Microplates can sometimes be used, or heavy resorbable sutures at the lower border of the mandible. Beware of the white eye blowout fracture in the child; an operation is advisable within 48h.

Post-operative care Scrupulous OH is required. Three doses of IV antibiotics are often required. The main problems are presented by IMF, and the risk to the airway post-operatively. IMF requires a liquidized diet of at least 2500 calories (2000 for F) and 3L of fluid daily. Do not discharge until this can be maintained at home. ORIF requires a soft diet for up to 3 weeks (semi-rigid fixation). Some claim immediate return to function with true rigid (bicortical) fixation.

Complications *Mandible*: infection, paraesthesia, damage to teeth, TMJ pain, malunion, delayed union, non-union, bony sequestration, plate and wire infection. *Maxilla*: post-operative deformity, epiphora, diplopia, late enophthalmos, anosmia. Failure of union is very rare, although malunion is a problem with poor reduction or late referral. *Malar*: diplopia, retrobulbar haemorrhage, enophthalmos, paraesthesia. *Nasal*: deformity, nasal obstruction.

Composite tissue loss Gunshot wounds have led to more facial # presenting as composite defects of hard and soft tissue with tissue loss. These patients need to be stabilized, often with surgical debridement and external fixation prior to free-tissue transfer as part of definitive Rx.

Facial soft tissue injuries

The face is highly visible and, once cut, no one can make the scar disappear. You can, however, give the patient the best possible scar by following certain principles. Definitive closure of soft tissue wounds should be done in tandem with fixation of bones or after exclusion of underlying bony injury.

Assessment ABCs, mechanism of injury, allergies, and PMH, need for tetanus and rabies prophylaxis. Wounds should be closed within 24h.

Examination Type of patient, type of wound (cut, burst, flap, tissue loss), special anatomy, eye, eyelid, lip, cranial nerves V/VII, and parotid/lacrimal duct.

Investigation X-ray for foreign body.

Plan treatment Clean simple wounds in a cooperative patient are best closed under LA. Otherwise admit for GA in theatre.

Clean wound Irrigate clean wounds with saline or aqueous chlorhexidine. Bites or dirty wounds with ingrained FB need aggressive scrubbing with 50:50 water:povidone iodine. Minimal or no excision of tissue for debridement. Explore all wounds for FB, #, nerve, duct, or vessel damage. Get haemostasis.

Wound closure In layers, mucosa, and muscle: resorbable 3/0–4/0; skin: monofilament 4/0–6/0 (⊃ Suturing, p. 388). Avoid tension on skin edge.

Types of wound

Simple lacerations Close in layers with accurate anatomical apposition. Approximate, don't strangulate. Use minimum number of sutures to achieve intact wound with slight eversion. Remove facial sutures in 6 days.

Crush lacerations Skin has burst: minimal edge excision, deep closure, and light skin approximation. Tends to swell. Remove sutures at 3–4 days.

Slicing/shelving lacerations Convert to simple where possible by excision, as tends to 'trap door' otherwise. If excision would be excessive, tack down carefully.

Avulsion If flap, and seems viable: reposition and avoid haematoma. If complete: skin graft or local flap.

Penetrating injuries Penetrating injuries especially through platysma should be explored by a senior surgeon in theatre, phone your next in line.

Anatomical sites

Eye Exclude globe injury.

Ear Drain haematoma if present to avoid 'cauliflower'.

Septum Drain haematoma to prevent perforation/collapse.

Eyelid, pinna, eyebrow, and vermilion Require precise matching. Test prior to anaesthetic for facial and trigeminal nerve function.

Special wounds

Abrasions Heal spontaneously but must be cleaned thoroughly; dress with chloramphenicol ointment.

Bites Easily get infected. Use co-amoxiclav, clean very carefully, and close primarily. Small twist or finger drain helpful.

Burns Need specialist referral.

Tissue loss Nasal tip, pinna, and lip commonest. Skin graft or local flap repair will succeed. Stitching severed part back on will not.

Gunshot wounds → Composite tissue loss, p. 501.

Surgery and the temporomandibular joint

TMD See ➔ Temporomandibular pain—dysfunction/facial arthromyalgia, p. 484.

Ankylosis May be true or false.

True ankylosis True ankylosis is restriction of movement caused by a pathological joint condition, usually due to trauma (intracapsular # in childhood) or infection. Extreme limitation of movement and X-rays will confirm degree of bony union. In fibrous union, exercises are of value. In bony union, interpositional arthroplasty or condylectomy with reconstruction is needed. Post-operative exercise is crucial.

False ankylosis Restriction of movement imposed by extra-articular abnormalities is very rare. Rx depends upon cause. *Trismus* (interincisal opening ~<40mm, is often due to limitation of movement due to spasm of muscles of mastication), this may be confused with ankylosis but does not affect the joint. It is much more common and complicates many oral surgical procedures; may follow trauma or infection, may be a manifestation of occult malignancy, or a response to treatment, e.g. radiotherapy.

Trauma Condylar #, see ➔ Common #, p. 494.

Intracapsular # Essentially a childhood injury (relatively shorter, thicker condylar neck), keep in function to prevent ankylosis. Condyle # are the subject of UK clinical guidelines (➔ Condylar #, p. 500).

Dislocation Occurs in normal joints due to exceptional circumstances, or in lax joints where dislocation is recurrent. May be unilateral or bilateral. Condyle can be palpated anterior to articular eminence, X-rays confirm position, mouth is gagged open. Rx: immediate reduction; the vast majority can be performed with LA around the dislocated joint &/or sedation. Place thumbs over molar teeth and exert downward and backward pressure (if LA is used, less force is needed and thumbs can be placed in buccal sulcus, avoiding the risk of being bitten). Advise jaw support when yawning, etc.; this is usually enough, and avoids IMF. In chronically recurring dislocations, patients can be taught to self-reduce. Exercises are of limited benefit but may avoid surgery. Sclerosant injections are unpleasant and no longer used. Operations are legion; capsular plication, pins to augment articular eminence, Dautrey down-fracture of zygomatic arch, obliteration of upper joint space, eminectomy, high condylectomy. No one operation has gained pre-eminence although eminectomy is probably the most favoured.

Condylar hyperplasia Rare. Rx: high condylectomy if active (bone scan, but interpretation variable and condylar replacement, e.g. with costochondral cartilage, is unpredictable) or wait for it to 'burnout', then definitive orthognathic surgery.

Tumours Rare. Rx: ablation, reconstruction, and radiotherapy if malignant.

Arthritides Rheumatoid, psoriatic, and gouty arthritides all manifest in the TMJ but in <15% of patients with the systemic disease. The signs and symptoms are joint stiffness, pain, tenderness, and crepitus. Δ: knowledge of systemic disease and local signs. Rx: treat systemic condition. Symptomatic Rx of joint with appliances, physiotherapy, exercises, NSAIDs and intra-articular steroids. Main long-term problem is limitation of function.

Osteoarthrosis A distinct entity of the TMJ, with a different clinical course from that seen in other joints. Appears to be a degenerative condition of articular cartilage. Δ: crepitus, limitation, and pain on movement, tenderness over condyle, often with X-ray evidence of condylar erosions. Most have symptoms for ~1yr which gradually ↓ over the next 2yrs. X-rays show condylar remodelling to a flat smooth surface. Patients then enter a long period of remission. Rx is therefore aimed at pain relief, using standard TMD measures (➲ Temporomandibular pain—dysfunction/facial arthromyalgia, p. 484). Those remaining unresponsive may benefit from intra-articular steroids (➲ Intra-articular steroids, p. 602), which probably accelerate natural remodelling. A small group will remain with pain 3–4 months after steroids, usually with X-ray abnormalities. They should be considered for high condylar shave or high condylectomy. Rarely, total joint replacement is appropriate.

Joint replacement A handful of specifically designed customized condyle and fossa replacements are available. These should be reserved for severe symptomatic end-stage joint disease in the hands of those with a sub-specialist interest.

Major pre-prosthetic surgery

Minor procedures, ➔ Minor pre-prosthetic surgery, p. 426; implantology, ➔
Introduction to implantology, p. 361. The aim is to enable an edentulous patient to live comfortably with functioning dentures, therefore surgery without
liaison with an understanding and competent prosthodontist is pointless.
All procedures for improving the denture-bearing area of the jaws are dependent on the use of a denture with a modified fitting surface (stent), which
is placed at operation and must be worn virtually permanently for up to 8
weeks post-operatively, the fitting surface being modified at intervals with a
soft acrylic lining material. There are many who would claim these procedures
do not work, and indeed there is little scientific support for them.

▶ Warn all patients undergoing lower jaw procedures about post-operative
mental nerve damage.

Epithelial inlay (vestibuloplasty) This is basically a skin graft to the
alveolar surface of the jaw, creating a deeper sulcus. Important points: excise all areas of scarred or hyperplastic tissue, dissect off any strands of
mentalis in the lower jaw, ensure preservation of the alveolar periosteum,
ensure the stent extends to the new sulcus depth, and ensure the skin–
mucosa junction lies on the labial surface.

Combination mucosal flap and epithelial inlay Usually suffices
in the maxilla due to its ↑ potential for denture retention.

Mental nerve repositioning Mental nerve compression by a denture flange following alveolar resorption is a common problem, producing a
sensation like an electric shock but with a background ache which ↑ during
the day and ↓ overnight. Leaving the −/F out for several days ↓ the pain.
The mental nerve is repositioned by creating a new foramen under its present position or laterally transposing the entire nerve into the soft tissues in
grossly atrophic mandibles. Peizosurgery is useful here as using this tool to
remove bone may be less likely to cause nerve damage.

Alveolar augmentation Problems with osseous donor site morbidity and length of procedure in elderly patients put these operations
out of favour. The use of 'sandwich' procedures (where the augmenting
material is literally sandwiched between horizontally osteotomized jaw),
coupled with effective bone substitutes and tunnelling procedures (➔ Ridge
augmentation, p. 426), have made augmentation, even in the comparatively
frail elderly, a far better proposition. Younger, fit patients with severe jaw
atrophy or those with incipient or actual pathological # may still benefit
from split rib grafting.

Vertical distraction osteogenesis A pre-prosthetic component
to this well-accepted technique for 'growing' bone by osteotomizing and
gradually moving bone apart (1–2mm/day) will probably replace all major
augmentation procedures.

Sinus lift A popular procedure combined with simultaneous or delayed
implants. After raising subperiosteal buccal flaps, a window is created to
expose antral lining. Lining of the floor and walls is elevated intact and this
space is filled with bone from the iliac crest, tibia, or chin to provide retention for implants.

Clefts and craniofacial anomalies

▶ 20% of cases of congenital facial malformation are accompanied by a second or third systemic malformation.

Cleft lip and palate

See also ⊃ Cleft lip and palate, p. 170.

▶ The aim is to replace anatomical structures in their correct position; the price is scarring, which will restrict growth to some degree. It is important to recognize that the stigmata of surgery is due to growth of the patient. Taking folic acid at the start of pregnancy reduces the risk of cleft lip and palate fourfold.

Lip closure Two main philosophies: *'plastic' approach*—performed neonatally or up to 3 months; flaps transgress skin boundaries and use supraperiosteal dissection. Gives good early aesthetic results (e.g. Millard). *'Functional' approach*—all skin boundaries are respected; uses subperiosteal dissection. Immediate aesthetics are less good due to pout caused by muscle repair but ↑ function and growth potential (e.g. Delaire). In the UK, a trend is emerging to blend the techniques of these philosophies.

Palatal closure Extensive surgery restricts maxillary growth, therefore use minimal simple repair which recreates a functioning soft palate (e.g. Von Langenbeck or Delaire).

Alveolus Vomer flap to close anterior alveolus and gingivoperiosteoplasty are 1° procedures advocated by some and decried by others.

Ears Preschool audiology. Many will benefit from grommets.

Nasal deformity Perhaps the greatest surgical challenge. 1° functional lip/nose repair may alter this.

Secondary surgery Lip revision (simple or complex). Sometimes required preschool or at time of alveolar bone graft.

Alveolar bone graft See ⊃ Alveolar bone graft, p. 171.

Speech, nasendoscopy, and pharyngoplasty All cleft palate patients have impaired speech. Fibre-optic nasendoscopy allows visualization of the palate during speech and aids assessment. Pharyngoplasty narrows the velopharyngeal opening to ↓ hypernasal speech. Successful palate repair ↓ need for pharyngoplasty.

Orthognathic surgery See ⊃ Orthognathic surgery, p. 510.

Craniofacial anomalies

A broad group of conditions involving the craniomaxillofacial region. A simple classification is shown in Table 12.2.

These patients need craniofacial teams (minimum: craniofacial surgeon, neurosurgeon, and anaesthetist). Coronal flaps to deglove the face are the mainstay of access, followed by craniotomy and osteotomy as required. Main risks are cerebral oedema, infection, damage to optic nerves and vessels; and, in neonates and children, paediatric fluid balance.

Table 12.2 Classification of craniofacial anomalies

Congenital	Acquired
Orbital malformations (hypertelorism, orbital dystopia)	Tumours (benign or malignant)
Craniosynostoses (premature fusion of cranial sutures)	Dysplasias (fibro-osseous) Neurofibromatosis
Craniofacial synostoses (Apert syndrome, ⮑ Apert syndrome, p. 782; Crouzon syndrome, ⮑ Crouzon syndrome, p. 783)	Post-trauma deformity
Encephaloceles	
Others (Treacher Collins syndrome, hemifacial microsomia, hemifacial hypertrophy and atrophy)	

Orthognathic surgery

This is the surgery of facial skeletal deformity and merges with cleft and craniofacial surgery. 1° indications are functional: speech, eating. 2° indications are aesthetic.

▶ Patients may not see these as quite such separate issues. Their reasons and motivation for seeking surgery must be understood and the limitations of surgery made absolutely clear before embarking on protracted and complex Rx.

Diagnosis and treatment planning See ⟐ Orthodontics and orthognathic surgery, p. 168.

Mandibular procedures

Involve ramus, body, alveolus, or chin.

IO vertical subsigmoid osteotomy Used to push back the mandible. EO approach used when suitable equipment for IO not available. The IO procedure is straightforward, performed via an extended third-molar type incision. Bone cuts are made with a right-angled oscillating saw from sigmoid notch to lower border. Technique is very instrument dependent.

Sagittal split osteotomy (Fig. 12.5 and Fig. 12.6.) Can move mandible backwards or forwards. IO incision similar to intra-oral vertical subsigmoid osteotomy. Bone cuts made from above lingula, across retromolar region, down buccal aspect to lower border. Split sagittally with an osteotome followed by spreaders. Main complication is paraesthesia of IDN.

Inverted L- and C-shaped osteotomy Usually EO approach. Rarely used; can lengthen ramus if used with bone graft.

Body ostectomy Shortens body of mandible. Need to gain space orthodontically or remove tooth. Watch mental nerve.

Subapical osteotomy Used to move dento-alveolar segments. Technically more difficult than it looks. Risk to tooth vitality.

Genioplasty The tip of the chin can be moved pretty much anywhere; the secret is to keep a sliding contact with bone and a muscle pedicle. Fixation should be kept away from areas of muscle activity as this leads to bone resorption. Effective treatment for obstructive sleep apnoea.

Maxillary procedures

Segmental Can be single-tooth, or bone and tooth blocks, e.g. Wassmund procedure, which involves tunnelling incisions in buccal sulcus and palate to move premaxilla. Problems are finding space for bone cuts and avoiding damaging teeth.

Le Fort I Mainstay procedure. Standard approach is the 'down-fracture' with horseshoe buccal incision, bone cuts at Le Fort I level, and segment pedicled on the palate. The freed maxilla can be moved up, down, or forward. Posterior movement more problematic. In cleft palate cases, concern over the adequacy of the palatal blood supply has led to some surgeons using tunnelled buccal incisions to make the bone cuts, thus preserving some of the buccal blood supply to the maxilla. Fixation is a problem when using this technique.

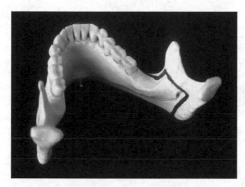

Fig. 12.5 A medial view of the bone cuts for the sagittal split osteotomy, note the position of the lingula and the medial bone cut.

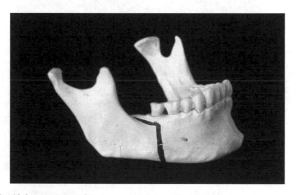

Fig. 12.6 Lateral view of the bone cuts for the sagittal split osteotomy.

Le Fort II Usually used for mid-face advancement. Bilateral canthal and vestibular incisions allow bone cuts at the Le Fort II level.

Le Fort III Really a subcranial craniofacial operation using a coronal flap plus vestibular and orbital incisions to move the entire mid-face and malar complex.

Malar osteotomy Used for post-traumatic defects. Approach via coronal incisions. Risk to infra-orbital nerve from maxillary bone cut. Augmentation is an alternative (◐ Aesthetic facial surgery, p. 524).

Rhinoplasty The correction of isolated nasal deformity. Usually done intranasally, supplemented by tiny incisions over the nasal bones to allow bone cuts. 'Open rhinoplasty', which involves degloving the nasal skeleton via a columella incision, is popular particularly for cleft patients.

Stability ↑ use of mini-plates in the fixation of the osteotomized segments has ↓ the reliance on bone grafts. Pre-surgical orthodontics (➲ Pre-surgical orthodontics, p. 168) makes a significant contribution to ↓ rate of relapse. IMF &/or elastic traction remains vital for long-term success. Good dental interdigitation, and planning movements within the capacity of the soft tissues, are probably the best anti-relapse measures.[4]

Distraction (➲ Distraction osteogenesis, p. 169.) The same principle coupled with conventional orthognathic osteotomies.

4 D. Tuinzing et al. 1993 *Surgical Orthodontics*, VU University Press.

Salivary gland tumours

Diseases See also → Salivary gland disease—1, p. 458; → Salivary gland disease—2, p. 460.

Classified by WHO into epithelial tumours, non-epithelial tumours, and unclassified tumours.

Common benign tumours Pleomorphic adenoma, → Salivary gland tumours, p. 460. *Monomorphic adenoma*—adenolymphoma (Warthin's tumour) affects M > F; rare <50yrs. Bilateral in 10%. Feels soft and cystic. Benign, very unlikely to recur despite being multifocal, associated with smoking.

Carcinomas Rare. *Adenoid cystic carcinoma*—characteristic 'Swiss cheese' appearance histologically. Spreads locally, particularly along perineural spaces. Can be compatible with long-term survival despite propensity for secondaries in lungs, although rarely cured. *Adenocarcinomas*—there are a wide range of these malignant tumours, ranging from the highly aggressive (terminal duct carcinoma) to the relatively indolent (polymorphous low-grade adenocarcinoma). It is essential that adequate histological Δ is made early (expert head and neck pathologist needed). Other carcinomas are rare, but may arise in a pre-existing pleomorphic adenoma or *de novo*. 5yr survival widely variable; poor prognosis—aggressive salivary cancers <10%, good prognosis—low-grade cancers >80%.

Other epithelial tumours Include *acinic cell tumour* and *mucoepidermoid tumour*. Both have variable, unpredictable behaviour, can recur locally and metastasize, and can occur at any age. On average, both compatible with ~80% survival.

Non-epithelial tumours Include haemangioma, lymphangioma, and neurofibroma. Account for 50% of salivary tumours in children.

Unclassified group Includes lymphomas, secondaries, lipomas, and chemodectomas.

Parotid History and examination are the prime diagnostic tools. Long history, no pain, and no facial nerve involvement suggest benign tumour. Facial palsy, pain, and rapid growth suggest malignancy. Chance of malignancy much greater in tumours >4cm. The feel of many tumours are characteristic. CT, FNAC, USS, &/or MRI may help. This is particularly important if 'extracapsular dissection' is the planned treatment rather than conventional segmental parotidectomy.

Submandibular Less common tumours. Pleomorphic adenoma remains most common. Malignant tumours account for up to 30%. Rx of most is gland excision via a skin crease in the neck. Modified neck dissection (to include level I, II, and III and any locally involved structures such as skin) for malignant or recurrent tumours.

Sublingual and minor glands >50% of tumours are malignant (mostly adenoid cystic) and require extensive surgery and reconstruction similar to floor of mouth cancer. Beware the 'mucocele' of the upper lip—it is almost certainly a tumour.

Surgery of the salivary glands

Surgery of the major salivary glands is primarily for tumours, obstruction, and, less commonly, inflammatory conditions. The minor glands are most commonly removed for mucoceles (➲ Mucoceles, p. 415) and more rarely for tumours. With the exception of lymphomas *all* salivary gland tumours should have surgery initially, patient permitting.

Parotidectomy The principles are complete excision of a tumour with a margin of healthy tissue and preservation of facial nerve. Clinically benign tumours in the superficial lobe have either 'extracapsular dissection', segmental superficial parotidectomy, or conventional superficial parotidectomy. In the deep lobe, total conservative parotidectomy. Malignant tumours require radical excision and radiotherapy. Radiotherapy alone is almost never curative. Whether or not to sacrifice the facial nerve adjacent to a malignant parotid tumour is a complex decision. Many would accept *nerve clinically affected*—pre-operatively, sacrifice, and reconstruct; *nerve clinically intact*—pre-operatively, preserve, and rely on post-operative radiotherapy.

Salivary duct calculi History is of recurrent pain and swelling in the obstructed gland, particularly before and during meals. Plain X-rays (lower occlusal for submandibular, cheek for parotid) reveal radio-opaque calculi, but do not exclude the radiolucent calculi and mucous plugs. Sialography reveals a stricture or obstruction. Commonest in the submandibular duct. Rx: *submandibular duct* for calculi lying anterior in duct—remove by passing a suture behind the calculus to prevent it slipping further down the duct, dissect the duct from an IO approach, and lift out stone; either marsupialize the duct or reconstruct. Posterior calculi—excise gland and duct. Rx: *parotid duct*—expose duct via IO approach for anterior stones or via a small skin flap onto a probe in the duct for more posterior calculi. Otherwise, selective superficial parotidectomy is the only safe approach.

Sialoendoscopy ± laser lithotripsy is available in some centres for proximal calculi in patients wishing to avoid gland excision and calculi <3mm.

Recurrent sialadenitis Severe recurrent infection of the parotid or submandibular glands leads to dilatation and ballooning of the ducts and alveoli called sialectasis. Sialography is the investigation of choice and often therapeutic, inducing long remissions between episodes of infection. Interventional sialography with specialized balloon/basket catheters is now being used to dilate or retrieve obstructions but has not replaced open surgery. Sialoendoscopy (visualizing and carrying out limited surgery via endoscopic examination of the ductal tree) has its enthusiasts. Diagnostically similar to information from conventional imaging. Treatment often requires multiple out-patient visits.

Conservative Rx Massage and repeated antibiotics (amoxicillin if not allergic) or irrigation of gland with tetracycline solution. When remission periods are short or intolerable, or the patient requires *definitive* Rx: submandibular gland excision or total conservative parotidectomy with removal of 90% of the duct. *Surgery for drooling*: in severe cases it is possible to re-site the parotid ducts into the hypopharynx &/or perform bilateral submandibular gland excision to control drooling without impairing lubrication for swallowing and oral health (Wilkes procedure). A more physiological approach is to reposition submandibular ducts and excise sublingual glands, as these are a major source of pooled saliva at rest. Intraglandular botulinum toxin injected either under USS control or simply following anatomical guidelines is becoming an increasingly useful conservative temporary tactic. Has to be repeated at intervals of 6–12 months.

Mucoceles See ➔ Mucoceles, p. 415.

Facial skin cancer

Skin cancer (❍ Skin neoplasms, p. 550.) The common facial skin cancers are basal cell carcinoma (BCC), SCC, and malignant melanoma. They may be preceded by actinic keratosis, carcinoma *in situ*, or lentigo maligna.

The 'best buy' Rx is usually excision with repair by 1° closure, skin graft, or local flap. Electron beam radiotherapy, topical photodynamic therapy, and topical 5-FU cream are alternatives.

Margins A margin of normal skin around the cancer of 5mm for BCC, 10mm for SCC, and 10–30mm for melanoma, dependent on site. The British Association of Dermatologists (BAD) produces a useful set of guidelines.

Techniques Mark out the periphery of the tumour, line of excision, and any flap repair *before* injecting LA (if used). Cut at 90° to skin through dermis and excise at level of fat layer. *Always* obtain good haemostasis (bipolar diathermy). Mark specimen to orientate for pathologist.

Repair

Primary closure Try to design excision in natural crease or resting skin tension line. Excise in an ellipse, undermine both sides, and close by halving the length of the wound. Use deep sutures to minimize tension. Excise any 'dog ears'.

Wedge excision Allows 1° closure of lip, eyelid, and helix.

Split skin grafts Are thin and take well, but tend to shrink and are a poor colour match. Taken with a Humby/Watson knife or a dermatome they leave a raw donor site which can take weeks to heal. Useful for scalp defects.

No skin graft will take on bare bone, tendon, or cartilage. Grafts will fail if they move, develop a haematoma, or become infected, as this prevents plasmatic imbibition and capillary ingrowth.

Full-thickness skin grafts Thicker and more robust, they do not take as easily. They are taken with a scalpel and the donor site is closed primarily. Better colour match.

Grafts are sutured to periphery of wound and immobilized with a bolster of antiseptic cotton or sponge and tie-over sutures for 7–10 days. The thicker the graft, the longer to take.

Local flaps These have their own blood supply and work by a combination of geometry and widespread undermining.

The flap is marked out at the same time as excision before LA. It is held in the new position by deep and skin sutures. Do not use pressure dressings. Haematoma is the biggest cause of failure in adequately designed flaps: take sutures out to ↓ pressure and ↑ flap circulation with delayed re-suture.

Common local flaps

Transposition flap Simple switch over of skin.

Rhomboid flap Very useful; relies on lax skin at donor site. Some studies show this flap to be used in 80% of facial skin cancers. (See Fig. 12.7 and Fig. 12.8 for examples of a rhomboid flap.)

Bi-lobed flap Transfers circles 80% and 60% to created defect.

Subcutaneous advancement flap A teardrop of skin is advanced on a subcutaneous fat pedicle.

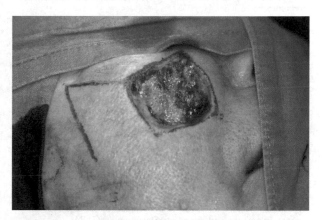

Fig. 12.7 Excision of facial BCC and outline of rhomboid flap.

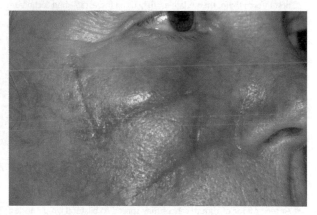

Fig. 12.8 Result after suture removal from the patient in Fig. 12.7: redness fades and scar softens over an 18-month period.

Oral cancer

Aetiology, epidemiology, Δ, and staging, ➲ Oral cancer, p. 452; neck lumps, ➲ Cervicofacial lymphadenopathy, p. 480; salivary tumours, ➲ Salivary gland tumours, p. 508.

Various parameters affect the choice of Rx for patients with oral cancer; not least among these, but often forgotten, are the patients themselves, their general health, understanding of their disease, geographical location, and social and domestic commitments. Classically, broad Rx principles are based on tumour staging, using the Tumour, Node, Metastasis (TNM) classification, and the patient's fitness for surgery (this tends to imply that if they can't cope with surgery, they can cope with travelling for and side effects of radiotherapy, which is not always the case). In many instances of oral cancer, combined surgery and radiotherapy constitutes optimal Rx.

Suggested management plan This will vary according to the surgeon concerned:

- Establish provisional Δ. History, examination, and get to know patient. FBC, U&Es, LFTs (including albumin), bone biochemistry, blood group, ECG, DPT.
- Arrange tissue Δ. By biopsy—usually under LA. Flexible nasendoscopy, head, neck, thorax, imaging (CT/MRI). This is to exclude synchronous 1° tumour in upper aerodigestive tract (present in, at most, 15% of cases). Palpate the neck for nodes. Stage tumour (TNM).
- Unless patient has made it very obvious they do not want to know the Δ, first inform them, then relatives, fully using the established techniques of breaking bad news with a cancer nurse specialist present.
  - T1–N0. Surgery or radiotherapy (including brachytherapy-radioactive implants) offers a similar cure rate. Surgery is often simpler and with less side effects.
  - Tumour close to bone having radiotherapy: safest to remove associated teeth to prevent osteoradionecrosis.
  - T2 but imaging N0. Have a 30% incidence of occult metastases; debate exists over watch and wait or selective neck dissection. Majority favour dissection.
  - T2 and T3. >50% of patients will have occult metastases; prophylactic radiotherapy (works for occult but not for obvious bulky nodes); or prophylactic selective neck dissection. In presence of imaging or palpable nodes, latter usually best.
  - For large tumours, close or +ve margins, and extracapsular spread, radiotherapy given post-operatively.
  - Vastly ↑ access is obtained for resection by osteotomizing the mandible (position plate beforehand).
  - Anterior floor of mouth cancer may spread to bilateral lymph nodes; bilateral selective neck dissection is indicated.
  - Presence or absence of extracapsular spread in cervical lymph nodes is strongest prognostic indicator of poor outcome.

- HPV-16 and -18 have become important causes of oropharyngeal cancer. In non-smokers, stage for stage these cancers have a very much better prognosis when treated with conventional techniques. It is probably sexually transmitted (although the exact nature and why most people clear oral HPV infection within a year are not fully understood). It is entirely preventable by vaccination of pre-sexual children with the same vaccine girls are receiving to prevent cervical cancer in most developed countries.

Simultaneous chemotherapy and radiotherapy can have a dramatic effect on poorly differentiated SCCs, especially those originating from post-nasal space, tonsil, and tongue base. This treatment has become increasingly popular and a little indiscriminate in some centres. The morbidity (osteoradionecrosis, trismus, dysphagia, mucositis, neutropenia) and mortality of treatment has ↑ as a consequence.

5yr survival 90% for T1–N0, but 30% for T2/3–N1 and worse for T4; however, this does *not* mean that extensive combination therapy and reconstruction is pointless in those with advanced oral cancers.

Several centres are reporting better-than-average 5yr survival figures with aggressive combination treatment regimens and identification of HPV-driven cancers means much of the previously widely held beliefs with regard to survival (often quoted as there has been no improvement in the last 50 years) should be reconsidered as they are simply incorrect.

Death comes in many ways, and a fungating uncontrolled cancer of the head and neck is one of the less pleasant. Attempted surgical 'cure' which alleviates local disease and symptoms and allows the patient a few more years of life and a gradual demise due to carcinomatosis or another disease is still worthwhile from all viewpoints. (Palliative surgery with curative intent.)

Chemotherapy There is, as yet, no proven role for cytotoxics in oral cancer, other than in combination with radiotherapy or in palliation. Other oncocytic, particularly biological agents, drugs are under investigation.

Immunotherapy This is the most significant emerging modality for head and neck cancer. Immunotherapeutic agents are increasingly under investigation in recurrent, metastatic, and 1° head and neck cancer.

Neck lumps

▶ Do not leave chronic cervical lymphadenopathy undiagnosed.
▶ A 1° head and neck malignancy must be excluded visually, by imaging or histology (or all three) before biopsy.

Children An exception; inflammation is common and tumour is rare, so a watch-and-wait policy is reasonable.

Diagnosis Listen to the story, look at the patient and lump. Palpate it. If needed, carry out a full head and neck examination. Most diagnoses will be made by then.

Investigation USS, aspiration cytology, and biopsy.

Causes Think (i) anatomy, (ii) pathology, and (iii) oddity.

Skin Lesions lie superficially.

Sebaceous cyst Look for punctum; is within skin. Excise.

Lipoma Soft, often yellowish. Excise.

Sublingual dermoid cyst Lies in floor of mouth, often under mylohyoid. Arises from trapped epithelium during embryonic fusion; contains keratin. Rx: total excision.

Lymph nodes Deep to platysma. Try to diagnose before biopsy. Opening of malignant nodes ↓ survival (➔ Oral cancer, p. 452).

Infection (➔ Cervicofacial lymphadenopathy, p. 480.) Nodes are large and tender. Causes: viral (e.g. glandular fever, HIV), bacterial (e.g. mycobacterial (which can calcify), actinomycosis), or reactive to other head and neck infection.

Malignancy Either metastatic from head and neck primaries (hard, rock-like nodes) or lymphoma/leukaemia (large rubbery), see ➔ Cervicofacial lymphadenopathy, p. 480. FNAC unhelpful in lymphoma; core or open biopsy needed. This creates a real conflict as haematologists want an urgent diagnosis and we want to prevent opening a neck and risking dissemination of cancer in SCC.

Glandular Think anatomically.

Salivary (➔ Salivary gland tumours, p. 508). Submandibular/lower pole of parotid: abscess, sialadenitis, obstruction, sarcoidosis, Sjögren syndrome. Sublingual: ranula, tumour.

Thyroid Benign and malignant tumours, goitre, thyroglossal cyst (may lie anywhere between foramen caecum of tongue and thyroid, tract goes behind, around, or through hyoid bone, moves with swallowing).

Arterial Don't biopsy!

Carotid aneurysm (Pulsatile.)

Carotid body tumour Found around carotid bifurcation. Usually firm, not hormonally active, 5% malignant. Rx: excise if symptomatic.

Schwannoma/neurofibroma All major nerves in neck can develop painless masses. Rx: subadvential excision, preserving healthy fibres if possible.

Pharynx

Diverticulum (Or pharyngeal pouch.) Fills on swallowing. Evert endoscopically or excise.

Larynx

Laryngocele Rare. Mainly M >60yrs. 80% unilateral. Excise.

Sternomastoid
- 'Sternomastoid tumour'—congenital ischaemic fibrosis causing torticollis.
- *True muscle tumours*—rare.

Bone Cervical rib, prominent hyoid bone.

Infections See also ➔ Dento-facial infections, p. 408. Ludwig's angina, submasseteric abscess, retropharyngeal abscess, parapharyngeal cellulitis, collar stud abscess (TB), infected cysts or pouches.

Oddities

Branchial cyst This is either a remnant from second and third branchial arches or degeneration of lymphoid tissue. It is an epithelial lined cyst which presents as a deep-seated swelling lying anterior to sternomastoid at or above the level of the hyoid. Prone to infection. Rx: total excision.

Branchial fistula A fistula from the tonsillar fossa to the skin overlying anterior lower third of sternomastoid. Present at birth; discharges intermittently. Rx: total excision of tract.

Cystic hygroma Presents in infancy and is a form of lymphangioma which appears as endothelium-lined multilocular cysts containing lymph. May be found anywhere in head–neck but classically behind lower end of sternomastoid. May suddenly ↑ in size if bled into or ruptured. Rx: total excision as soon as child is fit for operation. Cystic areas may be sclerosed using a modified streptococcal antigen, Picibanil®. Macrocystic lymphangiomas are relatively easy to dissect, microcystic are almost impossible.

Flaps and grafts

A *graft* is transferred tissue dependent on the recipient site capillaries for its survival. A *flap* is transferred tissue independent, at least initially, of the recipient site capillaries for survival.

It is the possibility of functional reconstruction of the head and neck in conjunction with the potential for cure that justifies the mutilation of radical surgery for oral cancer; however, head and neck reconstruction is used in other aspects of maxillofacial surgery, particularly trauma.

Mucosal grafts See ➔ Mucogingival surgery, p. 218.

Skin grafts May be split thickness or full thickness. Split thickness (taken by knife or dermatome from thigh or inner arm) take quickly and become wettable in the mouth. They are 'quilted' in place with sutures or compressed with bolsters. Full-thickness grafts (supraclavicular, post-auricular, or abdominal) provide a mediocre colour match when repairing skin defects of the face. Full-thickness donor sites are closed primarily.

Free bone grafts From rib, iliac crest, or calvarium. Rib, which is partially split at 1cm intervals, can be bent to conform to the shape of the mandible. Iliac crest supplies cortical or cancellous bone and can be cut to a template, but ↑ risk of DVT. Various synthetic mesh containers as a mould for cancellous bone exist. Calvarial bone has the theoretical advantage of being membranous bone and should resorb less when implanted in the face. Very few use cadaveric free bone grafts.

Nasolabial flap Random pattern pedicle flap based above and lateral to the upper lip; useful local flap. Requires division ~3 weeks later. Can be based inferiorly for intra-oral reconstruction or superiorly for nasal reconstruction.

Tongue flaps Random pattern pedicle flap for lip and palate repair. Requires division and inset 3 weeks later.

Forehead flap Based on anterior branch of superficial temporal artery; very safe flap, rarely used because of the poor donor site defect. Requires division later.

Masseter muscle flap Limited in size; can be used IO.

Temporoparietal fascial flap Pedicle or free flap based on superficial temporal vessels. Long flexible reconstruction. Difficult to raise. Tends to fibrose IO.

Temporalis flap Inferiorly based on deep temporal branches of maxillary artery. Limited use due to size and tendency to fibrose.

Deltopectoral flap Based on perforating internal mammary vessels. Thin skin suitable for skin or mucosa repair. Usually divided and inset after 3 weeks. Lateral donor site needs skin grafting.

Pectoralis major myocutaneous flap Also described with bone, but the bone is really a free rib graft. Based on acromiothoracic axis. Usually tunnelled after neck dissection. Very bulky flap; covers carotids after radical neck dissection. Workhorse head and neck pedicle flap. Useful as a salvage flap.

Latissimus dorsi myocutaneous flap Bulky flap based on thoracodorsal vessels. Needs to be tunnelled through axilla if pedicled. More commonly used as a free flap in the head and neck.

Free tissue transfer by microvascular re-anastomosis This has been the biggest advance in reconstruction. The following are useful and commonly used flaps.

Radial forearm flap A fasciocutaneous flap based on the radial artery. The skin available is thin and supple and can conform to the complex anatomy of the mouth (skin is often hairless, which is a big bonus). A thin segment of up to 10cm (length) 40% thickness of radius can also be transferred for bony reconstruction but the radius should be plated to prevent #.

Lateral upper arm flap Small vessel, thicker alternative to radial forearm free flaps. Radial nerve palsy a possible complication.

Deep circumflex iliac artery flap Based on the deep circumflex iliac artery. Sufficient good quality thick bone to reconstruct the dentate mandible. Internal oblique muscle usually transferred for soft tissue—good where non-mobile soft tissue repair needed. Skin transfer possible but less useful due to poor venous drainage.

Free fibula flap 25cm of fibula can be excised within a muscle cuff supplied by the peroneal vessels. Excellent length and thickness of bone for mandibular reconstruction. Skin transfer for mobile soft tissue available. Probably the most useful osseocutaneous flap for the head and neck.

Free rectus abdominus Bulky skin/muscle flap based on inferior epigastric vessels. Useful for massive facial defects but often limited by fat volume.

Anterolateral thigh free flap Soft tissue flap from thigh based on descending branch of lateral circumflex femoral artery. Skin thickness can limit usefulness infra-orally although thinning possible.

Subscapular system flaps Several skin, fat, and bone flaps can be harvested from these vessels; disadvantage is need to turn patient perioperatively.

Temporoparietal fascial flap Fascia-only flap from scalp which can be used free or pedicle with or without outer table of skull bone.

Perforator flaps A wide range of definitions. Probably the best is a skin flap based and anastomosed on an unnamed vessel perforating fascia and supplying a defined area of skin. Using that definition the demands and uses of the technique become more obvious. The anterolateral thigh flap is described as a perforator flap because the final vessel supplying the skin is a single main perforator through fascia but in reality most people anastomose the descending branch of the lateral circumflex femoral vessels.

Craniofacial implants Prosthetic eyes, ears, and noses can be securely fixed to the facial skeleton with implants using techniques similar to oral implants. Probably the best available ear and total nose reconstruction.

Aesthetic facial surgery

An increasingly popular area of surgery in the developed world. The mainstay procedures are described.

Browlift The older coronal excision is now rare being replaced by endoscopic browlift; approached through three vertical incisions using an endoscope and suspension sutures. Aim is to reduce frown furrows and elevate brow.

Blepharoplasty Upper and lower eyelid surgery. Traditionally involved the removal of skin, fat, and muscle, this often produced a sunken 'operated' appearance. Now the upper lid has skin and muscle excised but fat is simply cauterized producing shrinkage. The lower lid can be approached from the skin or the conjunctiva depending on whether skin excision is needed and fat may be removed, cauterized, or repositioned.

Otoplasty This is the correction of an external ear deformity, aims are to recreate the antihelix and reduce the angulation between the concha and the skull. Cartilage scoring and permanent sutures are the popular techniques.

Rhinoplasty The surgery of nasal deformity and function. The essential prerequisite is realistic expectations from the patient (beware young men seeking 'nose jobs'). Open rhinoplasty is performed through an incision in the columella skin, closed through nasal mucosa. Both aim to maintain or improve the airway and improve aesthetics by reshaping rather than removing constituent parts of the nose.

Rhytidectomy The facelift has several variants but the commonest is currently the superficial musculoaponeurotic system (SMAS) lift. This includes a diffuse layer of connective tissue which runs from the platysma in the neck to the temporoparietal fascia in the temple which is claimed to reduce relapse. The incision runs in the preauricular sulcus round the lobe and into the mastoid hairline. The jowl area is undermined, advanced up and back, excess removed, SMAS plicated, and skin closed.

Liposculpture This is the selective removal of fat. The area to be reduced is infiltrated with a solution of normal saline, lidocaine 0.1%, adrenaline 1:1,000,000, and bicarbonate and suction performed with a blunt cannula under vacuum (0.5–1 atmosphere—can be generated by a syringe).

Botulinum toxin Multiple different versions are available, 'Botox®' is actually the trade name of one of them (Xeomin®, Vistabel®, Neurobloc®, and Dysport® are others). It is a temporary (3–6 months) paralysing agent which when injected into muscles of facial expression can remove 'dynamic' wrinkles particularly around the forehead, lateral eyes, upper lip, and midline neck. Has therapeutic role in masseteric hypertrophy, blepharospasm, facial tics, drooling, gustatory lacrimation, gustatory sweating, torticollis, and some forms of trismus.

Fillers Temporary fillers made of collagen and hyaluronic acid and poly-L-lactic acid are popular to augment soft tissue of the face. They are injected into the lips, nasolabial folds, wrinkles, depressions, or areas of fat atrophy (seen in HIV). Autologous fat can also be used. Avoid 'permanent' fillers. Never use silicone.

Laser resurfacing, dermabrasion, and chemical peels These are all ways of improving the surface texture of skin basically by removing the surface layers either by evaporation, mechanical abrasion, or chemical burn. There is a risk of skin depigmentation and patients must avoid excessive sunlight afterwards.

Medicine relevant to dentistry

Principal sources *BNF* https://bnf.nice.org.uk/. E. Grimes 2013 *Medical Emergencies: Essentials for the Dental Professional* (2e), Pearson. D. Mitchell and A. Kanatas 2014 *An Introduction to Oral and Maxillofacial Surgery* (2e), OUP. C. Scully 2014 *Medical Problems in Dentistry* (7e), Churchill Livingstone. I. B. Wilkinson et al. 2017 *Oxford Handbook of Clinical Medicine* (10e), OUP.

NB: all drug doses relate to fit, adult patients ~70kg in weight. Always check doses for children, the elderly, and those with other medical conditions.

Anaemia

Anaemia is a ↓ in the level of circulating haemoglobin (Hb) to below the normal reference range for a patient's age and sex. It indicates an underlying problem and, as such, the cause of the anaemia should be diagnosed *before* instituting Rx.

▶ Never rush into transfusing patients presenting with a chronic anaemia. Perform basic blood investigations before giving iron or transfusing. Elective surgery in patients with an Hb <10g/dL is rarely appropriate.

Clinical features These are notoriously unreliable, but may include general fatigue, heart failure, angina on effort, pallor (look at conjunctivae and palmar creases, but unreliable), brittle nails &/or spoon-shaped nails (koilonychia), oral discomfort &/or ulceration, glossitis, and classically angular cheilitis.

Syndromes See Chapter 20.

Types of anaemia
Microcytic (MCV <78fL.) Iron deficiency anaemia is by far the commonest cause. Causes: chronic blood loss (gastrointestinal or menstrual), inadequate diet. FBC and biochemistry show microcytic, hypochromic anaemia with a low serum iron and a high total iron binding capacity (TIBC). ↑ RBC zinc protoporphyrin is a fast and sensitive early test. Thalassaemia and sideroblastic anaemia are rare causes of microcytosis.

Normocytic Commonly, anaemia of chronic disease. Other causes: pregnancy, acute blood loss, haemolytic anaemia, and aplastic anaemia. Once pregnancy is excluded, the patient needs investigation by an expert. The TIBC is usually ↓.

Macrocytic (MCV > 100fL.) Low vitamin B_{12} &/or low folate are the common causes. Vitamin B_{12} is ↓ in pernicious anaemia (deficit of intrinsic factor), alcohol abuse, small gut disease, and chronic exposure to nitrous oxide. Low folate is usually dietary, but may be caused by illness (e.g. coeliac disease, skin disease) or drugs such as phenytoin, methotrexate, trimethoprim, and co-trimoxazole.

Management In all cases the cause must be sought; this may necessitate referral to a haematologist. Drugs used in iron deficiency: ferrous sulfate 200mg tds. Transfusion of packed cells covered with furosemide 40mg PO if elderly or ↓ cardiac function, indicated rarely for severe microcytic anaemia. Lifelong IM hydroxocobalamin 1mg 3-monthly is used to treat vitamin B_{12} deficiency, and folic acid 5mg od for folate deficiency.

▶ Never use folate alone to treat 'macrocytosis' unless it is proven to be the only deficiency. NB: folic acid is *not* the same as folinic acid.

Note on sickle cell anaemia A homozygous hereditary condition causing red cells to 'sickle' when exposed to low O_2 tensions, resulting in infarctions of bone and brain. In sickle cell trait (heterozygous form), the cells are less fragile and sickle only in severe hypoxia. Management: perform Hb electrophoresis (or Sickledex® if result needed urgently) on all Afro-Caribbean (and consider Mediterranean, Middle Eastern, and Indian) patients planned for GA.

Haematological malignancy

Leukaemias A neoplastic proliferation of white blood cells. Acute leukaemias are characterized by the release of primitive blast cells into the peripheral blood and account for 50% of childhood malignancy. Acute lymphoblastic leukaemia, the commonest childhood leukaemia, now has up to 90% cure rate in favourable cases. May present as gingival hypertrophy and bleeding. Acute myeloid leukaemia is the commonest acute leukaemia of adults, with high remission rates possible but a tendency to relapse. Chronic leukaemias have cells that retain most of the appearance of normal white cells. Chronic lymphocytic leukaemia is the commonest and has a 5yr survival of >50%. Chronic myeloid leukaemia is characterized by the presence of the Philadelphia chromosome, a fact beloved by examiners. Affects the >40s. Rx: interferon &/or bone marrow transplantation or stem cell transplantation. Remissions are common, although a terminal blast crisis usually supervenes at some stage.

Myeloproliferative disorders Proliferation of non-leucocyte marrow cells, with a wide range of behaviour and presentation, including anaemia, bleeding, and infections.

Monoclonal gammopathies such as multiple myeloma are B-lymphocyte disorders characterized by production of a specific immunoglobulin by plasma cells. Multiple myeloma is also a differential Δ of lytic lesions of bone, particularly the skull. Δ: monoclonal paraprotein band on plasma electrophoresis, Bence Jones proteins in urine.

Lymphomas Solid tumours arising in lymphoid tissue. Their classification is confusing; previously divided into Hodgkin's or non Hodgkin's lymphomas, the latter group was so diverse as to be meaningless. The current (2016) WHO classification attempts to define them by cell type, and recognizes four broad categories—mature T cell, mature B and NK cell, Hodgkin's, and histiocytic and dendritic neoplasms. Prognosis is highly variable and type dependant. Lymphoma should always be considered in the differential Δ of neck swellings.

Cytotoxic chemotherapy This has been the mainstay of Rx for these diseases. It is essential to remember that any patient receiving these drugs will be both immunocompromised and liable to bleed.

Hints In haematological malignancy, anaemia, bleeding, and infection are the overwhelming risks. Look for and treat anaemia. Avoid aspirin, other NSAIDs, trauma, and IM injections. Prevent sepsis, and if it occurs, treat very aggressively with the locally recommended broad-spectrum antibacterials and antifungals, e.g. piperacillin/tazobactam 2.25g and gentamicin 80mg IV tds plus fluconazole up to 100mg daily. Liaise with haematologist urgently.

Amyloidosis Characterized by deposits of fibrillar eosinophilic hyaline material in a wide range of organs and tissues. Two types: *1° amyloidosis* (AL amyloid), a plasma cell dyscrasia. Signs and symptoms include peripheral neuropathy, renal involvement, cardiomyopathy, xerostomia, and macroglossia. Rx: immunosuppression (rarely helps). *2° amyloidosis* (AA amyloid). It reflects an underlying chronic disease: infection, rheumatoid, neoplasia. May respond to Rx of underlying disease. Δ: biopsy of rectum or gingivae—stain with Congo red.

Other haematological disorders

For the practical management of a bleeding patient, see ⊃ Post-operative bleeding, p. 386.

Bleeding disorders

Platelet disorders May present as nosebleeds, purpura, or post-extraction bleeding. Remember that aspirin is the most common acquired cause, its effect being irreversible for 1 week. Other causes include diseases such as Von Willebrand's disease; immune thrombocytopenic purpura (ITP); virally associated (especially HIV) thrombocytopenic purpura; thrombocytopenia 2° to leukaemia; cytotoxic drugs; or unwanted effects of drugs, notably aspirin and chloramphenicol. Management: ensure platelet levels of >50 × 10^9/L, preferably 75 × 10^9/L for anything more than simple extraction or LA. If actively bleeding, use a combination of local measures (⊃ Post-operative bleeding, p. 386), tranexamic acid, and platelet transfusion. Platelet transfusions are short-lived and if used prophylactically must be given immediately prior to or during surgery. Liaise closely with the laboratory. The quality of preparation varies by locality. Tranexamic acid mouthwash may ↓ oral bleeding.

Coagulation defects Present as prolonged wound bleeding &/or haemarthroses. Causes include the haemophilias, anticoagulants, liver disease, and von Willebrand's disease.

Others Less common causes include hereditary haemorrhagic telangiectasia, aplastic anaemia, chronic kidney disease, myeloma, SLE, disseminated intravascular coagulation, and isolated deficiency of clotting factors.

Haemophilia A (factor VIII deficiency) The commonest clotting defect. Inherited as a sex-linked recessive, it affects males predominantly, although female haemophiliacs can occur. All daughters of affected males are potential carriers. Usually presents in childhood as haemarthroses. Bleeding from the mouth is common. Following trauma, bleeding appears to stop, but an intractable general ooze starts after an hour or so. Severity of bleeding is dependent on the level of factor VIII activity and degree of trauma.

Haemophilia B (factor IX deficiency) Clinically identical to haemophilia A; also known as Christmas disease.

Von Willebrand's disease A combined platelet and factor VIII disorder affecting males and females. Mucosal purpuras are common, haemarthroses less so. Wide range of severity. May improve with age &/or pregnancy.

Management The haemophilias and Von Willebrand's disease should always be managed at specialist centres. Check the patient's warning card for the contact telephone number.

Anticoagulants

Heparin Given IV or high-dose SC for therapeutic anticoagulation. Its effect wears off in ~8h although it can be reversed by protamine sulfate in an emergency. Measure in activated partial thromboplastin time (APTT).

Warfarin Given orally; effects take 48h to be seen. Normal therapeutic range is an international normalized ratio (INR) of 2–4. Simple extractions are usually safe at a level within therapeutic range. Reverse the effects of warfarin with vitamin K &/or fresh frozen plasma if needed, but consider why the patient is anticoagulated in the first place. See ➔ Prophylaxis, p. 586.

Low-molecular-weight heparin Given SC, these are small fractions of heparin salts commonly used for short-term prevention of deep vein thrombosis or, in higher doses, for full anticoagulation. Measuring or reversing activity are rarely required but differ from heparin—anti-factor Xa assay is used to measure activity and reversal with protamine sulfate is only partially effective.

Cardiovascular disease

This is the commonest cause of death in the UK.

Clinical conditions

Hypertension A consistently raised BP (>140 mmHg systolic, >90 mmHg diastolic >3 months) and is a risk factor for ischaemic heart disease, cerebrovascular accidents, and renal failure. Up to 95% of hypertension has no definable cause: essential hypertension. 5% is 2° to another disease such as renal dysfunction or endocrine disorders.

Ischaemic heart disease ↓ of the blood supply to part of the heart by narrowing of the coronary arteries, usually by atheroma, causing the pain of angina pectoris. If myocardial cells die as a result, acute coronary syndrome (myocardial infarction (MI)) occurs (➜ Acute chest pain, p. 559).

Heart failure The end result of a variety of conditions, not all of them cardiovascular. Basically, the heart is unable to meet the circulatory needs of the body. In right heart failure, dependent oedema and venous engorgement are prominent. In left heart failure, breathlessness is the principal sign. The two often coexist. There is an ever-present risk of precipitating heart failure, even in treated patients, by ↑ the demands on the heart, e.g. by fluid overload or excessive exertion.

Hypovolaemic shock Collapse of the peripheral circulation due to a sudden ↓ in the circulating volume. If this is not corrected there can be failure of perfusion of the vital organs, resulting in heart failure, renal failure, and unconsciousness ending in death.

Murmurs Disturbances of blood flow which are audible through a stethoscope. They may be functional or signify structural disorders of the heart. Echocardiography will differentiate. They are of great relevance to dentists as their presence warns of the potential for colonization of damaged valves by blood-borne bacteria. Such a bacteraemia can be caused by dental procedures.

Dental implications

Patients with a PMH of rheumatic fever are very likely to have some damage to a heart valve, usually the mitral valve. Traditionally, advice has been to provide antibiotic prophylaxis for invasive dental procedures, but more recent guidance has advised against this.[1] The risk of precipitating heart failure or MI in patients with compromised cardiovascular systems is ever present. Prevent by avoiding GA, especially within 3 months of an MI, using adequate LA with sedation if necessary, and avoid excessive adrenaline loads. Consider potential drug interactions (➜ Alarm bells, p. 620) and remember some of these patients will be anticoagulated.

Exclusion of septic foci may be requested in patients at high risk from bacteraemia, e.g. heart transplant recipients, those with prosthetic valves or valvular damage, or those with a history of infective endocarditis. It is prudent to err on the side of caution with these individuals and some will need dental clearances.

---

1 NICE 2008 (updated 2016) *Prophylaxis against Infective Endocarditis* (⅗ http://www.nice.org.uk/CG64).

Respiratory disease

Disease of the chest is an everyday problem in developed countries. The principal symptoms are cough, which may or may not be productive of sputum, dyspnoea (breathlessness), and wheeze. The coughing of blood (haemoptysis) mandates that malignancy be excluded.

Clinical conditions

Upper respiratory tract infections Include the common cold, sinusitis, and pharyngitis/tonsillitis (which may be viral or bacterial), laryngotracheitis, and acute epiglottitis. All are C/I to elective GA in the acute phase. Sinusitis (⊃ Maxillary sinusitis, p. 422). Penicillin is the drug of choice for a streptococcal sore throat. Avoid amoxicillin and ampicillin, as glandular fever may mimic this condition and these drugs will produce a rash, of varying severity, in such a patient. Epiglottitis is an emergency, and if suspected the larynx should *NEVER* be examined unless expert facilities for emergency intubation are to hand.

Lower respiratory tract infections Both viral and bacterial lower tract infections are debilitating and constitute a C/I to GA for elective surgery. Bear in mind TB and atypical bacteria, e.g. *Legionella, Mycoplasma*, and *Coxiella*. Open TB is highly infectious and cross-infection precautions are mandatory (⊃ Cross-infection prevention and control, p. 750).

Chronic obstructive pulmonary disease (COPD) A very common condition usually caused by a combination of bronchitis (excessive mucus production, persistent productive cough >3 months per year for 3yrs) and emphysema (dilation and destruction of air spaces distal to the terminal bronchioles). Smoking is the prime cause and must be stopped for Rx to be of any value. Be aware of possible systemic steroid use.

Asthma Reversible bronchoconstriction causes wheezing and dyspnoea. Up to 8% of the population are affected; there is often an allergic component. Patients complain of the chest feeling tight. May be precipitated by NSAIDs. Penicillin and aspirin allergies are more common. Management of acute asthma, ⊃ Management, p. 571.

Cystic fibrosis An inherited disorder whereby viscosity of mucus is ↑. Patients suffer pancreatic exocrine insufficiency and recurrent chest infections. Δ: by history and sweat sodium measurement.

Bronchial carcinoma Causes >20% of cancer deaths. Principal cause is smoking. ↓ incidence in females, though not by much. Symptoms are persistent cough, haemoptysis, and recurrent infections. 2yr survival is only 10%. Mesothelioma is an industrial disease caused by asbestos exposure.

Sarcoidosis Most commonly presents as hilar lymphadenopathy in young adults. Oral lesions can occur. Erythema nodosum common.

Dental implications

Avoid GA. Use analgesics and sedatives with caution; opioids and sedatives ↓ respiratory drive; NSAIDs may exacerbate asthma. Advise your patients to stop smoking (and if you are a smoker, stop). Refer if suspicious, especially in the presence of confirmed haemoptysis.

Gastrointestinal disease

The mouth and its mucosal disorders and disorders of the salivary glands are covered in Chapter 11.

Oesophagus Presents symptoms which can be confused with those originating from the mouth, the most important being *dysphagia*. Difficulty in swallowing may be caused by conditions within the mouth (e.g. ulceration), pharynx (e.g. foreign body), benign or malignant conditions within the oesophagus, compression by surrounding structures (e.g. mediastinal lymph nodes), or neurological causes. It is a symptom which should be taken seriously and investigated by at least CXR, barium swallow, &/or endoscopy. Reflux oesophagitis is a common cause of dyspepsia, sore throat, cough, and bad taste.

Peptic ulceration and gastric carcinoma (Duodenal malignancy rare.) May present with epigastric pain, vomiting, haematemesis, or melaena.

Peptic ulceration Commonly due to infection with *Helicobacter pylori* and usually responds to *H. pylori* eradication therapy (combination of proton pump inhibitor/broad-spectrum antibiotic/anaerobicidal, i.e. metronidazole). Other causes include stress ulceration in critically ill or major surgical patients, and elderly people on NSAIDs. Prophylaxis is with H_2 antagonists or proton pump inhibitors to reduce acid secretion or sucralfate, a mucosal protectant, which maintains the protective gastric pH barrier but is a problem practically as it clogs fine-bore nasogastric tubes. Symptomatic relief of dyspepsia without significant ulceration is with antacids and alginates. Persisting epigastric pain or other symptoms *must* be investigated as gastric carcinoma requires early surgery and carries a poor prognosis.

▶ Endoscopic investigation of patients >40yrs with persisting epigastric symptoms is mandatory.

Non-malignant, *Helicobacter*-negative ulceration (oesophagitis, gastritis, duodenitis) clears with 1 month of proton pump inhibitor Rx (e.g. omeprazole 10–20mg od) and can often be maintained with H_2 antagonists (ranitidine or cimetidine).

Small bowel This has a multitude of associated disorders which tend to present in a similar manner; namely, malabsorption syndromes, diarrhoea, steatorrhoea, abdominal pain, anaemia, and chronic deficiencies. Coeliac disease and Crohn's disease are the best known conditions. Coeliac disease is a hypersensitivity response of the small bowel to gluten and is treated by strict avoidance. A number of oral complaints are related, typically 'cobblestoning' of the mucosa. Crohn's disease may affect any part of the gastrointestinal tract but has a preference for the ileo-caecal area. It is a chronic granulomatous disease affecting the full thickness of the mucosa and may result in fistula formation. Ulcerative colitis is often mistaken for Crohn's disease initially, but affects the colorectum only. Treatment with systemic steroids and other immunosuppressants is common.

Large bowel Diverticular disease is a condition with multiple outpouching of large bowel mucosa which can become inflamed, causing diverticulitis. The irritable bowel syndrome is a condition associated with ↑ colonic tone, causing recurrent abdominal pain; there may be some psychogenic overlay.

Colonic cancer is common in older patients; it may present as rectal bleeding, a change in bowel habit, intestinal obstruction, tenesmus (wanting to defecate but producing nothing), abdominal pain, or anaemia. It is treated surgically, with up to 90% 5yr survival if diagnosed early (Dukes A stage). Familial polyposis coli is associated with the Gardener syndrome (⊙ Gardener syndrome, p. 783). Antibiotic-induced colitis results from overgrowth of toxigenic *Clostridium difficile* after use of antibiotics, commonly ampicillin and clindamycin. It responds to oral vancomycin or metronidazole.

The pancreas Malignancy has the worst prognosis of any cancer and most Rx is essentially palliative.

Acute pancreatitis Often a manifestation of alcohol abuse. Aetiology is not entirely clear. Causes acute abdominal pain. Amylase levels are a guide but not infallible. Patients need aggressive rehydration, maintenance of electrolyte balance, and analgesia, in high-dependency or ICU setting.

Hepatic disease

The main problems presented by patients with liver disease are the potential for ↑ bleeding, inability to metabolize and excrete many commonly used drugs, and the possibility that they can transmit Hep B, C, &/or D (Hep A and E are spread by faecal–oral route). The liver is also a site of metastatic spread of malignant tumours. Patients in liver failure needing surgery, especially under GA, are a high-risk group who should have specialist advice on their management.

Jaundice The prime symptom of liver disease. It is a widespread yellow discoloration of the skin (best seen in good light, in the sclera), caused by the inability of the liver to process bilirubin, the breakdown product of haemoglobin. This occurs either because it is presented with an overwhelming amount of bilirubin to conjugate (e.g. haemolytic anaemia), or it is unable to excrete bile (cholestatic jaundice). Cholestatic jaundice in turn may be either intrahepatic or extrahepatic.

Intrahepatic cholestasis Intrahepatic cholestasis represents hepatocyte damage; this is reflected by ↑ aspartate transaminase levels on LFTs, and results in impaired bile excretion, as indicated by ↑ plasma bilirubin. Causes include alcohol and other drugs, toxins, and bacterial and viral infections. A degree of hepatitis is present with these causes, whereas 1° biliary cholangitis and anabolic steroids cause a specific intrahepatic cholestasis without hepatitis.

Extrahepatic cholestasis Extrahepatic cholestasis is caused by obstruction to the excretion of bile in the common bile duct by gallstones, tumour, clot, or stricture. Carcinoma of the head of the pancreas, or adjacent lymph nodes, may also compress the duct, and must be excluded.

Surgery in patients with liver disease
- Ascertain a Δ for the cause. Do hepatitis serology. Cross-infection precautions (➲ Cross-infection prevention and control, p. 750).
- Perform a coagulation screen. May need correction with vitamin K or fresh-frozen plasma.
- *Always* warn the anaesthetist, as it will affect the choice of anaesthetic agents.
- If a jaundiced patient must undergo surgery, correct fluid and electrolyte balance, and ensure a good peri-operative urine output by aggressive IV hydration with 5% glucose and mannitol diuresis to avoid hepato-renal syndrome (➲ *Oxford Handbook of Clinical Medicine*).
- Do not use IV saline in patients in fulminant hepatic failure, as there is a high risk of inducing encephalopathy.

Liver disease patients in dental practice
- Know which disease you are dealing with. If Hep B or C, employ strict cross-infection control (⊃ Cross-infection prevention and control, p. 750).
- Be cautious in prescribing drugs (consult the *BNF*/DPF) and with administering LA.
- *Do not* administer GAs.
- Take additional local precautions against post-operative bleeding following simple extractions (⊃ Post-operative bleeding, p. 386). A clotting screen should be obtained for anything more advanced, and in all patients with severe liver disease.

Renal disorders

The commonest urinary tract problems, infections, are of relevance only to those who manage in-patients. Rarer conditions such as renal failure and transplantation are, surprisingly, of more general relevance because these patients are at ↑ risk from infection, bleeding, and iatrogenic drug overdose during routine Rx.

Urine This is tested in all in-patients. 'Multistix' will test for glycosuria (diabetes, pregnancy, infection), proteinuria (diabetes, infection, nephrotic syndrome), ketones (diabetic ketoacidosis), haematuria (infection, tumour), and bile as bilirubin and urobilinogen (cholestatic jaundice).

Urinary tract infections A common cause of toxic confusion in elderly in-patients, especially females. Send a mid-stream urine (MSU) for culture and sensitivity, then start trimethoprim 200mg bd PO or ampicillin 250mg qds PO and ensure a high fluid intake. Minimal investigations of renal function are U&Es, creatinine, and ionized Ca^{2+}.

Nephrotic syndrome A syndrome of proteinuria (>3.5g/day), hypoalbuminaemia, and generalized oedema. Facial oedema is often prominent. Glomerulonephritis is the major precipitating cause and investigations should be carried out by a physician with an interest in renal medicine.

Acute kidney injury (formerly acute renal failure) A medical emergency causing a rapid rise in serum creatinine, urea, and K^+. It may follow surgery or major trauma and is usually marked by a failure to pass urine. *Remember* the commonest causes of failing to pass urine post-operatively are under-infusion of fluids and urinary retention. Rx: ↑ IV fluid input and catheterize (◐ Catheterization, p. 581). If acute kidney injury is suspected, get urgent U&Es, ECG, and blood gases. Obtain aid from a physician. Control of hyperkalaemia, fluid balance, acidosis, and hypertension are the immediate necessities.

Chronic kidney disease (formerly chronic renal failure) Basically the onset of uraemia after gradual, but progressive renal damage, commonly caused by glomerulonephritis (inflammation of the glomeruli following immune complex deposits), pyelonephritis (small scarred kidneys due to childhood infection, irradiation, or poisoning), or adult polycystic disease (congenital cysts within Bowman's capsule). It has protean manifestations, starting with nocturia and anorexia, progressing through hypertension and anaemia to multisystem failure. Continuous ambulatory peritoneal dialysis, haemodialysis, and transplants are the mainstays of Rx.

Main problems relevant to dentistry

- ↑ risk of infection, worsened by immunosuppression.
- ↑ bleeding tendency.
- ↓ ability to excrete drugs.
- Veins are sacrosanct; never use their arteriovenous fistula.
- Bone lesions of the jaws (renal osteodystrophy, 2° hyperparathyroidism).
- Generalized growth impairment in children.
- Potential carriage of Hep B, HIV.

Renal transplantation An increasingly common final Rx of renal failure, and when successful renal function may reach near-normal levels. Kidneys are, however, immunosuppressed and at greatly ↑ risk from infection. They may share the problems associated with chronic kidney disease depending on the level of function of the transplant.

Hints

- Take precautions against cross-infection (◆ Cross-infection prevention and control, p. 750).
- Treat all infections aggressively and consider prophylaxis.
- Use additional haemostatic measures (◆ Post-operative bleeding, p. 386).
- Be cautious with prescribing drugs (◆ Prescribing, p. 596).
- Never subject these patients to out-patient GA.
- Remember: veins are precious.
- Try to perform Rx just after dialysis if possible.

Endocrine disease

Addison's disease 1° hypoadrenocorticism. Atrophy of the adrenal cortices causes failure of cortisol and aldosterone secretion. 2° hypoadrenocorticism is far commoner, due to steroid therapy or ACTH deficiency (◑ Management of patients requiring steroid supplementation, p. 590). All need steroid cover.

Conn syndrome 1° hyperaldosteronism causes hypokalaemia and hypernatraemia with hypertension.

Cushing's disease/syndrome These are due to excess corticosteroid production. The disease refers to 2° adrenal hyperplasia due to ↑ ACTH, whereas the syndrome is a 1° condition, usually due to therapeutic administration of synthetic steroid or adenoma. Classical features are obesity (moon face, buffalo hump) sparing the limbs, osteoporosis, skin thinning, and hypertension.

Diabetes insipidus Production of copious dilute urine due to ↓ antidiuretic hormone secretion or renal insensitivity to antidiuretic hormone. May occur temporarily after head injury.

Diabetes mellitus Persistent hyperglycaemia due to a relative deficiency of insulin (◑ Management of the diabetic patient undergoing surgery, p. 588).

Gigantism/acromegaly Excess production of growth hormone, before and after fusion of the epiphyses, respectively.

Goitre A large thyroid gland, of whatever cause.

Hyperthyroidism Symptoms of heat intolerance, weight loss, and sweating occur. Signs are tachycardia (may have atrial fibrillation), lid lag, exophthalmos, and tremor. Commonest cause is Graves disease (◑ Graves disease, p. 784). Functioning adenomas are another cause.

Hypothyroidism Can be 1° due to thyroid disease, or 2° to hypothalamic or pituitary dysfunction. 1° disease is often an autoimmune condition. Symptoms are poor tolerance of cold, loss of hair, weight gain, loss of appetite, and poor memory. Signs are bradycardia and a hoarse voice.

Hyperparathyroidism 1° is caused by an adenoma. 2° is a response to low plasma Ca^{2+}, e.g. in renal failure, and 3° follows on from 2° when the parathyroids continue ↑ production, even if Ca^{2+} is normalized.

Hypoparathyroidism Usually 2° to thyroidectomy, when parathyroid glands inadvertently removed. Plasma Ca^{2+} ↓, resulting in tetany. Chvostek's sign is +ve if spasm of facial muscles occurs after tapping over the facial nerve.

Hypopituitarism Can lead to 2° hypothyroidism or 2° hypoadrenocorticism.

Inappropriate antidiuretic hormone secretion Caused by certain tumours (e.g. bronchial carcinoma), head injury, and some drugs. Hyponatraemia, overhydration, and confusion occur.

Lingual thyroid May be the only functioning thyroid the patient has; do not excise lightly. Do pre-operative isotope scan.

Phaeochromocytoma A very rare tumour of the adrenal medulla, secreting adrenaline and noradrenaline. Symptoms are recurring palpitations and headache with sweating. Simultaneous hypertension with a return to baseline on settling of symptoms is a good marker.

Pituitary tumours May erode the pituitary fossa (seen on lateral skull X-ray) and can cause blindness via optic chiasma compression.

Endocrine-related problems

▶ Always ask yourself: 'Is she, or can she be, pregnant?'

Pregnancy Pregnancy is a C/I to elective GA, the vast majority of drugs (➔ Prescribing, p. 596), and non-essential radiography (the most vulnerable period being in the first 3 months). Elective Rx is best performed in the mid-trimester.

Menopause The end of a woman's reproductive life and her periods. It is often associated with hot flushes/flashes and other physical problems. Emotional disturbances may coexist, and the incidence of psychiatric disorders ↑ at this time.

Related problems

Suxamethonium sensitivity Around 1:3000 people have an inherited defect of plasma cholinesterase. These families are absolutely normal in every respect except in their ability to metabolize suxamethonium. This leaves them unable to destroy the drug which, normally wearing off in 2–4min, produces prolonged muscle paralysis. This paralysis requires ventilatory support until the drug wears off, which, in the homozygote, may take as long as 24h.

Malignant hyperpyrexia A rare, potentially lethal reaction to, usually, an anaesthetic agent. Characterized by ↑ pulse, muscle rigidity, and ↑ temperature. Dantrolene sodium and cooling may be life-saving.

Rare endocrine tumours

Glucagonomas Secrete glucagon causing hyperglycaemia.

Insulinomas Secrete insulin. Causes sporadic hypoglycaemic episodes.

Gastrinomas Secrete gastrin causing duodenal ulcers and diarrhoea (Zollinger–Ellison syndrome).

Multiple endocrine neoplasia (MEN) syndromes A rare group of endocrine tumours. MEN IIb is medullary thyroid cancer, phaeochromocytoma, and oral mucosal neuromas.

Bone disease

Pathology of the bones of the facial skeleton is covered in Chapter 10.

Osteogenesis imperfecta (brittle bone disease) An auto-somal dominant type 1 collagen defect. Multiple # following slight trauma with rapid but distorted healing is characteristic. Associated with blue sclera, deafness, and dentinogenesis imperfecta (➔ Dentinogenesis imperfecta (hereditary opalescent dentine), p. 72). The jaws are *not* particularly prone to # following extractions.

Osteopetrosis (marble bone disease) There is an ↑ in bone density and brittleness, and a ↓ in blood supply. Prone to infection which is difficult to eradicate. Bone pain, #, and compression neuropathies may occur. Anaemia can complicate severe disease. Facial characteristics are frontal bossing and hypertelorism.

Achondroplasia An inherited defect in cartilaginous bone formation, usually autosomal dominant. Causes skull bossing; many have no other problems. Best known current representative would be Tyrion Lannister, a character from *A Game of Thrones*.

Cleidocranial dysostosis An inherited defect of membranous bone formation, usually autosomal dominant. Skull and clavicles are affected. Multiple unerupted teeth with retention of 1° dentition is characteristic.

Disorders of bone metabolism

Rickets/osteomalacia Failure of bone mineralization in, respectively, children and adults. Can be caused by deficiency, failure of synthesis, malabsorption, or impaired metabolism of vitamin D, and also hypophosphataemia or ↑ Ca^{2+} requirement in pregnancy.

Osteoporosis A lack of both bone matrix and mineralization. Important causes are steroid therapy, post-menopausal hormone changes, immobilization, and endocrine abnormalities. Hormone replacement therapy in post-menopausal women appears helpful. Results in ↑ incidence of #, especially femoral neck and wrist. Bisphosphonates are being aggressively promoted in the treatment of osteoporosis resulting in some of the noted ↑ in BRON (➔ Dento-alveolar surgery: bisphosphonates, denosumab, or anti-angiogenic medication, p. 390).

Fibrous dysplasia Replacement of a part of a bone or bones by fibrous tissue with associated swelling. It usually starts in childhood and ceases with completion of skeletal growth. Termed monostotic if one bone is affected, polyostotic if more than one bone, and Albright syndrome if associated with precocious puberty and *café au lait* areas of skin hyperpigmentation.

Cherubism A bilateral variant of fibrous dysplasia.

Paget's disease of bone A common disorder of the elderly, where the normal, orderly replacement of bone is disrupted and replaced by a chaotic structure of new bone, causing enlargement and deformity. The hands and feet are spared. Complications include bone pain and cranial nerve compression, or, more rarely, high output cardiac failure or osteosarcoma. Another condition that is treated with bisphosphonates.

Diseases of connective tissue, muscle, and joints

Connective tissue diseases

These are mainly vasculitides (inflammation of vessels).

Cranial arteritis (temporal arteritis) Giant cell vasculitis of the craniofacial region. Presenting symptom is unilateral throbbing headache. Signs are high ESR with a tender, pulseless artery. Major complication of temporal arteritis is optic nerve ischaemia causing blindness, so start high-dose steroids (60mg prednisolone PO od) and monitor using ESR. Biopsy confirms.

Polymyalgia rheumatica More generalized vasculitis affecting proximal axial muscles. Accounts for 25% of cases of cranial arteritis. Responds to steroids; gradual improvement with time.

Disease of muscles

Muscular dystrophy A collection of inherited diseases characterized by muscle degeneration. Duchenne's is the most common and is usually fatal in early adulthood.

Myotonic disorders Distinguished by delayed muscle relaxation after contraction. They are genetically determined in a complex fashion.

Polymyositis A generalized immune-mediated inflammatory disorder of muscle. If a characteristic rash is present the condition is known as *dermatomyositis* and has an association with occult malignancy.

Joint disease

Osteoarthritis 1° degeneration of articular cartilage, cervical and lumbar spine, hip and knee joints, commonly affected or 2° to trauma or other joint disease, resulting in pain and stiffness. Osteophyte formation and subchondral bone cysts, which collapse leading to deformity, are characteristic. Physiotherapy, weight loss, and analgesia are the mainstays of Rx. Joint replacement is definitive Rx.

Rheumatoid arthritis Immunologically mediated disease where joint pain and damage are the most prominent symptoms. Morning pain and stiffness in the hands and feet, usually symmetrical, is characteristic. There may be systemic upset and anaemia. Ulnar deviation of the fingers is pathognomonic. Rx includes NSAIDs, steroids, and physiotherapy. Second-line or disease-modifying antirheumatic drugs (DMARDs) may favourably influence outcome at expense of unwanted effects, e.g. penicillamine, antimalarials, immunosuppressants (including TNFα chimeric monoclonal antibody—infliximab). Dry eyes and mouth may be associated with rheumatoid arthritis (➔ Sjögren syndrome (secondary Sjögren syndrome), p. 460). TMJ symptoms are rare in rheumatoid arthritis, although up to 15% of patients have radiographic changes in the joint.

Juvenile rheumatoid arthritis (juvenile idiopathic arthritis, Still's disease) Rarer form of the disease affecting children. It can be much more severe than the adult condition and can cause TMJ ankylosis.

Psoriatic arthritis Associated with the skin condition and affects the spine and pelvis. It is usually milder than rheumatoid arthritis and has no serological abnormalities. The TMJ can be affected, but symptoms are usually mild despite some isolated case reports to the contrary.

Gout Urates are deposited in joints, causing sudden severe joint pain, often in the great toe. Affected joints are red, swollen, and very tender. Gout 2° to drugs, radiotherapy, or haematological disease is commoner than that caused by an inborn error of metabolism.

Ankylosing spondylitis Affects the spine, usually in young men. Inflammation involves the insertion of ligaments and tendons. It is associated with HLA B27. Later, kyphotic deformity and ↑ risk of cervical fractures.

Reiter syndrome Seronegative arthritis, urethritis, and conjunctivitis, usually in response to an infection. Oral lesions are often present. Genital and intestinal variants.

Perthes' disease Osteochondritis of the femoral head in, mainly, boys aged 3–11yrs. No systemic implications.

Neurological disorders

Cranial nerves

- *I: olfactory.* Sense of smell is rarely tested, although damage is quite common following head &/or mid-face trauma.
- *II: optic.* Examine the pupils for both direct and consensual reflex; assess the visual fields; check visual acuity and examine the fundus with an ophthalmoscope (→ Eyes, p. 10).
- *III: oculomotor.* The motor supply to the extra-ocular muscles except lateral rectus and superior oblique. It supplies the ciliary muscle, the constrictor of the pupil, and levator palpebrae superioris. A defect therefore causes impairment of upward, downward, and inward movement of the eye, leading to diplopia, drooping of the upper eyelid (ptosis), and absent direct and consensual reflexes.
- *IV: trochlear.* Supplies superior oblique, paralysis of which causes diplopia; worst on looking downward and inward.
- *V: trigeminal.* The major sensory nerve to the face, oral, nasal, conjunctival, and sinus mucosa, and part of the tympanic membrane. It is motor to the muscles of mastication. Sensory abnormalities are mapped out using gentle touch and pin-prick. Motor weakness is best assessed on jaw opening and excursion.
- *VI: abducens.* Supplies lateral rectus. A defect causes paralysis of abduction of the eye.
- *VII: facial.* Motor to the muscles of facial expression. Supplies taste from the anterior two-thirds of tongue (via chorda tympani) and is secretomotor to the lacrimal, sublingual, and submandibular glands. It innervates the stapedius muscle in the middle ear. The lower face is innervated by the contralateral motor cortex, whereas the upper face has bilateral innervation. Assess by demonstrating facial movements.
- *VIII: vestibulocochlear.* Is sensory for balance and hearing. Deafness, vertigo, and tinnitus are the main symptoms.
- *IX: glossopharyngeal.* Supplies sensation and taste from the posterior one-third of the tongue, motor to stylopharyngeus, and secretomotor to the parotid. Lesions impair the gag reflex in conjunction with X.
- *X: vagus.* Has a motor input to the palatal, pharyngeal, and laryngeal muscles. Impaired gag reflex, hoarseness, and deviation of the soft palate to the unaffected side are seen if damaged. The vagus has a huge parasympathetic output to the viscera of the thorax and abdomen.
- *XI: accessory.* Is motor to sternomastoid and trapezius, causing weakness on shoulder shrugging and on turning the head away from the affected side.
- *XII: hypoglossal.* Motor supply to the tongue. Lesions cause dysarthria (impaired speech) and deviation towards the affected side on protrusion.

Headache

The vast majority of headaches are benign; the secret is to pick out those which are not. Read on.

Tension headache Commonest type. Due to muscle tension in occipitofrontalis. Usually worse as the day progresses; may feel 'band-like'. Responds to reassurance, anxiolytics, and analgesics.

Migraine A distinct entity characterized by a preceding visual aura (fortification spectra). Severe, usually unilateral headache with photophobia, nausea, and vomiting. Thought to be due to cerebral vasoconstriction, followed by reflex vasodilation (the latter is the cause of the pain). 5-HT agonists, e.g. sumatriptan (C/I: ischaemic heart disease, cerebrovascular disease) abolish an attack if used early, and many drugs are used to prevent attacks (such as propranolol or pizotifen). F > M, the oral contraceptive being a contributing factor. There are many variants of classical migraine.

Migrainous neuralgia (cluster headache) Rarer than migraine and causes localized pain, usually around the eye, with associated nasal stuffiness. M > F. There is a typical time of onset, often in early morning, which recurs for several weeks: 'clustering'. Alcohol is a common precipitant. 5-HT agonists (sumatriptan) to treat and calcium channel blockers (verapamil) for prophylaxis.

Raised intracranial pressure A cause of headache demanding urgent further investigation. Pointers are headache, worse on waking, irritation, ↓ level of consciousness, vomiting, sluggish or absent pupillary reflexes, and bulging of the optic disc (papilloedema). *Rising BP and slowing pulse* are late premorbid signs of ↑ intracranial pressure.

Medication misuse headache Affects up to 1:50. Presents as daily headache due to excessive or regular use of OTC analgesics (especially codeine-containing) and some antimigraine preparations. Pain pathways may be altered and after withdrawal of the drug the headache may be slow to resolve.

Rare and wonderful headaches Ice-cream headache, post-coital headache, needle-through-eye headache, and many other distinctive and benign headaches are described.

More neurological disorders

CNS infections

Bacterial meningitis Must be considered in the differential Δ of headache with photophobia and neck stiffness. Organisms are *Haemophilus influenzae, Neisseria meningitidis* (meningococcus), *N. gonorrhoeae*, and *Streptococcus pneumoniae*. In children, the meningococcus is especially important and classically associated with a non-blanching purpuric rash. This is one of the very few indications for instituting immediate blind antibiotic therapy (parenteral penicillin).

Viral meningitis Usually mild and self-limiting. Distinguished from bacterial meningitis by lumbar puncture.

Herpetic encephalitis A rare manifestation of infection with the herpes simplex virus. Can be distinguished from drunkenness or dementia by history and rapid onset. Parenteral aciclovir can be curative.

CNS tumours Most brain tumours are 2° deposits. Although both benign and malignant 1° tumours are found, they are rare. Despite this, they are the commonest cause of cancer death in children after leukaemia.

Epilepsy An episodic outflow from the brain causing disturbances of consciousness, motor function, and sensory function. Most causes are idiopathic but those with onset in adult life must be investigated for local or general cerebral disease. Major or *grand mal* epilepsy is characterized by an aura and loss of consciousness, and followed by tonic and clonic phases. Incontinence is a good guide to a genuine seizure. The fit rarely lasts >5min; if it does, the patient has entered status epilepticus (◑ Fits, p. 569).

Petit mal (absence attacks) These are epileptic attacks usually confined to children, taking the form of a short absence when movement, speech, and attention cease.

Temporal lobe epilepsy Characterized by hallucinations of the special senses.

Localized (Jacksonian) epilepsy Affects limbs in isolation. Patients with established epilepsy (once any treatable cause has been excluded) must be maintained on adequate levels of antiepileptic drugs.

Febrile convulsions Fits, usually in children >5yrs old, 2° to pyrexia.

Cerebrovascular accidents (strokes) A very common cause of death in the elderly. A stroke is basically death of part of the brain following cerebral ischaemia, either due to bleeding into the brain or occlusion of vessels. It is often clinically difficult to distinguish these different types of stroke. As for acute coronary syndromes, rapid thrombolysis may be indicated, as may interventional endovascular procedures.

Multiple (disseminated) sclerosis A disorder characterized by demyelination in multiple 'plaques' throughout the CNS. Symptoms are multiple and disseminated in both time and place. It is the commonest neurological disease of young adults, and the most common form is relapsing/remitting. Parenteral interferon treatment can reduce recurrences.

Myasthenia gravis Muscle weakness due to inadequate response to, or levels of, acetylcholine. Extra-ocular muscles are often first affected.

Parkinson's disease A disease affecting the basal ganglia associated with a ↓ in the local levels of dopamine. Characterized by a 'pill-rolling' tremor, 'cog-wheel' rigidity, and bradykinesis with a shuffling gait.

Skin neoplasms

▶ The skin of the face is the commonest site of curable skin cancers, so look and think (➔ Skin cancer, p. 488).

Basal cell carcinoma (epithelioma, rodent ulcer) An indolent skin cancer which very rarely metastasizes. If it kills, it usually does so by local destruction. Chronic exposure to sunlight is a major aetiological factor. There are various forms, the commonest being an ulcerated nodule with raised pearly margins and a telangiectatic surface. Rx: excision (micrographic or conventional), radiotherapy (especially electron beam), cryotherapy, curettage, topical immune modulation, photodynamic therapy, and electrodessication.

Squamous cell carcinoma SCC of the skin is surprisingly indolent in comparison to SCC of mucosa but beware the external ear which can be aggressive in 40%. Presents as an ulcerated lesion with raised edges. Keratin horns may be present, and it may arise in areas of previously sun-damaged skin or in gravitational leg ulcers. Surgical excision or radiotherapy is Rx of choice.

Malignant melanoma This condition is being increasingly diagnosed, with a doubling of the incidence in the last 20yrs. The prognosis is dependent primarily on the depth of the tumour (Breslow thickness), as the thicker the lesion, the poorer the prognosis. Early metastasis is common. Sunlight is a major aetiological factor, possibly due to burning at an early age. Suspect if a pigmented lesion rapidly enlarges, bleeds, ulcerates, shows 'satellite' lesions, or changes colour. Prompt referral for specialist management is needed. Lots of 'sun aware' campaigns emphasize prevention.

Naevi Areas of skin containing a disproportionate number of melanocytes.

Lentigo simplex A freckle.

Dysplastic naevi Premalignant lesions often found in patients with malignant melanoma. They should be excised and patients advised to use high-factor sunscreens.

Lentigo maligna A premalignant pigmented lesion of the elderly.

Carcinoma *in situ* (Bowen's disease) Presents as a scaly, red plaque. It is basically a squamous carcinoma which has not yet penetrated beyond the basal layer.

Actinic keratosis Persistently sun-damaged areas of skin in which cancer may arise.

Kaposi's sarcoma A purple, vascular, multifocal malignant tumour typically seen in AIDS and other immunocompromised patients. Also seen intraorally.

Metastatic deposits Metastatic deposits to the skin occur most frequently from breast, kidney, and lung, but skin secondaries from oral cancer are increasingly being seen.

Dermatology

Psoriasis A common, relapsing proliferative inflammatory skin disease. Appears as a red plaque with a silvery scale, chiefly on extensor skin of knees and elbows, although any area can be affected. Can be associated with systemic disease, particularly arthropathy (◑ Diseases of connective tissue, muscle, and joints, p. 544). Rx is mainly topical: steroids, coal tar, dithranol &/or ultra-violet (UV)-B radiation, or psoralen-sensitized UVA radiation (PUVA). Rarely, methotrexate can be used.

Eczema Also called dermatitis. Has several variants according to aetiology.

Atopic eczema Starts in the first year of life with a red symmetrical scaly rash. Emulsifying ointments help prevent fissuring, although steroids are sometimes needed. Up to 90% grow out of it by age 12yrs.

Exogenous eczema Can be produced in anyone exposed to a sufficient irritant. The hands are the usual target, with blistering, erythema, and cracking of skin.

Allergic contact eczema A genuine allergic response, e.g. to nickel.

Seborrhoeic eczema A fungal infection mainly affecting the scalp ('cradle cap') in neonates.

Skin infections Fungal infections are particularly common, causing angular cheilitis, athlete's foot, paronychia, vaginitis, etc. Furuncles are staphylococcal boils. Erysipelas is a streptococcal cellulitis. Viruses cause herpes zoster and simplex infections, molluscum contagiosum, and warts.

Infestations Infestations of the skin bring a shudder to most people, but they are also a hazard of working closely with patients! Head lice respond to malathion. Flea bites, as well as being unpleasant, can spread plague, among other serious diseases. Scabies is an infestation with a mite which creates a characteristic itchy burrow in the finger webs.

Acne Acne vulgaris is characterized by the blackhead (comedone), and is an inflammatory condition caused by ↑ sebum secretion. It is hormone dependent, although superinfection with the acne bacillus is a contributing factor. Tends to scar. After proprietary lotions, low-dose tetracyclines help. Co-cyprindiol, a combined oral contraceptive, is a useful alternative in women. The teratogenic retinoid, isotretinoin, is particularly useful in severe and late-onset acne unresponsive to other Rx.

The skin and internal disease The skin, like the mouth, acts as an outside indicator for many internal diseases.

Erythema nodosum Painful, red, nodular lumps on the shins.

Erythema multiforme Circular target lesions.

Erythema marginatum Vanishing and recurring pink rings. These are all non-specific markers for a variety of diseases.

Vitiligo An autoimmune hypopigmentation, associated with other auto-immune conditions.

Pyoderma gangrenosum Blue-edged ulcers, especially on the legs; associated with ulcerative colitis and Crohn's disease.

Granuloma annulare Subcutaneous circular thickening and *necrobiosis lipoidica* (yellow plaques on the shins) are associated with diabetes.

Dermatitis herpetiformis Vesicular rash of knees, elbows, and scalp. Associated with coeliac disease.

Pretibial myxoedema Red swellings above the ankle. Associated with hyperthyroidism.

Skin diseases associated with malignancy These include *acanthosis nigricans* (rough, pigmented, thickened areas of skin in axilla or groin) and *thrombo-phlebitis migrans* (tender nodules within blood vessels which move from site to site).

Psychiatry

One way of getting to grips with a new subject—and to virtually all dentists psychiatry as opposed to psychology is new—is to categorize. The major adult psychiatric diagnoses are listed in order of severity. This is known as the 'hierarchy of diagnosis'.

Organic brain syndromes

Acute organic reaction (delirium, toxic confusion) Clouding of consciousness and disorientation in time and place are major symptoms. Mood-swings are common, and visual hallucinations, rare in other psychiatric conditions, can be present.

▶ There is an underlying, frequently treatable cause to this condition (infection, hypoxia, drugs, dehydration, alcohol withdrawal, etc.). Rx: find the cause and correct it, using sedation until the cause is identified and Rx has taken effect.

Chronic organic reaction (dementia) A global intellectual deterioration highlighted by a worsening short-term memory. *Never* label someone as demented until all other possible causes, including depression, have been excluded. They may require evaluation by a psychiatrist. Alzheimer's disease and multi-infarct dementia are the commonest causes. There is no cure, although effective support services and psychosocial interventions can improve the quality of life considerably. Anticholinesterase inhibitors, e.g. donepezil, and memantine, may slow the rate of cognitive decline.

Mental disabilities See ➔ Dentistry for people with disabilities, p. 46.

Psychosis Contact with reality is lost and normal mental processes do not function. There is loss of insight. If an organic condition is excluded, the Δ is one of four:

Schizophrenia A disorder where the victims live in an incomprehensible world full of vivid personal significance. First-rank symptoms are a good guide to Δ: delusions, thought insertion, broadcasting and withdrawal, passivity feelings, and visual and auditory hallucinations.

Affective disorders Mania, hypomania, manic-depressive psychosis, and depression. Mania and hypomania are characterized by euphoria, hyperactivity, overvalued ideas or grandiose delusions, and pressure of speech. They differ only in degree. Cyclical mania and depression is known as bipolar affective disorder. Rx is with major tranquillizers and prophylaxis with lithium carbonate.

Depression May be either psychotic or neurotic. Markers of major depressive illness are anhedonia (failure to find pleasure in things which once did please), anorexia, especially with weight loss, early morning wakening, tearfulness, inability to concentrate, feelings of guilt and worthlessness, and suicidal ideation.

Paranoid states Paranoid states are psychoses where paranoid symptoms predominate and, despite lack of insight, other diagnoses do not apply.

▶ The commonly abused drugs can all mimic or precipitate psychotic states, as can giving birth—puerperal psychosis.

Neuroses A neurosis is a maladaptive psychological symptom in the absence of organic or psychotic causes of the symptom and after exclusion of a psychopathic personality. Insight is present.

Anxiety neurosis This frequently coexists with depression. These patients often have physical symptoms for which there is no physical explanation.

Obsessional neurosis Intrusive thoughts or ideas which the subject recognizes as coming from within themselves, but resents and is unable to stop. May be associated with *compulsive behaviour* where repeated purposeless activity is carried out due to an inexplicable feeling that it must be done.

Phobia This is the generation of fear or anxiety out of proportion to the stimulus. Numerous stimuli exist, including dentists.

Anorexia nervosa/bulimia nervosa This is the development of weight reduction as an overvalued idea. Associated with weight ↓ of >25% of ideal body weight and obsessive food avoidance. Commonest in females, it is also associated with amenorrhea. Has a significant mortality rate; binge-eating followed by vomiting &/or laxative abuse can occur. Bingeing without weight loss is bulimia nervosa. Dental effects, ➋ Erosion, p. 252.

Personality disorders These are not illnesses but extremes of normal personality traits, e.g. obsessional, histrionic, schizoid (cold, introspective), and borderline (black-and-white thinking). The most important is the psychopathic (sociopathic) individual who has no concept of affection, shame, or guilt, and is characterized by antisocial behaviour. They are often superficially personable, highly manipulative, and totally irresponsible. They have insight and are responsible for their own actions ('bad not mad').

The immunocompromised patient

These are a group of individuals who present special problems because of defects in, or suppression of, their immune system. The condition with the highest profile among these is AIDS.

The chief effect of being immunocompromised is an ↑ susceptibility to infection, often due to opportunistic organisms. Anything which changes the host environment in favour of opportunistic pathogens (e.g. surgery, broad-spectrum antibiotics) can lead to potentially fatal infection with rare or otherwise innocuous organisms.

Drugs Drugs which suppress the immune response, e.g. corticosteroids, ciclosporin, azathioprine, cytotoxics, etc., are now in common use therapeutically. Cross-infection, → Cross-infection prevention and control, p. 750. Aggressive Rx of infections and antimicrobial prophylaxis are needed, → Principles of antibiotic prophylaxis, p. 586.

Congenital immunodeficiency states There are at least 18 of these. The commonest is selective IgA deficiency, which affects ~1:600; it has a wide spectrum of severity but may remain asymptomatic.

Acquired immunodeficiency

Autoimmune disease Autoimmune disease (e.g. SLE, rheumatoid arthritis) carries a minor ↑ risk of infection.

Chronic kidney disease (→ Chronic kidney disease (formerly chronic renal failure), p. 538.) Moderately ↑ risk.

Deficiency states Examples include anaemia. Carry a minor ↑ risk.

Diabetes mellitus Common and carries a moderate ↑ risk of infection.

Infections Severe viral infections, TB, AIDS (specific defect).

Neoplasia All haematological malignancies severely ↑ risk of infection.

AIDS AIDS is caused by infection with HIV. A CD4 T-lymphocyte defect ensues with failure of (mostly) cell-mediated immunity. The HIV antibody is useful as a marker of infectivity but its absence does not guarantee there is no infection present. Infection causes a short flu-like illness, then a variable latent period while CD4 cells ↓ in number. Full-blown AIDS develops when CD4 levels fall critically low. Infections characteristic of AIDS are *Pneumocystis jirovecii* pneumonia and disseminated mycobacterial infection. Kaposi's sarcoma is the tumour most often associated with the condition. The mode of transmission is, essentially, exchange of bodily fluids: unprotected sex, as a recipient of contaminated blood or blood products, or mother-to-fetus transmission. Treatment is with HAART and measures to prevent opportunistic infections. Oral manifestations of AIDS, → Oral manifestations of HIV infection and AIDS, p. 478. Practical procedures for control of cross-infection, → Cross-infection prevention and control, p. 750.

Prophylaxis after needlestick injury This depends on estimation of the likely HIV exposure risk. Triple therapy guidelines in the US. Local implementation via genito-urinary consultant in UK.

Useful emergency kit

Every practice should possess portable apparatus for delivering high-flow O_2. In addition, the facility to deliver nitrous oxide and O_2 mixture, e.g. via an anaesthetic or relative analgesia machine, can be invaluable.

The following should be readily available[2]:

- Automated external defibrillator.
- Basic set of oro-pharyngeal airways, with a self-inflating bag and mask system, e.g. ambu-bag.
- Non-rebreathing oxygen mask with tubing.
- Pocket mask with oxygen port.
- Portable high-vacuum suction.
- 'Spacer' device for inhaled bronchodilators.
- Automated blood glucose measuring device.
- Disposable syringes (2mL, 5mL, and 10mL), needles (19G and 21G), and a tourniquet. Butterfly needles and IV cannulae are great assets to those familiar with their use.
- Alcohol wipes.

Drugs

- Adrenaline, 1:1000 solution (1mg adrenaline in 1mL saline). Auto-injectors (0.3mg) often held by high-risk patients. Salbutamol aerosol inhaler (100 micrograms/actuation).
- Midazolam 10mg buccal.
- Oral glucose solution/tablets/gel/powder.
- Flumazenil 100 micrograms/mL 5mL ampoule (only if providing IV sedation).
- Glucagon 1mg IM injection.
- Aspirin dispersible (300mg).
- Glyceryl trinitrate (GTN) spray (400 micrograms/dose).

This list of drugs really is a *minimum* for any professional performing invasive Rx. Ideally, all public areas, let alone dental practices, should have access to an automated external defibrillator as this is the most valuable single piece of equipment in a cardiac arrest (→ Cardiorespiratory arrest, p. 560). All drugs should be in pre-filled syringes where possible. In hospital, check your 'crash cart' and be amazed at its contents.

▶ If you buy something, learn how to use it!

2 Resuscitation Council (UK) 2013 (updated 2017) *Primary Dental Care – Quality Standards* (ℜ http://www.resus.org.uk/pages/MEdental.pdf).

Fainting

Fainting (vaso-vagal syncope) is innocuous providing it is recognized. It is easily the most common cause of sudden loss of consciousness, with up to 2% of patients fainting before or during dental Rx. The possibility of vaso-vagal syncope while under GA, and hence failure to recognize the condition and correct cerebral hypoxia, is the major reason for recommending the supine position.

Predisposing factors: pain, anxiety, fatigue, relative hyperthermia, and fasting. Characteristic signs and symptoms: a feeling of dizziness and nausea; pale, cold, and clammy skin; a slow, thin, thready pulse which rebounds to become rapid; and loss of consciousness with collapse, if unsupported.

A faint may mimic far more serious conditions, most of which can be excluded by a familiarity with the patient's PMH. These include strokes, corticosteroid insufficiency, drug reactions and interactions, epileptic fit, heart block, hypoglycaemia, and MI.

Prevention
- Avoid predisposing factors.
- Treat patients in the supine position unless specifically contraindicated (e.g. heart failure, pulmonary oedema).

Management
- Lower the head to the level of, or below, the heart. Best achieved by laying the patient flat with legs slightly elevated.
- Loosen clothing (in the presence of a witness!).
- Monitor pulse. If recovery does not occur rapidly, then reconsider the Δ.
- Determine the precipitant and avoid in the future.
- If bradycardia persists with no evidence of recovery to rapid full pulse, try tiny dose of atropine (100 micrograms IV). Dose may be repeated up to 600 micrograms.

Acute chest pain

Severe, acute chest pain is usually the result of ischaemia of the myocardium. The principal differential Δ is between stable angina and an acute coronary syndrome/MI. Both exhibit severe retrosternal pain described as heavy, crushing, or band-like. It is classically preceded by effort, emotion, or excitement, and may radiate to the arms, neck, jaw, and, occasionally, the back or abdomen. Angina is usually rapidly relieved by rest and glyceryl trinitrate (0.5mg) given sublingually, or spray (400 micrograms per spray), which most patients with a history of angina carry with them.

Failure of these methods to relieve the pain, and coexisting sweating, breathlessness, nausea, vomiting, or loss of consciousness with a weak or irregular pulse, suggest an infarct.

Management depends on your immediate environment, but always ensure the patient is placed in a supported *upright* position if conscious, as the supine position increases pulmonary oedema and hence breathlessness.

Management

In dental practice Summon help (ambulance). Administer analgesia; the most appropriate form available here will be nitrous oxide/O_2 mixture (50% O_2). Don't panic. Be prepared should cardiac arrest supervene. Give aspirin 300mg PO. Tell ambulance staff what you have done.

In hospital Nurse upright. Give O_2. Establish IV access and give an opioid analgesic if available (2.5–5mg of diamorphine is most useful). Get ECG, U&Es. Summon help; in units integrated into general or teaching hospitals this may best be achieved by contacting the medical on-call team via the switchboard urgently, as thrombolysis or 1° endovascular intervention, if appropriate, improve outcome.

Cardiorespiratory arrest

▶ Don't await 'expertise'. *ACT*.

Ninety per cent of deaths from cardiac arrest occurring outside hospital are due to ventricular fibrillation (VF). This is also the commonest arrest pattern seen in hospital. It is potentially reversible by prompt (<90sec) defibrillation. The commonest underlying cause is ischaemic heart disease, but other causes may exist, especially in younger people. Acute asthma, anaesthesia, drug overdose, electrocution, immersion, or hypothermia often precipitate pulseless electrical activity (PEA) arrests. These are treatable conditions and potentially reversible.

In certain instances properly performed cardiopulmonary resuscitation (CPR) can sustain life for up to an hour while a precipitating condition is being treated.

Diagnosis and management These proceed simultaneously (Fig. 13.1).

Approach and assess Protect yourself! Do not become another casualty, whether in the street, practice, or hospital environment. Gently 'shake and shout' to assess the person's level of consciousness. If there is no response, shout for help (and ask whoever goes for help to come back to tell you if help is coming). *Then*:

• In witnessed and monitored arrests a single sharp blow over the heart (precordial thump) is worthwhile.
• Airway—carry out a chin lift or jaw thrust, and clear oropharynx. Remove loose dentures, but retain if they are well fitting (it gives a better mouth seal).
• Breathing—look, listen, and feel for breathing for no more than 10sec (if hypothermia suspected, up to 1min). If the person is breathing normally, place in recovery position. If not, get help even if this means leaving the patient yourself to do it.
• Commence chest compressions, at the middle of the lower half of the sternum, delivering 30 compressions in the first instance, before providing 2 rescue breaths.
• Remember, statistically the patient's best chance at survival once absence of breathing is confirmed is defibrillation; therefore, getting early help may be the most useful thing you can do. Children and victims of trauma or drowning are exceptions and may benefit from 1min of resuscitation before you leave to get help.

Rates of compression/ventilation

• CPR, single and two rescuers: 30 compressions to 2 ventilations.
• Aim for 100–120 compressions/min.

For those working in an environment where facilities for advanced life support (defibrillation, intubation/ventilation) exist, the 2015 UK Resuscitation Council/International Liaison Committee on Resuscitation (ILCOR) guidelines are reproduced in Fig. 13.2 and Fig. 13.3.

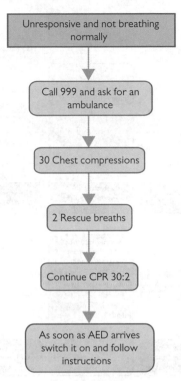

Fig. 13.1 Adult basic life support. AED, automated external defibrillator.
Reproduced with the kind permission of the Resuscitation Council (UK).

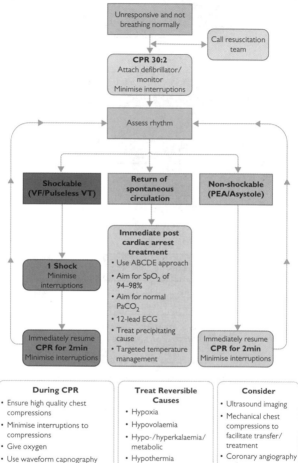

Fig. 13.2 Algorithm for advanced cardiac life support.
Reproduced with the kind permission of the Resuscitation Council (UK).

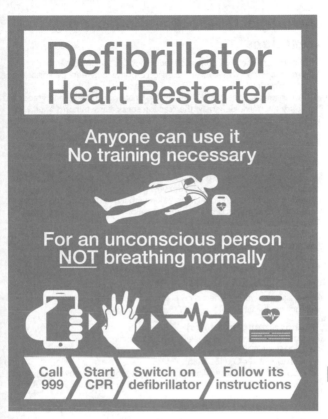

Fig. 13.3 Regarding the use of automated external defibrillators, the process is usually straightforward with modern devices.

Reproduced with the kind permission of the British Heart Foundation.

Anaphylactic shock and other drug reactions

Penicillins are the commonest offender, but it is worth remembering that there is a 10% cross-over in allergic response between penicillins and cephalosporins.

An anaphylactic reaction is not an all-or-nothing response, and grades of severity are seen. Generally, the reaction starts a few minutes after a par-enteral injection, and not immediately as does a simple faint. Some caution should be exercised, though, as the quicker the onset of an anaphylactic reaction the more severe it is likely to be. Some patients with known severe allergic reactions/previous anaphylaxis will carry an auto-injector (0.3mg adrenaline) to self-administer at the first sign of symptoms.

Principal symptoms are facial flushing, itching, numbness, cold extrem-ities, nausea, and sometimes abdominal pain. Signs include wheezing, facial swelling and rash, and cold clammy skin with a thin, thready pulse. Loss of consciousness may occur, with extreme pallor which progresses to cyanosis as respiratory failure develops.

It can be difficult to distinguish anaphylaxis from acute asthma in, e.g. an asthmatic given an NSAID they are allergic to. Don't panic, just go through management for acute asthma, then start on management for anaphylaxis (Fig. 13.4). Adrenaline is a bronchodilator anyway.

Angio-oedema Angio-oedema is sudden onset, with severe face and neck allergic swelling. The airway is at risk and therefore should be managed as for anaphylaxis.

Management (in adults)
- Place patient supine with legs raised, if possible.
- Check ABCDE (Airway, Breathing, Circulation, Disability + Exposure) and administer O_2 (15L/min).
- 0.5mL of 1:1000 adrenaline IM. Repeat after 5min, then every 5min until improved. Do not give IV—this concentration will induce ventricular fibrillation.
- If in practice, an ambulance should be called and the patient transferred to hospital, where the following may be carried out:
  - Fluid challenge—500–1000mL rapidly—the type of fluid isn't important, just plenty and fast.
  - 200mg of hydrocortisone IV.
  - 10mg of chlorphenamine slowly IV (if available).
  - O_2 by mask.
  - Salbutamol 0.5mg/mL (1mL) as IM or SC injection in patients on non-cardioselective beta-blockers if no response to adrenaline.

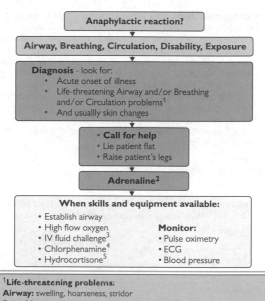

Anaphylactic reaction?

Airway, Breathing, Circulation, Disability, Exposure

Diagnosis - look for:
- Acute onset of illness
- Life-threatening Airway and/or Breathing and/or Circulation problems[1]
- And usually skin changes

- **Call for help**
- Lie patient flat
- Raise patient's legs

Adrenaline[2]

When skills and equipment available:
- Establish airway
- High flow oxygen
- IV fluid challenge[3]
- Chlorphenamine[4]
- Hydrocortisone[5]

Monitor:
- Pulse oximetry
- ECG
- Blood pressure

[1]**Life-threatening problems:**
Airway: swelling, hoarseness, stridor
Breathing: rapid breathing, wheeze, fatigue, cyanosis, SpO_2 < 92% confusion
Circulation: pale, clammy, low blood pressure, faintness, drowsy/coma

[2]**Adrenaline** (give IM unless experienced with IV adrenaline)
IM doses of 1:1000 adrenaline (repeat after 5 min if no better)
- Adult   500 micrograms IM (0.5 mL)
- Child more than 12 years: 500 micrograms IM (0.5 mL)
- Child 6–12 years: 300 micrograms IM (0.3 mL)
- Child less than 6 years: 150 micrograms IM (0.15 mL)

Adrenaline IV to be given only by experienced specialists
Titrate: Adults 50 micrograms; Children 1 microgram/kg

[3]**IV fluid challenge:**
Adult - 500–1000 mL
Child - crystalloid 20 mL/kg

Stop IV colloid
if this might be the cause
of anaphylaxis

	[4]Chlorphenamine (IM or slow IV)	[5]Hydrocortisone (IM or slow IV)
Adult or child more than 12 years	10 mg	200 mg
Child 6–12 years	5 mg	100 mg
Child 6 months to 6 years	2.5 mg	50 mg
Child less than 6 months	250 microgram/kg	25 mg

Fig. 13.4 Treatment for anaphylaxis algorithm.
Reproduced with the kind permission of the Resuscitation Council (UK).

Other drug reactions and interactions While there are a multi-tude of drug interactions which the dental surgeon should be aware of as a prescriber, the drugs most liable to present an emergency problem to the dentist are those which we administer as LAs.

Although it is possible to achieve toxic levels of lidocaine, adrenaline, prilocaine, or felypressin without intravascular injection, this gener-ally requires a particularly cavalier attitude to the administration of LA. Commonly, this effect is due to intravascular injection of a substantial pro-portion of a cartridge of LA. Confusion, peri-oral tingling, drowsiness, agi-tation, fits, or loss of consciousness may occur. Do not use more than 10 × 2.2mL cartridges of lidocaine/adrenaline (440mg lidocaine). In practice, you will rarely consider coming near this amount.

Management
- Stop procedure! (They won't be numb.)
- Place supine.
- Maintain airway, give O_2.
- Await spontaneous recovery (in ~30min) unless tragically a serious event such as MI supervenes, in which case treat as indicated.

Collapse in a patient with a history of corticosteroid use

The use of corticosteroids therapeutically or otherwise for whatever cause may suppress the adrenal response to stress. The longer the course of Rx and the higher the dose used, the more likely this is to occur. It is almost certain that a large number of people have unnecessary 'prophylaxis' with hydrocortisone and many would now argue that without evidence (short Synacthen® test) of adrenocortical insufficiency it is unnecessary. However, we take the view that you are less likely to cause harm by a brief supplementation of steroid than you are by ignoring the potential problem because it happens to be rare in reality.

It is worth remembering that virtually all serious steroid unwanted effects are from chronic usage (acute steroid-induced psychosis being the exception—a risk from the high-dose orthognathic regimens).

The prime aim is to prevent the occurrence of stress-induced collapse; therefore, if patients have received steroids in the past year or are on steroids at present, cover any stressful procedure, anaesthetic, infection, or episode of trauma with 25–50mg hydrocortisone IM (IV if under GA) 30min prior to elective stress. Seriously ill patients require IV qds doses covering the period of admission. It is a fallacy to believe you are ↓ risk of steroid unwanted effects by trying to avoid giving prophylactic steroids. Doubling the oral dose may work but is rather hit and miss. Calculating an 'exact' dose is unnecessarily complicated and risks people 'forgetting'. Stick to sticking them with 25–50mg hydrocortisone IM unless you have a very valid reason to change.

In patients presenting acutely, treat immediately. If collapse occurs in such a patient, Δ is established by pallor, rapid, thin pulse with a profound and sudden ↓ in BP, and loss of consciousness.

Management
- Place in supine position. Maintain airway. Give O_2. Obtain IV access.
- 200mg hydrocortisone IV immediately.
- Ensure help (i.e. an ambulance) is requested.
- Exclude other causes of collapse.

Fits

The majority of epileptic fits do not require active intervention as the patient will usually recover spontaneously. All that is needed is sensible positioning to prevent the patient from damaging themselves. Fits may be precipitated in a known epileptic by starvation, flickering lights, certain drugs such as methohexital, tricyclics, or alcohol, or menstruation. They may also follow a deep faint.

Diagnosis Many epileptics have a preceding aura followed by sudden loss of consciousness with a rigid extended appearance and generalized jerking movements. Frequently, they are incontinent of urine and may bite their tongue. There is a slow recovery with the patient feeling sleepy and dazed. There may be a *cause* for the fitting: trauma, tumour, and alcohol withdrawal are common. There are numerous others, any adult should have a first fit fully investigated by a neurologist.

▶ Should the fitting be repeated or last >5min, the patient has entered the state of status epilepticus. This is an emergency and requires urgent control.

Management Get help. In a simple major fit, the patient should be placed in the recovery position when practicable and allowed to recover. If they enter status epilepticus, 10mg midazolam IV/buccal/nasal usually aborts the fit; beware respiratory depression. Assess cardiorespiratory function; clear and maintain airway, and give O_2 if available. It is worthwhile considering placing an IV cannula or a butterfly in any epileptic patient with less than perfect control, as stress is an important precipitant. Status epilepticus should not be allowed to continue for >20min as the mortality rate (up to 30%) and chance of permanent brain damage ↑ with the length of attack.

Management in hospital Get help. After giving IV benzodiazepines (lorazepam 4mg, midazolam or 10mg diazepam as emulsion 10–20mg) and maintaining an airway, give an IV bolus of up to 50mL of 20–50% glucose unless you are certain blood glucose is >5mmol/L. Establish a 0.9% saline infusion and repeat the benzodiazepines if necessary. If the fits are not controlled it may be necessary to use a phenytoin infusion or induce anaesthesia with thiopental, an IV barbiturate, paralyse, and ventilate.

Hypoglycaemia

Hypoglycaemia is the diabetic emergency most likely to present to the dentist. It is an acute and dangerous complication of diabetes and may result from a missed meal, excess insulin, or ↑ calorific need due to exercise or stress. Most diabetics are expert in detecting the onset of hypoglycaemia themselves; however, a small number may lose this ability, particularly if changed to a new form of insulin. Recognition of this state is essential and an acutely collapsed diabetic should be assumed hypoglycaemic until proven otherwise, e.g. by blood glucose monitoring sticks or blood glucose levels.

Diagnosis Disorientation, irritability, increasing drowsiness, excitability, or aggression in a known diabetic, suggest hypoglycaemia. They often appear to be drunk.

Treatment

- If conscious, give glucose orally in any available form. Repeat if necessary every 10–15min. Get help.
- If impaired consciousness, give buccal glucose gel &/or 1mg of IM glucagon.
- If unconscious, protect airway and place in recovery position. If the correct kit is available, establish IV access and give up to 50mL of 20–50% glucose.

Acute asthma

An acute asthmatic attack may be induced in a patient predisposed to bronchospasm by exposure to an allergen, infection, cold, exercise, or anxiety. Characteristically, the patient will complain of a *tight chest* and shortness of breath. Examination will reveal breathlessness, with widespread expiratory wheezing. The accessory muscles of respiration may be used to support breathing. If the patient is unable to talk, you are dealing with a potentially fatal episode.

Management Make use of the patient's own anti-asthmatic drugs, such as salbutamol inhalers. Ideally, this should be administered in the form of a nebulizer using 24% O_2 and nebulized salbutamol. A do-it-yourself spacer can be fabricated from the patient's own inhaler pushed through the base of a paper cup. Repeated depressions of inhaler plunger will create an aerosol inside the cup which the patient can inhale. This will relieve most reversible airways obstruction. Steroids should be administered either as oral prednisolone, if the patient carries these with them, or as IV hydrocortisone up to 200mg IV, if available. This combination of salbutamol, steroids, and O_2 will often completely resolve an attack; however, in individuals who do not respond, an urgent hospital admission is required. Patients who are only partially responsive must have underlying irritants such as a chest infection either excluded or treated.

▶ Be aware of the possibility of anaphylaxis mimicking acute asthma. Remember adrenaline 0.5mL 1:1000 IM.

Management in dental practice
- Keep the patient upright.
- Administer salbutamol by inhaler and a spacer device. Repeat every 10min until resolved (or ambulance arrives).
- Give O_2.

If a complete response takes place, it is reasonable to allow the patient to return home. If there is any doubt, arrange for the patient to be seen at the nearest emergency department.

Management in hospital
- Nurse patient upright.
- Give nebulized salbutamol 5mg (with O_2) at 15–30min intervals, continuously if necessary.
- Give nebulized ipratropium 500 micrograms (with O_2).
- Establish IV access and give up to 200mg hydrocortisone IV or prednisolone 40mg PO.
- Monitor peak expiratory flow, arterial blood gases, and pulse oximetry.
- Obtain a CXR; exclude infection, pneumothorax.
- If incomplete response, obtain expert help rather than embarking on alternative Rx such as aminophylline.

Inhaled foreign bodies

The combination of delicate instruments and the supine position of patients for many dental procedures inevitably ↑ the risk of a patient inhaling a foreign body. Patients with facial trauma often have missing teeth—always think where could they be? Two basic scenarios are likely, depending on whether or not the item impacts in the upper or lower airway.

Upper airway This will stimulate the cough reflex, which may be sufficient to clear the obstruction. A choking subject should be bent forward to aid coughing. If the obstruction is complete or there are signs of cyanosis in:

- *Conscious patient*—support chest with one hand, strike between the scapulae with the heel of your other hand. Repeat up to five times if needed. If this fails, carry out abdominal thrusts (Heimlich manoeuvre) by encircling the victim with your arms from behind and delivering a sharp upward and inward squeeze to create sudden expulsion of air. Repeat up to five times. Alternate five back blows with the five abdominal thrusts. The first attempt is most likely to succeed and they may vomit.
- *Unconscious patient*—CPR should be commenced; this will provide circulatory support as well as help dislodge the foreign body.[3]

If all else fails, cricothyroid puncture may preserve life if the obstruction lies above this level.

Lower airway As only a segment of the lungs will be occluded, this presents a less acute problem. It is also easier to miss. Classically, this involves a tooth or tooth fragment slipping from the forceps and being inhaled. With the patient in a semi-upright position, the object ends up in the right posterior basal lobe. Should this happen, inform the patient and arrange to have a CXR taken as soon as possible. If the offending item is in the lungs (Fig. 13.5), removal by a chest physician by fibre-optic bronchoscopy is indicated, as failure to remove the tooth is inevitably followed by collapse and infection distal to the obstruction. Rarely, lobectomy may be needed.

3 Resuscitation Council (UK) 2015 *Adult Basic Life Support and AEDs* (⅏ https://www.resus.org.uk/resuscitation-guidelines/).

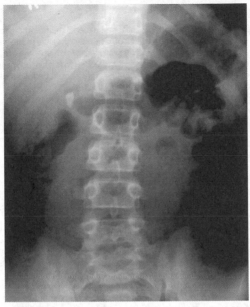

Fig. 13.5 When a lost tooth cannot be located, it must be searched for; ingestion is not a real problem but inhaled teeth must be removed.

If in doubt

When presented with a suddenly collapsed patient, the first thing to assess is your own response. Don't panic.[4] You are only of value to the patient if you can function rationally. Always instigate a call for help—we are all useless without it. If presented with a case of sudden loss of consciousness, in the absence of an obvious Δ, the following steps should be followed.

• Maintain the airway and provide O_2 if available.
• Place in the supine position. If the patient has simply fainted they will recover virtually immediately.
• Are they breathing? If not then get help before starting CPR (➔ Cardiorespiratory arrest, p. 560). If they are breathing normally:
  • If in dental practice, give glucagon 1mg IM.
  • If in hospital, establish IV access and give up to 20mL 20–50% glucose IV.
  • Give hydrocortisone up to 200mg IV.
  • If unable to get access, use glucagon 1mg IM.

These measures will usually resolve most cases of sudden, non-traumatic loss of consciousness.

If the patient is acutely distressed and breathless they should be treated in an upright position and given O_2 while you try to differentiate between an acute asthmatic attack, anaphylaxis, and heart failure, and treat as indicated.

Always ensure that someone has requested assistance in the form of an ambulance or, if in hospital, that the appropriate staff have been contacted. If at all possible, try to speak to the receiving doctor *yourself*.

Immediately after resolution of an emergency there tends to be a period of numb inactivity among the staff involved. Use this period to review your management of the situation and carefully document what happened. If the patient has been transferred to hospital or another department, a brief, legible account of proceedings must accompany them. Include drugs used, their dosages, and when they were given. Try to ensure that a friend or relation of the patient is aware of the situation.

4 Thank you Douglas Adams!

Management of the dental in-patient

The vast majority of in-patients will experience considerable anxiety on being admitted for operation, including about those procedures which are in themselves 'routine'. In addition, as dentists have little training in medical clerking and ward work, there is a substantial risk of compounding an already stressful situation by being overly stressed yourself. Minimize this by preparation. Learn about the ward(s) you will work on before taking up a post. Never be afraid to ask nursing staff if you are unsure, and try to know a day in advance what cases are coming in.

Pre-operation

All patients attending as in-patients for operation must (i) be examined and 'clerked' and (ii) have consented to surgery. In addition, many will require a variety of pre-operative investigations; these vary widely from consultant to consultant, so get to know the local variations. Common investigations and their indications are listed in the following paragraphs (Sampling techniques, ➲ For sampling, p. 578; samples, ➲ Investigations—general, p. 14).

Clerking This basically consists of taking a complete medical and dental history from the patient, including any drugs they are taking at present (which you must remember to continue while in hospital by writing up in the drug 'kardex'), a family history for inherited disease, and a social history for problems related to smoking, alcohol, drug abuse, and ability to cope at home post-operatively. This is followed by a systematic clinical examination (➲ Medical examination, p. 8). Any special investigations are then arranged, and the results of these should be seen before the patient goes to theatre. Any problems uncovered should be relayed to the anaesthetist, who is the only person capable of saying whether or not the patient is 'fit for anaesthesia'. Any required pre-, peri-, or post-operative drugs are written up (➲ Prescribing, p. 596).

Consent All patients undergoing GA or sedation must give written, informed consent. It is advised that patients receiving interventions under LA also do so. Every hospital has its own surgical consent form which you complete. After having the procedure and its likely potential risks explained, the patient also signs. It is essential that you are happy in your own mind that you understand what the operation entails, current UK regulations suggest the surgeon who will operate or someone who is capable of doing the operation should take the consent. Obtain consent only for procedures with which you are familiar.

Investigations

See ➲ Investigations—general, p. 14.

Full blood count Elderly patients. Any suspicion of anaemia.

Sickle cell test All Afro-Caribbeans for GA. Consider also those of Mediterranean, Arabic, or Indian origin. There may be a local policy but usually not. Ask your anaesthetist.

Urea and electrolytes All patients needing IV fluids, on diuretics, diabetics, or with renal disease. Have a low threshold for doing this test.

Coagulation screen All major surgery, any past history of bleeding disorders, liver disease, or history of ↑ alcohol, anticoagulants.

Liver function tests Liver disease, alcohol, major surgery.

Group and save/cross-match Major surgery, trauma, shock, anaemia.

ECG heart disease All major surgery, most patients >50yrs.

CXR trauma Active chest disease, possible metastases.

Hepatitis B and C and HIV markers Varies; usually at-risk groups only; pre-test counselling now considered mandatory. Check local hospital policy.

Post-operation
Immediately post-operation, patients are resuscitated in a recovery room adjacent to theatre, with a nurse monitoring cardiorespiratory function. Once recovered, unless they are to be monitored in the ICU/HDU, they will be returned to the ward. In all patients, ensure a patent airway and consider the following:

Analgesia May take the form of LA (should be given post-anaesthetic/ pre-surgery), oral or parenteral NSAIDs, or oral or parenteral opioids. Immediately post-operatvely, analgesia is best given parenterally. Antiemetics such as cyclizine 50mg oral, IM, or IV, or ondansetron 4mg IM or IV should be given if nausea or vomiting is present. Many anaesthetists consider this their responsibility—ask.

Antimicrobials Given in accordance with the selected regimen (→ Principles of antibiotic prophylaxis, p. 586). Certain patients may benefit from corticosteroids pre- and post-operatively to ↓ oedema; regimens vary.

Nutrition A problem principally for patients undergoing major head and neck cancer surgery (→ Oral cancer, p. 452), who should have had a dietetic assessment pre-operatively and a decision made about post-operative feeding (nasogastric tube, gastrostomy) but it is worthwhile reminding nursing staff to order soft diets for all oral surgery patients who can feed by mouth and to have liquidizers available for patients in IMF.

Fluid balance Covered in → Intravenous fluids, p. 579.

Post-operative airway Special consideration needs to be given to patients in IMF and those with tracheostomies. Immediate post-operative rigid IMF is now rare; however, post-operative elastic IMF is common. These patients need to be specially attended by a nurse looking after that patient only, for the first 12–24h ('specialed'). Lighting, suction, and the ability to place the patient head-down if they vomit, is mandatory. Other techniques include tongue suture, prolonged retention of a nasopharyngeal airway, elective prolonged intubation, and tracheostomy. Avoiding this situation, see → Treatment of facial fractures, p. 500. Tracheostomy is a great aid to secure airway management, but enormously inconvenient for patients and has its own complications. If indicated it is essential to care for the tube by suction and humidification to ensure patency.

Venepuncture and arterial puncture

Venepuncture To become proficient in the skills of venepuncture you must practise the art in all its forms. To develop the skill of placing IV cannulae, cultivate a sympathetic anaesthetist, as anaesthetized patients are venodilated and will not feel pain! When carrying out cannulations and arterial punctures on patients in the ward, a drop or two of 2% plain ligno-caine deposited SC with a fine needle will aid both your peace of mind and the patient's comfort. While most hospitals have phlebotomy services you will be asked to get blood and cannulate out of hours and when the phle-botomists fail, so learn as soon as you can.

Tools of the trade Tourniquet, alcohol wipes, cotton wool. Green (21G) needles and butterflies are commonly used. Many hospitals have adopted sealed 'vacutainer' systems which are convenient but fiddly to use. Learn the basics first, then your hospital's system. Sometimes finer needles or butterflies are needed, e.g. blue (23G). Many hospitals now have sealed sterile 'cannulation packs' for bedside use. Patients who are difficult to can-nulate can have fluids and certain drugs through fine (20G) or even 22G IV cannulae; most have 18G. Shocked patients or those needing blood should have at least a 16G and preferably a 14G cannula inserted. Note that gauges and colours are not consistent between needles and cannulae.

Sites of puncture

For sampling First choice is the cubital fossa. Inspect and palpate; veins you can feel are better than those you can only see. Insert the needle at a 30–40° angle to the skin and along the line of the vein. If no veins are found in the cubital fossa, try the back of the hand with a butterfly and use a similar approach. The veins of the dorsum of the foot are a last resort before the femoral vein lying just medial to the femoral artery in the groin.

For infusion Single-bolus injections; use a 21G butterfly in a vein on the back of the hand.

For IV fluids or multiple IV injections place a 18G IV cannula in a straight segment of vein in the forearm, hand, or just proximal to the 'anatomical snuffbox'. Try to avoid crossing a joint as the cannula tissues more quickly if subjected to repeated movements. When inserting the cannula ensure the skin overlying the vein is fixed by finger pressure; pierce the skin, and move the stylet along the line of the vein until it enters the vein and blood flows into the cannula. As soon as you enter the vein, pull the stylet back into the cannula to minimize the risk of going through the vein. Insert the full length of the cannula into the vein and secure. Keep patent with saline flush.

Arterial puncture Whenever possible, obtain an arterial sampling syr-inge. Use LA unless the patient is anaesthetized. The syringe and needle must be flushed with heparin. Use radial, brachial, or femoral arteries. Palpate, prepare area with alcohol wipe, and insert needle at 30–60° to skin. When the needle enters the artery, blood pulsates into the syringe. Only 1–2mL are needed. All ITUs have a blood gas analyser and some other areas of your hospital will have one too; find out where it is and how to use it. If not, the specimen goes in a chilled bag to the biochemist. The puncture site needs to be firmly pressed on for 2–3min to prevent formation of a painful haematoma.

Intravenous fluids

Principles The maintenance of daily fluid requirements plus replacement of any abnormal loss by infusion of (usually) isotonic solutions. Normal requirements are ~2.5–3L in 24h. This is lost via urine (normal renal function needs an absolute minimum of 30mL/h, but aim for 60mL/h, faecal loss, and sweating. Where possible replace with oral fluids; IV fluids are a second best.

Common IV regimens 1L normal saline (0.9%) and 2L 5% glucose in 24h ('2 sweet and 1 salty'). Add 20mmol potassium chloride per litre after 36h, unless U&Es suggest otherwise. Hartmann's solution/Plasma-Lyte 148 are more expensive but the most physiological crystalloids. Increase these in the presence of abnormal losses, burns, fever, dehydration, polyuria, and in the event of haemorrhage or shock.

Special needs
- For burns, start with Hartmann's and be guided by the burns centre.
- For fever, use saline.
- For dehydration or polyuria, use 5% glucose, unless hyponatraemic. Exception is ketoacidosis: use saline.
- Haemorrhage demands replacement whole blood if available (it rarely is); packed cells are what you will be offered in most hospitals in most countries.
- Shock needs, crystalloid challenge (not 5% glucose—use saline/ Hartmann's), blood and control of haemorrhage. Be guided by the pulse, BP, urine output, haemoglobin, the haematocrit, and the U&Es.

↓ fluid load in heart failure, and avoid saline. Shock and dehydration are rare complications of maxillofacial trauma or any other condition principally presenting to the dentist; therefore in their presence consider damage to other body systems and seek appropriate advice.

Polyuria Post-operatively, is usually due to over-transfusion. Review anaesthetic notes, and if this is the case simply catheterize and observe.

Oliguria Post-operatively, is usually due to under-transfusion or dehydration pre- or peri-operatively. First, palpate abdomen for ↑ bladder and listen to chest to exclude pulmonary oedema. Then catheterize the patient to exclude urinary retention and allow close monitoring of fluid balance. Then ↑ rate of infusion of fluid (max 1L/h) *unless* the patient is in heart failure or bleeding. The former needs specialist advice, the latter needs blood or an operation. In an otherwise healthy post-operative patient, if this does not produce a minimum of 30mL/h of urine, a diuretic (20–40mg furosemide PO/IV) may be tried. Take care when using fluid challenges, as if failure to pass urine is renal it is possible to fluid overload the patient quickly. Review the fluid balance and U&Es over several days for an overview.

Blood transfusion

▶ Group and save—you won't get blood; group and cross-match—you will get blood in ~1h; type specific group—you will get blood urgently.

Blood may be required for patients in an acute (e.g. traumatized) situation, electively (e.g. peri-operatively) during major surgery, or to correct a chronic anaemia (🔁 Anaemia, p. 578). In practice, the former two are much more commonly encountered by junior dental staff.

Whole blood Indicated in patients who have lost >20% blood volume, exhibit signs of hypovolaemic shock, or in whom this appears inevitable.

▶ Remember maxillofacial injuries *alone* only rarely result in this degree of blood loss (🔁 Bleeding, p. 490).

Always take blood for grouping in severely traumatized patients, and proceed to cross-match as indicated by the clinical signs. Always use cross-matched blood, except in utter extremis when O-rhesus –ve blood can be used. Massive transfusions create problems with hyperkalaemia, thrombocytopenia, and low levels of clotting factors; therefore in patients with severe haemorrhage, simultaneous fresh frozen plasma (4–6 units) and platelets (6 units) will be needed. Most laboratories only provide packed cells.

Autologous blood Blood donated by a patient prior to elective surgery for use only on themselves. It avoids risks of cross-infection but requires a specially interested haematology department, so check locally. Autotransfusion is sometimes used in vascular surgery.

Packed cells Used for the correction of anaemia if too severe for correction with iron, or if needed prior to urgent surgery. This ↓ the fluid load to the patient, but elderly individuals and those in heart failure should have their transfusion covered with a small dose of furosemide PO or IV.

Useful tips
- Cross-match one patient at a time and be sure you are familiar with local procedures.
- Nurse will perform regular observations of temperature, pulse, respiration, and urine output during transfusion—look at them!
- Don't use a giving set which has contained glucose, as the blood will clog.
- Except in shock, transfuse slowly (1 unit over 2–4h; >4h the cannulae start to clog).
- 1 unit of blood raises the Hb by 1g/dL = 3% haematocrit.

Complications
- ABO incompatibility. Causes anaphylaxis; manage accordingly (🔁 Anaphylactic shock and other drug reactions, p. 564).
- Cross-infection.
- Heart failure can be induced by over-rapid transfusion.
- Milder allergic transfusion reactions are the commonest problem; Rx by slowing the transfusion. If progressive or temperature >40°C stop transfusion and inform laboratory to check cross-matching. IV hydrocortisone 100mg and chlorphenamine 10mg are useful standbys.
- Citrate toxicity is a hazard of very large transfusions and can be countered by 10mL of calcium gluconate with alternate units.

Catheterization

This is not a topic normally covered by the dental syllabus, but the dental graduate may find him- or herself confronted with a patient needing urethral catheterization if working on an oral and maxillofacial surgical ward. The only procedure they are likely to need to be able to perform is temporary urethral catheterization. This is indicated for urinary retention (almost always post-operatively), for precise measurement of fluid balance, or, rarely, to avoid use of bedpan or bottle. Avoid catheterization if a history of pelvic trauma is present, as an expert is needed. Catheters are associated with a high incidence of urinary tract infections, and the presence of a urinary tract infection is a relative C/I.

Equipment Most wards have their own; ask for it and ensure you have an assistant available. It should contain a tube of local anaesthetic gel, a dish with some aqueous chlorhexidine, swabs, a waterproof sheet with a hole in the middle, sterile gloves, a 10-mL syringe filled with sterile water, and a drainage bag. In most cases a 14–16 French gauge Foley catheter will suffice. Use a silicone catheter if you anticipate it being *in situ* for more than a few days.

Procedure Explain what you are going to do and why. If catheterizing for post-operative fluid balance, do it in the anaesthetic room after intubation (ask the anaesthetist first!). The operating theatre is the best place to learn. The procedure can be made aseptic by wearing two pairs of disposable gloves; one pair is discarded after achieving analgesia, which is done by instillation of lidocaine gel (also acts as a lubricant). Find the urethral opening and, using the nozzle supplied, squeeze in the contents of the tube. In the female, finding the opening is the only significant problem and most women are catheterized by female nursing staff. In the male, it is necessary to massage the gel along the length of the penis and leave *in situ* for several minutes before progressing. Once analgesia is obtained, the female urethra is easily catheterized; if you have been unable to find the meatus to instil LA you should not proceed but get help instead. In the male, hold the penis upright and insert the tip of the catheter; pass it gently down the urethra until it reaches the penoscrotal junction, pull the penis down so that it lies between the patient's thighs, thereby straightening out the curves of the urethra, and advance the tip into the bladder until urine flows.

Once urine flows, the catheter balloon can be inflated with sterile water. In the conscious patient it should be painless; if not, deflate the balloon and reposition the catheter. In the anaesthetized patient, insert the catheter all the way, inflate, then pull back. Connect the drainage bag and remember to replace the foreskin over the glans to avoid a paraphimosis.

▶ If, in the presence of adequate analgesia, you are unable to pass the catheter *do not* persist, but get expert assistance.

Enteral and parenteral feeding

The main role for this type of feeding, as far as dental staff are concerned, is in the care of debilitated patients and those undergoing surgery for head and neck cancers. In view of the latter, it is worthwhile having a basic understanding of the subject.

Enteral feeding Enteral feeding is providing liquid, low-residue foods either by mouth, fine-bore nasogastric tube, or gastrostomy. A range of proprietary products are available for these feeds. Be guided by the local dietitian, who has expertise in this area which you will lack. The major problem is osmotic diarrhoea, which can be ↓ by starting with dilute solutions.

Fine-bore nasogastric tubes These are the mainstay in enteral nutrition for patients undergoing major oropharyngeal surgery. In many institutions, nurses are not allowed to pass these tubes, although they are allowed to pass standard nasogastric tubes for aspirating stomach contents. You can therefore find yourself asked to pass such a tube by someone who is more proficient but forbidden to do so. Gastrostomy tubes are placed by the relevant specialists (and have higher complication rates).

Technique Wear gloves. Explain the procedure to the patient and have them at 50–60° upright with neck in neutral position. Place a small amount of lidocaine gel in the chosen nostril after ensuring it is patent. Keep a small drink of water handy. Select a tube; check the guidewire is lubricated and does not protrude. If a tracheostomy tube is present, the cuff should be deflated to allow passage of the tube. Lubricate the tube and introduce it into the nostril; pass it horizontally along the nasal floor. There is usually a little resistance as the tube reaches the nasopharynx; press past this and ask the patient to swallow (use the water if this helps). The tube should now pass easily down the oesophagus, entering the stomach at 40cm. Secure the tube to the forehead with sticky tape and only now remove the guidewire, being careful to shield the patient's eyes. Inject air into the tube and listen for bubbling over the stomach. Confirm position with a CXR. (Some systems require leaving a radio-opaque guidewire in prior to X-ray: check the tube you are using.)

Problems
- Nasal patency. Select the least narrow nostril, use a lubricant, and, if necessary, a smaller tube and topical vasoconstrictor.
- Gagging/vomiting. Press ahead; all sphincters are open.
- Tube coiling into mouth. Cooling the tube makes it more rigid and often helps. As a last resort, topical anaesthesia and direct visualization with a laryngoscope or nasendoscope, while an assistant passes the tube, may be necessary.
- Tube pulled out by patient. If they must have the tube, consider a nasogastric tube 'bridle' designed for this problem or a stitch to the septum or soft tissue of the nose.

Parenteral feeding Hazardous and expensive. Central or peripheral lines are required and need to be maintained. Neither as safe nor efficient as enteral feeding. Avoid if at all possible.

Refeeding syndrome Patients who have been starved for >5 days and are then fed enterally or parenterally risk this electrolyte and fluid imbalance characterized by severe hypophosphataemia with other biochemical disturbances. Avoid by supplementation with B vitamins and gradated biochemical correction.[5]

Percutaneous endoscopic gastrostomy (PEG) Feeding tube placed directly in stomach through abdominal wall at endoscopy.

Radiologically inserted gastrostomy (RIG) X-ray (or US)-guided version of a PEG. Needs nasogastric tube in place to inflate stomach.

5 E. Reber et al. 2019 *J Clin Med* 13 8.

Pain control

LA (→ Local analgesia—tools of the trade, p. 626); RA (→ Sedation—relative analgesia, p. 632); IV sedation (→ IV sedation, p. 634); cryoanalgesia (→ Cryosurgery, p. 634).

Pain control aims to relieve symptoms while identifying and removing the cause; the exception is when the cause is not treatable, as in palliative and terminal care. Then, the approach is to deal with the symptoms to enable the patient to have a quality to their life.

Acute and post-operative pain May often be well controlled by LA (→ Local analgesia—tools of the trade, p. 626), but it is often necessary to use systemic analgesics. Useful analgesics in this situation include paracetamol (1000mg PO/PR/IV 4-hourly) and ibuprofen (400–600mg 8-hourly). Both these can be combined with codeine (8–30mg). NSAIDs such as diclofenac (50mg PO 8-hourly or 75mg IM perioperatively, followed by one further dose of 75mg IM). These drugs are all simple analgesics and, with the exception of paracetamol, have the advantage of an anti-inflammatory action which is at least as important as their central analgesic effect. In *post-operative* pain, opioid analgesics are helpful when used parenterally and short term. Morphine 10mg 3–4-hourly combined with an antiemetic such as metoclopramide (10mg IM/IV) is useful in the immediate post-operative period. Patient-controlled analgesia (PCA) systems (see p. 585) after major surgery are commonly used. They are set up by the anaesthetists.

Pain following maxillofacial trauma This is a problem, as these patients must be assessed neurologically for evidence of head injury which C/I opioids. The addition of codeine phosphate (60mg IM) to a NSAID is often effective and does not significantly interfere with neurological observations. Alternatively, PR or IM diclofenac sodium may suffice. There is often a hospital acute pain team who will be happy to advise in difficult cases.

Facial pain Facial pain not of dental or iatrogenic origin is covered in → Facial pain, p. 464. These conditions often require the use of co-analgesics such as antidepressants, antiepileptics, and anxiolytics.

Pain control in terminal disease An important subject in its own right. Points to note include aim for continuous control using oral analgesia; use regular, not on demand, analgesia titrated to the individual; and diagnose the cause of each pain and prescribe appropriately (e.g. steroids for liver secondaries or ↑ intracranial pressure, NSAIDs &/or radiotherapy for bone metastases, co-analgesics for nerve root pain, etc.). Remember that psychological dependence is very rare in advanced cancer patients using long-term opioids, and analgesic tolerance slow to develop. When starting patients on opioid analgesia, always consider using an antiemetic (→ Antiemetics, p. 605) and a laxative. OH may be incredibly difficult for patients with oral cancer or following head and neck surgery. Use of chlorhexidine gluconate and metronidazole (200mg bd) ↓ the smell associated with wound infection or tumour fungation even when there is no prospect of eliminating it entirely. Patients rarely develop the disulfiram reaction to metronidazole on this regimen that occurs with higher doses.

Pre-emptive analgesia Surgery is painful. Providing LA (consider the long-acting agent bupivacaine/levobupivacaine) or systemic analgesia before surgery begins may ↓ overall requirements for analgesia.

Patient-controlled analgesia The optimal technique for severe post-operative pain. A small machine delivers a bolus (1–2mg morphine) when the patient presses a button. Can be repeated as needed.

Two variables: (i) bolus dose; (ii) 'lock out time' time during which machine will not respond (allows time for opioid to achieve maximum effect and prevents overdosage).

Prophylaxis

Prophylaxis is the prevention of an occurrence. In surgery this is usually infection or thromboembolism. Prophylaxis used to prevent the occurrence of bacterial infection is quite different from treating an established infection. There are two broad categories of patients requiring antibiotic prophylaxis: (i) those who have it to prevent a minor local bacteraemia causing a serious infection out of all proportion to the procedure, e.g. the immunocompromised; and (ii) those who receive it to prevent local septic complications of the procedure, e.g. wisdom-tooth removal.

Principles of antibiotic prophylaxis The regimen should be short, high dose, and appropriate to the potential infecting organisms. The aim is to prevent pathogens establishing themselves in surgically traumatized or otherwise at-risk tissues; therefore the antimicrobial must be in those tissues prior to damage or exposure to the pathogen. It must not, however, be present too long before this, as there is then a risk of pathogen resistance and damage to commensal organisms. The regimen should therefore start immediately pre-operatively (i.e. <6h) or peri-operatively (e.g. with anaesthetic induction) and should be continued for 24–48h maximum. When practicable, select an antimicrobial as specific to the common pathogens for that procedure as possible, except in the immunocompromised, where broad-spectrum prophylaxis is appropriate.

Prophylaxis against infective endocarditis is no longer indicated on a routine basis.[6]

Examples
- Immunocompromised (e.g. severe leucopenia)—2.25g piperacillin/tazobactam plus 120mg gentamicin IV pre-operatively. Repeat qds for 24h.
- Dento-alveolar surgery—simple extractions need not be covered but third-molar surgery often is. Regimens: metronidazole 400mg PO (500mg IV) pre-operatively followed by 400mg tds for 24h, amoxicillin 1g PO/IV followed by 500mg tds for 24h.

Prophylactic anticoagulation Prevention of DVT &/or pulmonary embolus in susceptible patients (e.g. women on the pill, prolonged surgery, iliac crest grafts) can be achieved using daily low-molecular weight heparin SC od (various types available—check which one your hospital favours).[7] Thromboembolic antiembolism (TED) stockings will also ↓ DVT. Rx of pulmonary embolus, ➔ DVT, p. 592.

---

6 NICE 2008 (updated 2016) *Prophylaxis against Infective Endocarditis* (℗ http://www.nice.org.uk/CG64).

7 NICE 2018 (updated August 2019) *Venous Thromboembolism in over 16s: Reducing the Risk of Hospital-acquired Deep Vein Thrombosis or Pulmonary Embolism* (℗ http://www.nice.org.uk/NG89).

Management of the diabetic patient undergoing surgery

▶ Many hospitals have a diabetic team who will advise on the management of these patients. Find out if this happens in your locality and make use of them. Type 2 diabetics are an increasing group in the developed world and have a plethora of health problems.[8]

Guidelines
- Know the type and severity of the diabetes you are dealing with.
- Inform the anaesthetist (and diabetic team if available).
- Remember these patients are more likely to have occult heart disease, renal impairment, and ↓ resistance to infection, so get an ECG, U&Es, and use antibiotics prophylactically.
- If nursing staff are experienced with blood glucose estimation using blood glucose testing strips or similar, 2–4-hourly tests will suffice for monitoring control. Otherwise pre-, peri-, and post-operative blood glucose estimation is needed.
- If in doubt and you are on your own (although you never should be), use a glucose, potassium, insulin (GKI) infusion (➔ Management: insulin-dependent, p. 588).
- Always have diabetics first on the operating list, in the morning if possible. Admit to hospital the day before surgery if insulin regimen is to be used.

Management: non-insulin dependent
If anything other than a minor, short procedure, treat as insulin dependent. If random blood glucose is >15mmol/L treat as insulin dependent.

Patients being treated under LA, or LA and sedation should maintain their carbohydrate intake and any oral hypoglycaemic drugs as normal. Plan surgery to fit their regular mealtimes. Have carbohydrate readily to hand if needed, and ensure adequate post-operative analgesia, as pain or trismus can easily interfere with their usual intake. Remember antibiotic prophylaxis.

Patients for GA Halve the dose of oral hypoglycaemic 24h prior to surgery and omit on day of surgery. Do blood glucose pre- and post-operatively (if >15mmol/L go to GKI). Halve normal dose of oral hypoglycaemic until able to take normal diet, then back to normal dose. Keep an eye on the K^+ concentration (U&Es pre- and post-operatively) and keep well hydrated. If in doubt, manage as for insulin dependent.

Management: insulin dependent
Admit 24–48h pre-operatively to optimize control. If glycaemic control poor, involve diabetic team early. Examine the patient carefully. Get an ECG, FBC, U&Es, and random blood glucose. Look for heart and respiratory disease, leucocytosis indicating infection, anaemia, hypo- or hyperkalaemia, and renal impairment. If these are acceptable, normal insulin/carbohydrate intake up to and including evening meal the day before

8 A. T. Kharroubi & H. M. Darwish 2015 *World J Diabetes* 6 850.

surgery. Omit long-acting insulin on the day before surgery. Starve following this, and place on an IV infusion of glucose (glucose 5–10% 500mL), potassium (10mmol K^+ injected into bag of glucose) infused via a controlled rate device over 5h, i.e. 100mL/h. This is infused via a three-way tap into a peripheral cannula. Simultaneously, *short-acting insulin* is infused via a pump through the three-way tap into the same cannula at a rate indicated by the sliding scale (Table 13.1). The insulin is normally made up as 49.5mL N saline with 50IU of short-acting insulin giving 50mL = 50IU insulin, but always check your local nurses' policy.

The original GKI had a fixed amount of insulin injected into the 500mL of glucose but the flexibility of sliding scale delivery has made this technique the most frequently used.

The scale details will vary according to the type of fingerprick glucose tests available in your locality; numbers are *not* absolute but the principle will always work. Choice of crystalloid is variable; 10% glucose ↑ carbohydrate and anabolism but tends to tissue veins quickly.

Once the patient can eat and drink, resume normal insulin regimen and discontinue infusion as blood glucose levels normalize.

Table 13.1 Sliding scale

Blood glucose (mmol/L)	Insulin (IU/h)
>22	8
18–22	6
14–18	4
10–14	3 Target zone
6–10	2
2–6	1
<2	Stop and give glucose

Management of patients requiring steroid supplementation

Principle These patients are unable to respond to the stress of surgery due to depletion or absence of their endogenous corticosteroid response.

Groups Patients with Addison's disease, patients prescribed corticosteroids for modulation of the immune system, and steroid abusers from various 'sports'.

Addison's disease This is the rarest of these groups but requires the most aggressive supplementation as sufferers are entirely reliant on prescribed steroids. Minor surgery can safely be covered with IM hydrocortisone sodium succinate 100mg qds the day of surgery. Major surgery should be covered for 3 days using the same regimen. IV administration is kinder over the longer period.

Patients prescribed steroids Do you know why they are on these drugs? Consider the underlying disease and whether it has any bearing on your Rx plan; e.g. a patient receiving steroids as part of a cytotoxic regimen will also be at risk from bleeding and infection. In an uncomplicated case before minor surgery, all that is needed is a single IM injection of hydrocortisone 50mg 30min prior to the procedure. Alternatives are an IV injection immediately pre-operatively followed by double the normal oral dose of steroid. Another way is to ask the patient to take a double dose on the day of the operation, normal dose plus 50% the day after, and normal plus 25% on the third day, thereafter returning to their usual dose. Those undergoing major surgery should have the IM/IV regimen over 24h or longer.

Steroid abusers Unfortunately these are a real and ↑ problem.[9] Although these drugs are taken for their androgenic effect, few 'sportspersons' have access to appropriate advice or drugs and many users will have a degree of suppressed steroid response. It is probably safest to cover procedures using the IM regimen as for those on prescribed steroids, although this could be considered overkill. Remember the risk of shared needles.

9 J. Mcveigh & E. Begley 2016 *Drugs Educ Prev Policy* **24** 278.

Common post-operative problems

General

Pain Use appropriate analgesia (⊃ Analgesics in hospital practice, p. 600).

Pyrexia A small physiological ↑ in temperature occurs post-operatively. Other causes: atelectasis, infection (wound, chest, urine), DVT, incompatible transfusion, allergic reactions.

Nausea and vomiting Antiemetics, e.g. IM/IV cyclizine 50mg. Prochlorperazine 12.5mg or metoclopramide 10mg. Ondansetron for the recalcitrant (4mg IV/IM, 8mg PO).

Sore throat Common after intubation; needs reassurance and simple analgesia. Cold water ↓.

Muscle pain Often follows suxamethonium use in anaesthetic induction. Again, reassurance and simple analgesics.

Hypotension Usually caused by autonomic suppression by a GA. Treat by placing 'head-down'. If necessary, speed up IV infusion for a short while.

Chest infection CXR, culture sputum, and start on ampicillin or cefuroxime until culture results available.

Confusion A symptom, therefore look for the cause, e.g. infection, electrolyte imbalance, alcohol withdrawal, hypoxia, or dehydration, and correct. Only consider sedation, e.g. haloperidol 1–5mg (care in the elderly), after action has been taken to deal with the cause and the patient constitutes a threat to themselves or others.

Rarer general complications

Urinary retention Comparatively rare, even after major maxillofacial surgery. Early mobilization and adequate analgesia helps; if not, use temporary catheterization (⊃ Catheterization, p. 581).

Superficial vein thrombosis Follows 'tissued' cannulae or irritant IV injections. Observe for infection, treat pain, and consider supportive strapping.

DVT Signs are painful, shiny, red, swollen calf, usually unilaterally but may be bilaterally. 'At risk' are immobile patients especially following pelvic surgery, patients with cancer, women on the pill, the elderly, and the obese. Confirm by Doppler USS or ascending venography. Prevent by using a low-molecular-weight heparin (dalteparin, enoxaparin) pre-operatively and 5 days post-operatively &/or pressure stockings, and ensure early mobilization. Stop the pill prior to any major surgery. Rx: bed rest, leg strapping and elevation, analgesia and heparinization (give 5000 units stat IV followed by 50,000 units in 50mL normal saline by syringe driver infusion starting at 1000 units/h (1mL/h) and adjust according to the kaolin–cephalin clotting time (KCT)/APTT, keep between 1.5–2.5 times the control values). The major risk of DVT is the development of pulmonary embolus. This classically presents 10 days post-operatively when the patient has been straining at stool and may occur despite no apparent DVT. Symptoms are pleuritic chest pain, dyspnoea, cyanosis, haemoptysis, and an ↑ jugular venous pressure. Signs of shock are often present, ranging from very little in the young who can compensate, to cardiac arrest! Usually a clinical Δ, confirmed after heparinization, analgesia, and O_2 have been instituted, by CXR, blood gases, spiral CT, or lung ventilation—perfusion scan &/or pulmonary angiography. ECG will sometimes show deep S waves in I, pathological Q waves in III, and inverted T waves in III (SI, QIII, TIII). Must be followed up by 3–6 months anticoagulation with warfarin, so involve a haematologist.

Less serious but more common are post-phlebitic limb, varicose veins, limb swelling, and skin discoloration. May lead to varicose eczema.

Local complications following oral surgery

Local pain, swelling, infection, and trismus are the commonest. Antral complications may follow maxillary surgery. These are considered in the relevant chapters.

Chapter 14

Therapeutics

Relevant pages in other chapters Chapter 13: Medicine relevant to dentistry; Chapter 15: Analgesia, anaesthesia, and sedation; asepsis and antisepsis, ⟶ p. 380; antiseptics and antibiotics in periodontal disease, ⟶ Treatment with antimicrobials, p. 208; fluoride, ⟶ p. 28; sugar-free medications ⟶ p. 118.

Principal sources BMA/Royal Pharmaceutical Society of Great Britain March 2014 *BNF* 67. Consumers Association *Drugs and Therapeutics Bulletin*. MedicinesComplete ℜ https://about.medicinescomplete.com/. Scottish Dental Clinical Effectiveness Programme (SDCEP) 2015 guidance on anticoagulants and SDCEP 2016 *Drug Prescribing for Dentistry* (3e) ℜ http://www.sdcep.org.uk. *BNF* ℜ http://www.bnf.nice.org.uk. NB: although available on the Internet, ℜ https://www.bnf.org/ is not recommended for use in clinically critical situations. The *BNF* has an amalgamated *BNF*/Dental Practitioners' Formulary (DPF).

Definitions

Generic Pharmaceutical name.

Proprietary Trade name. Depending on patents, a generic drug may have more than one proprietary name.

Poisons information UK National Poisons Information Service: ✆ 0344 892 0111 (medical professionals use ℜ http://www.toxbase.org).

Medicines information services

Birmingham	✆ 0121 424 7298	Cardiff	✆ 029 2074 2979; 029 2074 2251
Bristol	✆ 0117 3422867		
Ipswich	✆ 01473 704 431	Aberdeen	✆ 0122 455 2316
Leeds	✆ 0113 2065377	Dundee	✆ 01382 632 351; 01382 660 111 Extn 32351
Leicester	✆ 0116 258 6491		
Liverpool	✆ 0151 794 8113/7/8		
London	✆ 020 7188 8750; 020 7188 3849; 0207188 3855	Edinburgh	✆ 0131 242 2920
		Glasgow	✆ 0141 211 4407
		Belfast	✆ 028 9504 0558
Newcastle	✆ 0191 2824631	Dublin	✆ 01473 0589; 01453 7941 Extn 2348
Southampton	✆ 023 8120 6908/9		

UK Medicines Information (UKMi) Specialist Pharmacy Service ℜ https://www.sps.nhs.uk/.
UK Drugs in Lactation Advisors Service (UKDILAS) ✆ 0116 258 6491 or ✆ 0121 424 7298.

Prescribing

The following topic is a brief guide to the clinical use of some of the more commonly used and useful drugs in hospital and general dental practice. Doses are for healthy adults. (See Table 14.1 for abbreviations.)

Prescribing in general dental practice Extremely useful information is available in the *BNF*, which is updated every 6 months in print and monthly online. Use this as the first line of enquiry when unsure about any topic concerning drugs. Drugs listed in the DPF (found at the back of the *BNF*) can be prescribed in the UK within the NHS on form FP10 D (GP14 in Scotland, WP10 D in Wales, HS47 in Northern Ireland). Any other required drugs must be prescribed privately or via the patient's GMP. Many are available more cheaply over the counter (OTC) at pharmacies.

Prescribing in hospital The *BNF* is the definitive reference and should always be available for consultation. Use this to check dose alterations in children (*BNF for Children*) and the elderly, and for more detailed tables of drug interactions, C/Is, and unwanted effects. Any drug in the hospital pharmacy may be prescribed by a hospital dentist for in-patients, patients being discharged, and out-patients. The only exception is controlled drugs for those with dependency, which must be prescribed by specially licensed doctors, usually a psychiatrist.

In hospitals, there are three methods of prescribing: (i) a hospital prescription chart recording both prescriptions and dispensing, kept on the ward for in-patients; (ii) a take-home prescription form redeemable only at the hospital pharmacy for patients being discharged from the ward; and (iii) hospital out-patient prescriptions, used in emergency departments and some out-patient clinics, redeemable at outside pharmacies.

Good prescribing Avoid abbreviations and write drug names legibly, using the generic name whenever possible. Always describe the strength and quantity to be dispensed. When describing doses, use the units micrograms, milligrams, or millilitres when possible. Do not abbreviate the term microgram or unit (when prescribing insulin) as these are easily misinterpreted.

Controlled drugs Each prescription must show the name and address of the patient, and the form, strength, dose, and total quantity of the drug to be dispensed, in both words and figures. When writing in general practice, the prescription must also incorporate the phrase 'for dental treatment only'.

Prescribing in the elderly Doses may need adjustment and are often substantially lower than for adults (often 50% lower).

Prescribing for children Children differ markedly from adults in their response to drugs, especially in the neonatal period when all doses should be calculated in relation to body weight. Older children can usually be prescribed for in age ranges, usually up to 1yr, 1–6yrs, and 6–12yrs. All details of dosages should be checked in the *BNF* or *BNF for Children*.

Table 14.1 Dose and route abbreviations

Dose		Route	
od	once a day	IM	intramuscular
mane	in the morning	INH	inhalation
nocte	at night	IV	intravenous
bd	twice daily	NEB	nebulization
tds	three times daily	PO	by mouth
qds	four time daily	PR	per rectum
prn	as required	PV	per vagina
		SC	subcutaneous
		SUB	sublingual
		TOP	topical

Prescribing in liver disease (➔ Hepatic disease, p. 536.) As most drugs rely on hepatic metabolism, it is prudent to seek medical advice before prescribing for patients with severe liver disease.

Prescribing in renal impairment (➔ Renal disorders, p. 538.) Doses almost always need to be ↓ and some drugs are C/I completely. Medical advice should be sought.

Prescribing in pregnancy (➔ Endocrine-related problems, p. 542.) Avoid if possible.

Prescribing in terminal care See ➔ Pain control in terminal disease, p. 584.

Analgesics in general dental practice

▶ Consult the *BNF* for dosages in children. See also ➔ Prescribing for children, p. 596. Most dental pain is inflammatory in origin and hence is most responsive to drugs with an anti-inflammatory component, e.g. aspirin and the NSAIDs.

Of the peripherally acting analgesics in the DPF, aspirin, paracetamol, and ibuprofen are available cheaper direct to the public from pharmacies.

Aspirin Used in mild to moderate pain, it is also a potent antipyretic, which should *not* be used in children <12yrs (due to the rare but serious risk of Reye syndrome). Avoid in bleeding diathesis, gastrointestinal ulceration, and concurrent anticoagulant therapy. Ask about aspirin allergy, particularly in asthmatics. Often causes transient gut irritation (as do all NSAIDs). *Dose:* 300–900mg 4–6-hourly PO. Maximum 4g per day. Topical salicylate gels are now C/I in those aged <16yrs.

Ibuprofen Popularly used for mild to moderate pain; has a moderate antipyretic action. Risks and side effects are similar to those of aspirin but less irritant to the gut. *Dose:* 300–600mg qds PO.

Paracetamol Similar in analgesic efficacy to aspirin but has no anti-inflammatory action and is a moderate antipyretic. Does not cause gastric irritation or interfere with bleeding times. Overdosage can lead to liver failure. *Dose:* 1000mg 6-hourly PO (maximum dose 4g/24h in adults).

The addition of *codeine* to the minor analgesics, while never being proven to be of advantage, may have marginal benefits in some cases. No combination analgesics are currently prescribable on the DPF.

There are very few indications for the use of opioid analgesics in general dental practice. Although *dihydrocodeine* remains in the DPF, it is statistically inferior to ibuprofen 400mg in post-operative pain relief.[1]

Carbamazepine (➔ Carbamazepine, p. 618.) Prescribable in the DPF.

NB: while all NSAIDs *may* exacerbate asthma and there is a higher incidence of NSAID allergy in asthmatics, the Committee on Safety of Medicines recognizes that this *does not* constitute a C/I for the use of these valuable analgesics. Frank allergy to NSAIDs or proven exacerbation of asthma *is* a C/I.

---

1 J. E. Edwards et al. 2000 *Cochrane Database Syst Rev* 2 CD002760.

Analgesics in hospital practice

In addition to those available in the DPF, some drugs available only within hospitals are of considerable value.

Diclofenac sodium

Diclofenac sodium is available in tablet, IM injection, suppository, and in od, slow-release form. It is a mid-potency NSAID, and a useful alternative to high-dose lower-potency NSAIDs or an opioid which has no anti-inflammatory effect. Immediate-release medicines 75–100mg daily in 2–3 divided doses. Soluble tablets are available. Naproxen is being recommended as a less cardiotoxic alternative but has no soluble equivalent.

Opioid analgesics

The opioids act centrally to alter the perception of pain, but have no anti-inflammatory properties. They are of value for severe pain of visceral origin, post-operatively (acting partly by sedation), and in terminal care. However, they all depress respiratory function and interfere with the pupillary response, and are C/I in head injury. All opioids cause cough suppression, urinary retention, nausea, constipation by a ↓ in gut motility, and tolerance and dependence. The risk of addiction is, however, greatly overstated when these drugs are used for short-term post-operative analgesia and in the terminal care context. Fear of creating drug dependence should *never* cause you to withhold adequate analgesia.

Codeine phosphate A moderate opioid analgesic useful for short-term analgesia and less likely to mask a head injury; 30–60mg 4-hourly PO. (Rarely IM as this is a controlled form.) May be some advantage when used in combination (8/15/30mg) with simple analgesics or NSAIDs.

Morphine In oral form (tablets, elixir, or slow-release tablets or capsules), the drug of choice in the management of terminal pain. Always prescribe a laxative. (Macrogol laxatives are popular.) Lactulose (an osmotic laxative) may be preferred as it is a smaller volume to take. This can be combined with senna (a stimulant laxative): see *BNF.*) Dose: dependent on previous analgesia, but often starts at 10mg morphine 4-hourly or 30mg slow-release morphine sulfate bd. When used IM or IV for acute or post-operative pain: slow IV 5mg every 4h; give an antiemetic.

Buprenorphine A mixed agonist/antagonist with similar problems to pethidine and pentazocine. Unique in that it can be given sublingually. Sublingual 200–400 micrograms every 6–8h. IM or slow IV 300–600 micrograms every 6–8h. This is often used in opioid withdrawal.

Diamorphine hydrochloride (heroin) A very potent opioid which should be reserved for severe pain in an in-patient setting. Like morphine it is reversed by naloxone. IM/SC 5mg every 4h. Slow IV 1.25–2.5mg 4-hourly.

Tramadol An opioid which acts by two central methods. Lower side effect profile. IM/IV 50–100mg every 4–6h. Immediate-release PO initially 100mg, then 50–100mg 4–6-hourly, maximum 400mg/24h. Can cause nausea and vomiting, especially IV.

▶ Chronic and post-operative pain require *regular*, not as-required, analgesia, given in adequate amounts and within the therapeutic half-life of the drug.

Gabapentin A gamma-aminobutyric acid analogue that was developed for use in treatment of epilepsy. Stabilizes nerve cell membranes. It is also licensed for use in neuropathic pain in adults. 300mg PO od, ↑ to bd then tds. Subsequent ↑ in dose may be required to a maximum of 3.6g a day in three divided doses (maximum per dose 1.6g).

Pregabalin Was designed as a more potent successor to gabapentin. Also intended as an anticonvulsant it is used for treatment of neuropathic pain and in generalized anxiety disorder. 150mg in 2–3 divided doses, ↑ to a maximum of 600mg daily. There is some potential for abuse and pregabalin is a controlled drug in the US.

PCA (⮀ Patient-controlled analgesia, p. 585.) A computerized system for post-operative pain control allowing patients to deliver small regular doses of IV/SC morphine/diamorphine. Gold standard post-operative analgesia for severe pain.

Anti-inflammatory drugs

These are among the groups of drugs that may be either analgesics or co-analgesics (drugs which are not analgesic in themselves but may aid pain relief either directly or indirectly). The two major groups are the NSAIDs (➲ Analgesics in general dental practice, p. 598) and the corticosteroids.

Steroids are used in various forms, topical, oral, intralesional, and parenteral, and all have uses in dentistry.

Topical steroids

Hydrocortisone mucoadhesive buccal tablets 2.5mg lozenges dissolved in the mouth qds.

Benzydamine A topically active NSAID. Used as a spray or mouthwash to ↓ pain from inflammatory mucosal conditions. 0.15% benzydamine hydrochloride mouthwash or spray, 4–8 sprays every 1.5–3h or 15mL gargle every 1.5–3h. Can dilute with an equal amount of water if stinging, not usually required for >7 days.

Betamethasone Prepared as a 0.5mg betamethasone phosphate soluble tablet dissolved in 20mL water. Rinse around mouth qds, don't swallow.

Hydrocortisone 1% and oxytetracycline 3% Ointment is a useful Rx for aphthae and related conditions seen in hospital. Hydrocortisone 1% cream is also available with miconazole 2% in the DPF.

Intralesional steroids

Triamcinolone acetonide 1mL (40mg) injected into lesion. Needs LA. Used in granulomatous cheilitis, intractable lichen planus, keloid scars, and painful postsurgical trigger spots.

Intra-articular steroids

These can be used to induce a chemical arthroplasty in arthrosis of the TMJ (➲ Surgery and the temporomandibular joint, p. 496).

Hydrocortisone acetate 5–10mg single injection.

Triamcinolone (40mg/mL.) Can be used intra-articularly.

Systemic steroids

Main indication is prophylaxis in those with actual or potential adrenocortical suppression. Occasionally used in erosive lichen planus, severe aphthae, e.g. Behçet's disease (➲ Behçet's disease, p. 782), or arteritis (➲ Connective tissue diseases, p. 544).

Hydrocortisone sodium succinate This is used for prophylaxis; dose 100mg IM 30min pre-operatively. Doubts exist about the need for this unless the patient has demonstrated adrenocortical insufficiency (short Synacthen® test).

Prednisolone 10–20mg PO as enteric-coated tablets given with food. Regimen dependent on the condition treated.

Methylprednisolone 2–40mg daily by mouth, 10–500mg IM/IV. Various regimens described for control of oedema, post major surgery.

Dexamethasone (4mg/mL.) Various regimens described for control of oedema, post surgery.

Other immunosuppressants

Azathioprine and thalidomide These are sometimes used in specialist centres. Topical tacrolimus in carboxymethylcellulose base is used for erosive lichen planus.

Antidepressants

This is another group of drugs which can be used as co-analgesics. In conditions such as atypical facial pain they may be used as the sole 'analgesic'. However, there are no antidepressants prescribable in the DPF.[2]

In the past, there has been considerable debate about the potential interactions between the commonest antidepressants, the tricyclics, and the monoamine oxidase inhibitors (MAOIs), and adrenaline contained in LA (which constitutes the most commonly professionally administered drug anywhere). To date, there is *no clinical evidence* of dangerous interactions between the adrenaline in LA preparations commonly used in dentistry and the tricyclics or the MAOIs. In hospital practice, the two most commonly used antidepressants are amitriptyline (a sedative tricyclic antidepressant) and dosulepin (a related compound).

Amitriptyline also used for neuropathic pain Use with caution in patients with cardiac disease (as arrhythmias may follow the use of tricyclics) and avoid in diabetics, epileptics, and pregnant or breastfeeding women. It can precipitate glaucoma, ↑ the effect of alcohol, and cause drowsiness (which can impair driving). In common with other tricyclics it can cause sedation, blurred vision, xerostomia, constipation, nausea, and difficulty with micturition, although tolerance to these side effects tends to develop as Rx progresses. There is often an interval of 2–4 weeks before these drugs reach a level that exhibits a clinically evident antidepressant effect. *Dose*: 10mg od, ↑ if necessary to 75mg od nocte. Higher doses to be given on specialist advice. Children and elderly, half-dose.

Dosulepin Similar properties and unwanted effects to amitriptyline, however not routinely used. It has, however, been demonstrated to be of value in the Rx of 'facial arthromyalgia' (a composite group of TMD and atypical facial-pain patients).[3] *Dose*: initially 75mg nocte, ↑ to 150mg daily if needed. Half-dose in elderly.

Nortriptyline A less sedating tricyclic. *Dose*: 10mg od nocte; can be ↑ if necessary to 75mg daily.

Tranylcypromine A MAOI that may be of value in treating facial pain unresponsive to tricyclics. *Dose*: 10mg bd before 15.00h. Can be ↑ to 10mg morning and 20mg afternoon. MAOIs can precipitate a hypertensive crisis induced by dietary and drug interactions (sympathomimetics, opioids, especially pethidine, and foods containing tyramine, e.g. cheese, meat, or yeast extracts). LA is, however, safe.

Selective serotonin re-uptake inhibitors (SSRIs) SSRIs are much less sedative antidepressants, given as a single dose mane. Fluoxetine is best known (20mg daily) and also abused (overprescribing and used to prolong effects of MDMA or 'Ecstasy', ⊃ Ecstasy, p. 797). Paroxetine 20mg mane, sertraline 50mg mane, and citalopram 20mg mane, are similar.

2 DPF 2019 *BNF* **78** (⬧ http://bnf.nice.org.uk).

3 C. Feinmann & M. Harris 1984 *Br Dent J* **156** 205.

Antiemetics

There are no antiemetics prescribable in the DPF; however, they form an essential part of in-patient hospital prescribing. The common indication is the control of post-operative nausea and vomiting, which may be due to the procedure, anaesthetic, post-operative analgesia, or blood in the stomach.

Prochlorperazine This is a phenothiazine antiemetic which acts as a dopamine antagonist and acts at the chemoreceptor trigger zone. Avoid in small children as the drug's major side effect, the production of extrapyramidal symptoms, is especially common in this group. *Dose for prevention*: 5–10mg 2–3 times per day PO or 12.5mg deep IM (can repeat with PO dose at 6h). *Dose for acute attack*: 20mg PO then 10mg PO 2h later, deep IM 12.5mg then PO dose 6h later. Not licensed for IV use.

Metoclopramide This has both peripheral and central modes of action. It ↑ gut motility, thus emptying the stomach. Acute dystonic reactions may occur, especially in young women and children; a bizarre acute trismus is sometimes seen as one of the manifestations. *Dose*: 10mg tds PO, 10mg IM 8-hourly. High-dose intermittent and continuous IV regimens are used for antiemesis in centres using cytotoxic chemotherapy.

Domperidone This is less likely to cause central unwanted effects such as sedation and dystonia, as it does not cross the blood–brain barrier. Acts on the chemoreceptor trigger zone and is particularly useful for chemotherapy patients. *Dose*: 10mg tds. Maximum dose 30mg per day. May be used as part of a combination regimen, e.g. domperidone, prednisolone, and nabilone (a synthetic cannabinoid).

Ondansetron This is a selective $5-HT_3$ receptor antagonist that is very effective in prevention and Rx of post-operative nausea and vomiting. *Prevention dose*: 16mg PO 1h before anaesthesia or 4mg IV/IM at induction. *Treatment dose*: 4mg IM/IV one dose. Granisetron and tropisetron are similar $5-HT_3$ receptor antagonists.

Hyoscine, antihistamines, and major tranquillizers all have antiemetic properties but are rarely indicated. If unable to control emesis with one agent use two, acting at separate sites *after* excluding intestinal obstruction, e.g. due to opioid constipation.

Cyclizine This is an antihistamine and is often combined with opioid preparations as an antiemetic—however, it can aggravate heart failure. Cheap. *Dose*: 50mg tds IV/PO/IM.

Do not forget the benefits of a nasogastric tube in preventing nausea and vomiting from a distended or irritated stomach. Constipation can also cause nausea—remember to exclude it as a cause.

Anxiolytics, sedatives, hypnotics, and tranquillizers

The short-term control of fear and anxiety associated with dental Rx is an entirely appropriate use of the benzodiazepines. It should not be confused with the long-term control of anxiety which is rife with problems of dependence and drug withdrawal. A benzodiazepine may also be a valuable adjunct in the management of TMD, where it acts as both a muscle relaxant and an anxiolytic (➔ Temporomandibular pain—dysfunction/facial arthromyalgia, p. 484). IV and oral sedative techniques prior to surgery ➔ Benzodiazepines—techniques, p. 636.

Diazepam This has a long half-life and is cumulative on repeated dosing. Like all benzodiazepines, it can cause respiratory depression, therefore patients should be warned not to drive or operate machinery while on this drug. *Dose for anxiety/TMD*: 2mg tds, maximum 30mg in divided daily doses. *Dose for sedation with LA*: 5–10mg PO 1–2h before procedure.

Paradoxical disinhibition may occur in children and its use in those <16yrs is not advised. Diazepam in lipid emulsion (Diazemuls®) has traditionally been used in status epilepticus (➔ Fits, p. 569). A rectal preparation is popular for paediatric sedation in some countries (➔ Certain drugs interact, p. 634).

Midazolam This is a water-soluble benzodiazepine of about double the potency of diazepam. Its main use is in IV sedation (➔ Midazolam, p. 636). Midazolam may be given in an oromucosal solution form (or the IV preparation) by buccal topical administration. Also popular as a paediatric sedative for suture removal. *Dose for sedation*: slow IV initially 2–3.5mg 5–10min before procedure at 2mg/min, ↑ in 1mg steps if required. Usually total dose 3.5–5mg. Maximum 7.5mg per course. For status epilepticus by buccal administration, 10mg then 10mg after 10min if required.

Nitrazepam A long-acting hypnotic which tends to cause a hangover effect. *Dose*: 5–10mg nocte.

Temazepam A shorter-acting hypnotic. *Dose for conscious sedation*: 15–30mg 30–60min before procedure orally. Main indication is pre-operatively or as pre-medication. An out-patient sedation technique is described ➔ Diazepam, p. 636. Gelatin capsule preparations should no longer be used as they can be melted down for IV abuse.

In hospital practice The following may also be prescribed:

Chlordiazepoxide Sometimes used instead of diazepam in TMD. It has the same side effect profile. *Dose*: 10mg tds, ↑ to maximum of 100mg daily, in divided doses. It is the drug of choice in the stabilization of alcohol-dependent patients.

Lorazepam Sometimes used as a pre-medication by anaesthetists. *Dose for sedation*: procedures 2–3mg PO the night before procedure, 2–4mg 1–2h before operation. Alternatively, slow IV injection of 50 micrograms/kg 30–45min prior to operation. *Dose for anxiety*: 1–4mg PO in divided doses.

Clomethiazole A hypnotic sometimes used to ↓ severe insomnia in the elderly. Main indication is in management of alcohol withdrawal.

Zaleplon, zolpidem, and zopiclone
These are non-benzodiazepine hypnotics. Not licensed for long-term use, there is still potential for dependence.

Zaleplon
10mg at bedtime (reduced in the elderly), is shorter acting than similar drugs.

Zolpidem
10mg taken at bedtime. Should reduce dose by half in elderly. Similar short-acting effect to zopiclone.

Zopiclone
Dose: 7.5mg nocte. Problems similar to benzodiazepines. May be of practical help when local policy controls use of temazepam.

Haloperidol Very useful in control of acute psychosis, also used for nausea and vomiting. *Dose:* 1–2mg IM. Less painful than, and does the same job as, chlorpromazine, but main problem is extrapyramidal side effects.

Flumazenil A specific benzodiazepine reversal agent (Ⓓ Flumazenil, p. 635). Dosages should be ↓ in elderly. Avoid in children.

Alimemazine An antihistamine; a useful sedative for children.

Chloral hydrate (Chloral Elixir Paediatric.) 5mL used as a sedative for removing facial sutures. Oral midazolam is an alternative.

Antibiotics—1

Principles of antibiotic use

When prescribing, consider (i) the patient, (ii) the likely organisms, and (iii) the best drug. Patients influence choice, in that they may be allergic to various drugs, have hepatic or renal impairment, be immunocompromised, be unable to swallow, be pregnant or breastfeeding, or taking an oral contraceptive; consider also the age and severity of the infection. The infecting organism should ideally be isolated, cultured, and its sensitivity to antibiotics determined, but this is only feasible in hospital practice. In reality, most infections are treated blind, therefore it is essential to know the common infecting organisms in your field, and their sensitivities. You also need to know the drugs' modes of action, absorption, unwanted effects, development of resistance, interactions, and techniques available for delivery. The best drug is the one which is safe in that patient, specific to the infecting organism, and can be given in a reliable convenient form. Remember prophylaxis (➜ Principles of antibiotic prophylaxis, p. 586) differs from Rx with antibiotics, and antibiotics do not replace the drainage of pus in abscesses.

Benzylpenicillin

Inactive orally and only used IM or IV. *Dose*: 600–1200mg IV/IM qds. Drug of choice in streptococcal infections. Like all penicillins it is bactericidal: it interferes with cell-wall synthesis. Good tissue penetration except for CSF. Most important unwanted effect is hypersensitivity, which is usually manifested as a rash, rarely as fatal anaphylaxis. Patients allergic to one penicillin will be allergic to all; theoretically 10% will be allergic to cephalosporins as well. A history of atopy (e.g. asthma) ↑ risk.

DPF prescribable antibiotics

Phenoxymethylpenicillin Oral equivalent of benzylpenicillin. *Dose*: 250–500mg qds PO. Has a narrow spectrum, but is now largely superseded by:

Amoxicillin This has a broad spectrum similar to *ampicillin*, but is better absorbed and achieves higher tissue concentrations. *Dose*: 500mg tds PO. Both ampicillin and amoxicillin cause a maculopapular rash in patients with glandular fever, lymphatic leukaemia, or possibly HIV infection (this is *not* true penicillin allergy). Amoxicillin was the drug of choice in prophylaxis against infective endocarditis (➜ Principles of antibiotic prophylaxis, p. 586). May interfere with the action of oral contraceptives. All penicillins ↓ excretion of methotrexate, therefore ↑ risk of toxicity.

Tetracycline One of a group of broad-spectrum antibiotics with a problem of ↑ bacterial resistance. It is likely to promote opportunistic infection with *Candida albicans*, particularly when used topically, as has been recommended for the Rx of aphthae. Other problems are the deposition of tetracyclines in growing bone and teeth, causing staining and hypoplasia (therefore avoid in children <12yrs and pregnancy) and erythema multiforme. It is also particularly likely to render the oral contraceptive ineffective. *Dose*: 250–500mg qds PO. Absorption inhibited by chelation with milk, etc., therefore should be taken well before food. May be of value in periodontal disease (➜ Chronic periodontitis, p. 208). Doxycycline 200mg day 1, then 100mg od PO and oxytetracycline 250–500mg qds PO are prescribable.

Erythromycin A similar spectrum to penicillin, but bacteriostatic. Active against penicillinase-producing organisms. Formerly an alternative to amoxicillin for endocarditis prophylaxis (superseded by clindamycin). Nausea is a major problem. *Dose:* 250–500mg qds PO/IV.

Oral cephalosporins Of little value in dental practice, but cefalexin 250mg qds or 500mg bd PO and cefradine 250–500mg qds PO are prescribable. Clindamycin and metronidazole are also in the DPF (see ➔ Antibiotics—2, p. 610).

Antibiotics—2

Clindamycin Should be used cautiously in the management of dental infections, due to the risk of antibiotic-induced colitis. Useful in staphylo coccal osteomyelitis in conjunction with metronidazole (which inhibits overgrowth with *Clostridium difficile*). Has replaced erythromycin for single-dose prophylaxis of infective endocarditis (⊃ Principles of antibiotic prophylaxis, p. 586) when indicated. *Dose:* 150mg qds.

Metronidazole An anaerobicidal drug, and as such effective in many acute dental and oral infections. Classical dose for NUG is 200mg tds PO for 3 days. For other anaerobic infections is more often used as 400mg bd/tds (depending on severity) PO. Available as tablets, IV infusion, or suppository. Main problem is severe nausea and vomiting if taken in conjunction with alcohol (disulfiram reaction). Remember, it is *not* effective against aerobic bacteria.

Antibiotics of use in hospital practice In addition to the aforementioned:

Flucloxacillin A penicillin active against penicillinase-producing bacteria. *Dose:* 250–500mg qds PO/IV. Can be combined with ampicillin as co-fluampicil.

Co-amoxiclav Co-amoxiclav is amoxicillin plus clavulanic acid. The latter destroys beta-lactamase (penicillinase) and hence widens the range of amoxicillin to include the commonest cause of resistance in infections of the head and neck. Now included in the DPF. *Dose:* 375mg or 625mg (same amount of clavulanic acid but double amoxicillin) tds PO or 600–1200mg tds IV. Problems as for amoxicillin.

Cefuroxime A parenteral broad-spectrum cephalosporin often used in combination with metronidazole for surgical prophylaxis in contaminated head and neck procedures. *Dose:* 250–500mg bd PO, 750–1500mg tds IV.

Gentamicin A bactericidal aminoglycoside antibiotic, active mainly against Gram –ve organisms. Complementary to the penicillins and available as a topical (ear use), parenteral preparation or impregnated in some temporary and resorbable implants used in surgical site infection. Major problem is dose-related ototoxicity and nephrotoxicity (monitor levels if used for >24h). *Dose:* up to 5mg/kg monitored use local guidelines. Endocarditis prophylaxis, ⊃ Principles of antibiotic prophylaxis, p. 586.

Co-trimoxazole This has few indications in the head and neck which have not been replaced by trimethoprim alone. It is used, however, in ear, sinus, and urinary infections, but is C/I in pregnancy and folate deficiency (as it is a folate antagonist). *Dose:* 960mg bd PO.

Chloramphenicol Useful topically in bacterial conjunctivitis (0.5% eye drops, 1% eye ointment, apply 3-hourly). Systemic use is strictly limited due to toxicity. Ointment is an excellent wound dressing.

Vancomycin A unique bactericidal antibiotic. Two main uses are orally in the Rx of antibiotic-induced colitis (125mg qds 10 days PO), and for prophylaxis of patients at high risk from infective endocarditis (⮕ Principles of antibiotic prophylaxis, p. 586). Ototoxic, nephrotoxic, prone to cause phlebitis at infusion sites, and makes people feel generally unwell, therefore not to be used lightly.

Teicoplanin This is similar to vancomycin. Lasts longer. Can be given IV or IM. Fewer unwanted effects and kinder on patient, but more expensive.

Antifungal and antiviral drugs

Antifungals

The main fungal pathogen in the mouth is *Candida albicans* (➲ Oral candidosis (candidiasis), p. 438).

Nystatin Available as mixture. *Dose:* 100,000 units qds using 1mL of the mixture and holding it in the mouth before swallowing.

Miconazole This is a useful drug, particularly in management of angular cheilitis, as it is active against streptococci, staphylococci, and *Candida*. Miconazole oral gel 24mg/mL is of use in chronic mucocutaneous and chronic hyperplastic candidosis. *Dose:* 2.5mL qds 20mg/g gel. Apply a pea-sized amount after food qds. Can be applied to dentures also. Miconazole cream is used topically for angular cheilitis.

Fluconazole Available in both PO and IV formulations for severe mucosal candidosis in both normal and immunocompromised patients as a second-line treatment to topical preparations. Avoid in pregnancy. *Dose:* 50mg od PO for 7–14 days. Itraconazole, posaconazole, and voriconazole are other antifungal drugs.

There are recognized potentially serious interactions between miconazole, fluconazole, and related drugs and antibacterials, anticoagulants, antidiabetics, antiepileptics, antihistamines, anxiolytics, cisapride, ciclosporin, and theophylline. Check what your patient is currently taking. Candidal resistance to fluconazole is now recognized—get C&S if Rx not working.

Antivirals

Most viral infections are treated symptomatically. Herpes labialis is the viral condition most often seen and treated by dentists.

Aciclovir Active against herpes simplex and zoster; relatively non-toxic and can be given systemically or topically. *Dose:* herpes labialis: apply 5% aciclovir cream to site of prodromal or early lesion 4-hourly for 5 days; herpetic stomatitis: 200mg PO (400mg in immunocompromised) five times daily for 5 days; herpes zoster: 800mg PO five times daily for 7 days.

Penciclovir Penciclovir as a 1% cream applied 2-hourly for 4 days is prescribable according to the DPF for herpes labialis.

Other anti-herpes drugs include: *idoxuridine, famciclovir,* and *valaciclovir. Ganciclovir* is active against all herpes viruses, EBV, and CMV; however, it is very toxic and therefore has no indications in dentistry.

HIV infection There is no known cure but combinations of drugs slow or even halt disease progression. It possible they can reduce viral load to 'undetectable levels'. HAART is described in ➲ Rx, p. 479. Used (unlicensed) for postexposure prophylaxis. Get immediate expert advice if in this situation. Lipodystrophy syndrome is associated with antiretroviral therapy. *Inosine pranobex* is licensed for use in treating mucocutaneous herpes simplex in conjunction with podophyllin. *Interferon* is an interesting drug, with no indications in dentistry.

Antihistamines and decongestants

Antihistamines

Rarely used in the usual range of dental practice. Sometimes indicated in the management of allergy, especially hayfever, for pre-medication and sedation in children, occasionally as antiemetics, possibly in the management of over-active gag reflex, and as part of the emergency Rx of angio-oedema and anaphylaxis (→ Anaphylactic shock and other drug reactions, p. 564). Main differences between the antihistamines are duration of action and degree of accompanying sedation and antimuscarinic effects.

Chlorphenamine A sedative antihistamine. *Dose:* 4mg qds PO.

Promethazine Also a sedative antihistamine. *Dose:* 10–20mg bd/tds PO or 20–30mg nocte when used as a hypnotic. On sale to the public as a hypnotic.

The sedative effects of these drugs potentiate alcohol and ability to drive or operate machinery safely. They should be used with caution in glaucoma, prostatic hypertrophy, and epilepsy.

Although these drugs are available in the DPF, probably the most useful antihistamines are not. These include a wide range of non-sedating antihistamines; e.g. cetirizine and loratadine are available as OTC generics to the public, replacing terfenadine due to its greater unwanted effects.

Alimemazine A sedative antihistamine which may be of some value in the itching of uraemia, and occasionally used by anaesthetists as a pre-medication in children. *Adult dose:* 10mg bd/tds; paediatric pre-medication: 2.5–10mg, dependent on age.

Decongestants

These are valuable in the management of sinusitis and particularly in the closure of oro-antral fistulae.

Ephedrine nasal drops These produce vasoconstriction of mucosal blood vessels and ↓ the thickness of nasal mucosa, thus relieving obstruction. Avoid in patients taking MAOIs. Other problems: prolonged use leads to a rebound vasodilatation and a recurrence of nasal congestion, and long-term use results in tolerance and damage to nasal cilia. *Dose:* ephedrine nasal drops 0.5–1%, 1–2 drops into the relevant nostril qds for 7–10 days. For symptomatic nasal decongestion and as an adjunct to the management of oro-antral fistulae (→ Oro-antral fistula, p. 422) inhalation of menthol and eucalyptus is valuable. *Dose:* 1 teaspoonful of menthol and eucalyptus inhalation BP (British Pharmacopoeia) is added to a pint of hot water, and the warm, moist air is inhaled with a towel over the head.

Xylometazoline and oxymetazoline nasal drop Xylometazoline and oxymetazoline nasal drop and spray 0.1% are a more potent alternative to ephedrine, but more likely to cause a rebound effect. Systemic decongestants are of dubious value and contain sympathomimetics. They do not, however, cause rebound also known as rhinitis medicamentosa. For prescribed, short-term use, thereby avoiding risk of rebound, xylometazoline or oxymetazoline are drugs of choice; spray into relevant nostril tds.

Oral anticoagulants and antiplatelets

Warfarin Many regions' oral and maxillofacial surgery routine practice is to perform extractions as normal for patients on warfarin with an INR <4. The INR should ideally be checked within 24h of the procedure starting. If multiple extractions are required, a single extraction should be carried out first. Subsequent extractions of two or three teeth at any time may be carried out if recovery is uneventful. Patients with an INR >4 should be referred to their anticoagulant clinic or physician. Patients requiring multiple extractions or with other significant co-morbidities should be seen in an area which can provide a higher level of care. Local haemostatic measures should be taken to achieve haemostasis following extractions, such as packing the socket with oxidized cellulose and suturing gingivae with local pressure.

Novel oral anticoagulants (NOACs) While warfarin is still one of the most widely used anticoagulants, there is now a group of newer oral anticoagulants including dabigatran (direct inhibitor of thrombin, a coagulation factor), apixaban, and rivaroxaban (inhibit factor Xa of the coagulation cascade). Monitoring is not normally required for these newer drugs and an INR pre-treatment is not required. However, as with warfarin, local measures should still be taken to achieve haemostasis.

Patients taking a NOAC undergoing a dental procedure with a higher risk of bleeding complications may be advised to miss (apixaban/dabigatran) or delay (rivaroxaban) their morning dose on the day of treatment.

Antiplatelets Two new-generation antiplatelet drugs include prasugrel and ticagrelor, both alternatives to clopidogrel. It is advised that treatment is completed without interrupting antiplatelet medication. Local guidelines should always be consulted and if unsure the patient's GMP or specialist should be contacted for advice.

Precautions According to the SDCEP anticoagulants guidance (2015), the following precautions should be taken:
- Consultation with GMP or specialist.
- If time-limited course of medication, delay non-urgent, invasive procedures until no longer taking the medication.
- Stage treatment, starting with a single extraction.
- Treat early in the day and week (allowing time for management of prolonged bleeding).
- Atraumatic technique.
- Local measures for haemostasis (e.g. suture, oxidized cellulose pack, pressure).
- Provide verbal and written post-treatment advice and emergency contact details.

Bisphosphonates These are a range of drugs which act on osteoclasts and reduce the rate of bone turnover. They bind to hydroxyapatite and their effect is therefore extremely long term (possibly up to 10yrs). They are an important group of drugs in the prophylaxis and treatment of osteoporosis, steroid-induced osteoporosis, Paget's disease, bone metastases (particularly breast, myeloma, and prostate), and hypercalcaemia of malignancy.

They come in differing degrees of potency, non-nitrogen-containing oral preparations being the least potent and nitrogen-containing IV preparations being the most potent. Osteoporosis tends to be managed with less potent drugs and hypercalcaemia and bone metastases with the most.

Bisphosphonate-related osteonecrosis of the jaws (BRONJ aka BRON aka anti-resorptive-related osteonecrosis of the jaws (ARONJ)) is a condition where alveolar bone is exposed in the mouth in patients taking these drugs (Fig. 10.2). The condition appears to be progressive and there is no established effective treatment although several are being investigated. Bone necrosis without mucosal breach is also described. The incidence is variable but is probably much less than 1% for patients treated with low-potency drugs for osteoporosis, up to 30% for myeloma survivors at 10yrs who have received highly potent drugs and who have had extractions.

Prevention is the most useful management strategy and all patients prior to starting bisphosphonates should have optimum dental health established such that it is highly unlikely they will ever need to have a tooth removed in the future. This is a shift away from the 'benefit of the doubt' approach most dentists are currently trained in. The nearest comparable approach is in the prevention of osteoradionecrosis. See Table 14.2.

Table 14.2 Bisphosphonate preparations currently available and their relative potency

	Primary indication	Nitrogen containing	Dose	Relative potency
Disodium etidronate	Paget's disease	No	5mg/kg Daily for 6 months	1
Sodium clodronate	Myeloma Bone metastases (breast)	No	1600mg Daily	10
Tiludronic acid	Paget's disease	No	400mg daily For 3 months	50
Alendronic acid	Osteoporosis	Yes	10mg/day 70mg/week	1000
Risedronate sodium	Osteoporosis	Yes	5mg/day 35mg/week	1000
Ibandronic acid	Osteoporosis Bone metastases	Yes	150mg PO/month 3mg IV/3-monthly 50mg PO od 6mg IV/3-weekly	1000
Disodium pamidronate	Bone metastases	Yes	90mg/3 weeks	1000–5000
Zoledronic acid	Bone metastases	Yes	4mg/3 weeks	10,000+

Denosumab is a human monoclonal antibody that inhibits osteoclast formation, function, and survival. It is used in the treatment of osteoporosis, bone metastasis, and a number of other conditions that result in ↑ bone turnover. It is only available in IV form and is considered a million times more potent than etidronate. Denosumab and other non-bisphosphonate drugs such as anti-angiogenic drugs bevacizumab, sunitinib, and aflibercept still have the potential to cause bone necrosis. This is known as 'medication-related osteonecrosis of the jaw' or 'MRONJ'.

Management of established MRONJ, ⊃ Treatment of established MRONJ, p. 390.

Miscellaneous

A number of drugs not fitting into any specific category are important in managing oral and dental disease. These include the following:

Carbamazepine Primarily an antiepileptic drug which is of considerable value in the management of trigeminal and glosso-pharyngeal neuralgia. C/I in those sensitive to the drug, patients with atrioventricular conduction defects, porphyria, and should be used with extreme caution in patients on MAOIs, who are pregnant, or who have liver failure. May interfere with the oral contraceptive. Common unwanted effects are gastrointestinal disturbances, dizziness, and visual disturbances. Rarely, rashes may occur, as can leucopenia. Do a FBC soon after starting carbamazepine: blood dyscrasias usually occur in the first 3 months. *Dose:* 100–200mg bd; can be ↑ gradually to 200mg tds/qds. Maximum 1600mg daily in divided doses. It is important to be sure of your diagnosis before starting patients on long-term carbamazepine (➜ Facial pain, p. 464). A slow-release preparation with fewer unwanted effects is available.

Vitamins There is no indication for first-line Rx with vitamins in dental practice. Deficiency due to inadequate dietary intake in the UK is exceedingly rare. Although it can occur in the elderly and alcoholics, these people should be fully investigated and not treated empirically. Severe gingival swelling, stomatitis, glossitis, or pain should be fully investigated before using vitamin supplements.

Artificial saliva Valuable adjunct in the management of xerostomia, especially after radiotherapy and in Sjögren syndrome. A slightly viscous, inert fluid which may have a number of additives, such as antimicrobial preservatives, fluoride, flavouring, etc. Useful preparations are Glandosane® and Saliva Orthana®, aerosol sprays sprayed sublingually 4–6 times per day. The latter contains fluoride. Saliva Natura® is an 'organic' alternative. Regular sips of water may be of more practical long-term help. *Use:* all should be sprayed into the floor of mouth area to act as a 'puddle' for redistribution. Do not spray all over mucosa. Use qds. In addition, the DPF states the following may only be prescribed for patients having undergone radiotherapy or suffering from sicca syndrome: AS Saliva Orthana®, Glandosane®, Biotene Extra Gel Mouthspray®, Biotene Extra Moisturising Gel®, Saliveze, and Salivix®.

Topical anaesthetics Two main uses:
1. For preparation of a site prior to injection, e.g. of LA. Lidocaine 5% ointment or spray is the most useful. Flavoured benzocaine pastes are available in some countries.
2. EMLA® and tetracaine (Ametop®) can be used on mucosa. Carmellose gelatin paste acting as a mechanical barrier is useful in areas where it will adhere. Many OTC agents are available; few are of great potency. To ↓ pain from minor oral lesions (e.g. for HSV-1 or aphthae). Benzydamine rinse is a mainstay.

Fluorides Fluoride supplementation is discussed in ➋ Fluoride, p. 28. It is important when using rinses, and particularly gels, that the fluid is not swallowed, since there is a risk of toxicity (➋ Planning fluoride therapy, p. 30).

Retinoids These are used in some centres to manage erosive lichen planus and leucoplakia; they have proved disappointing.

Alarm bells

When prescribing any drug for patients already compromised by concomitant disease or drug therapy, it is essential to exclude possible interactions. This can be achieved fairly quickly by consulting the comprehensive *BNF*.

Interactions with the most commonly given drug (LA) are covered in ⇒ Local analgesia—tools of the trade, p. 626.

The lists in Table 14.3 are not comprehensive and some of the drugs mentioned can be used in a suitably modified dose or under specific circumstances. These tables are designed to ring alarm bells, and encourage you to both think and consult the *BNF*.

Adverse reactions Almost any drug can produce these, and many are missed. Try to avoid polypharmacy, and never prescribe without being aware of a patient's full medical history. Always enquire about drugs, including self-prescribed medication. See Table 14.4 for emergency drugs.

Table 14.3 Contraindications of common drugs

Common drugs with relative C/Is in renal disease	Common drugs with relative C/Is in liver failure
Aspirin	Aciclovir (↓ dose)
All benzodiazepines	All penicillins (↓ dose)
All opioids	All opioids
All sedatives	Amphotericin
All antihistamines	Cephalosporins (↓ dose)
All NSAIDs	Co-trimoxazole (↓ dose)
Erythromycin	Benzodiazepines (↓ dose)
Metronidazole (↓ dose)	NSAIDs
Paracetamol	Tetracyclines
Tetracyclines	
Fexofenadine	
Common drugs with relative C/Is in pregnancy	Common drugs with relative C/Is in breastfeeding
Aspirin	Antihistamines
Benzodiazepines	Aspirin
Carbamazepine	Benzodiazepines
All opioids	Carbamazepine
Co-trimoxazole	Co-trimoxazole
NSAIDs	Metronidazole
Metronidazole	Tetracyclines
Tetracyclines	

Table 14.4 Emergency drugs

Oxygen	Cylinder size D (3401) or E (6801) plus reducing valve, flow meter, tubing, and oxygen mask
Adrenaline	1mg in 1mL (1:1000) solution (IM injection)
Hydrocortisone sodium succinate	100mg powder, plus 2mL water for injection (IM injection)
Chlorphenamine maleate	10mg in 1mL solution (IM injection)
Glucagon	1mg powder, plus 1mL water for injection (IM injection)
Glucose or sugar	Drink, tablets, or gel (PO administration)
Salbutamol inhaler	0.1mg per dose (INH administration)
Glyceryl trinitrate	0.5mg tablets (rarely kept as has short shelf-life) or 0.4mg per dose spray (sublingual administration)
Aspirin	300mg tablets (PO administration)
Midazolam	10mg in 2mL solution (IV/IM injection)

Report suspected adverse reactions to the Medicines and Healthcare products Regulatory Agency (MHRA) website: http://yellowcard.mhra.gov.uk/; email: yellowcard@mhra.gov.uk; 0800 731 6789, or in writing to:

Freepost Yellow Card Scheme
MHRA
10 South Colonnade
Canary Wharf
London
E14 4PU

Report:
• *All* serious adverse reactions.
• *Any* reactions to 'black triangled' drugs in the *BNF*/DPF.

Analgesia, anaesthesia, and sedation

NB Since the report of the GDC in 2001, the status of general anaesthesia in dental practice, and inevitably the medico-legal aspects of anaesthesia and sedation in the UK, have altered considerably. This varies widely from country to country. General principles, however, remain the same.

Relevant pages in other chapters Local analgesia for children, p. 82; emergencies in dental practice, Useful emergency kit, p. 557.

Principal sources D. A. Mitchell & A. N. Kanatas 2015 *An Introduction to Oral and Maxillofacial Surgery* (Chapter 4) (2e), CRC Press. SDCEP 2017 *Conscious Sedation in Dentistry: Dental Clinical Guidance*. The Dental Faculties of the Royal Colleges of Surgeons and the Royal College of Anaesthetists 2015 *Standards for Conscious Sedation in the Provision of Dental Care*.

Definitions
General anaesthesia (GA) A state of unrousable unconsciousness to which analgesia and muscle relaxation is added to produce 'balanced anaesthesia'.

Analgesia The absence of pain.

Sedation An altered level of consciousness in which the patient, although awake, has a ↓ level of fear and anxiety.

Indications, contraindications, and common sense

When dealing with LA, GA, and sedative techniques, indications and C/Is are often relative, and the following should be thought of as guidelines rather than immutable laws.

Local anaesthesia The technique of choice for simple procedures or when a GA is C/I. LA is C/I in:
- Uncooperative patients (of any description).
- Infection around the injection site.
- Patients with a major bleeding diathesis.
- Most major surgery.

Adverse reaction to LA is a C/I, but in reality once allergy to preservatives in the solution is excluded, LA allergy probably does not exist.

Conscious sedation This is an extension of the LA technique using drugs and patient-management techniques. It is of benefit to anxious or mildly uncooperative patients and is a kind supplement to apicectomy or third-molar removal. C/Is include:
- Cardiorespiratory, renal, liver, or psychiatric pathology.
- An unescorted patient or one unable or unwilling to conform to the requirements of conscious sedation (➲ Benzodiazepines—techniques, p. 636).
- A demonstrated adverse reaction to sedative agents.
- Pregnancy, during which benzodiazepines should be avoided.

General anaesthesia Indicated when LA or LA and sedation is ineffective or inappropriate (as described earlier in this section). C/Is include:
- All those for conscious sedation.
- Presence of food or fluid in the stomach (most anaesthetists require at least 6h fasting after food and 4h after fluid).

The anaesthetist usually prefers hospital admission for patients with the following:
- Cardiovascular or respiratory disease (especially MI <6 months ago).
- Uncorrected anaemia, sickle cell trait or disease.
- Severe liver or renal impairment.
- Uncontrolled thyrotoxicosis or hypothyroidism.
- Poorly controlled diabetes, adrenocortical suppression.
- Porphyria.
- Pregnancy.
- Neurological disorders, e.g. myopathy or multiple sclerosis.
- Cervical spine pathology such as rheumatoid arthritis or cervical spondylosis.
- Certain drugs, e.g. steroids, antihypertensives, MAOIs, anticoagulants, narcotic analgesics, antiepileptics (need to avoid using methohexital), lithium, alcohol.
- Malignant hyperpyrexia, scoline apnoea, and other unwanted reactions to anaesthetic agents.

- Causes of upper airway obstruction such as angio-oedema, submandibular cellulitis, Ludwig's angina, and bleeding diathesis affecting the neck. (In fact, these are indications to secure the upper airway.)
- Previous problems with anaesthesia.

Ask about previous GA and any problems.

While all these conditions create problems with anaesthesia they may not preclude it absolutely within the hospital setting. They do, however, indicate the need for careful assessment and early prior consultation with the anaesthetist.

Local analgesia—tools of the trade

While any disposable needle and syringe system can be used to give LA, the vast number of LAs given in dental practice (>50,000/dentist/lifetime) has led to some very useful modifications.

LA cartridges Two sizes, 1.8mL and 2.2mL, come pre-sterilized. Commonest solution used is lidocaine 2% with adrenaline 1:80,000. Most formulations are now latex free.

Cartridge syringes Use with LA cartridges, resterilizable. Used with ultra-fine disposable needles. Major advantage is the ability to perform controlled aspiration during LA injection (although the consistency with which this is achieved has been questioned).

Disposable 'safety' syringes These are a single-use system designed to reduce the risk of needlestick injury. Once the needle has been used, an integral safety sheath is permanently slid over the needle.

Lidocaine/adrenaline Most commonly used preparation (2% lidocaine 1:80,000 adrenaline), gives effective pulpal analgesia for 1.5h and altered soft tissue sensation for up to 3h. Extremely safe; maximum dose 3mg/kg lidocaine without adrenaline, 7mg/kg with adrenaline. Also available in ampoules 1% + 2% lidocaine plain or with 1:200,000 adrenaline. There are theoretical criticisms that the maximum dose is too high, but these have not been borne out in practice, nor has the demonstrated effect of a change in serum potassium levels after lidocaine/adrenaline injection in the mouth.

Prilocaine/octapressin Similar but slightly less duration and effect compared to lidocaine/adrenaline. May cause methaemoglobinaemia in excess. Maximum safe dose (adult) 600mg (8 × 2.2mL cartridges). In reality, there are few hard indications for the use of prilocaine over lidocaine.

Mepivacaine Short-acting LA advocated for restorative work but has not really caught on. Maximum safe dose 400mg.

Bupivacaine Long-acting LA (6h plain, 8h with adrenaline); useful as a post-operative analgesic. Maximum safe dose 2mg/kg. Only available in ampoules. Levobupivacaine is a similar drug.

Articaine This is now widely used (4% articaine 1:100,000 adrenaline) At least as effective as lidocaine; said to diffuse through bone better. No hard evidence of superiority.

Topical analgesics Lidocaine is the only really useful topical analgesic among those just listed. It is available as a spray or a paste which is applied to mucosa several minutes prior to injecting. There is a high incidence of contact eczema in people frequently exposed to these preparations, so do not apply with bare fingers. Benzocaine in lozenge or paste form is used for mucosal analgesia. Tetracaine is a topical analgesic for use on mucous membranes. Cocaine 4% solution is used as a nasal mucosal analgesic and vasoconstrictor.

EMLA® cream, a eutectic mix of lidocaine and prilocaine, is an invaluable skin topical analgesic, used prior to venepuncture in children. Apply to puncture site and cover with Opsite® or equivalent dressing for at least 30min. Tetracaine (Ametop®) is similar and has a quicker onset of action.

Handling equipment One cartridge and needle per patient. Discard cartridge if a precipitant is seen in the solution or if air bubbles are present. Store in a cool dark place and use before expiry date. Warm cartridge to ↓ discomfort and load into the syringe immediately prior to use. Aspirate before injecting. The ↑ risk associated with needlestick injuries has spawned a number of devices to aid re-sheathing the needle. It is simpler to hold the cover in a pair of artery forceps.

Local anaesthetic toxicity Any clinician administering local anaesthetic should be aware of the signs of toxicity and understand its immediate management. It is important to note that local anaesthetic toxicity may occur some time after the initial injection. The Association of Anaesthetists guidelines on management of severe local anaesthetic toxicity can be found online.[1]

Signs
- Circumoral numbness.
- Dizziness/lightheadedness.
- Metallic taste.
- Drowsiness and disorientation.
- Visual and auditory disturbances.
- Sudden alteration in mental status.
- Severe agitation or loss of consciousness with or without tonic–clonic convulsions.
- Cardiovascular collapse.

1 ⏾https://www.aagbi.org/publications/guidelines/management-severe-local-anaesthetic-toxicity-2-2010-a4-sheet

Local analgesia—techniques

Local infiltrations and the inferior dental block are the mainstay of LA technique; however, numerous others are available as alternatives, supplements, and fallbacks.

Infiltrations Can be used in most instances.[2] The aim is to deposit LA supraperiosteally in as close proximity as possible to the apex of the tooth to be anaesthetized. The LA will diffuse through periosteum and bone to bathe the nerves entering the apex. Reflect the lip or cheek to place mucosa on tension and insert the needle along the long axis of the tooth aiming towards bone. At approximate apex of tooth, withdraw slightly and deposit LA slowly. For palatal infiltrations, achieve buccal analgesia first and infiltrate interdental papillae; then penetrate palatal mucosa and deposit small amount of LA under force.

IDB (inferior alveolar block) May be used to anaesthetize mandibular molars; also effective for premolars, canines, and incisors (the latter if supplemented by infiltration). Aim is to deposit solution around the inferior alveolar nerve as it enters the mandibular foramen underneath the lingula. The patient's mouth must be widely open. Palpate the landmarks of external and internal oblique ridges and note the line of the pterygomandibular raphe. With the palpating thumb lying in the retromolar fossa, the needle should be inserted at the midpoint of the tip of the thumb slightly above the occlusal plane lateral to the pterygomandibular raphe. The needle is inserted ~0.5cm and if a *lingual nerve block* is required, 0.5mL of LA is injected at this point. The syringe is then moved horizontally ~40° across the dorsum of the tongue and advanced to make contact with the lingula. Once bony contact is made the needle is withdrawn slightly and the remainder of the LA injected. It should never be necessary to insert the needle up to the hub. Note that the mandibular foramen varies in position with age (for children, see ⊃ Local analgesia for children, p. 82). In the edentulous, the foramen, and hence the point of needle insertion, is relatively higher than in the dentate.

Gow-Gates technique Blocks sensation in Vc by depositing LA at head of condyle.[3] Akinosi approach: LA deposited above lingula.[4]

Long buccal block The long buccal nerve is anaesthetized by injecting 0.5–1mL of LA posterior and buccal to the last molar tooth.

Mental nerve block The mental nerve emerges from the mental foramen lying apical to and between the first and second mandibular premolars. LA injected in this region will diffuse in through the mental foramen and provide limited analgesia of premolars and canine, and to a lesser

---

2 D. H. Awal et al. 2017 *Dent Update* **44** 838 (ℜ https://www.dental-update.co.uk/issuesThreeArticle.asp?aKey=1734).

3 G. A. Gow-Gates 1973 *Oral Surg Oral Med Oral Pathol* **36** 321.

4 J. O. Akinosi 1977 *BJOS* **15** 83.

degree, incisors on that side. It will provide effective soft tissue analgesia. Place the lip on tension and insert the needle parallel to the long axis of the premolars angling towards bone, and deposit the LA. *Do not* attempt to inject into the mental foramen as this may traumatize the nerve. LA can be encouraged in by massage.

Sublingual nerve block An anterior extension of the lingual nerve can be blocked by placing the needle just submucosally lingual to the premolars; use 0.5mL of LA.

Posterior superior alveolar block A rarely indicated technique. Needle is inserted distal to the upper second molar and advanced inwards, backwards, and upwards close to bone for ~2cm. LA is deposited high above the tuberosity after aspirating to avoid the pterygoid plexus.

Nasopalatine block Profound anaesthesia can be achieved by passing the needle through the incisive papilla and injecting a small amount of solution. This is extremely painful (for hints on how to overcome pain on palatal injections, see ◑ Pain on injection, p. 630).

Infra-orbital block Rarely indicated. Palpate the inferior margin of the orbit as the infra-orbital foramen lies ~1cm below the deepest point of the orbital margin. Hold the index finger at this point while the upper lip is lifted with the thumb. Inject in the depth of the buccal sulcus towards your finger, avoid your finger, and deposit LA around the infra-orbital nerve.

Intraligamentary analgesia Individual teeth can be rendered pain free by injecting small amounts of LA along the periodontal membrane via a specially designed system (high-pressure syringe and ultra-fine needles). Has the advantage of rapid onset and specific analgesia to isolated teeth; it is a useful adjunct to conventional LA and in some hands may replace it for minor procedures. Disadvantages include post-injection discomfort due to temporary extrusion and an apparent ↑ incidence in 'dry socket'.

Intraosseous analgesia A recently reintroduced technique which produces profound single-tooth analgesia. Needs specialized equipment and technique.

▶ When developing LA technique there is no alternative to seeing, doing, and doing again.

Local analgesia—problems and hints

Failure of anaesthesia

There are enormous differences in the individual response to a standard dose of LA, both in the speed of onset, duration of action, and the depth. Soft tissue analgesia is more easily obtained, needing a lower degree of penetration of solution into nerve bundles, than does analgesia from pulpal stimulation. A numb lip does not therefore indicate pulpal anaesthesia.

Causes of failure are:

- Poor technique and inadequate volume of LA.
- Injection into a muscle (will result in trismus which resolves spontaneously).
- Injection into an infected area (which should not be done anyway as this risks spreading the infection).
- Intravascular injection; clearly of no analgesic benefit. Small amounts of intravascular LA cause few problems. Toxicity, ◑ Other drug reactions and interactions, p. 564.
- Dense compact bone can prevent a properly given infiltration from working. Counter by using intraligamentary or regional LA.
- Infrequently, anastomosis from either aberrant or normal nerve fibres not transmitted with a blocked nerve bundle.

Pain on injection

This is to a certain degree inevitable, but can be ↓ by patient relaxation; application of topical LA; stretching the mucosa; and slow, skilful, accurate injection of slightly warmed solution in reasonable quantities. Causes of pain include:

- Touching the nerve when giving blocks, resulting in 'electric shock' sensation and followed by rapid analgesia (it is extremely rare for any permanent damage to occur).
- Injection of contaminated solutions (particularly by copper ions from a pre-loaded cartridge). Avoid by loading the cartridge immediately prior to use.
- Subperiosteal injections are painful and unnecessary, therefore avoid.

Other problems with administration

Lacerated artery May be followed by an area of ischaemia in the region supplied, or painful haematoma. Rare.

Lacerated vein Followed by a haematoma which resolves fairly quickly.

Facial palsy Can be caused by incorrect distal placement of the needle tip, allowing LA to permeate the parotid gland. The palsy lasts for the duration of the LA.

Post-injection problems

Lip and cheek trauma Tell patient to avoid smoking, drinking hot liquids, and biting lip or cheek. Assure them the sensation will pass in a few hours and that their face is not swollen (whether adult or child). If the advice goes unheeded and they return with traumatized mucosa, Rx: antiseptics/antibiotics and simple analgesia.

Needle-tract infection Rare. Broad-spectrum antibiotic if needed.

General points

Thick nerve trunks require more time for penetration of solution and more volume of LA. In nerve trunks, autonomic functions are blocked first, then sensitivity to temperature, followed by pain, touch, pressure, and motor function. Concentration of analgesic ↑ rapidly around the nerve at first and provides soft tissue analgesia; however, this is reached substantially before the levels needed for pulpal analgesia, which takes several minutes and will wear off first (usually within an hour of a standard lidocaine/adrenaline LA). Disinfection of mucosa prior to LA is not required in reality; however, sterile disposable needles are absolutely mandatory due to risks of cross-infection. LA for children, ➔ Local analgesia for children, p. 82. Faints, ➔ Fainting, p. 558.

Sedation—relative analgesia

Relative analgesia (RA) is the most commonly used and safest form of sedation in dentistry. It has two aspects: (i) the delivery of a mixture of nitrous oxide and O_2; (ii) a semi-hypnotic patter from the sedationist. In dentistry, two different techniques of nitrous oxide sedation have been described: (i) inhalational sedation with a fixed concentration of nitrous oxide; (ii) RA in which nitrous oxide is titrated to the patient. In the authors' view, RA is the most useful.

Nitrous oxide

This has both sedative and analgesic properties; the former is the most useful. The analgesic effect requires high levels of nitrous oxide. It is an inert gas which does not enter any of the body's metabolic pathways and is distributed as a poorly soluble solution. This allows very rapid distribution; peak saturation is reached within 5min and is similarly eliminated (90% in 10min). Usually administered as a 50% mixture with oxygen (Entonox®) by paramedics, for analgesia the technique was modified for dentistry using one of two techniques: RA or inhalational sedation.

Indications It is of particular value in anxious patients undergoing relatively atraumatic procedures and in children, for whom the benzodiazepines are less suitable.

Contraindications Few, but include upper airway obstruction, e.g. a cold. Pregnancy (risk of teratogenicity and miscarriage to both the patient and staff), first trimester makes the procedure difficult and pre-existing vitamin B_{12} deficiency would C/I its use. It is good practice to confirm the date of the last menstrual period and/or risk of pregnancy prior to use. Other C/ I, e.g. complex medical history, are relative and may limit nitrous oxide use in practice but not in hospital. There is also a risk of nausea and vomiting when using nitrous oxide gas.

Nitrous oxide pollution This is the major problem associated with RA. It is essential to have a scavenging system in place as nitrous oxide accumulation can lead to vitamin B_{12} deficiency and demyelination syndromes. There is a real potential hazard to pregnant staff working in confined conditions with this gas.

Aim

To produce a comfortable, relaxed, *awake*, patient who is able to open their mouth on request with no loss of consciousness or the laryngeal reflex. During the procedure patients will experience general relaxation, a tingling sensation often in the fingers or toes, and describe feeling mildly drunk. There is often a sense of detachment and distortion of the sense of time. Rarely, patients may dream despite being awake, and these can be sexual fantasies, which is another reason for always having a second person in the surgery.

Technique

An RA machine will not deliver <30% O_2. Start by delivering 100% O_2 via a nasal mask and set flow control to match their tidal volume (flow rates 6–8L/min for adult, 4L/min for child). Then give 10% nitrous oxide for 1min, ↑ (if needed) to 20% for 1min, ↑ to 30% (if needed) for 1min, and so on. Most patients achieve adequate levels of sedation at 20–30%; some may require less, a few rather more. Remember that RA relies on the reassuring banter of the operator more than any of the other sedation techniques, and many view this as hypnosedation. Give LA and carry out Rx. To discontinue, turn flow to 100% O_2 and oxygenate patient for 2min. Then remove mask and get the patient to sit in a recovery room for 10min, by which time 90% of nitrous oxide will have been blown off and they will be safe to leave the surgery.

Sedation—benzodiazepines

General pointers, problems, and hints

Benzodiazepines These are both sedative and hypnotic drugs which are useful for sedation of patients. Two techniques are generally used: oral and IV.

Elderly patients tend to be very sensitive to benzodiazepines and doses are best halved in the >60yrs age group initially. Interestingly, children show not only resistance to these drugs but sometimes paradoxical stimulation, and benzodiazepine sedation is not recommended for the <16s.

Post-operative drowsiness is perhaps the biggest problem, as patients may be influenced by, e.g. diazepam, for up to 24 h after administration (this time is ↓ with midazolam). There is also a re-sedation effect (with oral benzodiazepines) caused by enterohepatic recirculation (first-pass effect).

Poswillo Committee Its report redefined 'sedation' as the 'single injection of a single drug'. In terms of IV sedation in an out-patient setting this is the surest way to avoid problems provided the 'single injection' is titrated and incremental.

IV sedation The most efficient and effective method of extending the use of LA in dental Rx; however, it requires substantial skill and confidence in venepuncture and administration of the drugs; therefore an inexperienced operator, or a patient with needle phobia, form relative C/Is. As do inability to be accompanied, the need to be in a responsible position within 24h of sedation (e.g. looking after young children on own, driving, etc.), patients with liver or renal impairment, glaucoma, psychoses, pregnancy, or a demonstrated allergy to the benzodiazepines.

Certain drugs interact These include cimetidine, disulfiram, anti-parkinsonian drugs, other sedatives, narcotic analgesics, antiepileptic drugs, antihistamines, and antihypertensives. Patients on these may be best treated (and then cautiously) in a hospital environment. Patients addicted to alcohol or other drugs may require a substantial dose modification; usually a big ↑. Those being sedated need to give written informed consent. Always provide written post-operative instructions because the patients will not remember verbal ones. The role of operator sedationist is a perfectly sound and legal occupation, but note that a second appropriate person, i.e. one trained in CPR, must be present. At no time should the patient lose consciousness during IV sedation. There is no need to starve patients prior to being sedated, although many local policies dictate this and oral medication should be continued. Rectal sedation is popular in some countries using a prepackaged solution of diazepam given PR dose 2–10mg. Nasal inhalation techniques are also being introduced.

Alternative techniques In many countries, multiple drug techniques are only carried out by trained anaesthetists although in the US oral surgeons are trained in these techniques. These techniques include:
- Any form of conscious sedation for patients <12yrs (other than RA).
- Benzodiazepine and any other IV agent e.g. opioid, propofol, ketamine.
- Propofol alone or with any other agent.
- Inhalational sedation using any agent other than nitrous oxide.
- Combined routes (IV/inhalational) except using nitrous oxide for cannulation.

American oral surgeons recognize these techniques which are now the subject of a prospective new training programme in conscious sedation in dentistry.[5]

Flumazenil A specific benzodiazepine reversal agent. *Dose*: 200 micrograms IV over 15sec followed by 100 micrograms at 60sec intervals until reversal occurs. NB: this drug has a shorter half-life than the drugs it will reverse, therefore multiple doses may be required. Patients *should never* be reversed and then left unsupervised. This is an essential emergency drug for IV sedationists.

Guidelines exist highlighting the recommended standards of monitoring during anaesthesia and recovery.[6]

5 D. C. Craig et al. 2007 *Br Dent J* 203 621.

6 Association of Anaesthetists of Great Britain and Ireland 2016 *Anaesthesia* 71 85.

Benzodiazepines—techniques

Oral sedation

This is of use for managing moderately anxious patients. There are problems, however, with absorption time and the risk of sedation occurring too early or too late. There is again a risk of patients having sexual fantasies under the influence of these drugs. Two drugs are used:

Temazepam 30mg, 1h pre-Rx produces a degree of sedation similar to that seen with IV techniques.

Diazepam Either divided regimen, 5mg night before, 5mg morning of Rx, and 5mg 1h pre-Rx; or as 10–15mg 1h prior to Rx. Both drug and technique are highly variable in consistency and quality of sedation achieved. Both doses may have to be modified depending on the size and age of the patient.

IV techniques

A far greater control of the duration and depth of sedation can be consistently achieved with this approach. Gives excellent sedation with detachment for ~30min with amnesia for the duration of Rx. The major disadvantage is a potential for respiratory depression, post-Rx drowsiness, and amnesia (a reversal agent is available but not suitable for routine reversal of conventional sedation ➲ Flumazenil, p. 635). Skill with venepuncture is a prerequisite of the technique. Diazepam has been entirely superseded by diazepam in lipid emulsion (Diazemuls®) as diazepam is not water-soluble and is very irritant.

Midazolam A water-soluble benzodiazepine of roughly double the strength of diazepam. Has a much shorter half-life, with no significant metabolites, creating a quicker and smoother recovery, and it is more amnesic than diazepam. It is supplied in 5mL ampoules, containing 5mg midazolam, allowing 1mg/increment. Drug of choice.

Diazepam in lipid emulsion Diazepam is metabolized to desmethyldiazepam, which has a long half-life. It is presented in a 2mL ampoule containing 10mg diazepam, given in slow IV increments (usually 2.5mg via a butterfly) until signs of sedation are observed. Suggested maximum dose 20mg.

IV technique Relax the patient and have them sitting in the chair. Place a tourniquet around the most convenient arm and ask them to dangle the arm at their side. Any useful veins on the dorsum of the hand will become quickly evident. While this is happening, get your equipment ready: cannula, 0.9% saline flush, dressing, disinfectant wipe, and drug in syringe.

Look at the hand: is there a reasonable straight segment of vein? (If not, cut your losses and look elsewhere.) If there is, secure the hand with your non-dominant hand, palmar surface to palmar surface, with your thumb in a position to tense the skin overlying the selected vein. Stroke the back of the hand and tap the vein to engorge it. Prepare the skin with disinfectant wipe; get your 'second appropriate person' to help remove the needle cover and inform the patient there will be a slight scratch. Introduce the cannula tip at a shallow angle through skin, then ↓ the angle further and move along the line of the vein until it has entered, as revealed by a flashback into the extension tubing. Then introduce the length of the needle along the vein carefully, so as to avoid cutting through, and secure with tape/dressing (Fig.

15.1). Release tourniquet and flush the cannula with a small amount of 0.9% saline. Place the patient in the supine position and give a small bolus (2–3mg diazepam, 1–2mg midazolam). Wait for 1min and then give further increments until adequate level of sedation is achieved. Leave the cannula in to maintain venous access. Loss of laryngeal reflex constitutes oversedation and means you must stop and ensure the airway is patent, only proceeding if there is no respiratory depression and the airway can be protected.

Monitoring A 'second appropriate person' must be present. Pulse and BP should be monitored. Pulse oximetry is mandatory. An itchy nose is an early sign of 'complete' sedation. Hiccups constitute oversedation.

Post-sedation
Allow time for recovery (30–60min) in calm surroundings. The patient must be accompanied home and forbidden to drive or assume a responsible position for 24h.

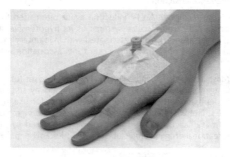

Fig. 15.1 A cannulated hand.
Courtesy of Tim Zoltie, University of Leeds, UK.

Anaesthesia—drugs and definitions

General anaesthesia is a triad of unconsciousness, muscle relaxation, and analgesia.

IV anaesthetic agents

Propofol (dose 2.5mg/kg) A true ultra-short-acting anaesthetic and is completely metabolized within 5h. Less irritant than the others and the drug of choice for day-case anaesthesia.

Thiopental (dose 4mg/kg) Although an ultra-short-acting barbiturate anaesthetic, its half-life is 6–12h. It is a poor analgesic and relatively sparing to the laryngeal reflexes, requiring a greater depth of anaesthesia to prevent laryngospasm. Highly irritant on injection but cheap and very popular as an in-patient induction agent. It will abolish epileptic seizures in induction doses. Has been mainly superseded by propofol but is still occasionally used for rapid sequence inductions.

Etomidate (dose 0.3mg/kg) An IV induction agent often used for patients with compromised cardiovascular systems as its hypotensive side effect is less than other agents. Can be associated with involuntary movements, cough, and hiccup. Is rarely used now due to its association with adrenal suppression.

Ketamine (dose 1–2mg/kg) Can be given IM at higher doses (unique among anaesthetic agents for this). Tends to maintain the airway and causes little respiratory depression. It is a good anaesthetic agent for use in the 'field' where there is limited equipment. Its use is limited by a high incidence of severe nightmare hallucinations in adults, which are eased by midazolam. Popular recreational drug in some club scenes (⊃ Ketamine, p. 798).

Inhalational anaesthetics

Nitrous oxide Excellent analgesic but cannot be used as a sole agent. It is mainly used to supplement other inhalational anaesthetics or in RA. Problem created by its rapid excretion if used for peri-anaesthetic analgesia; wears off rapidly so no post-operative analgesic benefits.

Halothane No longer used in UK. Causes hypotension and dysrhythmias. Can cause VF if used with adrenaline. Hepatotoxic.

Enflurane Less likely to produce dysrhythmias or hepatitis. Avoid in epileptics. Rarely used now.

Isoflurane Close relation of enflurane but more potent. Causes less cardiac problems than halothane. Commonly used hospital agent, may cause coughing with inhalational induction.

Sevoflurane Newer agent with rapid onset and recovery. Good for inhalation induction and increasingly becoming inhalational agent of choice.

Desflurane Another rapid-onset inhalational agent. Can cause coughing.

All inhalational agents cause some degree of muscle relaxation.

Muscle relaxants

Used to create laryngeal relaxation for intubation; this stops patients breathing, and they must then be ventilated until the agent wears off or is reversed.

Suxamethonium Used for emergency cases for rapidly securing airway. Short-acting depolarizing muscle relaxant; quick, good recovery but cannot be reversed. Main problems for the patient are muscle pains, which arise 24–48h after administration. These can be very severe and are more likely in the ambulant. It can also cause severe bradycardia, especially on repeat dose in children. Metabolized by plasma cholinesterase, absence of which can lead to suxamethonium sensitivity (⊙ Suxamethonium sensitivity, p. 542). Causes an ↑ in K^+, therefore know U&Es in all but very routine cases.

Pancuronium, atracurium, vecuronium, and rocuronium All non-depolarizing muscle relaxants; slower acting and longer lasting, but can be reversed using neostigmine.

Mivacurium A short-acting, non-depolarizing agent which, it was hoped, would fill the role of suxamethonium. Disappointing in practice.

Analgesics Opioids are mainstay and include:
- Diamorphine—soluble potent morphine salt (heroin, ⊙ Diamorphine (heroin), p. 600).
- Morphine—long acting, mainly used for post-operative analgesia.
- Fentanyl—first of the short-acting opioids. Provides 1–2h of postoperative analgesia.
- Alfentanil—purely used as anaesthetic opioid due to short duration.
- Remifentanil—continuous infusion needed because of ultra-short duration; ideal for anaesthesia but not post-operative pain relief.

All opioids cause some degree of respiratory depression.

Anaesthesia and the patient on medication

Certain drugs should ring alarm bells when patients require a GA. These include the following:

Monoamine oxidase inhibitors Should be stopped 2 weeks prior to GA.

Antiepileptic drugs Must be continued up to, during, and after GA.

Antihypertensives Should be continued, but ensure the anaesthetist is aware they are being taken.

Bronchodilators Should be continued. Give inhaler with pre-medication and ensure nebulizer is available post-operatively.

Cardioactive drugs Should all be continued. Warn the anaesthetist, as these patients often benefit from a pre-operative anaesthetic assessment.

Cytotoxics Patients on these rarely need GA, but if they do they need FBC, U&Es, and LFTs. Suxamethonium should be avoided.

Diabetic drugs For management, see ◑ Management of the diabetic patient undergoing surgery, p. 588.

Lithium Measure levels. Omit prior to major surgery.

Oral contraceptives Think about DVT prophylaxis, although experience suggests the risk is remote. *BNF* recommends discontinuing 4 weeks prior to major elective surgery; this is generally unnecessary for maxillofacial/oral surgery. Be guided by local policy. Hormone replacement therapy does *not* need to be stopped.

Sedatives and tranquillizers If the patient takes a regular dose these can be maintained, but warn the anaesthetist.

Corticosteroids Patients on long-term steroids require supplementation, ◑ Endocrine-related problems, p. 542; ◑ Collapse in a patient with a history of corticosteroid use, p. 568; ◑ Management of the dental in-patient, p. 576.

Oral anticoagulants Stop and heparinize for all major surgery. Monitor clotting. INR for warfarin. Kaolin–cephalin clotting time (KCT) for heparin.

Anaesthesia—hospital setting

With the exception of the out-patient GA service provided by some hospitals, GA in a hospital setting is similar to that for any other surgical service. The provision for, and the care of, the patient immediately prior to, during, and after the anaesthetic is the domain of the trained anaesthetist. The input from the hospital trainee is the same, whether in a dental or surgical specialty, and is mainly covered in ➔ Management of the dental in-patient, p. 576. The fundamental problem for any dental, oral, or maxillofacial anaesthetic is that the surgeon and anaesthetist both need to have access to the same anatomical site: the shared airway. The means by which this is overcome in hospital practice is usually by endotracheal, particularly nasoendotracheal, intubation, muscle relaxation, and ventilation.

Endotracheal intubation Secures and isolates the airway by placing a tube into the trachea via the nose, mouth, or a tracheostomy. This tube has an inflatable cuff which prevents aspiration of debris and is connected to an anaesthetic machine to allow delivery of O_2, nitrous oxide, or air, and an inhalational anaesthetic. Most anaesthetists also use a throat pack to supplement the cuff, *which must be removed at the end of the operation*. Intubation is a specialist skill and must be learned by practice; skilled practitioners can perform blind and fibreoptic nasoendotracheal intubation, which is of enormous value in cases with trismus; most cases are, however, performed by direct vision of the vocal cords using a laryngoscope with the patient's neck fully extended. The major risk of intubation is intubating the oesophagus *and not recognizing it*. Other complications include traumatizing teeth; vocal cord granulomata; minor trauma to the adenoids; and rarely, pressure necrosis of tracheal mucosa and laryngeal stenosis.

The laryngeal mask airway (LMA) The LMA has become an acceptable method of maintaining the airway. Structurally, it is a curved tube with a large cuff at its end. It is a device which is inserted orally without direct vision following the normal curve of the pharynx. Its onward progression is stopped by the upper end of the oesophagus and at this point the cuff is inflated, forming a seal around the entrance to the larynx. Patients must be starved as it does not protect against aspiration. It occupies a substantial volume in the mouth. The necessity of movement of the LMA to allow surgical access may displace the cuff, possibly causing laryngeal obstruction. Expensive and are autoclavable up to 40 times, however many are now single use. It requires quite deep anaesthesia both to pass and maintain the LMA, which may prolong anaesthesia inappropriately.

The LMA should only be used by those trained in intubation.

Muscle relaxation Essential for successful tracheal intubation in elective patients. For most oral surgery, once intubated ventilation is aided by small doses of non-depolarizing muscle relaxant. An alternative is a continuous infusion of a very short-acting opioid (e.g. remifentanil).

Ventilation May be hand or mechanical. The latter is more precise and convenient for the anaesthetist. It involves a machine providing intermittent positive pressure ventilation. If LMAs are used, the patient maintains spontaneous ventilation.

Monitoring There are increasingly sophisticated non-invasive techniques available: pulse oximetry to measure the percutaneous saturation of haemoglobin with O_2 (a normal person breathing air will have a saturation >95%); capnograph to measure end-tidal CO_2 (normal: 5.2kPa or 40mmHg); ECG and automatic BP machines. It must be stressed, however, that these machines do not replace, only ↑, the ability of the anaesthetist to use clinical observation of pulse, colour, skin changes, and ventilatory pattern. Minimum standard of monitoring in the UK set by Royal College of Anaesthetists is BP, ECG, SaO_2, and end-tidal CO_2.

Malignant hyperpyrexia See ⮑ Malignant hyperpyrexia, p. 542.

Anaesthesia—practice setting

Since the GDC's 2001 amendment to *Maintaining Standards: General Anaesthesia and Resuscitation*, the administration of GAs in dental practice setting has been effectively abolished in the UK. This has seen a huge pressure to ↑ the number of specialist (particularly) paediatric day units concentrating on paediatric exodontia and minor oral surgical work. This is often integrated with the community service for special-needs dentistry patients in the out-patient (ambulatory) setting.

The ideal team to provide exodontia under GA is a small skilled group, e.g. anaesthetist, dentist, operating department practitioner and nurse, who have received appropriate postgraduate training, and have suitable facilities.

Out-patient anaesthesia is given to healthy patients; the majority of anaesthetics, from induction to recovery, are a few minutes. The LMA is frequently used as an airway adjunct for day-case extraction, avoiding the need for muscle relaxation and intubation.

Controversial points

Pollution with anaesthetic gases In the hospital environment it is possible to scavenge the majority of gases as patients are either intubated, or have an LMA or a relatively leak-proof face mask. This is not the case in a dental surgery, as the patients are breathing through a nasal mask and, invariably, through their mouths.

Hazards of inhaling anaesthetic gases These are not well established. It is true that patients continuously breathing nitrous oxide for 24h or so begin to have suppression of the bone marrow and that chronic recreational abuse can cause subacute combined degeneration of the spinal cord. The short-term and intermittent long-term effects of exposure to inhalational anaesthetic agents are, however, simply not known. It remains common sense that no one should work in a polluted atmosphere. The current guidelines are HC (76) 38.

Selected principal recommendations of the Poswillo Committee

Sedation

- Sedation be used in preference to GA whenever possible.
- For sedation by inhalation, the minimum concentration of O_2 be fixed at 30%.
- Flumazenil be reserved for emergency use.
- IV sedation be limited to the use of one drug with a single titrated dose to an endpoint remote from anaesthesia.
- The use of IV sedation in children be approached with caution.
- Dentists must be aware of the significance of pulse oximetry readings.
- All patients treated with the aid of sedative techniques be accompanied by a responsible person.
- Undergraduates should have experience of managing at least five cases of IV sedation and ten cases of inhalation sedation, and be proficient in venepuncture.
- Interested dentists should complete a recognized course in IV sedation within 2 years of qualification.

2009 GDC recommendations on GA and dentistry

These reinforce and extend the Poswillo recommendations. A *referring* or treating practitioner who breaches these recommendations will now be liable to a charge of serious professional misconduct.

Points to note
Referring
- A full PMH must be taken.
- A full explanation of risks and alternatives must occur before referral.
- Justification for the use of GA must be made in the referral letter.
- A copy of the letter must be retained.

Dental treatment under general anaesthesia
Dental treatment under GA should only be carried out when it is judged to be the most clinically appropriate method of anaesthesia; and only take place in a hospital setting that has critical-care facilities.

General anaesthesia
GA may only be given by someone who is on the specialist register of the General Medical Council as an anaesthetist; a trainee working under supervision as part of a Royal College of Anaesthetists' approved training programme; or a non-consultant career-grade anaesthetist with an NHS appointment under the supervision of a named consultant anaesthetist, who must be a member of the same NHS anaesthetic department where the non-consultant career-grade anaesthetist is employed.

The anaesthetist should be supported by someone who is specifically trained and experienced in the necessary skills to help monitor the patient's condition and to help in any emergency.

The Department of Health (England) publication 'A Conscious Decision—a review of the use of general anaesthesia and conscious sedation in primary dental care' (July 2000) provides the basis for these recommendations.

Dental materials

Principal sources J. F. McCabe & A. W. G. Walls 2008
Applied Dental Materials, Blackwell Publishing.

Properties of dental materials

Definitions

Coefficient of thermal expansion The extent to which a material expands upon heating. The fractional ↑ in length for each degree of temperature ↑.

Creep The slow plastic deformation that occurs with the application of a static or dynamic force over time, after the material has set.

Elastic modulus A measure of the rigidity of a material, defined by the ratio of stress to strain (below elastic limit).

Fatigue When cyclic forces are applied, a crack may nucleate and ↑ by small increments each time the force is applied. In time the crack will ↑ to a length at which the force results in # through the remaining material.

Hardness Resistance to penetration. A number of hardness scales are in use (e.g. Vickers, Rockwell, Mohs'). Between these scales, hardness values are not interchangeable.

Resilience The energy absorbed by a material undergoing elastic deformation up to its elastic limit.

Stiffness An indication of how easy it is to bend a piece of material without causing permanent deformation or #. It is dependent upon the elastic modulus, size, and shape of the specimen.

Strain Change in size of a material that occurs in response to a force. It is the change in length divided by the original length.

Stress Internal force per unit cross-sectional area acting on the material. Can be classified according to the direction of the force: tensile (stretching), compressive, or shear.

Thermal conductivity Ability of a material to transmit heat.

Thermal diffusivity Rate at which temperature changes spread through a material.

Toughness The amount of energy absorbed up to the point of #. A function of the resilience of the material and its ability to undergo plastic deformation rather than #.

Wear The abrasion (mechanical or chemical) resistance of a substance.

Wettability Ability of one material to flow across the surface of another, determined by the contact angle between the two materials and influenced by surface roughness and contamination. The contact angle is the angle between solid/liquid and liquid/air interfaces measured through the liquid.

Yield strength (Or elastic limit.) The stress beyond which a material is permanently deformed when a force is applied.

Evaluation of a new material

Before it reaches the dental supply companies a new material should have undergone the following tests:

- *Standard specifications* (i.e. physical properties), e.g. compressive strength, hardness, etc. The actual values obtained are mainly of value in comparing the new material with those already in use and which are performing satisfactorily. Compliance with an international (International Organization for Standardization (ISO)) standard indicates fitness for dental use.
- *Laboratory evaluation.* Should be relevant to the clinical situation, but this is easier said than done!
- *Clinical trials.* Usually conducted under optimal conditions. Many materials have been less successful under the conditions imposed by clinical practice, particularly those with demanding placement techniques.

Clinically, the important questions to ask a representative selling or promoting any dental material include:

- Details of the chemical constituents.
- Handling characteristics, e.g. presentation, mixing, working time, setting time, and dimensional changes on setting.
- Performance in service.
- Cost.
- Shelf life.
- Does the material meet the relevant ISO standard?

Then decide whether this new material has any significant advantages over the material you are familiar with.

Restoration of teeth

When restoring or replacing teeth it should be remembered that the teeth themselves are composed of enamel, dentine, and pulpal tissues each with quite different properties that must be taken into account when selecting a material with which to restore them. In addition, the teeth emerge from a complex dentogingival junction and are supported in alveolar bone by the viscoelastic periodontal ligament. All of these features are difficult to reproduce with current dental materials and most likely will not be until teeth themselves or their individual tissues are able to be bioengineered.

Amalgam

Dental amalgam is made by mixing together mercury (Hg) with a powdered silver–tin alloy (mercury around 50% by weight) to produce a soft mass that can be packed into a preparation before setting.

Types of amalgam There are two ways of classifying amalgam:
- *Particle shape*—can be lathe-cut (irregular), spheroidal, or a mixture of the two. Spheroidal particles give a more fluid mix which is easy to condense, can be carved immediately, and take 3h to reach occlusal strength (compared to >6h for lathe-cut amalgams). Spheroidal amalgams are preferable for pinned restorations.
- *Particle composition*—the first (conventional) alloys introduced had a low copper content (5%). The weakest (Sn–Hg or λ-2) phase of the set amalgam could be eliminated by ↑ the proportion of copper, so a variety of high copper (10–30%) amalgams have been introduced that react to eliminate it. These are more expensive, but superior in terms of corrosion resistance, creep, strength, and durability of marginal integrity. There are two types of high-copper alloy: (i) a single composition alloy of silver–tin–copper; (ii) a blended (dispersion) mix of silver–tin and copper–silver alloys. Of these, (i) is the most resistant to tarnishing.

Types of amalgam currently available Conventional lathe-cut, conventional spherical, high-copper dispersion lathe + spherical, high-copper single spheroidal, and high-copper single lathe-cut amalgam (Table 16.1).

Handling characteristics

Mixing or trituration This is carried out mechanically, in one of two ways:
- Pre-encapsulated by manufacturer, with automatic vibrator—preferred method.
- Using an amalgamator that dispenses Hg and alloy in correct proportions and mixes them. However, the amalgamator requires refilling by hand which ↑ likelihood of Hg spillage occurring. The duration of trituration varies from 5 to 20sec.

Condensation Carry out incrementally by hand instruments (lathe-cut or spheroidal). Preparations should be overfilled so that the Hg-rich surface layer is removed by carving.

Carving With spherical alloys this can be commenced immediately; burnishing is recommended in an attempt to prevent marginal leakage.

Polishing Polished amalgams look good, but whether polishing is necessary is still the subject of debate. NB: maximum strength takes 24h to develop, so it is advisable to recommend patients do not chew on the restored tooth for this time where possible.

Table 16.1 Composition of amalgams

	Average composition (%)			
	Silver	Tin	Copper	Zinc
Conventional	68	28	4	0–2
High copper	60	27	13	0

Marginal leakage While amalgam corrosion products will form a marginal seal in time, microleakage can be ↓ by the use of either a conventional cavity varnish (e.g. Copalite®) or a bonding agent (e.g. Amalgambond® or Panavia-21™) in the interim. The latter (an anaerobic resin adhesive) also bonds to set amalgam.[1] Alternatively, sealing over the completed restoration with a fissure sealant has been suggested, and this is a possible solution to the 'ditched', but caries-free amalgam.

Toxicity Despite toxicity scares and the introduction of posterior composites, amalgam is still widely used, mainly because of its ease of handling. In Norway, Denmark, and Sweden, dental amalgam is banned for environmental reasons. The Control of Mercury (Enforcement) Regulations 2017 stipulate there should be no use of amalgam in the treatment of deciduous teeth, in children under 15yrs or pregnant or breastfeeding women, except when strictly deemed necessary by the practitioner on the grounds of specific medical needs of the patient.[2] It is likely further phasing down will occur (possibly to a full ban!). These regulations aim to reduce mercury in the environment and are not a reflection on any specific safety concerns about amalgam.

In addition, there is a link between allergy to constituents of dental amalgam and lichenoid eruptions in the oral cavity in certain individuals.

The greatest actual risk appears to be related to the inhalation of Hg vapour and as such, the dental team as well as patients are theoretically at risk.

Attention should be paid to the following:
- Avoid spilling Hg if non-encapsulated system employed.
- Waste amalgam should be stored appropriately to prevent mercury vapour release.
- When removing old amalgams, safety glasses, masks, and high-volume aspiration are a wise precaution.
- Amalgam separation devices should be in use as per Hazardous Waste Directive (91/689/EEC). Should comply with British Standard Dental Equipment—amalgam separators (BS EN ISO 11143:2008) (℠ http://www.bsigroup.com).

---

1 D. C. Watts et al. 1992 *J Dent* 20 245.

2 ℠ https://www.legislation.gov.uk/uksi/2017/1200/contents/made.

Composite resins—constituents and properties

The modern composite resin is a mixture of resin and particulate filler, the handling characteristics of which are determined largely by the size of the filler particles and method of cure.

Constituents

Resin Most composite resins are based on either Bis-GMA (addition product of bisphenol A and glycidylmethacrylate) or urethane dimethacrylate plus a diluent monomer, triethylene glycol dimethacrylate (TEGMA).

Filler (E.g. quartz, fused silica, glasses such as aluminosilicate and borosilicate.) Confers the following benefits on the composite resin:
- Compressive strength, abrasion resistance, modulus of elasticity, and # toughness.
- Thermal expansion and setting contraction.
- Aesthetic qualities.

Composite resins can be subdivided according to particle size:

Macrofilled (Or conventional.) Contains particles of radio-opaque barium or strontium glass 2.5–5μm in size, to give 75–80% by weight of filler. Good mechanical properties, but hard to polish and soon roughens.

Microfilled Contains colloidal silica particles 0.04μm in size and 30–60% by weight. Retains a good surface polish, but is unsuitable for load-bearing situations, has poor wear resistance, and ↑ contraction shrinkage.

Nanofilled By combining nanometric particles and nanoclusters in a conventional resin matrix, manufacturers claim to offer ↑ wear resistance as well as polishability and lustre.

Hybrid Contains a mixture of conventional and microfine particles designed to optimize both mechanical and surface properties. Contains 75–85% by weight of filler, of which the bulk is conventional (1–50μm). Some manufacturers achieve up to 90% filler loadings by using blended sizes of filler particles.

Packable (condensable) Developed to simulate the 'condensation' of amalgam although no ↓ in volume as compressed therefore not strictly condensed. Resin and ceramic fillers are incorporated into a network of ceramic fibres. Claim to have ↑ wear resistance and less polymerization shrinkage.

Initiator/activator
- Chemically cured: benzoyl peroxide (or sulfinic acid) initiator + tertiary amine activator.
- Light cured: amine + diketone activated by blue light (460–70nm).

Other constituents These include pigments, stabilizers, and silane coupler to produce bond between particles and filler.

Composites may also be classified as:
• Microfilled.
• Posterior composite.
• All-purpose.
• Flowable.
• Condensable/packable.

Important properties of composites
• Polymerization shrinkage of 1–4%.
• Thermal expansion is significantly greater than enamel or dentine, and without an acid-etch bond can result in marginal leakage.
• Elastic modulus should be high to resist occlusal forces. Modulus of hybrid type is greater than other composite resins, amalgam, or dentine. However, composite resins are still brittle and # if used in thin section.
• Wear resistance is greatest in hybrids.
• Radio-opacity is particularly useful, especially for posterior resin composites.
• ? Toxicity. Resins have been found to be toxic in cell culture. Also controversy surrounding the oestrogenicity of composite resins.

Newer developments include hydroxyl ion-releasing composite resin to counteract demineralization during periods of low pH in the restoration. Also use of fibre reinforcement to fabricate posts and cores as well as bridges/splints.

Composite resins—practical points

Method of polymerization

Chemical (self-cure) No additional equipment required, but mixing of two components introduces porosity and the working time is limited.

Light activation Provides long working time, command set, and better colour stability, but requires a light source, has a limited depth of cure, and the temperature ↑ during setting can be as high as 40°C. Three types of light source are currently available: quartz tungsten halogen (QTH), plasma arc light (PAC), and light-emitting diode (LED). PAC and LED lights confer theoretical advantages in, e.g. speed and depth of cure, portability (not PAC), lifetime, and reliability of light source. LED models are becoming most widely used replacing QTH. PAC light sources claim quicker curing times due to ↑ intensity but are more expensive.

Dual-cure Curing is initiated by a conventional light source, but continues chemically to help ensure polymerization throughout the restoration.

Practical tips for light activation
- Replace bulbs every 6–12 months. Some lights correct for the effects of bulb ageing.
- Air attenuates light beam, ∴ position as close to tooth as possible.
- Preparations >2mm depth should be cured incrementally.
- Precautions are necessary to protect eyes from glare, ∴ use safety shield, get the patient to close their eyes, and the DN to look away.
- The efficiency of the light source can be tested by curing a block of composite. Practical depth of cure is half the thickness of set material.
- The greater the intensity of the light source, the greater the depth of cure.

Finishing Ideally, a mylar strip to produce the contour of the restoration. Then refine with microfine diamond or multi-bladed tungsten carbide finishing burs (under water spray), finishing strips, and then polish with aluminium oxide-coated discs (e.g. Sof-Lex™). Shofu points or finishing pastes (Shofu CompoSite™ finishing kit) are useful for inaccessible concave surfaces.

Problems with composite resins

- Difficult to obtain satisfactory contact points and occlusal stops. Modern placement techniques have made improvements in this regard, e.g. using sectional contoured matrix bands.
- Post-operative sensitivity.
- Polymerization shrinkage.
- The C-factor (configuration) is the ratio of bonded to unbonded surfaces in a cavity. The higher the C-factor, the more likely the risk of effects of polymerization shrinkage (bond failure, cuspal deflection, post-operative sensitivity).
- Depth of cure of light-cured materials is limited. This is a particular problem in posterior teeth.

Indirect composite inlays may circumvent the last two problems (→ Indirect resin composite or porcelain inlays/onlays, p. 225).

Fissure sealants Composite resins containing little or no filler, which are either self- or light-cured. Clear or opaque types are available, the former having better flow characteristics (whether this is an advantage depends upon the position of the tooth). Success depends upon being able to achieve good moisture control for the acid-etch bond.

Flowable composite resins Predominantly resin with a reduced percentage of filler particles, and consequently shrink considerably on curing. Some advocate using them as liners or in the bottom of proximal preparations, but the high shrinkage precludes this. RMGIC is preferable in proximal preparations, which are below the cemento-enamel junction (bonded-base approach); however, they have a place in the marginal repair of restorations and some advocate their use for facial cervical margin restorations.

Flowable technology has led to further developments in the ability to bulk fill with the addition of several new materials such as SDR® flow+ from Dentsply with a 4mm depth of cure. In addition, the data from this material and similar suggests ↓ polymerization shrinkage and cusp deflection.

Pink composite (E.g. Amaris® Gingiva by Voco.) These pink-coloured composite restoratives can be used chairside and some, e.g. GC Gradia® gum shades, are compatible with their laboratory microceramic composite namesake.

Enamel and dentine bonding

Research would suggest that:
- Success depends upon adequate moisture control, as contact with saliva for as little as 0.5sec will contaminate the etch pattern.
- A prophylaxis prior to etching is not required unless abundant plaque deposits are present.
- 30–50% buffered phosphoric acid provides the best enamel etch pattern.
- An etching time of 15–20sec is adequate for both 1° and permanent enamel, and 15sec for dentine is recommended.
- The etch pattern is easily damaged; using a probe to aid etchant penetration of pits and fissures, or applying etchant by rubbing vigorously with a pledget of cotton wool, is C/I.
- There is no difference in bond strength whether an etchant solution or gel is used. Gels take twice as long to rinse away but have the advantage of greater viscosity and colour contrast.
- Rinse for at least 15sec.
- Remineralization of etched enamel occurs from the saliva, and after 24h it is indistinguishable from untreated enamel.
- Etched enamel is porous and has a high surface energy.

The etch pattern consists of three zones (from surface inwards):
- Etched zone (enamel removed): 10µm.
- Qualitative zone: 20µm.
- Quantitative porous zone: 20µm.

Composite resin tags may penetrate up to 50µm into enamel to give micromechanical retention.

NB: many of the newer dentine adhesive systems do not have a separate acid-etch stage. These systems use a combination of acidic primers and bonding resins, either as a single stage or applied separately (➲ Dentine-adhesive systems (dentine bonding agents), p. 658).

Dentine-adhesive systems (dentine bonding agents)

The advantages of bonding to dentine (e.g. preservation of tooth tissue) have fuelled considerable research effort. The problems that have had to be overcome include the high water and organic content of dentine; the presence of a 'smear layer' after dentine is cut; and the need for adequate strength immediately following placement, to withstand the polymerization contraction of composite resin. These difficulties have been approached in a number of ways, making the topic of dentine bonding confusing, a situation that has been exacerbated by the pace of new developments and by the claims of the manufacturers.

Indications
- Marginal seal where preparation margin is in dentine or cementum, e.g. cervical (Class V), proximal (Class II) box.
- Retention and seal of direct resin-composite restorations.
- Retention and seal of indirect porcelain and composite inlays.
- Dentine adhesives have also been used for repairing # teeth, cementing ceramic crowns and veneers, and as an endodontic sealer.

The smear layer This consists of an amorphous layer of organic and inorganic debris, produced by cutting dentine. It ↓ sensitivity by occluding the dentine tubules and prevents loss of dentinal fluid. The smear layer is partially or completely removed &/or modified during dentine bonding.

Mechanism of dentine bonding
Most dentine adhesive systems aim to modify and partially remove the smear layer, by the application of an acidic primer. This demineralizes the underlying surface, exposing the collagen and opening up the dentinal tubules. It is important to keep this surface moist to prevent the collagen becoming flattened (*not* with saliva, though!). This layer is then infiltrated using a resin with bi-functional ends: one hydrophilic end, which is able to bond to wet dentine, and one hydrophobic end capable of bonding to the composite resin. In this infiltrated hybrid layer molecular entanglement of the collagen and resin occurs, providing the basis for the bonding system.

Practical points
- Follow manufacturer's instructions.
- For better results, use a matched resin-composite and adhesive system.
- When a dentine adhesive is used, polymerization shrinkage of composite resin is more likely to result in cuspal deformation and post-operative pain. An incremental filling and curing technique will help to solve this problem.
- Pre-curing the adhesive bonding agent before placing the composite ↑ bond strength to dentine.[3]
- No technique produces zero microleakage.

3 J. Chapman et al. 2007 *Quintessence Int* **38** 637–41.

Techniques

Etch and rinse
- *Three step* (acid etch, primer, and adhesive)—37% phosphoric acid usually used to remove the smear layer and demineralize the surface dentine. A primer is then applied, often containing a solvent such as acetone to eliminate water in the dentine that is then filled by resin tags. Another method is to use an aqueous primer solution. Benefit of ease of use as well as stronger acid etching of the enamel.
- *Two step* (etchant and primer/adhesive).

Self-etching
- *Two step*—a weaker acid is used to solubilize the smear layer and at the same time act as the difunctional primer (hydrophilic and hydrophobic ends). Second stage is adhesive.
- *One step*:
  - Self-etching one-step mix. The resin bonding agent is mixed in the same liquid as the etch and primer. Often unidose presentation.
  - Self-etching, no mix 'one-bottle system'.

If enamel is present, it is usually better to undertake etch and rinse whereas at the other extreme when dentine only is present, e.g. a crown preparation, then the weaker acid of the self-etching technique may be preferable. Self-etching possibly leads to less post-operative sensitivity.

Bonding to metals and ceramics

The described bonding systems may be used in conjunction with preparation of metal or ceramic surfaces to allow bonding of materials other than composite resin to the tooth surface. Metal surfaces are usually sandblasted to provide roughness for micromechanical retention then prepared with a 4-META-derived conditioner before application of a composite luting cement. Ceramic surfaces are usually etched then silanated before luting. This allows for a great variety of clinical uses including orthodontics as well as fixed prosthodontics.

Glass ionomers

Glass ionomer = *polyalkenoate*.

Setting reaction

Alumino-silicate glass powder + polyalkenoic acid → calcium + aluminium polyalkenoates (base + polyacid → polysalt + water).

The set material consists of unreacted spheres of glass surrounded by a silicaeous gel, embedded in metal polyalkenoates. Fluoride is uptaken and released from the cement to give theoretical cariostatic properties.

Presentation

- Powder + liquid.
- Powder (with anhydrous acid) + water.
- Encapsulated.

Tartaric acid is added to lengthen working time. In some products, polymaleic acid replaces polyacrylic and Diamond Carve™ is hand-mixed glass polyphosphonate.

'High-viscosity' or reinforced GIs, e.g. GC Fuji IX GP™, are claimed to have improved earlier physical properties and resistance to dissolution.

Properties

Adhesion To enamel and dentine by: (i) ionic displacement of calcium and phosphate with polyacrylate ions; (ii) possible absorption of polyalkenoic acid onto collagen. Some authors recommend pre-conditioning the dentine, e.g. with 10% polyalkenoic acid (GC Dentin Conditioner™) for 30sec. Whether this ↑ adhesion is controversial. GIC also bonds to the oxide layer on SS and tin.

Cariostatic Due to fluoride release throughout the lifetime of the restoration. GIs are also able to take up fluoride when the IO concentration is raised, the 'reservoir effect'. However, the therapeutic benefit of fluoride release has yet to be proven to be clinically significant.

Thermal expansion Similar to enamel and dentine.

Strength Brittle material. Tensile strength is only 40% of composite resin.

Radiolucent Except for the cermets, which are rarely used.

Abrasion/erosion resistance Poor, but improving with newer materials, especially with the high-viscosity versions.

Biocompatibility This has been questioned following reports of pulpal inflammation when used as a luting cement and pulp response studies have shown conflicting results. However, literature has demonstrated no such reports of pulp reactions after cementation of cast restorations with GIC.[4]

---

4 S. Sidhu and G. Schmaiz 2001 *Am J Dent* **14** 387.

Applications

GIs are unable to match the aesthetics and abrasion resistance of the composite resins, and brittleness limits their use to non-load-bearing situations. However, their adhesive and fluoride-releasing properties have resulted in a range of applications and matching formulations.

Type I Luting cements for crowns, bridges, and orthodontic bands.

Type II Restorative cements. There are two subtypes: (i) aesthetic and (ii) reinforced. Can also be used as a fissure sealant, for the restoration of 1° teeth (➜ Material selection for intracoronal restorations, p. 84) and for repairing defective restorations.

Type III Fast-setting lining materials. Defer placement of amalgam for at least 15min and composite for 4min. In load-bearing situations or where lining is exposed to the oral environment (e.g. in sandwich technique), use of a type II reinforced cement or RMGIC is preferable.

Type IV Includes the light-cure and dual-cure GI (use of a light source optimizes the properties of the dual-cure materials, although they will self-polymerize without). 3M Vitremer™ is an example of a so-called tri-cure GI where, in addition to the acid–base reaction and the photoinitiated free radical methacrylate cure there is also a further dark methacrylate cure that can occur in the absence of light.

Forms of true GI can also be used for fissure sealants, orthodontic cements, core build-ups, and for restoration of deciduous teeth.

Practical tips

- A dry field is essential.
- Encapsulated systems ensure optimal mixing and allow placement via a syringe tip, e.g. Ketac-Fil™.
- Cement should be inserted before its sheen is lost.
- GI sticks to instruments, ∴ use powder as a separator if powder-liquid.
- Cellulose or soft metal strips provide the best finish.
- Water balance during setting is critical. Absorption of water results in dissolution, and dehydration leads to crazing, ∴ cement must be protected with waterproof material, e.g. light-cured bonding resin, which acts as a lubricant for finishing and can then be cured.
- Although most manufacturers claim that trimming can be started 10–15min after placement, it is better to defer for >24h.

Other glass ionomer/composite-based products

Resin-modified glass ionomers These allow 'command' setting and help overcome the moisture sensitivity and low early mechanical strength associated with conventional GI. The acid–base reaction of GI is supplemented by the addition of 75% resin (hydroxyethyl methacrylate Bis-GMA). The initial set of the material is due to the formation of a polymerization matrix, which is strengthened by the acid–base reaction. They are easier to handle than conventional GIs and may be polished immediately after light-curing. Aesthetics approach those of resin-based materials, plus the advantage of fluoride release (although this is still of unproven clinical significance). These materials can be used in conjunction with composite resin for placement in deep proximal preparation where the deepest parts of the preparation are below the cemento-enamel junction. This type of open sandwich restoration fell into disrepute when restorations were placed with traditional GIC. Single-surface glass ionomer restorations have a relatively poor survival of <40% across 10yrs.[5] Also widely used as lining materials and luting cements.

Compomer Polyacid-modified composite resin. It combines the adhesive and fluoride-releasing properties of GI with the abrasion resistance of composite resin and is called, with a touch of originality, 'compomer'. Composed of a single hydrophobic resin filled with acid-leachable glass particles. Bonded with a bi-functional primer and light-cured. It is claimed that the chemical reaction takes place through uptake of water from saliva leading to fluoride ions leaching out. Popular in general practice due to ease of technique and especially useful for restoration of deciduous teeth.

Giomers This group of materials may be described as composite resins with active (GI) filler particles. The filler particles are based on pre-reacted surface or fully reacted GI filler particles (S-PRG) whereas the acid–base reaction process occurs after initial setting in acid-modified composites. Have been shown to be capable of sustained fluoride ion release in the absence of water (unlike GI and compomers that require water absorption before fluoride recharge can occur). Possibly useful for high-caries-risk individuals. E.g. Shofu Beautifil II™.

Ormocers Organically modified ceramics, e.g. Admira®. Made up of three components: organic polymers, ceramic glasses, and polyvinylsiloxane. Claimed to confer less polymerization shrinkage, good handling, marginal integrity, and biocompatibility (less free diluent monomer). Lack of clinical trials to date.

Cermets These are similar to GIs, except that the ion-leachable glass is fused with fine silver powder. Mixing with a polymeric acid gives a cement consisting of unreacted glass particles to which silver is fused, held together by a metal–salt matrix with the benefit of ↑ wear resistance. Cermets have been largely superseded by the RMGICs and are now generally discouraged.

5 J. F. J. T. Burke & P. S. K. Lucarotti 2019 *BDJ* 206 e2.

Ceromers Ceromers are second-generation indirect composite resins. Their main components are silanized microhybrid inorganic fillers embedded in a light-curing organic matrix. Ceromers have high filler content and so improved mechanical properties compared to traditional composites. They are, however, less wear resistant than enamel with potential problems in the long term in high loading sites. The material may be used as indirect onlays with benefits over porcelain in 'camouflaging' of shade as well as a fibre-reinforced crown or bridge material (Targis Vectris®) with variable success.

Cements

Types of cement

Based on zinc oxide eugenol (ZOE) Powder of pure zinc oxide is mixed (in a ratio of 3:1) with eugenol liquid to give zinc eugenolate and unreacted powder. Setting time is 24h. This is the weakest cement, but the eugenol acts as an obtundent and analgesic, ∴ used as a sedative dressing. The following modifications change the properties for various indications.

Accelerated ZOE (E.g. Sedanol®.) Addition of zinc acetate to the powder ↑ setting time to 5min.

Resin-bonded ZOE (E.g. Kalzinol®.) Addition of 10% hydrogenated resin to the powder ↑ strength.

EBA Addition of ortho-ethoxybenzoic acid (62%) to the liquid ↑ strength.

Zinc phosphate (E.g. DeTrey® Zinc.) The powder consists of zinc and magnesium oxides, and the liquid 50% aqueous phosphoric acid. The working time is ↑ by adding the powder in small increments. Popular in the past because of its strength. Although low setting pH theoretically C/I its use for vital teeth, in practice this does not seem to be a problem.

Zinc polycarboxylate (E.g. Poly-F Plus®, Durelon™.) The powder is a mixture of zinc and magnesium oxides and the liquid is 40% aqueous polyacrylic acid. Anhydrous acid formulations have been introduced, which are mixed with water or encapsulated. The powder should be added quickly to the liquid. The temptation to remove excess cement should be resisted until it has reached a rubbery stage. Adheres to dentine, enamel, tin, and SS. Often used as temporary cement where ↑ adherence required.

Calcium hydroxide Chemically curing types comprise two pastes which are mixed together in equal quantities. One paste contains the calcium hydroxide plus fillers in a non-reacting carrier, and the other polysalicylate fluid. The set material consists of an amorphous calcium disalicylate complex plus calcium hydroxide and has a pH of 11. In addition to being bacteriostatic, calcium hydroxide can induce mineralization of adjacent pulp. Light-cured formulations which are resin-based are available. Have ↓ bactericidal properties, but ↑ strength.

RMGIC This is a popular luting cement used for indirect cast restorations and for cavity lining.

Strength

Phosphate > EBA or polycarboxylate > resin-bonded ZOE > accelerated ZOE > calcium hydroxide.

Practical points

- Generally, the thicker the mix, the greater the strength.
- Heat ↓ setting time, ∴ a cooled slab is advisable.
- To stop cement sticking to the instruments during placement, dip in cement powder (except calcium hydroxide) or use non-stick instruments.
- When luting, apply cement to crown or inlay before tooth.

Choice of cement

Temporary restorations Choice depends upon how long the dressing needs to last and whether any therapeutic qualities are required. Pure ZOE is useful for a tooth with a reversibly inflamed pulp, but resin-bonded ZOE is stronger. GI is preferable for semi-permanent dressings and endodontic provisionalization because it seals the preparation margins.

Luting cement Zinc phosphate, GI, and polycarboxylate are all popular as luting cements. EBA cement is C/I because of ↑ solubility. Composite-based luting systems are often used in conjunction with dentine adhesive systems. Mandatory for cementing ceramic or porcelain inlays/onlays and ceramic veneers. Now available as one-step luting cements with no etching or bonding required.

Lining cement Choice of lining depends upon the depth of the preparation and the material being used to restore it:
- *Amalgam*—minimal: preparation sealer (Gluma® Densensitizer); moderate: RMGIC (Vitrebond™); deep: use a sub-lining of calcium hydroxide (direct or indirect pulp capping) and any of the cements listed. Typically RMGIC is recommended as it seals as well as lines the preparation.
- *Composite resin*—dentine adhesive system with direct or indirect pulp capping as indicated.

Pulp capping Hard-setting calcium hydroxide or MTA.

Sedative dressing ZOE &/or calcium hydroxide.

Bacteriostatic dressing Calcium hydroxide plus GI (stepwise excavation).

Impression materials

Classification See Table 16.2.

Elastomers Indicated when accuracy is paramount, e.g. crown and bridge work, and implants.

Condensation-cured silicone These materials are relatively cheap compared with other elastomers, but prone to some shrinkage and should be cast immediately. Addition-cured silicones are preferred.

Addition-cured silicone This type of silicone is very stable, which means that impressions can be posted or stored prior to casting. A perforated tray or rim lock tray is advisable as the adhesives supplied are not very effective. Up to five viscosities are manufactured, allowing a range of impression techniques. NB: powdered latex gloves (now rarely used) can retard setting of putty materials.[6] Can also be used for registering occlusion.

Polysulfide Messy to handle, but useful when a long working time is required. Use with a special tray and, although stable, cast within 24h. Not recommended except in complete denture cases.

Polyether (e.g. Impregum™) Popular because it uses a single mix and a stock tray. The set material is stiff, although newer products (e.g. Penta Soft™) have addressed this and removal can be stressful in cases with deep undercuts or advanced periodontitis. Absorbs water, ∴ do not store with alginate impressions. Can cause allergic reactions. Routinely used for implant cases and crown and bridge work, especially when there are multiple preps.

Hydrocolloids

Reversible hydrocolloid This is accurate, but liable to tear. Requires the purchase of a water bath and is not infection-control friendly.

Irreversible hydrocolloid (alginate) Setting is a double decomposition reaction between sodium alginate and calcium sulfate. Popular because it is cheap and can be used with a stock tray. However, it is not sufficiently accurate for crown and bridge work. Impressions must be kept damp and cast within 24h. Alginate can retard the setting of gypsum and affect the surface of the model.

Impression compound Available in either sheet form for recording preliminary impressions, or in stick form for modifying trays. The sheet material is softened in a waterbath with warm water (55–60°C) and used in a stock tray to record edentulous ridges. The viscosity of compound results in a well-extended impression, but limited detail. Admix impression material (mix of greenstick and impression compound) is useful for denture cases with severe resorption.

Zinc oxide pastes Dispensed 1:1 and mixed to an even colour. Used for recording edentulous ridges in a special tray or the patient's existing dentures, but C/I for undercuts. Setting time is ↓ by warmth and humidity. Fared worse in one particular RCT.[7]

---

6 W. W. L. Chee & T. E. Donovan 1992 *J Prosthet Dent* **68** 728.

7 J. F. McCord et al. 2005 *Eur J Pros Rest Dent* **13** 105.

Table 16.2 Classification of impression materials

	Elastic	
Non-elastic	Elastomers	Hydrocolloid
Compound	Silicone	Reversible
ZOE paste	Polysulfide	Irreversible
Wax	Polyether	

Impression techniques

(For crown and bridge work.)

▶Time spent recording a good impression is an investment, as repeating laboratory work is costly.

Special trays These help the adaptation of impression material and ↓ the amount required, i.e. ↑ accuracy and ↓ cost. Can be made in cold-cure acrylic or light-activated tray resin. Special trays are rarely used for crown and bridge work impressions, with stock trays used routinely. Usually the palate does not need to be included, so design the special tray accordingly or use a lower stock tray. For the opposing arch, alginate in a stock tray will suffice.

Monophase technique (E.g. polyether.) The same mix of medium-viscosity material is used for both a stock tray and syringe. Although less accurate than other methods, it is adequate for most tasks.

Double-mix technique (E.g. polysulfide, addition-cured silicone.) A single-stage technique necessitating the mixing of heavy- and light-bodied materials at the same time, and use of a special or stock tray.
● Apply adhesive to tray.
● Mix light- and heavy-bodied viscosities simultaneously for 45–60sec.
● Remove retraction cord or preferably leave in place and dry preparation, while nurse loads syringe with light-bodied material.
● Syringe light-bodied mix around prep. A gentle stream of air helps to direct material into crevice.
● Position tray containing heavy-bodied material.
● Support tray with light pressure until 2min after apparent set.

Putty and wash technique (E.g. silicone.) The putty and light-bodied viscosities can be used with a stock tray, either:
● *Single stage*—similar to the double-mix technique, or
● *Two stage*—this involves taking an impression of the prep with the putty, using a polythene sheet as a spacer. This is then relined with the light-bodied material, which is also syringed around the prep. Depending on circumstances and clinician preferences, different impression techniques and materials may be favoured, however there is limited evidence to prove superiority, particularly regarding denture fabrication. More high quality RCTs are needed to determine if any material or technique is advantageous.[8]

Cost In decreasing order:
● Addition-cured silicone using putty/reline.
● Polyether with special tray.
● Addition-cured silicone using double mix and special tray.
● Polysulfide with special tray.
● Condensation-cured silicone using putty/reline.
● Hydrocolloid.

8 S. Jayaraman et al. 2018 *Cochrane Database Syst Rev* 4 CD012256.

Automixing dispensers This double-cartridge presentation is exceptionally popular. The two pastes are extruded and mixed in the nozzle when the trigger is pressed. Appears expensive, but ↓ waste and the mixture is void free. Many manufacturers are now producing their materials in this format.

Disinfection of impressions Impressions should be rinsed to remove debris and then immersed in a solution of sodium hypochlorite (1000ppm available chlorine) or a glutaraldehyde-free proprietary disinfectant such as Perform® for 10min. In general, dimensional stability of impressions seems unaffected by current protocols.[9]

Intraoral scanning Various systems are now available that record impressions digitally and miss out messy conventional impressions altogether, digitally relaying the detail of a conventional impression. Current scanners are sufficiently accurate in capturing details required to fabricate most restorations including inlays/onlays, crowns, fixed bridgework, fixed partical dentures, copings, and frameworks.[10] These are becoming more commonplace in general practice and have the advantage that sections can be rescanned without the additional expense of a repeat impression. Other advantages include direct receipt by the laboratory reducing transportation costs and time as well as being better for the environment due to the lack of printed laboratory tickets, labels, and postage/packaging. They are often tolerated well by patients who find conventional impressions difficult to cope with and can be useful for patient education purposes.

Tips for IO scanning:
- Scan systematically to ensure no areas are missed.
- Use retraction cord around preparations unless supra-gingival margins.
- Ensure area being scanned is dry and the soft tissues are not obstructing the image.
- Practise scanning technique to ensure as efficient and comfortable for the patient as possible.
- Ensure a bite registration is recorded.
- Communicate clearly with the laboratory what is required.

9 E. Kotsiomiti et al. 2008 *J Oral Rehab* **35** 291.

10 F. Mangano et al. 2017 *BMC Oral Health* **17** 149.

Casting alloys

An alloy is a mixture of two or more metallic elements. The chemistry of alloys is too complicated for this book chapter (and its author), so for a fuller understanding, the reader is referred to the source text.

The properties of an alloy depend upon:
- The thermal treatments applied to the alloy (including cooling).
- The mechanical manipulation of the alloy.
- The composition of the alloy.

NB: the properties of an alloy may differ significantly from that of its constituents.

The main examples of alloys in dentistry include amalgam (➲ Amalgam, p. 650), steel burs and instruments, metallic denture bases, inlays, crowns and bridges, NiTi endodontic instruments, and orthodontic wires.

A warm, moist mouth provides the ideal environment for corrosion. To overcome this problem, dental casting alloys comprise an essentially corrosion-resistant metal (usually gold), with the addition of other constituents to enhance its properties. However, with the possible exception of titanium, all have the potential to affect hypersensitive individuals.

Additions to gold alloys

Copper ↑ strength and hardness, but ↓ ductility.

Silver ↑ hardness and strength, but ↑ tarnishing and ↑ porosity.

Platinum/palladium (As in type III/IV gold alloys.) ↑ melting point (which confers advantage for soldering).

Zinc or indium Scavenger, preventing oxidation of other metals during melting and casting.

Traditional dental casting gold alloys

ISO standard ISO standard is that the noble metal (gold, platinum, palladium, iridium, ruthenium, rhodium) content must be >75% with no less than 65% gold. Four types are defined by proof stress (stress required to cause a permanent deformation of a particular value (e.g. 0.2%)—similar to elastic limit) and elongation (ductility) values from type I (low strength for castings subject to low stress) to type IV (extra-high strength).

Clinically this means the type I and II alloys are used in low load-bearing situations such as inlays; type III where demands are higher such as full cuspal coverage onlays, crowns, and bridges; and type IV where rigidity is required for removable partial denture bases or clasps.

Dental casting semi-precious alloys These have 25–74% noble metal content.

Low gold alloys Similar to the traditional gold alloys, four types are defined by proof stress and elongation properties. High palladium content imparts 'whiteness'. Popularity ↑ with ↑ cost of gold.

Silver palladium Palladium (generally >25%), silver, gold, indium, and zinc. Cheaper than gold alloys and of equivalent hardness, but less ductile, more difficult to cast, and prone to porosity.

Base metal casting alloys Contain no gold, platinum, or palladium.

Nickel chromium 75% nickel, 20% chromium. Used in crowns and bridge work. In latter, ↑ rigidity compared to gold alloys is an advantage. However, castings are less accurate than gold, and nickel sensitivity can C/I its use.

Cobalt chromium 35–65% cobalt, no less than 25% chromium. Modulus of elasticity (rigidity) twice that of type IV gold alloys ∴ good for denture base but not as good for clasps. Proportional limit (ability to withstand stress without permanent deformation) high. A good polish is difficult to achieve, but durable. Used mainly for P/−.

Titanium Good biocompatibility; used for implants and their super-structure and in patients with allergies to other materials as a denture base material. In its use for implants, the titanium can be subjected to post-manufacture heat treatment to optimize the grain structure (small α grain size and well-dispersed β phase with a small α–β interfacial zone). This improves the properties with regard to cyclic fatigue and crack propagation. (Also see Chapter 6.)

Alloys for porcelain bonding Requirements:
- Higher melting point than porcelain.
- Similar coefficient of thermal expansion to porcelain (leucite used in the porcelain to bring it closer to that of the metal).
- Will not discolour the porcelain.
- High modulus of elasticity (rigidity) to avoid flexure and # of porcelain.
- Ability to bond to the porcelain to avoid detachment.

Indium is usually added to facilitate bonding to porcelain. Copper is C/I as it discolours the porcelain. A matched alloy and porcelain should be used.

High gold ↑ palladium or platinum content (to ↑ melting point) compared to non-porcelain alloys but need thick copings for strength ∴ bulky. Also costly.

Medium gold 50% gold, 30% palladium. Good properties and economical. Widely used.

Silver palladium Cheap, but care required to avoid casting defects.

Nickel chromium Very high melting point and modulus of elasticity, but casting more difficult due to shrinkage, voids. Also bond strength to porcelain via ceramic oxide weak. NB: some patients are sensitive to nickel.

Casting For gold (melting point <950°C):
- Wax pattern and sprue are invested in gypsum-bonded material.
- Wax burnt out by slowly heating investment mould to 450°C.
- Alloy melted either by gas/air torch or electric induction heating and cast with centrifugal force.
- Casting allowed to cool to below red-heat.
- Quenched. Some alloys are used as cast and others heat-hardened.
- Cleaned with ultrasonics and acid immersion.

For nickel chromium and cobalt chromium alloys (melting points 1200–1500°C), need silica or phosphate bonded investment and either oxyacetylene torch or electric induction heating.

Casting faults A casting may:
• Be dimensionally inaccurate (depends on balancing out of casting contraction and investment expansion on setting).
• Display finning (due to overheated and cracked investment material) and bubbling (due to surface porosities in the investment material).
• Be porous/contaminated (broken pieces of investment or dirt falling down the sprue) or incomplete (sprue problem, premature solidification of the molten metal, insufficient centrifugal force, back pressure effects from poor escape of gases, cooling shrinkage).

Wrought alloys

Wrought alloys are hammered, rolled, drawn, or bent into the desired shape when they are solid.

Stainless steel Steel is an alloy of iron and carbon. The addition of chromium (>12%) produces a passive surface oxide layer which gives SS its name. The SS used in dentistry is also known as austenitic steel (because the crystals are arranged in a face-centred cubic structure) or 18:8 steel (due to the chromium and nickel content). Available as:
- Preformed sheets for denture bases. The SS is swaged onto the model by explosive or hydraulic pressure. This produces a thin (0.1mm), light denture base resistant to #. Rarely used today.
- Wires are produced by drawing the SS through dies of ↓ diameter until the desired size is achieved. This work-hardens the wire, but heat treatments are carried out to give soft, hard, or extra-hard forms. Manipulation of SS wire also work-hardens the wire in the plane of bending, ∴ trying to correct a bend is more likely to result in #. Main applications are orthodontics and partial denture clasps. SS can be welded and soldered.

Soldering SS Requires use of a flux (e.g. Easy-flo™ flux) to remove the passive oxide layer (this reforms after soldering). Do not overheat as this can anneal and soften the components.
- Melt a small bead of low fusing silver solder (e.g. Easy-flo™ solder) onto the wire.
- Mix up the flux with water to a thick paste and apply to the item to be added.
- Heat up the solder so that wire underneath is a cherry red.
- Bring the fluxed wire into the molten solder and remove the flame at the same time.

This is not easy and requires practice, which explains the popularity of electrical soldering.

Cobalt chromium This has a similar composition to the cast form (**Ə** Casting alloys, p. 670).

Cobalt chromium alloys These are used in orthodontics as an archwire material. It has the advantage that it can be hardened by heat treatment after being formed. Also used for post fabrication in post and core crowns (Wiptam wire).

Titanium alloys Nickel and titanium alloy (nitinol) is useful in orthodontics as it is flexible, has good springback, and is capable of applying small forces over a long period of time. However, it is not easy to bend without #. Titanium molybdenum alloy (TMA) is also used for archwires and has properties midway between SS and nitinol.

Gold Mainly historical as expense limits the application of wrought gold alloys to partial denture clasp fabrication.

Alloys for dentures Cast cobalt chromium is the material of choice for partial denture connectors because of its high proof stress and modulus of elasticity: thin castings are strong, rigid, and lightweight. Although wrought gold alloys are more suitable for clasps, the advantage of being able to cast connector and clasps in one means that cobalt chromium is more commonly used (➲ Removable partial dentures—components, p. 294). Be aware of nickel allergy.

Dental ceramics

Ceramics are simple compounds of both metallic and non-metallic oxides. Although many of the materials used in dentistry are ceramics, the term is commonly used to refer to porcelain and its derivatives.

Dental porcelain has three basic requirements: function (durability, strength, and biocompatibility), form (ability to form complex shapes), and aesthetics (colour, translucency, and transmission of light).

Dental ceramics exist in a spectrum from exclusively non-crystalline amorphous glasses through a combination of glass and crystalline mixtures to all-crystalline. In general, the 'glassier' the ceramic: ↑ translucence, ↑ aesthetics, but ↓ fracture resistance.

Properties
- Firing shrinkage 30–40%, ∴ crown must be overbuilt.
- Chemically inert provided the surface layer is intact.
- Low thermal conductivity.
- Good aesthetic properties.
- Brittle. The main cause of failure is crack propagation which almost invariably emanates from the unglazed inner surface. This can be ↓ by:
  - Fusion of the inner surface to metal, as in the platinum foil and metal-bonded techniques.
  - The use of a strengthened porcelain core.
- High resistance to wear.
- Glazed surface resists plaque accumulation.

Porcelain jacket crown (PJC)
Now considered somewhat old-fashioned. For strength, a minimum porcelain thickness of 0.8mm is required and a 90° butt joint at the margin.

Conventional PJC construction involves placement of a platinum matrix on the die onto which a core of aluminous porcelain is laid down. First 'dentine' then 'enamel' porcelains are built up in layers, using porcelain powder and water mixed to form a slurry, until the desired shape is achieved. This is then compacted by water removal to ↓ firing shrinkage and then fired to ↓ porosity, which ↑ strength and ↑ translucency. Glazing produces a glossy outer skin which resists cracking and plaque accumulation. It can be added as a separate layer or by firing at a higher temperature after the addition of surface glazes. The platinum foil lining is unaffected by the firing and so should maintain accuracy of fit throughout. It is removed prior to cementation to give space for the cement lute (~25μm).

Metal ceramic
The porcelains used for bonding to a metal substructure have additional leucite added to ↑ the coefficient of thermal expansion to almost match the alloys used. Also, porcelain that fuses below the melting point of the alloy is required. Bonding to the metal occurs by a combination of:
- Mechanical retention.
- Chemical bonding to the metal oxide layer on the surface of the alloy.

The greater strength of porcelain bonded to metal crowns allows use in load-bearing areas and is due to:

- The metal substructure supporting the porcelain.
- ↓ crack propagation by bonding the inner surface of the porcelain to metal.
- The outer surface of porcelain being under tension, thus ↓ crack propagation.

But drawbacks are ↓ aesthetics, gingival staining, over-contouring cervically, and in some patients it may cause allergy.

Good success rates reported (94% at 8yrs).[11]

All-ceramic alternatives to metal ceramic restorations

Glass ceramic—glasses usually derived from silicone dioxide and with various amounts of aluminium form aluminosilicates or feldspaths. With addition of low levels of leucite they are commonly labelled as *feldspathic* porcelains.[12]

With high-leucite variants, extra strength is attained. Can be powder-liquid, machined, or pressed.

A specific popular variant has the usual aluminosilicate glass enhanced with lithium dioxide to give lithium disilicate glass in the form of IPS e.max®. The manufacturer claims ↑ flexural strength as well as ↑ optical properties via light transmission.

A further category of dental ceramics is a crystalline system infiltrated with lanthanum glass known as VITA In-Ceram®. This again provides ↑ strength. It is used as a core that is then layered with veneering porcelain to add characterization. VITA In-Ceram®, like many of its competitors, offers a wide range of applications ranging from aesthetics for anterior work to strength required for multiple unit bridges.

The final category is the polycrystalline form of dental ceramic. Unable to be pressed, the zirconium oxide used in this technique must be oversized initially to compensate for firing shrinkage. This is either done by machining an oversized framework for firing (e.g. 3M ESPE Lava™) or fabrication of an oversized die on which the framework is constructed for firing (Nobel Procera™).

Porcelain repairs

Can be carried out using composite and a silane coupling agent. A number of proprietary kits (e.g. Cojet™) are available.

11 B. Reitemeier et al. 2013 *J Pros Dent* **109** 149.

12 A. Shenoy & N. Shenoy 2010 *J Conserv Dent* **13** 195.

CAD/CAM

CAD—computer-aided design. CAM—computer-aided manufacture.

Implant dentistry has speeded the progress of 'digital solutions'. Intraoral scanners can be utilized to provide information pertaining to a preparation and the adjacent teeth and opposing arch to allow a laboratory scanner to allow for CAD. This then can be progressed to CAM and a prosthesis formed (or its substructure). Dental ceramics may be constructed in this way to provide all-ceramic solutions for fixed prostheses.

Porcelain veneers A thin shell of porcelain or castable ceramic ~0.5–0.8mm thick (➲ Veneers, p. 258). Their thin section limits their ability to hide underlying tooth discoloration. Amenable to CAD/CAM fabrication. Newer ceramics claim thicknesses of 0.3–0.4mm (e.g. Lumineers™) to be possible without ↑ fracture.

Porcelain inlays Useful material for specific inlay/onlay treatment indications. Only limited long-term studies available. Also amenable to CAD/CAM fabrication.

Denture materials—acrylic resins

Acrylic is the most commonly used polymer for denture bases. Not only can it be relined, repaired, and added to comparatively easily, but it is also aesthetic and lightweight. Acrylic is composed of a chain of methacrylate molecules linked together to give PMMA.

Presentation Usually comprises a liquid and a powder mixed together (Table 16.3). The liquid is stored in a dark bottle to ↑ shelf life.

Manipulation The powder and liquid should be mixed in a ratio of ~2.5:1 by weight. The mix passes through several distinct stages: sandy–string–dough–rubbery–hard (set). The dough stage is the best for handling and packing.

In denture fabrication, the wax pattern and teeth are invested in plaster. The wax is then boiled out and the plaster coated with sodium alginate as a separator. The resultant space is then filled to excess (to allow for contraction shrinkage of 7%) with acrylic dough under pressure. The acrylic is then polymerized.

Mode of activation

Self-cure Self-cure acrylics show less setting contraction, but more water absorption than heat-cure acrylics. This may result in the final item being slightly over-sized, thus ↓ retention. Self-cure acrylics are more porous, only 80% as strong, less resistant to abrasion, and contain a greater level of unreacted monomer compared to heat-cure acrylics. The main applications of self-cure acrylics are for denture repairs and relines, and orthodontic appliances, although for the latter the greater strength of heat-cure acrylics is preferable.

Heat-cure Conventionally, polymerization requires heating in a hot-water bath for 7h at 70°C, then 3h at 100°C. The flask should be cooled slowly to minimize stresses within the acrylic. However, resins with different curing cycles (fast heat-cure) are now available. Microwave energy can be used to cure acrylic resin, but (apart from lunchtime) has no advantage over a water bath.

Light-cure Light-cure resins are supplied as mouldable sheets. Used for denture bases or special trays.

Properties

- The glass transition (or softening) temperature of self-cure acrylic is 90°C, and for heat-cure acrylic 105°C.
- Poor impact strength and low resistance to fatigue #.
- Abrasion resistance not very good, but usually adequate.
- Good thermal insulator—undesirable as it can lead to the patient swallowing foods which are too hot.
- Low specific gravity (i.e. not too heavy).
- Radiolucent. Attempts to ↑ radio-opacity have not been very successful.
- Absorbs water, resulting in expansion. Drying out of acrylic should be avoided.
- Residual monomer (due to inadequate curing) weakens acrylic and can cause sensitivity reaction.
- Good aesthetics.

Table 16.3 Presentation of acrylic

Powder	Liquid
PMMA beads (<100mm)	Methyl methacrylate monomer
Initiator, e.g. benzoyl peroxide	Cross-linking agent
Pigments &/or fibres	Inhibitor, e.g. hydroquinone activator (self-cure only)

The strength of a denture depends upon:
- Design, e.g. adequate thickness, avoidance of notches.
- Strength of the acrylic, i.e. low monomer content, ↓ porosity, adequate curing. Can be ↑ by using high-impact resin.

Researchers are still evaluating methods of ↑ strength of denture resins. The addition of high-performance fibres (e.g. glass fibres) appears promising.

Denture materials—rebasing

Rebasing a denture base involves replacement of the fitting surface. Rebases can be either:
- Hard: heat- or self-cure, or
- Soft:
  - Permanent: heat-, self-, or light-cure.
  - Temporary:
    - Tissue conditioner: self-cure.
    - Functional impression material: self-cure.

The properties of self-cure materials are generally inferior, ∴ they should only be used as a temporary measure.

Hard rebases Heat-cure PMMA is preferred, but requires the patient to do without the denture while it is being added. A self-cure material has obvious advantages, but even the higher acrylics, e.g. butylmethacrylate, should only be used as a temporary measure as they are weaker than PMMA and discolour.

Soft liners These require a material with a glass transition temperature below or at that of the mouth so that it is soft and resilient. The majority of soft liners are either based on silicone or acrylic (polyethylmethacrylate or PMMA powder plus alkyl methacrylate monomer and a plasticizer) or polyphosphazene fluoroelastomer[13] (Table 16.4).

Heat-, light-, or self-cure types are available. The self-cure materials have inferior properties, but all require replacement during the lifetime of the denture.[14]

Tissue conditioners These usually comprise powdered polyethyl-methacrylate to which a plasticizing mix of esters and alcohol is added. No chemical reaction takes place, the liquids merely soften the powder to form a gel and leach out over time, resulting in hardening. To ensure maximum tissue recovery the lining should be a minimum thickness of 2mm and re-placed every few days, e.g. Coe-Soft®, Coe-Comfort™, Viscogel®. May be used when relining denture after implant placement for minimal loading during osseointegration.

Functional impression materials The tissue-conditioning mater-ials are usually used for this purpose, an impression being cast of the fitting surface after a few days of wear.

13 F. Kawano et al. 1992 *J Prosthet Dent* **68** 368.

14 E. R. Dootz et al. 1993 *J Prosthet Dent* **69** 114.

Table 16.4 Rebasing—soft liners

Plasticized acrylic	Silicone polymers
Good bond to denture	Bond with denture base not reliable
Harden over time	Maintain resilience
More readily distorted	Absorb water: *Candida* colonization
	More elastic

Safety of dental materials

Before a new material can be marketed it must successfully pass both laboratory and clinical trials to evaluate its safety. It is worth remembering that laboratory tests for cytotoxicity cannot always be extrapolated clinically and even cytotoxic materials can be utilized in the correct indication based on assessment of risk. Think of materials such as sodium hypochlorite, ZOE, and amalgam. In Europe, a CE mark would be issued to accredit its use in a certain clinical situation. Yet, some adverse effects only become apparent after the material has been in clinical use. Unless used with care, many materials may prove a hazard to the patient or the dental team.

Hazards to the patient

Systemic effects

Allergic reactions

- *Amalgam*—although genuine cases of amalgam allergy exist, these are rarer than the tabloid press would suggest. For proven cases, composite resin or cast restorations should be used.
- *Nickel*—as a constituent of some alloys can cause contact eczema. Sensitive patients often have a history of allergy to jewellery or watch casings. Alternative alloys are available.
- *Acrylic monomer*—can cause an allergic reaction and should be considered in a patient complaining of a 'burning mouth'. The concentration of monomer is ↑ in poorly cured acrylic and greater in self- than heat-cure. Extended curing, e.g. 24h, may ↓ concentration of monomer to an acceptable level; if not a cobalt chrome or SS denture base will be required.
- *Epimine*—in polyether impression material.

If an allergy is suspected, consider referral to a dermatologist.

Directly toxic

- *Beryllium*, present in some nickel alloys, is known to be a carcinogen. Provided the alloy is not ground, any risks are confined to the production laboratory. Beryllium-free alloys are becoming ↑ available.
- *Fluoride* in excess can be toxic (➲ Safety and toxicity of fluoride, p. 28).

Ingestion or inhalation of air-borne dust/aerosols must be avoided.

Local effects

Eye damage

Curing lamps can cause eye damage due to the glare. The simplest solution is to ask the patient to close their eyes and use a shield.

Thermal injury

Can result in injury:

- To the pulp, e.g. caused by exothermic setting reactions.
- To the mucosa, e.g. caused by dentures which are thermal insulators, as the patient may swallow drink/food that is too hot; or by the setting reaction of self-cure denture reline materials; or by overzealous heating of thermoplastic impression materials, e.g. greenstick.
- To the soft tissues, e.g. by hot instruments.

Chemical injury
Can be caused by noxious chemicals (e.g. etchant, hydrogen peroxide) being allowed to come into direct contact with the tissues.

Hypersensitivity reactions
Can occur in response to the materials that cause systemic allergy.

Hazards to staff

In the surgery
- Allergic reactions, e.g. topical anaesthetics, latex gloves, methyl methacrylate monomer, dentine adhesive systems.
- Eye damage from light sources. Use eye protection or shielding.
- Alginate dust.
- Mercury vapour.
- Nitrous oxide.

In the laboratory
- Cyanide solution for electroplating.
- Vapours from low-fusing metal dies.
- Siliceous particles in investment materials.
- Fluxes containing fluoride.
- Hydrofluoric acid used for etching porcelain veneers.
- Beryllium in some alloys.
- PMMA powders.
- Methyl methacrylate monomer.
- Casting machines.

Law and ethics

Relevant pages in other chapters Hiring and firing staff, ➋ p. 742.

Principal sources and further reading GDC 2013 *Standards for the Dental Team*. P. Heasman 2013 *Master Dentistry Volume 2: Restorative Dentistry, Paediatric Dentistry and Orthodontics* (2e), Churchill Livingstone. P. Lambden 2002 *Dental Law and Ethics*, Radcliffe Medical Press. R. Rattan & J. Tiernan 2004 *Risk Management in General Dental Practice*, Quintessence. Dental Protection advice booklets 'Handling Complaints' (available for different jurisdictions, ⌕ https://www.dentalprotection.org/uk).

Definitions
Claimant (Or in Scotland, *pursuer;* Northern Ireland, *plaintiff.*) The person bringing a claim in a civil action.

Defendant (Or in Scotland, *defender.*) The person against whom a claim is made.

Legislation A country's written law. In the UK laid down in Acts of Parliament (generally referred to as 'Primary legislation').

Secondary legislation The precise implementation of the general rules laid down in the Act (often published as Regulations or Statutory Instruments).

Litigation An action brought in a court of law.

Claim form A document setting out the details of a proposed action, which is served upon (delivered to) the defendant.

Affidavit A written statement made on oath.

On qualification Register with the GDC (➋ The General Dental Council and registration, p. 706). Get professional indemnity or professional insurance cover (➋ Professional indemnity and defence organizations, p. 702).

Consider taking out sickness and accident insurance.

Legal processes

England, Wales, Scotland, and Northern Ireland

Civil law Civil cases involve claims made by individuals against other individuals/organizations for a breach of civil rules, e.g. breach of contract, negligence, unpaid debt. Civil cases are decided on the balance of probability. The only remedy is financial recompense, the aim of which is to restore the injured party to the position they were in at the outset or, if this is not possible, to compensate them financially to the extent that they have been left in a worse position. The losing party is usually liable for the costs of both sides. Depending upon financial value, cases are allocated to:

- Small claims track: claims with value of <£10,000 (England/Wales), <£3000 (Northern Ireland/Scotland) or personal injury <£1000.
- Fast track.
- Multi track.
- County Court.
- High Court.

Appeals are referred to the Court of Appeal (civil division).

Criminal law Criminal prosecutions are undertaken when the 'law' has been broken, e.g. speeding, fraud, assault. The decision to proceed with a prosecution is made by the Crown Prosecution Service (CPS—England/Wales), Crown Office and Procurator Fiscal Service (COPFS—Scotland), or Public Prosecution Service (PPS—Northern Ireland).

In criminal law, the case must be proved 'beyond reasonable doubt' which is a higher level of proof than the 'balance of probability' used in civil proceedings. Depending upon the severity of the crime, cases are heard in a:

- Magistrates' Court. Appeals to Crown Court.
- Crown Court (with a judge and jury). Appeals go to the Court of Appeal (criminal division).

The UK Supreme Court is the highest court of appeal for both criminal and civil cases (taking over the role previously invested in the House of Lords).

Scotland

Civil law The Sheriff Court is the lowest civil court with appeals going to the Inner House of the Court of Session which sits at Parliament House in Edinburgh. The final court of appeal for civil cases is the UK Supreme Court.

Criminal law The decision to proceed with a criminal prosecution is made by the office of the Procurator Fiscal (PF). The PF is a qualified advocate/solicitor appointed by the Lord Advocate.

Depending upon the severity of the crime, criminal cases are heard in:

- Justice of Peace Courts.
- Sheriff Courts (cases heard by sheriff ± jury).
- High Court of Justiciary (cases heard by judge + jury) and the final appeal court for criminal cases.

Coroner's Court

This straddles the two systems and meets to consider unnatural and unexpected deaths, e.g. a death in the dental chair. The process is investigative (as opposed to the claimant versus defendant stance taken in the other courts).

Any unexpected death should be reported to the Coroner in England, Wales, and Northern Ireland, or to the PF in Scotland, either directly or through the police (the Registrar of Deaths will notify the authorities if this has not already been done).

Jury service

Dentists are not automatically exempt from jury service (except in Northern Ireland/Scotland). It is possible to apply for discretionary exemption or deferral of service using the form sent with the summons. Jury service can only be deferred once. Where a person has attended for jury service in the previous 2yrs they have a right to be excused service.

Complaints

A complaint is any expression of dissatisfaction about any aspect of a dental service or treatment that requires a response. It may be spoken or written in nature. It is part of the dental professional's role to deal with complaints properly and professionally.[1,2] All providers of dental services should have a complaints procedure with an appointed person responsible for dealing with complaints. All members of the team should be familiar with the complaints procedure. A written record of all complaints received should be retained. Practices working within the NHS are required to produce an annual report of complaints received.

Stages

Local resolution An NHS complaint may be made either to the practice or direct to the Health Board/NHS England. A private complaint can be made either to the practice or via the Dental Complaints Service.

Once a complaint is received:

• Acknowledge receipt/respond to the complaint within 3 working days of receipt[3] (2 days for an NHS complaint in Wales[4]). If the complaint is made in person, provide the patient with a copy of the complaint procedure. Advise in writing of the estimated response timetable. Aim to provide a full response within 10 working days (or 20 working days for a hospital/trust or NHS complaint in Scotland[5]).

• Update the complainant if it will not be possible to meet the planned deadline.

• Fully investigate the complaint. Contact defence society for advice if required. Investigation may require the complaint to be shared with the treating clinician and members of staff who are the subject of the complaint.

• Offer to meet to discuss the complaint with the patient in person, if appropriate.

• Provide a full written response to the complainant, ensuring all points raised by the complaint are addressed along with a solution or options for the complainant to consider where appropriate. Resolution may include refund/replacement of work (can be offered as goodwill gesture), an explanation, or an apology.

If the patient is still not satisfied, inform the patient of additional options for resolution:

• Ombudsman.

• Dental Complaints Service (private patients).

Cooperate fully with any formal enquiry into the treatment of a patient.

1 BDA 2007 Advice sheet (B10) 'Handling Complaints' (Ⅸ http://www.bda.org).

2 GDC 2013 *Standards for the Dental Team* (Ⅸ http://www.gdc-uk.org).

3 *Local Authority Social Services and NHS Complaints (England) Regulations 2009* (Ⅸ http://www. legislation.gov.uk).

4 *The National Health Service (Concerns, Complaints and Redress Arrangements) (Wales) Regulations 2011* (Ⅸ http://www.legislation.gov.uk).

5 *The National Health Service (General Dental Services)) (Scotland) Regulations 2010* (Ⅸ http:// www. legislation.gov.uk).

Time limits NHS complaints should be brought ≤12 months after the event or the complainant realizes there was a problem. However, this time bar may be extended if there is good reason for delay and the complaint can still be fairly investigated.

NHS England/Health Board
Can deal with an NHS complaint directly or, with the patient's consent, refer the complaint to the practice to address. Where a complaint is difficult to resolve it may:
- Offer mediation—a confidential, voluntary process which seeks to assist complaint resolution in a non-confrontational manner.
- Advise patient of their right to approach the Ombudsman.

Second stage
NHS Ombudsman
The Ombudsman is independent of the NHS and investigates complaints relating to NHS services within hospitals/trusts/health authorities/practice. The Ombudsman **may** not become involved in complaints where legal action is intended/has commenced, and will only deal with complaints that have failed to be resolved through local resolution. Can investigate the complaint and may recommend the following, where appropriate:
- Apology.
- Explanation of what went wrong.
- Change of decision made.
- Repayment of costs incurred as result of incident.
- Change in procedure.
- Improvement in facilities.
- Compensation which can take into account a patient being disadvantaged due to administrative failings.

Dental Complaints Service
An independent complaints service funded by the GDC which aids in the resolution of complaints regarding private dental treatment provided in the UK. When a patient contacts the service, they will encourage the complainant to try and resolve the issue with the practitioner directly through their complaints procedure. Where this has been tried, they will contact the practitioner and provide assistance to both parties to try and reach a fair resolution. When complaints cannot be easily resolved, the Dental Complaints Service may invite the clinician and patient to attend a complaints panel meeting after which recommendations for resolution are proposed. The Dental Complaints Service can also refer a complaint onwards to the GDC fitness to practise process if they feel it is necessary.

Other bodies
- Independent Complaints Advocacy Service (ICAS), England.
- Patient and Client Council (PCC), Northern Ireland.
- Patient Advice and Support Service (PASS), Scotland.

Although not part of the complaints process, ICAS, PCC, and PASS can give independent advice about the NHS process and assist a patient in making a complaint.

- Care Quality Commission (CQC). Regulates NHS and private practices in England.
- Health Inspectorate Wales (HIW). Regulates practices providing any element of private care in Wales.
- Regulation and Quality Improvement Authority (RQIA). Regulates practices providing any element of private care in Northern Ireland.
- Health Improvement Scotland. Regulates independent healthcare services.

These statutory bodies regulate the quality of healthcare and the service provided to patients. Although they have no direct role in the complaints process, they require providers of dental services to investigate complaints effectively and to show that they try to learn lessons from them. Review of complaints procedures may form part of a practice inspection by one of these bodies.

It is a legal requirement for all practices providing registered activities to ensure they are registered with the appropriate body.

'Disciplinary' procedures

NHS England/Health Boards have the right to investigate and take action if they have concerns regarding a clinician's performance. The decision to investigate may occur:

- Following a complaint from a patient or another clinician.
- Where a dentist is under investigation by a statutory body.
- Where a Board considers a dentist may be in breach of their terms of service/contract based upon a complaint, practice inspection, statistical data, or information from a regulatory body.

Commissioners of healthcare have the power to suspend a dentist to protect the interests of patients, staff, and the practitioner. The decision to suspend a dentist may be made while awaiting a decision from a statutory body or while an investigation is ongoing. Throughout the process, a practitioner may elect to receive support from a colleague or member of their Local Dental Committee. It is recommended that dentists seek advice from their indemnity provider who may provide support/legal representation.

If a registrant is charged with a criminal offence the police will usually report this to the GDC, as this may raise questions about the fitness to practise of the registrant.

Complaint by GDP against GDP The Local Dental Committee may be asked to arbitrate. Advice can also be sought from defence organizations. Clinicians have a professional duty to raise concerns when necessary to protect patients and should seek advice from their professional indemnity organization and take into account GDC guidance.[6]

---

6 GDC 2009 *Principles of Raising Concern* (⅋ http://www.gdc-uk.org).

Further reading

Department of Health, Social Services and Public Safety for Northern Ireland (DHSSPSNI) 2009 *Complaints in Health and Social Care: Standards and Guidelines for Resolution and Learning* (⌖ http://www.dhsspsni.gov.uk).

Valid consent

Valid consent is the voluntary and continuous permission of a capable patient to receive a particular treatment based on the patient being informed regarding the purpose, nature, and likely risks of the treatment, including the likelihood of its success and any alternatives to it. Permission given under any unfair or undue pressure is not consent. Consent is seen as a continual process and not a 'one-off' episode, so it is important to ensure communication throughout all stages of treatment is clear and ensures consent is still valid at all times. This is GDC Standard 3.3.

The ruling in Montgomery v Lanarkshire [2015] UKSC 11 declares that a material risk to *that* patient has to be considered when consenting a patient. This means that while it might not be necessarily a relevant (or material) risk to all patients undergoing the same procedure, in that particular case it may be a significant material risk to that patient, and therefore would determine if they undergo the procedure or not. For example, a professional trumpet player may well place a completely different material risk on a procedure that could involve paraesthesia (either permanent or transient) of the lip than someone else, given that this may be a material risk to their livelihood. It is therefore important to have robust conversations with patients about what they might reasonably see is a material risk to them as an individual. This requires you to have rapport and a genuine wish to truly understand your patient. This is effectively GDC Standard 3.1.3.

Treatment without any consent = assault/battery.

Treatment with general consent, but without explanation of what is involved may = negligence.

Consent should be obtained by the clinician in immediate charge of the treatment. Consultants must ensure that junior staff are appropriately trained and qualified to obtain consent.

Consent can be given in writing, verbally, or be implied.

Written consent This may be preferable, especially when extensive treatment is planned. It is a legal requirement for treatment involving conscious impairment such as sedation or GA. A signed form indicating that a patient agrees to treatment is not necessarily proof that consent is valid because the patient may not have understood the information provided at the time they gave their consent, or they may not have had enough information to make a proper decision, or enough time to consider their options.

Verbal consent This should be the minimum obtained for treatment. The benefits of having a third party present at all times are obvious. Information discussed as part of the consent process should be carefully recorded in the clinical records.

Implied consent Implied consent to a dental examination is given by attending an appointment and sitting in the dental chair; however, this does not cover provision of treatment.

Consent for children Those aged 16yrs and 17yrs are presumed to have the competence to give consent for their own treatment. Younger children who understand fully what is involved in the proposed procedure can also give consent (although their parents will ideally be involved). In other cases, someone with parental responsibility must give consent on the child's behalf, unless they cannot be reached in an emergency. If a competent child consents to treatment, a parent cannot override that consent (the 'Gillick competence' principle). Legally, the person with 'parental responsibility' (➲ Some specific problems, p. 696) can consent if a competent child refuses (except in Scotland), but it is likely that taking such a serious step will be rare. For children in care, consult an authorized representative of the local authority.

Consent for adults who are not competent to give consent The Mental Health Act[7] requires that it should be assumed that a patient over age 16yrs has the capacity to consent to treatment unless proved otherwise. However, there is an anomaly in GDC Standard 3.2.4 that states a 'clinician should not assume that a patient has the capacity to consent to treatment, but to relate to the relevant legislation' (which is the Mental Health Act. So, you have to assume, but not assume, all at the same time!).

Capacity to consent to treatment is based upon whether a patient can:
• Understand information provided regarding the proposed care.
• Retain the information provided.
• Use or weigh that information as part of the process of making the decision.
• Ask for further information if they need to, before reaching their decision.
• Communicate the decision (whether by talking, using sign language, or by any other means).

Under common law, no person can consent for a patient who lacks mental capacity; however, the Mental Capacity Act 2005[8] enables an individual with capacity to give another individual a lasting power of attorney (LPA) to make medical decisions on their behalf should their capacity become impaired. In Scotland, a welfare attorney or guardian may be appointed to act in the same way.

Where no LPA exists, a patient lacking capacity may receive treatment necessary to preserve life, health, or well-being provided that the treatment is in the best interests of the patient and no valid 'advance refusal' exists.

When considering whether treatment is in a patient's best interests:
• Encourage the person to take part in the decision.
• Identify all relevant circumstances (what the person would take into account if they had capacity), e.g. past/present views, beliefs/values (religious/cultural).
• Avoid discrimination.
• Assess whether the patient may regain capacity at a later time (this is relevant if treatment can be deferred until then).

7 *The Mental Health Act 2007* (⌘ http://www.legislation.gov.uk/ukpga/2007/12/contents).

8 *The Mental Capacity Act 2005* (⌘ http://www.legislation.gov.uk/ukpga/2005/9/contents).

- Consult others, e.g. anyone involved in caring for the patient, close relatives, LPA, deputy appointed by Court of Protection.
- An Independent Mental Capacity Advocate may be appointed where major medical treatment is being contemplated.

Treatment of patients lacking capacity must take into account the Mental Capacity Act Code of Practice.[9] The final 'decision-maker' regarding healthcare rests with the doctor/healthcare worker responsible for carrying out the particular treatment.

Some specific problems
- Treatment of an unconscious patient may be valid under the legal doctrine of 'necessity', but is limited to emergency care.
- If a patient's photographs are to be used for a lecture or presentation, written authority to do so should be obtained from the patient confirming their understanding of how/when images will be used.
- It is important to check that a person providing consent for a child's treatment has parental responsibility to do so. A child's mother will automatically have parental responsibility (unless this has been removed by a court). A father may not, depending upon his relationship with the mother at the time the child was born and whether his name appears on the birth certificate. Parental responsibility can be awarded by an order of the court to an individual who does not automatically have parental responsibility. Juvenile patients may be brought for treatment by grandparents and therefore it is important to ensure that valid consent has been obtained for any treatment planned.

---

9 Office of the Public Guardian 2013 *Mental Capacity Act Code of Practice 2007* (⅋ https://www. gov.uk/government/publications/mental-capacity-act-code-of-practice).

Contracts

A contract is a legally binding agreement between parties and can be verbal, written, or implied. In law, they are equally binding, but as the parties may have differing recollections of what was said, the advantages of a written agreement are apparent.

Between dentist/provider and commissioner of NHS services A dentist providing NHS general dental services in England/Wales will have a contract/agreement with the NHS England/Health Board. For clinicians providing NHS 1° dental care, the method of remuneration depends upon the jurisdiction being worked in and can be item of service, continuing care, or Units of Dental Activity (UDA) based. Compliance with clinical governance/quality assurance requirements is an integral part of the contract. Breach of contract/terms of service may lead to action being taken.

Between principals/providers and associates/performers, or partners Because of their importance, these should be written with the help of a solicitor. The BDA has sample agreements for partnerships, assistantships, associateships, performers, and for expense-sharing arrangements and, in cases of dispute, can arrange arbitration.

A binding-out clause This is a common inclusion designed to prevent unfair competition by a rival practice being set up in the near vicinity. However, these need to be fair (e.g. 1-mile radius in a busy suburban area for 1yr) to be enforceable. Arrangements for payment of fees for any remedial or replacement work also should be included and what will occur on termination of a contract regarding subsequent remedial treatment. Careful consideration should be given to include safeguards in case the practice runs into financial difficulties. For dentists providing UDAs/Units of Orthodontic Activity (UOAs), the contract should include details of how many UDAs/UOAs are allocated, how payment will be made, and how any discrepancy will be addressed.

Between dentist and staff Terms and conditions of employment should include a job description, pay, and holiday entitlements and arrangements. Additional information such as bonuses for additional qualifications and loyalty, sickness allowances, pensions, a confidentiality policy/clause, disciplinary rules, and termination procedures with details of notice required by each party may be contained within a staff handbook. The terms should lay out what is expected of an employee in relation to protection of confidentiality.

An employer must pay employees at least the national minimum wage. Advice sheets are available from the BDA.

Written treatment plans These are not intended to form the basis of a contract. Consent can be withdrawn at any point. GDC guidance states that whenever a patient is returning for treatment following an examination, a written treatment plan and cost estimate should be given.[10] Dentists providing NHS dental services are required to provide a written treatment plan advising of any NHS charges ± alternative options for private treatment under the terms of their contract.

The treatment plan and estimate should be signed by the patient if they wish to proceed with treatment and ideally should advise patients of the need to attend booked appointments, payment policy, and practice procedure for failed or missed appointments. As treatment progresses, patients should be informed of any changes to the original treatment plan and any effect on costs. In the event of any dispute over treatment or costs, the signed plan can be referred to.

A clinician is required to provide a reasonable degree of care and, subject to the dentist having done this, a patient would pay the agreed fee. Failure to provide goods, e.g. dentures, crowns that are 'satisfactory' and 'fit for purpose', may result in a patient successfully challenging breach of contract under the provisions of the Sale and Supply of Goods Act 1994.

Where fees are not paid and no response to telephone calls and written accounts is received (document all attempts to contact), the options for recovery of fees are (i) issue a County Court Summons (the Citizens Advice service has an explanatory leaflet), or (ii) employ a debt collection agency. The latter is considerably easier. It is important to be aware that it is not uncommon when bad debts are pursued, that a patient may bring a counterclaim citing negligence or breach of contract.

10 GDC 2013 *Standards for the Dental Team* (🔗 http://www.gdc-uk.org).

Negligence

Professional negligence is defined as a failure to exercise reasonable care, in one's professional capacity, which results in a patient suffering harm.

Often negligence cases hinge on what constitutes 'reasonable care'. If a dentist can show that their actions were in line with those of a large number of their colleagues, he/she is unlikely to be held negligent (Bolam test). However, if those actions were deemed to be illogical by the court, negligence may well be found in that situation even if others may have done the same (Bolitho test).

For a negligence case to win, the onus is on the claimant to prove:
• The dentist owed a duty of care to the patient.
• There was a breach of that duty.
• Damage occurred to the claimant as a direct result of that breach.

The ploy of attempting to shift the onus of proof onto the defendant by pleading res ipsa loquitur ('the facts speak for themselves') is rarely successful. If the case is proved, financial compensation will be awarded by the court, taking into account the damage that occurred and the steps necessary to put it right.

Where no demonstrable loss has occurred, a patient has no recourse in the law but may still voice a complaint to a regulatory body or via the practice complaints procedure.

Criminal negligence For criminal proceedings to be started the negligent action must be very serious and have some accentuating factor, e.g. the dentist was drunk or drugged, or blatantly disregarded well-known safety principles.

Contributory negligence When the actions of a patient have been partially (or completely) to blame for the damage that occurred, then contributory negligence can be pleaded, e.g. failure to follow post-operative instructions.

Vicarious liability An employer can be held responsible for any negligence by an employee that occurs during their employ. This means that a dentist is responsible for the actions or omissions of their staff, e.g. dental nurse, receptionist. However, as every individual is responsible for their own acts, a charge of negligence could be brought against both employee and employer. It is also possible to be held vicariously liable for acts and omissions of somebody who you do not employ if it can be demonstrated that an individual was acting under your control/direction, e.g. this could apply to self employed members of the team. This is a developing area of the law with recent rulings in the courts concerning Uber and Pimlico Plumbers, which have ruled that some forms of self-employment are more akin to worker status.

Time bar The period of limitation during which a patient must bring a claim is usually 3yrs but this does not begin to run until the patient knows, or ought to have known, of the damage that is said to have occurred. For children, the time bar does not start until 18yrs of age; there is no time bar in the case of mental disability. A patient may petition the Court to set aside the time bar if they can show reasonable grounds for this to be done.

The steps involved in a civil action for damages

- Usually the first intimation of trouble is a solicitor's letter (known as a letter before action). Advice should always be sought from an indemnity provider as soon as correspondence is received. All correspondence received should also be passed on. Failure to do so could compromise a clinician's position or affect an indemnity provider's ability to assist.
- If the patient's solicitor proceeds, a letter of claim or summons will be served. Civil claims protocols lay out the timescale by which a response should be provided.
- An indemnity organization will investigate a claim and, if necessary, obtain an expert report. Should the case appear not to be defensible, then the indemnity provider will try to settle the matter out of court. Where there is no evidence of negligence or it proves impossible for the two sides in the proceedings to agree whether or not negligence has occurred, the case may proceed to a full hearing.
- Prior to the trial, counsel for the defence will need to establish the full facts of the case. This can be time-consuming.
- At the end of the trial, the verdict will be given on the balance of probability, and the level of compensation set as appropriate.

There but for the grace of God go I? It must be remembered that doctors and dentists are human beings and not infallible. The law does realize that unforeseen accidents can happen. The defence organizations advise: 'when complications and errors do arise, you should be prepared to give your patients factual information about what has happened in a caring and supportive fashion. Saying that you are sorry that an incident has occurred is not necessarily an admission of guilt, fault or liability'.[11]

The importance of clear, concise, and contemporaneous notes cannot be over-emphasized. Good-quality record cards, radiographs, photographs, and study models (where appropriate) are invaluable in supplying evidence to support that appropriate care was provided.

11 Dental Protection Limited 2013 *Annual Review* (๙ http://www.dentalprotection.org/uk).

Professional indemnity and defence organizations

All GDC registrants are required to have adequate and appropriate indemnity cover to ensure that patients can claim compensation if they are entitled to it. The GDC presently recognizes arrangements provided by:

- Dental defence organizations.
- Professional indemnity insurance.
- NHS indemnity.
- Certain other forms of employer-provided indemnity such as 'crown indemnity' provided by the Ministry of Defence.

Registrants are required by the GDC to provide proof of cover if a complaint is made to the GDC about fitness to practise. Proof of indemnity provision is also a requirement when applying to join a list to provide NHS dental services and as part of practice clinical governance procedures.

Dental defence organizations

In the UK, there are three non-profit-making, mutual organizations:

- Dental Protection Limited (DPL—part of Medical Protection Society).
- Medical and Dental Defence Union of Scotland (MDDUS).
- Dental Defence Union (DDU—part of Medical Defence Union).

Their addresses are given in ➔ Useful addresses, p. 806.

As well as providing professional indemnity cover, these organizations provide their members with advice, information, and support in proceedings involving professional matters, e.g. GDC fitness to practise hearings, NHS performance investigations, and various other situations. In addition, they also contribute significantly to the social life of medical and dental students. It is important to note that the support of these mutual organizations in a case may be discretionary and therefore not necessarily guaranteed, although this discretion is said by them to be rarely used. Since they are not regulated in the same way as insurance companies this can make it difficult to contest a decision not to support a member, however rare that might be. On the other hand, insurance policies may have excesses that while they make the policy look cheaper than traditional indemnity, the cost to the dentist can still be high if they have to pay any excess.

Indemnity insurance

Provided directly by commercial insurance companies and also through service providers, cover is subject to the terms, conditions, and any exclusions of the insurance policy. Some professional organizations, e.g. British Association of Dental Nurses, include some degree of indemnity insurance as part of their membership subscription. Insurance-based indemnity provides cover for claims arising during the period that the policy is in force. 'Run-off' cover may also need to be purchased to cover claims arising outside of the insurance term if changing indemnity provider or retiring.

It is vitally important to check the terms and conditions of any insurance, especially with regards to run-off cover to ensure you are fully covered at all times, and any excess that applies to the policy. Some policies may also include retroactive cover to pick up claims that the previous insurer or indemnifier may not.

Some of the corporate bodies in dentistry also have their own products that are available to those who work within their organization. It is also possible to access bespoke policies from the general insurance market, but this can be more complex.

It is therefore vitally important to obtain the correct advice and look closely at the details of any policy or indemnity cover provided when deciding what type of indemnity is suitable for you.

NHS indemnity

Crown/NHS indemnity provides cover relating to acts or omissions of doctors and dentists working in NHS hospitals and salaried 1° care. Crown/NHS indemnity covers work undertaken within the NHS contract; it does not provide assistance for private treatment, regulatory issues (GDC/General Medical Council), fatal accident enquiries, or coroner's inquest. It is recommended that additional professional indemnity is taken out to cover involvement in such situations.

It is important to ensure that indemnity cover is sufficient to cover all aspects of work being undertaken, e.g. implants, maxillofacial surgery, cosmetic procedures.

Professional standards and ethics

Do as you would be done by.

Although ethics are not imposed by legislation, professional ethics are necessary to maintain the standing of the profession in the eyes of the public. Clinicians who behave unethically may have to account for their actions to the GDC.

The GDC expects dental professionals to abide by the following principles:

* Put patients' interests first and act to protect them.
* Respect the patient's dignity and choices.
* Treat information about patients as confidential and only use it for the purpose for which it is given. Breach of confidentiality may be justified only in exceptional circumstances if in the patient's or public interest.
* Cooperate with other team members and colleagues in the interests of the patient and respect their role in caring for patients.
* Do not make claims which could mislead patients. Be trustworthy.
* Maintain appropriate standards of personal behaviour in all walks of life so that patients have confidence in you and the public have confidence in the dental profession.
* Do not solicit patients from other dentists.
* When consulted for emergency treatment by a colleague's patient: treat as necessary to alleviate pain and refer the patient back with an explanation of what was done.
* Refer to suitably qualified colleagues cases which are beyond your competence and require specialist advice and/or treatment.

Advertising

All professional advertisements must still be legal, decent, truthful, and have regard for professional propriety. Advertising that is false, misleading, or has the potential to mislead patients is unprofessional and may lead to fitness to practise proceedings.

In accordance with European guidance, advertisements on websites must provide full details of all dental professionals named on the site including the professional qualifications, country from which they were obtained, and GDC registration numbers. The GDC takes the view that listing honorary qualifications or membership of professional organizations in advertising material may be misleading to members of the public.[12]

See also Chapter 18.

12 GDC 2013 *Standards for the Dental Team* (🖰 http://www.gdc-uk.org).

The General Dental Council and registration

The General Dental Council and registration

The GDC is a statutory regulatory body set up by the Dentists Act to regulate dental professionals in the UK. Anyone wishing to work in the UK as a dentist, therapist, dental hygienist, clinical dental technician, orthodontic therapist, dental technician, or dental nurse must be registered with the GDC or be 'in training' on an approved training scheme. The Council recently changed and now comprises 12 members (six dentists/dental care professionals (DCPs) and six lay members). At least one member has to work/reside wholly or mainly within each of England, Scotland, Wales, and Northern Ireland.

Functions of the GDC
- Maintain a register of qualified dental professionals.
- Set standards of dental practice/conduct.
- Assure quality of dental education.
- Protect patients and assist with complaints.

In addition to the Dentist and DCP registers, the GDC maintains 13 Specialist Lists covering oral surgery, paediatric dentistry, prosthodontics, oral medicine, dental and maxillofacial radiology, endodontics, restorative dentistry, oral microbiology, orthodontics, periodontics, dental public health, oral and maxillofacial pathology, and special care dentistry.

In addition to having the required qualifications, to be included on the register an applicant must pay the annual retention fee and complete the necessary CPD requirement (→ Continuing professional development, p. 772). Failure to satisfy the CPD requirement or pay the retention fee can lead to erasure from the list.

A dentist or DCP may risk having their name erased from the register if they are convicted of a criminal offence (even if unrelated to professional practice or arising from a time prior to registration) or it is found that their fitness to practise is impaired. If a registrant enters a plea of guilty in a criminal matter or accepts a caution for a charge, this will be taken as an admission of guilt by the GDC.

Fitness to practise proceedings
It is important to remember that a fitness to practise proceeding is *not* the same as a court case for negligence. It is possible to be negligent in the eyes of the law but this would not necessarily be a GDC fitness to practise matter, and likewise it could be that there is a fitness to practise matter that does not hinge on a negligent act. These are two separate entities: negligence is purely about righting a wrong, whereas fitness to practise is about protecting the public. However, a fitness to practise proceeding may also lead to a claim being made for negligence, and vice versa.

If the GDC receives information that raises questions about a registrant's fitness to practise it can investigate and, where necessary, impose conditions on an individual's registration. Fitness to practise may be alleged to be impaired due to:
- Misconduct, either professional or personal, including convictions/cautions received in UK or elsewhere.
- Deficient professional performance.
- Adverse health.

The GDC has a set procedure to investigate concerns about fitness to practise.

Caseworker/Case Examiner A caseworker considers information to assess if issues are raised regarding a registrant's fitness to practise. The registrant would be made aware of the complaint at this stage and asked to provide the clinical records. Where the complaint relates to clinical care, the relevant patient records may be reviewed by a clinical assessor. If a decision is made that the concerns do question a registrant's fitness to practise, the case is referred to a Case Examiner. A letter is sent to the professional advising them of the investigation and inviting them to respond to the allegations. The Case Examiner has various powers:

- To adjourn the case for further information.
- To close the case and take no further action.
- To issue a letter of advice to the registrant.
- To issue a warning to the registrant.
- To issue a warning to the registrant and direct that the warning should be published on the GDC website.
- To refer the case to the Interim Orders Committee.
- To ask the registrant to agree a series of undertakings on their registration.
- Or to refer the case to one of the three practice committees for a full inquiry.

The case examiner can also refer the case to an Interim Orders Committee (IOC) if it is felt that interim action on the registration of a clinician may be necessary to protect the public, while the investigation is undertaken.

Investigating Committee (IC) The IC meets in private and assesses all information relating to an allegation including the registrant's response. The IC can decide to:

- Take no further action.
- Issue advice or a warning either privately or public (attached to register entry).
- Refer to a Fitness to Practise Committee ± IOC.

Fitness to Practise Committees

The Professional Performance Committee
Considers allegations relating to deficient performance.

The Health Committee
Considers allegations which suggest that a registrant's fitness to practise may be impaired by some aspect of their health. Most of these cases relate to physical or mental health problems, e.g. motor function impairment, drug/alcohol dependency, depression, but registrants with communicable diseases of various kinds may also be referred to the Health Committee.

The Professional Conduct Committee (PCC)
May deal with cases arising from criminal convictions or misconduct. Misconduct may, however, also be used to cover cases arising from allegations of poor performance.

When the Committee decides that 'on the balance of probability', fitness to practise has been impaired it may impose the following sanctions:
- Erasure from the register for 5yrs (except for grounds of adverse health).
- Suspension from the register for up to 12 months.
- Conditions applied to registration for a period of up to 3yrs.
- Reprimand.

Wise precautions or how to avoid litigation

▶ **When in doubt, contact your defence organization**

- Good records are invaluable and should be concise, factual, and objective. They should contain details of any presenting complaint, assessment, diagnosis, treatment options (and what is discussed with the patient as part of the consent process), treatment provided, and any additional advice given. Any treatment the patient declines should be documented as well as cancelled or missed appointments. Do not record anything that you would not wish a patient to read (e.g. personal comments about a patient). The Data Protection Act 1998 allows patients to access copies of their medical records (Ⓓ Data Protection Act, p. 766).
- Take radiographs whenever clinically justified. Justification should ideally be documented in the records and be in accordance with contemporary guidance. It is a legal requirement to provide a radiographic report.
- Clinical records (including radiographs and models) should be kept for at least 11yrs. For children, they should be retained until age 25yrs, or for 11yrs, whichever is the longer. Where extensive work has been carried out or problems occurred, it may be wise to retain records indefinitely, however this may fall foul of the rules regarding data retention under General Data Protection Regulation, so it is important to seek guidance on this from your indemnifier.
- Always protect the patient's eyes and airway.
- Update the medical history at every recall and ensure this is recorded in the records.
- Keep up to date. Comply with CPD requirements. Continuing with outdated techniques could render a dentist liable to a charge of professional misconduct. Similarly, be familiar with the current evidence base and be wary of using controversial or unproven procedures or materials.
- The GDC require that you have a personal development plan (PDP) to ensure structured learning. Assistance with PDPs may be obtained through postgraduate deaneries and also via external sources.
- Always have a third person present during treatment to act as a chaperone. This is of paramount importance if using sedation, as reports of patients having erotic fantasies when sedated can no longer be regarded as amusing anecdotes.
- Refer a patient when it is in their best interests.
- Ensure that appropriate cross-infection policies are in place and are consistently adhered to (Ⓓ Cross-infection prevention and control, p. 750).
- Act in accordance with up-to-date guidance issued by the GDC (🔗 http://www.gdc-uk.org).
- Comply with the Ionizing Radiation Guidelines (Ⓓ Radiographs—the statutory regulations, p. 754).

If you are sued, immediately contact your defence society. When a complaint is received, deficiencies in records may be identified; however, *never* alter, amend, or rewrite the records. Any additions to a record should be clearly initialled and dated at the time the entry was made.

Advice lines

Dental Protection: ☏ 0845 608 4000 (UK), ☏ +44 (0)20 7399 1400 (outside UK). Email: enquiries@dentalprotection.org

Dental Defence Union: ☏ 0800 374 626 (UK), ☏ 1800 535 935 (Ireland). Email: advisory@theddu.com

Medical and Dental Defence Union of Scotland: ☏ 0845 270 2034. Email: advice@mddus.com

Taylor Defence Services: ✎ taylordefenceservices.co.uk

AllMedPro: ✎ allmedpro.co.uk. Email: info@allmed.co.uk

Professional Dental Indemnity: ✎ professionaldentalindemnity.co.uk

BDA Indemnity: 020 7535 5858
https://bda.org/indemnity
email indemnity@bda.org

Forensic dentistry

Theoretically, forensic dentistry encompasses all aspects of dentistry and the law, but here we will confine ourselves to the application of dental science to criminal investigations.[13]

Identification Dental tissues survive the effects of fire, water, and time well; information from the surviving dentition may be helpful in identification where other means of distinguishing a person have been lost. Teeth can be used to indicate the approximate age of a victim and may be compared to dental records to aid identification. Examination of the skull and jaw may also provide information relating to age, sex, racial origin, and time elapsed since death.

When comparing dental records with post-mortem records it must be remembered that dental treatment may have been carried out subsequent to the last dental chart and that missing teeth or additional restorations do not necessarily exclude identification. Comparative radiographs may be as individual as fingerprints. From a forensic point of view, the value of accurate, up-to-date records, and identification marks in dentures, are self-evident. Notes regarding IO piercing and tattooing may also prove valuable.

Occasionally, a practitioner may be requested by the police to release confidential information. The advice of a defence society should be sought before a decision is made to release any information. A registrant has a duty to protect confidentiality. Information may be disclosed if a Court Order is obtained.

Bite marks Bite marks in inanimate objects left at the site of a crime have on occasion contributed to the conviction of the perpetrator. If the 'evidence' is a perishable foodstuff, a permanent record can be made either by casting in stone or rubber base material, following photography with a linear scale.

Bite marks may be found on human skin, both on a victim of assault as well as on the perpetrator where a victim has bitten their assailant. Additionally, they may be seen in children who have been the victim of abuse. Good photographs, including a linear scale, are essential. If the victim/suspect is alive, photographs need to be repeated 24-hourly as the clarity of the bite may improve with time. A swab of the bite mark may provide a saliva sample which can be compared to a suspect's saliva.

---

13 K. Whittaker 1989 *A Colour Atlas of Forensic Dentistry*, Wolfe.

Useful contact information

The General Dental Council
37 Wimpole Street, London W1G 8DQ
☎ +44 (0)845 222 4141 or +44 (0)20 7887 3800
🔗 http://www.gdc-uk.org

The Dental Complaints Service
Stephenson House, 2 Cherry Orchard Road, Croydon CR0 6BA
☎ +44 (0)845 612 0540
🔗 http://www.gdc-uk.org/sites/dcs

Care Quality Commission
National Customer Service Centre, Citygate, Gallowgate, Newcastle upon
    Tyne NE1 4PA
☎ +44 (0)3000 616161
🔗 http://www.cqc.org.uk

Regulation and Quality Improvement Authority
9th Floor Riverside Tower, 5 Lanyon Place, Belfast BT1 3BT
☎ +44 (0)28 9051 7500
🔗 http://www.rqia.org.uk

Healthcare Inspectorate Wales
Bevan House, Caerphilly Business Park, Van Road, Caerphilly CF83 3ED
☎ +44 (0)29 2092 8850
🔗 http://www.hiw.org.uk

Professionalism and communication

Relevant pages in other chapters Complaints, ➲ p. 690; Valid consent ➲ p. 694; Professional standards and ethics, ➲ p. 704; The GDC, ➲ The General Dental Council and registration, p. 706; Management skills, ➲ p. 740; Hiring and firing staff, ➲ p. 742; Clinical governance, ➲ p. 772; Continuing professional development, ➲ p. 772; Clinical audit and peer review, ➲ Clinical audit, p. 773.

Principal sources GDC guidance on standards for dental professionals (updated) ℘ https://standards.gdc-uk.org. Royal College of Surgeons of England (RCSEng) *Good Surgical Practice* ℘ https://www.rcseng.ac.uk/standards-and-research/gsp/. RCSEng, various guidelines at ℘ https://www.rcseng.ac.uk/dental-faculties/fds/publications-guidelines/clinical-guidelines/.

What is professionalism?

A dictionary definition of 'professionalism'

'The occupation which one professes to be skilled in and to follow. A vocation in which a professed knowledge of some department of learning or science is used in its application to the affairs of others or in the practice of an art founded upon it. In a wider sense, any calling or occupation by which a person habitually earns his living.'

Professionalism in dentistry

How different from this broad definition is medical and dental professionalism? Do we individually profess special skill and knowledge? No—that is transparently defined by our peers by assessment, qualification, and registration to effectively prove that we have these properties. In the UK, the GDC holds registration lists for all dentists and certain specialists (General Medical Council for oral and maxillofacial surgeons) and similar legal structures exist throughout the world. Royal colleges, faculties, and specialist associations all see a major part of their role as 'standard setting' for their areas of expertise. Again, this is repeated throughout the world. It is this concept of a universal sense of commitment to a role that defines medical and dental professionalism, not any individual country's legal definition of it (which is why professions often constitute the major opposition to dictatorships or other extreme political systems).

A useful definition of medical and dental professionalism for our purposes is international and based on the work of Swick.[1] They:

- Show altruism (subordinate their interests to the interests of those in need).
- Adhere to high ethical and moral standards.
- Respond to the needs of society, behaviours reflect a social contract with their communities.
- Show the values of probity, compassion, empathy, and respect for themselves, patients, and colleagues (not just peers).
- Exercise accountability for themselves and colleagues.
- Recognize and act appropriately on conflicts of interest.
- Reflect critically on their practice and strive for improvement.
- Show a commitment to continuing professional development (in its widest sense).
- Can deal effectively with high levels of complexity and uncertainty.
- Respond positively to appropriate suggestions for improvement whatever the source.
- Demonstrate an appreciation of diversity.
- Adhere to the principles of 'duty of care'.

Individual and collective professional self-regulation lies at the heart of the concept of medical and dental professionalism. That is based on the precept that society trusts us with certain privileges by virtue of the job (in all its aspects) that we do and we maintain that trust by individual high standards of behaviour and collective regulation and remediation or censure of

1 H. M. Swick 2000 *Academ Med* **75** 612.

those who fail to live up to those standards. I suspect for many of you this concept is self-evident although you may not have considered it in quite these terms. Why does 'professionalism' now need to be transparently and didactically taught?

Although the concept of the doctor (and latterly the dentist) as a 'healer' goes back into antiquity, the concept of a dual-role 'healer' and 'professional' is relatively new with the emergence of the 'learned professions' in the middle ages. Until the 1960s, the role and commitment of the healing professional was largely implicit, evolving and supported by the majority of society. During the next 20yrs, an increasingly critical view of the professions developed among the social sciences, managerial echelons, and politicians, documenting failures and questioning its relevance to society. In the 1980s and onward, an increasing dominance of either state or corporate sector employers and a diminishing influence of the medical professional was seen. This tended to ↑ the value of systems to state or corporate sector over the values of healthcare professionalism. However, more recently it has been widely recognized that 'neither economic incentives, nor technology, nor administrative control has proved an effective surrogate for the commitment to integrity evoked in the ideal of professionalism'.[2] We therefore give more 'bang for their buck' by committing to being professional than any externally imposed system. Given that we, as healthcare professionals, have been disrespected and disenfranchised by these influential groups why should we adhere to the notion of professionalism? Clearly the great and good of the medical and dental political world see it as important   is this just to protect their own status?

Probably not. Individually or collectively we cannot do our jobs without a functioning system to work within. The best way to influence that is to wield the power that comes with the trust afforded by society in general in an organized, unified, and responsible fashion. Society needs healers, we are still far and away the most trusted of groups in society. The general public is not happy with their leaders. The bureaucrats (state or corporate) control the marketplace and are blamed for defects in the system. Being a professional is the best way to improve the system and genuinely being professional is what makes you want to improve it—for the betterment of all.

Therefore, a better definition might read:

> An occupation whose core element is work based on the mastery of a complex body of knowledge and skills. It is a vocation in which knowledge of some aspect of science or learning or the practice of an art founded upon it is used in the service of others. Its members are governed by codes of ethics and profess a commitment to competence, integrity and morality, altruism, and to the promotion of the public good within their domain. These commitments form the basis of a social contract between the profession and society, which in return grants the profession a monopoly over the use of its knowledge base, the right to considerable autonomy in practice and the privilege of self-regulation. Professions and their members are accountable to those served and to society.[3]

2 W. Sullivan 1999 Hastings Cent Rep 29 7.

3 S. Cruess et al. 1999 Academ Med 74 878.

Politics and the public

Social contract Social contract is a term derived from Gough:[4] 'the rights and duties of the state and its citizens are reciprocal and the recognition of this reciprocity constitutes a relationship which by analogy can be called a social contract'. It is a complex mix of the explicit (written, legal or paralegal codes, rules, and regulations) and the implicit (unwritten, individual and collective senses of obligation and purpose reflecting personal and group codes of ethics and morals). It can have universal and local components (i.e. those applicable internationally and those that are country or locality specific). Importantly, it is constantly evolving and seeks to balance society's expectations of medicine with medicine's expectations of society.

Professionalism Professionalism is the basis of dentistry's contract with society. In common with medicine it requires placing the interests of patients above those of ourselves (within reason), setting and maintaining standards of competence and integrity, and providing expert advice to society on matters of health.

For professionalism to have any effective basis in reality the public must trust in us individually and collectively, this depends on our integrity both individually and collectively. The fact that annual polls consistently place doctors and dentists at the very top of lists in which the public place their trust bears out the fact that this has been the case since the origin of our professions.

This in itself can create problems.

The patient, individually or as a community, is *not* the customer who is always right. Politicians elected or unelected do *not* always have the best interests of the population at heart. In situations where we as professionals see this to be the case we are obliged to speak out. This can carry with it accusations of paternalism or politicization.

Political implication It is illogical to believe that health is not a political issue—it affects the public good and is a right in most civilizations. It is therefore part of being a professional to express both concerns and potential solutions at systems that fail to deliver what they should for patients. What is counterproductive is the descent into party or partisan politics which is the rightful quagmire of the politician.

Equally, a desperate avoidance of the appearance of being paternalistic in the name of political correctness becomes counterproductive if we fail to advise patients what we feel is in their best interests. They are entitled to ignore that advice (providing they are competent to do so) and go elsewhere but they are not entitled to demand that we provide a treatment we genuinely believe is not in their best interest.

The fact remains that, as healthcare professionals, we are trusted and society needs us. The continuing commitment to the role of the healthcare professional is key to that.

4 J. Gough 1957 *The Social Contract*, OUP.

Standards

The GDC is the regulatory body of the dental profession in the UK. The principal standard setting bodies in the UK for dentistry are the GDC, the Specialist Dental Education Board, the Committee of Postgraduate Dental Deans, the Dental Faculties of the Royal Colleges of Surgeons, the Specialty Associations, the BDA, and the dental degree-awarding universities. Each of these has a different and sometimes conflicting role and each can be influenced to a greater or lesser degree by the government. Each country has its own bodies with variations on the same functions.

Principles All these bodies claim to seek to uphold standards and all to a greater or lesser degree speak for a constituent group. This has the inevitable problem of creating a potential conflict of roles. Each organization has to manage the conflict between altruism and self-interest, professional representation and state or corporate control, public good, and a union function.

Self-regulation It has been mentioned that self-regulation is a key principle of professionalism and one which is regularly attacked by state and corporate bodies. The preservation of collective self-regulation carries with it certain obligations on the individual: maintenance of competence, participation in the process of self-regulation, support for the relevant bodies, and behaviour that reflects integrity. The collective must demonstrate that individuals falling short of their obligations are corrected.

Re-establishing the primacy of the healthcare professional This will require a renegotiation of the social contract. There are legitimate worries on both sides and advantage is taken of serious failures in professional behaviour to disproportionately undermine the healthcare professional's viewpoint. The repeated use of Shipman (a GP serial killer) or Karadzic (a psychiatrist mass murderer) as examples reinforces this even though these individuals' monstrous personality disorders could not have been contained by conventional medical self-regulation. Because of these failures in self-regulation, the GDC is looking to follow its medical counterparts by introducing revalidation for dentists in four key domains. One of these key domains is 'professionalism'. Because of this, it is clear that dentists need to understand what professionalism entails.[5]

Balancing needs and wants Society wants (and needs) healers with a professional mindset. It has to have healthcare professionals using their knowledge and skill to heal, cure, and relieve suffering. It wants individuals' competence in discrete areas guaranteed. People want to be involved as patients. They want to see that those they trust behave to high ethical (and arguably moral) standards. It also needs accountability. Professionals want (and need) trust and respect and the acknowledgement that some failings are inevitable. Their expertise should be recognized and made appropriate use of. They should be sufficiently autonomous to act in the best interests

---

5 General Dental Council 2013 *Standards for the Dental Team* (🔗 https://standards.gdc-uk.org).

of patients (politicians dictating and lawyers second guessing helps no one). They need reasonable, reliable, validated, and trusted regulatory and training processes which they have ownership of. They need adequate resources to care optimally for patients. They need to work in a system which transparently promotes the values society wishes to see in its healthcare professionals: caring, altruism, courtesy, and competence.

The best way forward The best way forward is to ensure the balanced role of competent healer and caring professional in all training and practising dentists.

In 2013, the GDC issued a document called 'Standards for the Dental Team'.[6] This document is centred on the principles of practice in dentistry. It states that as a dental professional you are responsible for keeping to the following nine principles:

- Put patients' interests first, acting to protect them.
- Communicate effectively with patients.
- Obtain valid consent.
- Maintain and protect patients' information.
- Have a clear and effective complaints procedure.
- Work with colleagues in a way that is in patients' best interests.
- Maintain, develop, and work within your professional knowledge and skills.
- Raise concerns if patients are at risk.
- Make sure your personal behaviour maintains patients' confidence in you and the dental profession.

6 ꝏ https://standards.gdc-uk.org.

CanMEDS

The Royal College of Physicians and Surgeons of Canada have been involved for many years in a project, known as CanMEDS,[7] designed to describe the competencies required of a physician. As you can see, these include the role of 'professional' although their definition is narrower than that already used as it overlaps with the other CanMEDS roles. This descriptive system has been used extensively by the royal colleges in the UK in designing higher training curricula, the Modernising Medical Careers group, and the equivalent group for basic postgraduate training in dentistry in the UK.

It comprises:

- Medical expert—the central role based on clinical knowledge and skills but integrating with the other described 'competencies'.
- Communicator—valuing and being effective in the doctor–patient relationship including the continuous dynamic exchanges that occur before, during, and after the encounter.
- Collaborator—the idea being recognition of and respectful working within a healthcare team to achieve optimal patient outcome.
- Manager—accepting that we are all part of whichever healthcare organization we work in and the development and maintenance of sustainable practice, allocation of resources, and effectiveness of the system are part of our responsibility.
- Health advocate—using your professional status to improve the health and well-being of individuals, communities, and populations.
- Scholar—the demonstration of a lifelong commitment to reflective learning and the creation, dissemination, application, and translation of clinical knowledge and skills.
- Professional—a commitment to the health and well-being of individuals and society through ethical practice, profession-led regulation, and high personal standards of behaviour.

7 Based on the CanMEDS 2015 framework (& http://www.royalcollege.ca/rcsite/canmeds/canmeds-framework-e).

Commitments

Most of us never actually took a Hippocratic Oath although many think we did. The statement some of you may have read out at graduation will have been a modern-day version outlining your commitment to professionalism. It was none the worse for that because at the time it was a marker of how you felt about the profession you were entering. The genuinely wonderful *Oxford Handbook of Clinical Medicine* included in its ninth edition both the old and a new version (p. 1) so rather than repeat it I've included a synopsis of principles and commitments based on a physicians' charter.

Principles

- *Primacy of patient welfare.* We serve the interests of our patient(s).
- *Patient autonomy.* We must empower patients to make informed decisions about their treatment.
- *Social justice.* Discrimination has no place in healthcare. Resources should be fairly allocated.

Commitments

- *Professional competence.* Commitment to lifelong learning and maintenance of all relevant knowledge and skills.
- *Honesty.* With patients and peers in relation to consent and medical error.
- *Confidentiality.* Well recognized but of even greater significance in the electronic age.
- *Probity with patients.* Avoidance of any misuse of the relationship between professional and patient—for sexual, financial, or any personal advantage.
- *Improving quality of care.* Including working collaboratively with others to reduce error, ↑ patient safety, and optimize use of resources and patient outcome.
- *Improve access to care.* All healthcare systems should aim to have a uniform and adequate standard of care.
- *Scientific knowledge.* Demonstrate integrity in the creation and use of scientific knowledge.
- *Avoid conflicts of interest.* Be honest. Recognize and disclose conflicts of interest in practice, teaching, or research.
- *Professional responsibilities.* Set and maintain standards, show due respect, and work collaboratively in educating, assessing, and remediation of colleagues.

It should by now be becoming obvious that many groups are saying similar things about both the nature of professionalism and the perception of professionalism. The primacy of 'doing the right thing' for your patients, your colleagues, your society, and yourself is the key principle that shines through.

Understanding (and overcoming) systems

Introduction As we all work in systems of greater or lesser complexity we need to learn how to cope with, redesign, or overcome systems that prevent optimum outcome for our patients. In a general dental practice (a very small system), considerable power and autonomy is placed with the dentist and system design is important. In huge environments, like hospitals, many aspects of the system may be out of our control so learning how to overcome or adapt existing systems becomes crucial.

Process This describes the individual steps that constitute each point in a journey through a system from start to finish. The easiest way to understand this is to imagine a patient's journey in great detail. This is the process view and it is essential when implementing an error avoidance strategy. The first step is to identify the high-level view—an overall stepwise progression of the journey that highlights 15–20 key steps. Next, detailed process mapping takes place inviting the views of all the staff involved in the process (remember it is looking at the system first and individuals only if there is a defined problem with one individual's behaviour). Avoid rarities and personal anecdote. Look for waste in the process: of time, money, effort, goodwill, etc.

Process pathology This includes bottlenecks which may be real (a step performed by one person, at one time that takes longest) or functional (trying to do multiple non-consecutive tasks which waste time between each task). *Demand/capacity mismatch*, the failure to understand these terms are a root cause of much of the mismanagement of the UK health service. Demand is the need plus want for the service, i.e. all requests for the service, *activity* is what has been done (always retrospective), *capacity* is what the system could do under optimal conditions, and *backlog* is cumulative unmet demand. *Carve-out* is where overall capacity is reserved for particular demands (e.g. fast-track cancer referrals).

Responsibility/authority mismatch This is a core underlying problem in most systems and the major source of stress in most hospital environments—the person held responsible (i.e. blamed when things go wrong) does not have the necessary authority to prevent them from going wrong.

Understanding that a patient's journey is a system allows you to improve it and use the techniques for error avoidance outlined in 'Human factors' (◑ Human factors, p. 726). In the microcosm of a dental practice, the most difficult thing may be simply accepting this concept. In the huge, highly complex, externally interfered with hierarchical systems within hospitals, the emphasis has to be on adapting the aspects of the overall system so that you have authority over it to improve it, even if this effectively subverts imposed aspects of that system.

Human factors

Introduction Sometimes referred to as 'ergonomics', this consists of a group of topics concerned with human–human and human–system interaction with a particular relevance to the prevention of error. Popular over the last 25yrs or so in so-called high-risk industries—aviation, nuclear, petrochemical, and military—they have recently become recognized as being of potential value in healthcare, particularly in the Anglophone world.[8]

The blame culture A longstanding tradition of managing when things go wrong is to find out who is to blame and punish them. That's it. It is astonishing that it has taken so long to accept that this is not the most useful way of going about things.

Error and error avoidance We all make mistakes, this is inevitable and inescapable. What is important is that the potential for serious harm coming from those mistakes is minimized and that we and others learn from those mistakes. In order to do that, a move away from the blame culture has to take place. In some industries this has been achieved to a large extent (aviation). In healthcare there have been some notable attempts. These have been successful where the system is trusted, usually anonymized, and reliable feedback is given. They have largely failed where a system has been imposed by an outside body which is not trusted (government or corporate body), league tables devised, and feedback has been minimal or useless.

System failure The recognition that humans make mistakes (that are usually non-malicious) but that things go disastrously wrong only when these mistakes are compounded, led to an approach where the system was analysed for failure rather than an individual being blamed.

Swiss cheese This is an analogy for systems failure and error occurrence.[9] For something to go seriously wrong (e.g. a patient dies from taking the wrongly prescribed drug), multiple failings have to happen. Think of trying to thread a straw through multiple layers of Swiss cheese. It will only pass through if all the holes, which are in different places on each slice, line up. One slice out of place and it won't pass (i.e. the error won't happen). In the patient analogy, the wrong drug might be prescribed, but the dispensing pharmacist might recognize this, or the patient might realize they were allergic to it.

Red flags This is the term given to the signs and symptoms of an error in progress. Recognition of a 'red flag', e.g. a change in the order of an operating list, should make everyone more aware of the potential for an error to occur.

Situational awareness This is our capacity to be aware of multiple aspects of our immediate environment. A simple example would be driving behind a car which is travelling slower than you in the inside lane

---

8 J. Reason 2000 *BMJ* **320** 768.

9 J. Reason 1990 *Human Error*, Cambridge University Press.

of a three-lane motorway at the point of a junction which has another car travelling at the same speed coming on the motorway. The calculation you make to position yourself safely without losing speed is your situational awareness. Stress massively reduces this and effectively blinkers you to potentially important outside influences.

Root cause analysis (aka critical event analysis) This is supposed to happen after 'clinical incident' reporting, the idea being that the areas of system failure are identified and measures put in place to prevent failure at that point in the future. Obviously, this requires feedback and resource for change going to the people and places affected.

Effects of stress and personality As mentioned before, individual personalities and learning techniques exist for all of us. If we are put in a position where we have to work or learn in a way that is at odds with our preferred approach we become, to a greater or lesser extent, stressed. The effect of stress on situational awareness is described. If situational awareness is ↓, the potential for error ↑. This is one logical reason why certain types of professions have to be assessed under stress—we have to be competent and able to function under levels of stress that would cripple others.

Crisis intervention techniques If you are working in a hierarchy, how do you tell the boss he or she is doing something wrong? One excellent technique is the PACE approach.

Probe 'Is it me? I don't understand why we are doing [the wrong thing] this.' This is usually enough and saves face all round.

Assert 'I'm sorry but I don't think this is right. I'm not happy.' The ante has been raised but it is still non-confrontational. It takes real bull-headedness to press on in the face of this.

Confront 'Look, this isn't right. I know you're the boss but I am sure this is not what should be happening.' This is a point of no return but you are doing the right thing.

Emergency 'Stop. I am not going to let this happen.' An extreme situation where you intervene (possibly even physically) to prevent harm to a patient.

Leadership and followership The concept of leadership is often that of someone who is always in control, always knows what to do, is always right, and carries all the responsibility. Just reading that should make everyone realize it is nonsense. True leadership is about keeping things together, using the right people in the right place at the right time to achieve an agreed goal. Followership is acknowledging this and the leader who gives way (and becomes a 'follower' temporarily) to allow someone with a more appropriate skill set to lead is enabling that to happen.

Understanding personalities

We are all different. That seems self-evident but the fact that different personality types exist and that they have a direct bearing on the way we learn and act, does not seem to have permeated training structures or workplace management.

While no human being is completely stereotyped into a category with regard to both personality and learning preferences, most of us show tendencies towards various behaviour types. It is important to realize that no one type is better than another but that certain types are more suited to certain roles in life and certain ways of learning new information, skills, or behaviours and that being forced to act outside that type can lead to significant stress. We might not be able to change the environment we work, teach, or learn in but understanding that someone may be of a personality type where that environment produces counterproductive stress may help us modify the situation or them to accept that this is not a role they are suitable for.

Myers–Briggs type inventory This is one (there are others) way of assessing personality types. This is a quite lengthy questionnaire which categorizes 'preferences' in four main categories:

Introversion/extraversion Essentially this reflects the extent to which you engage the world in your head or the 'real world'.

Sensing/intuiting This is about how you gain information; do you rely on the five senses (are heavily factual) or have a sixth-sense feel for things?

Thinking/feeling Do you prefer a critical/analytical approach to decision-making or rely on instinct more heavily?

Judging/perceiving Do you seek order, sense, and predictability or are you happier to take things as they come?

This is a gross simplification of the process but gives you an idea of how people can differ, no one 'type' (indicated by the letters allocated to the different sections) is better than another but certain types cope better in certain situations, jobs, roles, and interpersonal relationships. Just going through the process aids in personal insight and reflective capability.

Learning types Just as there are four distinct personality traits which flow into each other so there are equivalent learning types. These also match the stages of learning and reflection and development of what has already been learned. The distinction between people is that they tend to prefer one stage more than another and can feel uncomfortable or even stressed if forced into an area they are less comfortable in.

Stage 1 Reflective observation (thinking about buying a computer, reading all the magazines).

Stage 2 Abstract conceptualization (reading the manual after buying it).

Stage 3 Active experimentation (bought it, chucked the manual away, plug it in, and start pressing buttons).

Stage 4 Concrete experience (got one that works and going to stick with it).

Change management

Change Change is an inevitable and ongoing process in our everyday lives and the workplace and is certainly no bad thing in itself. The intense resentment felt by most professionals towards change has come about by imposed change, with no or facile consultation, no evidence base, and no internal motivation for that change. The fact that most of these imposed changes fail, often due to the incredible power of healthcare professionals' inertia even in the absence of tacit opposition, is a lesson that those who would impose change continually fail to learn.

Change management Change management is a useful concept both because we may wish to change practices, systems, or treatments within our control for good reasons and because we may wish to oppose change where we feel it is potentially harmful, wasteful, lacking in evidence, or just plain wrong. To do that, it helps to understand a little of the processes.

What can change? In terms of our professional environment, three basic groups: individuals (ourselves, patients, colleagues), groups of individuals (nurses, trainees, those who are sharing a common experience), and organizations and systems.

Approaches There are two which are not mutually exclusive but tend to have different emphasis: changing attitudes in the relevant individuals and hoping that behavioural change will follow ('hearts and minds') and a more punitive approach emphasizing the legal and business reasons for change. While the latter has become increasingly popular it is unsurprisingly less effective with highly motivated and educated healthcare professionals.

Helpful concepts There is an unfortunate tendency for many trying to implement change to stick with conventional management theory which looks on organizations as machines with staff as components of that machine. This leads to the folly that a detailed plan for change can be worked out in advance (often by outsiders), people are told what to do and will both do it and do it consistently, and that this process will be automatically replicable from one area to another. A much more useful concept is that organizations are complex evolving ecosystems functioning on a series of interdependent nested systems.[10] This concept believes guidance from a few simple rules will allow permanent effective change generated by internal motivation. It is the theory behind 'post-it note' exercises—although all too often these are corrupted by those 'in charge' falling back on conventional practice.

Groups of individuals Groups of individuals need leaders but leaders do not have to be the font of all knowledge (⊃ Understanding personalities, p. 728)—acting as enablers or facilitators they can earn the support of the group by active listening, designing a plan of action, facilitating that plan (rather than doing it themselves), seeing what happens, and giving feedback (⊃ Feedback use, p. 737).

10 E. Mitleton-Kelly 2003 *Complex Systems and Evolutionary Perspectives on Organisations*, Elsevier.

Individuals For individuals to function effectively with change they need to develop emotional intelligence: 'the capacity for recognizing our own feelings and those of others, for motivating ourselves and for managing emotions well in ourselves and in our relationships'.[11] Discovering what motivates ourselves and others is the key technique in ensuring people feel they 'own' the change and the change process, the key aspect of successful change management.

11 E. Mitleton-Kelly 2003 *Complex Systems and Evolutionary Perspectives on Organisations*, Elsevier.

Verbal and non-verbal communication

We have two ears and one mouth, but they are rarely used in those proportions.

Learning to listen This is hard to do but hugely rewarding. Try to cultivate an active listening style; don't interrupt unless it is essential and if you do, always give the opportunity to come back to a point that may be vital to them at some time in the future.

Time Time is needed to learn these skills, to use them in imparting news (especially bad news) to people, and to allow people to absorb that news. Allocate it, allow it, and stick to it.

Preparation When communicating, it is helpful to be sure of the information you are imparting and that you want to impart it. Prepare what you want or have to say as well as how you will say it.

Words have power Saying 'sorry' can be taken as an admission of guilt or as a sincere form of empathy. Timing, intonation, and body language influence how the same word is understood by the person hearing it.

Honesty Honesty is best but does not mean burdening someone with extraneous detail which clears your conscience but unnecessarily harms someone else.

Questions People will have questions but may need time to refocus to ask them—suggest they write them down for next time. They will also have a legitimate need to have some answered—if you can, do so, but don't be afraid to admit you don't know. If you can't, but know someone who can, then that is a fair response. Equally you may ask questions; the most useful after breaking bad news, perhaps surprisingly, is 'How do you feel about that?' The number of different responses will astonish you and it is of huge importance to let people express themselves at this point.

Consistency Few things are more disorientating than being told different things by different people about the same subject, especially if that subject is your personal health or that of a loved one. Be sure of what has been said before—ask the person you are talking to as it is what they remember or understand that is important to the conversation. Try to ensure all team members do this before launching into some detailed explanation which may be at odds with what has gone before. If previous information is incorrect it must be corrected but include an explanation of how that 'misunderstanding' arose.

Empathy and compassion These are important components of communication but this does not mean you are a limitless source nor does it mean you are an emotional punchbag for upset individuals. Having boundaries in your role as a professional communicator is essential to prevent burn out.

Principles of neurolinguistic programming

Neurolinguistic programming (NLP) was first developed by a psychologist, Richard Bandler, and John Grinder, a linguist, in the 1970s. NLP is often referred to as the 'art and science of personal excellence'.

What is NLP?
It is a set of interpersonal skill techniques to improve the impact and effectiveness of communication.

- *Neuro* is associated with the brain and what happens in your mind. We all use our senses, Visual, Auditory, Kinaesthetic, Olfactory, and Gustatory (VAKOG), to interpret the world around us. In other words, what you see, hear, feel/touch, smell, and taste all impact your thought processes, interpretation of that information, and subsequent behaviour or response.
- *Linguistic* is associated with language and how you communicate and influence others. What you say, how you say it, and what you mean by it!
- *Programming* relates to patterns of behaviour which you learn and repeat (a learned behaviour). Internal thoughts and previous experiences have an influence on patterns of behaviour. Those patterns may help you make sense of situations, solve problems, and help make decisions.

Four key principles of NLP

Rapport When communicating with others, build rapport—this can be done through matching body language, eye contact, tone of voice (pace and leading), and active listening. Understand the situation from the other person's perspective, 'Seek first to understand, then to be understood'.[12]

Outcomes Know the outcome you want, 'Begin with the end in mind'.[13]
- Frameworks such as SWOT and SMART can assist in developing a 'well-formed outcome'.
- SWOT (Strengths, Weakness, Opportunities, and Threats).
- SMART (Specific, Measurable, Achievable, Realistic, and defined Time frame).

Senses Use all your senses—VAKOG—to interpret and make sense of the world around you. Be aware we all see, hear, and feel things differently.[14]

Flexibility Be flexible in your approach. Others may interpret situations/ the world differently. The more flexible you can be, the more options you create.

---

12 S. R. Covey 1994 *The Seven Habits of Highly Effective People*, Simon & Schuster.

13 S. R. Covey 1994 *The Seven Habits of Highly Effective People*, Simon & Schuster.

14 NB: we all live in our own unique worlds and have our own 'map of the world', check out the world of others before presuming/interpreting you are talking about the same experience/thing. You may be surprised!

Presentation skills

Presenting Presenting is not teaching, but it can be a useful tool in teaching. It can also be a nerve-wracking chore (job interview presentations) or a rite of passage exercise in survival at a national scientific conference. Regardless of its intended purpose, it can be made better and more pleasant (for you and your audience) by following some simple rules that are based around preparation, planning, and delivery.

Preparation What are you trying to say—this is essential, if you don't know what you want to say, how can you say it? No one wants to listen to you work it out on the spot—that is boring and embarrassing. It is also vital that you understand whether what you want to say agrees with what the audience wants to hear and what the organizers want you to say. It is not always the same thing. Why do they want you—do you have or have promised some special expertise or are you a replacement? Who are you speaking to and who has asked you to speak, are their agendas the same (some attendances are 'mandatory' which tends to produce a hostile audience which needs to be defused), what are their backgrounds, ages, degree of knowledge of the subject you are asked to speak on? What would they like to get out of it? How many people will be there? This has obvious implications for the choice of media—PowerPoint to five people is dull and ineffective, a flipchart to 100 is impossible. What is the context of your presentation—is it a 10min talk with 5min of questions wedged into a plethora of others; part of a structured course with experts before and after you; or just you with relative flexibility? This is essential for timing considerations; if you are allocated a finite time you must stick to it, which means starting and finishing to the minute. If you are allocated a vague time ('40min to an hour') set yourself a specific time and break it into 20min chunks (the attention span of most people for listening). Work out how you get to the venue, a backup plan, and who to contact if things go wrong, get there early, and ensure all audiovisuals are working before the audience arrives (getting your presentation to work while the audience sits there growing restless is a cardinal sin).

Planning Now that you have an idea of what is going to happen you can plan the presentation. It is crucial you know your subject and are up to date for the level of your prospective audience. Once you have a good idea of the relevant content, work out what is feasible to deliver (in the allocated time and to that particular audience). More really is often less in presentations. What sort of language are you going to use? What sort of attire will be right for that occasion? Is there a dress code? What technique are you going to use to deliver the presentation?

The message not the media The message not the media is the defining aspect of your presentation. Media include blackboards, whiteboard, flip chart, overhead projector, visualizer, 3-D objects (for smaller groups), and microphones and computers/LCD projectors for larger groups. Videos and handouts can be used for both. Be familiar with what you are actually going to use (it often won't be your own computer, many a video clip disaster has stemmed from this). Mastery of the older presentation techniques, which are often more suitable for smaller groups, requires greater skill and confidence than slide-based approaches which explains their popularity and overuse. Many presentations will use PowerPoint, while this has many advantages the misuse of the technology has created the well-recognized condition of 'death by PowerPoint'—too many flamboyant slides, rushing through multiple slides that contribute nothing and give the impression of bad preparation, and freezing of the system if multiple lines and pictures are added to the slide. Do not become obsessed with the media, it can distract the audience from what is important—your message. Design this like a story, know what the end is going to be then work out a way to get there. Now you know where you are going, work out the start—an interesting title and an outcomes slide coupled with a short, friendly introduction helps. Build into the bulk of your talk, avoiding abbreviations, keeping it short and simple, and re-emphasizing important points and why they are relevant to the audience. If your talk is longer than 20min build in 'energizers', these can be breaks where people move about and do things (for the brave and experienced) or interjecting questions into the audience.

Delivery Delivery using the set, dialogue, closure approach for teaching helps structure every presentation (➲ Structure of a learning episode, p. 736). Start on time, ensure your non-verbal communication (➲ Verbal and non-verbal communication, p. 732) is positive and open. Engage the audience and introduce yourself in a way that gains credibility, tell them what you are going to talk about and why it is important to them (or why they might enjoy it). Ensure text slides or overhead projector images are clear and legible with no more than seven words per line and five lines per slide. Do not read your slides to the audience, it's insulting, they can read too! It takes a minute to read a text slide. Use good-quality pictures and diagrams that are relevant, don't just show off. Avoid extra logos and pictures on a slide that will simply distract the audience. Ensure you have an aims and objectives slide at the beginning and summary slide at the end. Practise so that you know which slides are where and how far into the presentation you are.

When allowed by the structure of the environment, try to ask questions at the end before you summarize what you've talked about. This enables you to check the audience has understood you and to build anything missing into your summary and creates an opportunity for a definitive termination of the presentation (which prevents things dragging on and the audience remembering some daft question rather than your summary).

Teaching, learning, and assessing professionalism

Teaching In order to teach effectively you have to ensure others are enabled to learn.

Learning In order to learn you have to participate actively in different styles of teaching.

Domains of learning This is the term given to what can be learned. Usually three are described—cognitive (knowledge), psychomotor (skills), and affective (attitude). Some would argue (and I agree) that a fourth domain exists—interpersonal, as this is a group of abilities (verbal and non-verbal) that can be used for good and bad reasons. Each of these domains has more appropriate ways of teaching, learning, and assessing them (e.g. you don't assess operative skill with a multiple choice question (MCQ)).

Learning outcomes The current term for aims and objectives. Basically, this is working out what you are trying to learn or teach before you start trying to do it. From a teacher's perspective it is useless to start trying to teach something unless it can be feasibly learned in that episode. It helps to state what you are going to do in whatever period of time and with whatever learner(s) you have. From that you can work out how to do it. Think of it as knowing where you want to go, then working out the best way to get there on any given day and in any set of circumstances.

Structure of a learning episode Set, dialogue, and closure. This structure allows the efficient construction of any high-quality teaching episode.

Set This is the initial preparation of the episode, ensuring the environment is the best it can be, introducing yourself, discovering your audience, and agreeing your roles. Establish what you are going to do and how you are going to do it.

Dialogue This is the bulk of the teaching, the information imparted, or the skill taught. Interactivity with your learners is crucial and achieved by questions, eye contact, and direct involvement. Skills teaching involves a four-stage procedure during this phase:
- A silent demonstration.
- A talked stepwise demonstration.
- An opportunity for the learner to talk the skill through by directing the teacher to do the skill.
- A demonstration of the skill by the learner saying what they are going to do before they do it.

Closure The end is important as it is often the aspect best remembered by the learner. An effective closure consists of questions with explanations followed by a summary followed by a termination. A definitive stop prevents the process from becoming messy and the last (strongest) memory of the learners from being something irrelevant.

Teaching knowledge Books, journals, lectures, and the Internet are all sources of knowledge. Retention is improved by repetition and application. Simple acquisition of facts is only the first step in possessing useful knowledge. It is the integration of data and its application to variable information, i.e. working out a treatment plan from a series of signs and symptoms that is essential in a dentist.

Teaching skills The four-stage technique works but has specific challenges in carrying out procedures on conscious patients (need to agree code words) and in long complex procedures (which have to be broken down into smaller steps).

Teaching interpersonal skills The ability to relate effectively to other people can be taught and learned in a variety of ways, although the most effective is watching people in action and analysing what they are doing and what impact their words and actions are having on the people around them.

Teaching attitudes Attitudes are the essence of professionalism, they govern what drives us and are defined by what we do (not what we say). The only really effective way of teaching appropriate attitudes is by acting them out as role models who are valued by those who are learning.

Feedback use 'Pendleton's rules': ask what went well—if they struggle, tell them or if in a group, ask others, then ask them how they would improve or do things differently the next time, and ensure they are told about any significant points for improvement if they miss them (either personally or using others in a group).

In-workplace assessment tools

Given that what we do is the most crucial aspect of assessment and the workplace is the most real-life environment, these tools have been created to get as close to real life as possible.

Current popular tools These consist of two observational tools—mini clinical examination exercise (Mini-CEX) and direct observation of procedures (DOPS) or procedure-based assessment (PBA) (the names will change again but the principles are valid)—an interactive tool, case-based discussion (CBD), and a peer assessment tool, the multi-source feedback (MSF).

Mini-CEX This assesses an interaction with a patient using either a check-list or a global rating scale (depending on level of the assessment) and can assess knowledge, interpersonal skills, examination skills, and, to a certain extent, attitude.

DOPS/PBA The latter is a similar idea but intended to assess technical skills. There is a generic checklist built into the pro forma but it is important to understand that this tool was primarily intended to assess physicians carry out relatively simple technical skills (it originated from the Royal College of Physicians). The PBA adapted from DOPS by the Royal College of Surgeons of England is designed to assess more complex technical skills; however, the checklist approach is less appropriate in assessing higher skill levels than a global rating scale.

CBD An interactive discussion between assessor and assessee around case notes picked by the assessee, designed to assess a wide range of hard and soft thought process and skills (i.e. from technical quality of note keeping to ability to reflect on a mistake).

MSF (Aka 360-degree appraisal, multisource feedback, etc.). Assessee chooses 8–15 relevant people to complete a structured questionnaire. Statistically valid results are achieved if there are at least eight completed returns. Sceptics should try this one and it can be extremely useful in helping self-reflection and improvement on a range of subjects. Originally developed by the Royal College of Physicians and Surgeons of Canada (see CanMEDS, ➲ CanMEDS, p. 722).

LEPS This is an in-workplace tool for general dental practice developed by NHS Education Scotland.

Assessing the healthcare professional Clearly all the domains of learning or the subdivisions of these described in the CanMEDS document have to be assessed and a range of techniques are needed for this. While basic facts can be tested by rigid, simple tools like single best answer MCQs, assessing the higher levels of function demanded of a healthcare professional needs much more. A combination of the in-workplace assessment tools and externally validated conventional examinations (incorporating rigid but reliable assessments like MCQs and objective structured clinical examination (OSCE) as well as the more flexible and valid interactive techniques like structured vivas, moulages, and scenario-based assessments) are clearly necessary to ensure what both dentistry and society need—the competent healthcare professional.

Chapter 19

Practice management

Relevant pages in other chapters Contracts, ➔ p. 698; Biocompatibility of dental materials, ➔ Safety of dental materials, p. 684.

Principal sources and further reading The BDA have an excellent range of advice sheets covering many of the topics in this chapter (🔗 https://www.bda.org/). G. Bridges 2019 *Dental Reception and Supervisory Management* (2e), Wiley-Blackwell. GDC 2013 *Standards for the Dental Team*. R. Rattan 2007 *Quality Matters: From Clinical Care to Customer Services*, Quintessence Publishing.

Management skills

A happy practice environment is not only more pleasant to work in, but the bonhomie will also be transmitted to patients. One of the challenges of trying to manage a dental practice while also being a clinician within it is that of having enough dedicated time in which to do full justice to your management responsibilities. Practice management training courses are widely available and certainly worth investing in. They can help in developing systems leading to ↑ efficiency and job satisfaction and ↓ stress for the whole dental team.

Keys to successful management

Clear and effective communication Good communication skills are essential not only between the practice team and patients but equally between team members to ensure smooth running of the practice. Whatever the role in the dental team, communication should be clear and unambiguous and it should be remembered that good communication involves the ability to listen as well as talk. An effective complaints/feedback procedure should allow patients to raise concerns openly (however minor), thereby enabling the practice to learn from the issues raised and improve their service. Addressing problems with either staff or patients at the earliest opportunity and in an open, honest, and sympathetic manner will often prevent more significant complaints occurring at a later date.

Practice procedures should be in place to ensure messages (whether received by email, telephone, post, or in person) are documented and delivered to the correct team member promptly so they can be acted upon.

Delegation Delegate tasks that do not require your training and expertise. In addition to reducing stress and freeing time to concentrate on tasks that do require your skills, this also ↑ job satisfaction for ancillary staff, provided they are given the training and time to cope with new responsibilities, e.g. getting team members involved in collecting/auditing feedback. Due to the number of administrative and legislative requirements that need to be dealt with when running a dental practice, a practice manager has become an essential member of the dental team.

Teamwork Successful leadership involves encouraging staff to develop their potential both as individuals and as valued members of the team, as well as enabling discussion as to what the goals are to be and how to achieve them. This can be facilitated on either a group or individual level by staff meetings, appraisals, or audits and achieved by making sure that any outcomes are specific, measurable, attainable, relevant, and time-based ('SMART').

Motivation to work as a team can be fostered by financial incentives linked to the performance of the practice, but it is wise to identify what motivates individual members of the practice as money may not be the most important factor for all employees.

Staff meetings For teamwork to be successful, the opportunity for team members to discuss problems and ideas for improvements needs to be created. Regular structured staff meetings should be planned with an agenda prepared in advance to which all team members should be encouraged to contribute. Patient feedback, complaints, significant events, and changes in guidance/policies should be discussed. Minutes of the meeting should be kept, recording date of meeting, members present, matters discussed, and actions taken. The minutes should be accessible to all team members for future reference.

Staff training All new staff members should undergo induction training in practice procedures and policies. A record of training provided should be kept. Review of all staff training should be carried out annually and development of further skills encouraged allowing delegation of additional tasks where appropriate. To comply with GDC requirements, all dentists and DCPs must carry out relevant CPD (➲ Continuing professional development, p. 772). Practice owners should ensure reasonable opportunity is given to staff members to undertake CPD and ensure their skills and knowledge are updated.

A manual of practice procedures, routines, and policies should be kept which is freely available to all staff. All members of staff should be involved in periodically reviewing and updating this information and the date of any policy or procedure updates should be recorded and all relevant members of the team should sign to say they have read and understood the changes. In-house training days with speakers either from within the practice, or invited, are useful especially in areas such as dealing with medical emergencies and cross infection. Verifiable online training is widely available on a practice or individual basis and can often prove to be a more time- and cost-effective method of training larger numbers of staff.

Dentists and DCPs involved in the taking and development of radiographs should have received appropriate training and have this training updated (➲ Radiographs—the statutory regulations, p. 754). Documented evidence of appropriate training should be kept.

Pay Motivation can often be enhanced by financial incentives. Therefore, by structuring payment to comprise (i) a fixed hourly rate; (ii) an individual bonus, which is related to attendance, sickness record, and productivity paid as a percentage of the hourly rate; and (iii) a group bonus which is a fixed proportion of the profits of the practice, all staff have an inducement to reduce overheads and improve efficiency in the practice. Care must, however, be taken to ensure financial incentives are not seen to compromise patient care, e.g. by encouraging patients to opt for a particular treatment or product.

Hiring and firing staff

Hiring

- Identify what tasks the practice team would like the new member of staff to perform. Decide on the criteria for an ideal candidate (be realistic) as this will aid selection later.
- Draw up a job description and person specification. Consider including details of the practice, role of the new member in the team, required skills, training to be provided, hours of work, pay, and other benefits. Check with local colleges for availability on dental nurse training courses should this be applicable.
- Advertise post. Use local press/hospitals/Internet/professional magazines. Regarding dental nurses, colleges often have a list of suitable candidates who already have a place on a training course but who do not have a position in a practice. Remember to include a realistic closing date for applications.
- Shortlist candidates.
- Interview. Preferably have two or three people on the panel. The interview should be structured so that candidates are asked the same questions and given a score for each answer allowing a total to be recorded. Questions about any of the protected characteristics under discrimination law should be avoided (pregnancy, religion, race, etc.). While allowing the most suitable candidate to be identified, scoring also gives the process transparency should a complaint on the grounds of discrimination or unfair selection process be made against the practice by an unsuccessful applicant. Notes should also be made, because after several interviews the candidates may begin to merge! Hopefully a suitable person will be found and they should be offered the job in writing, subject to at least two references (including the most recent employment), proof of the right to work in the UK, and, where applicable, occupational health screening, proof of hepatitis B and tuberculosis inoculation, proof of registration, professional indemnity, and appropriate Disclosure and Barring Service (DBS) check. If no one is acceptable, go back and reassess requirements.
- Draw up the initial job offer outlining the basic terms and conditions of employment. Include the length of any trial period and how assessment is to be carried out at the end of the trial (usually 6–8 weeks is long enough). Both employee and employer should retain a signed copy. For non-registered dental nurses, apply for a place on a training programme. Terms and conditions may need to include provision for what happens if a trainee nurse fails to complete the training course/pass the exam.
- Orientate and train the new member of staff, giving plenty of time for feedback in both directions. Both employer and employee should keep a record of training given.
- Within 6 weeks of employment commencing you must notify the employee, in writing, of the terms of their enrolment in a qualifying workplace pension scheme, and their option to opt in or out dependent upon age/earnings.[1]

---

1 🖉 https://www.gov.uk/workplace-pensions.

- Towards the end of the trial period, if progress is satisfactory, draw up a written statement of terms and conditions (contract of employment). This must be provided within 2 months of an employee commencing work (➲ Between dentist and staff, p. 698).
- Ensure at all stages (advertising, assessing applicants, interviewing) there is no element of discrimination on grounds of disability, sex, age, religion or belief, race, pregnancy, maternity/paternity, marriage or civil partnership, gender reassignment, or sexual orientation.
- Ensure that an employee's rights to statutory sick pay, annual leave, minimum wage, PAYE, workplace pension, maternity benefits/rights, parental leave, adoption leave, &/or paternity leave are honoured.

Always put all matters regarding employment in writing.

The BDA advice sheets on the recruitment and employment of staff in dental practice are useful references.

Firing

Practically and emotionally, dismissal of staff is not easy and if taken to tribunal, can be expensive. The Trade Union and Labour Relations Acts allows for dismissal due to capability, conduct, contravention of the law, redundancy, or 'some other substantial reason'.

Employees may bring an unfair dismissal claim after 2yrs' employment (1yr in Northern Ireland). To defend a claim of unfair dismissal the practice should have followed a set disciplinary procedure:

- Investigate any allegations regarding performance/conduct to determine whether a formal disciplinary procedure is indicated.
- Notify the employee in writing of a formal hearing to discuss their conduct advising them of the allegation. The employee should be allowed to bring a fellow employee or union representative to the interview.
- At the formal meeting, allow the employee opportunity to give an explanation (e.g. inadequate training) and consider this explanation.
- Decide on what action to take:

Oral warning A note of the oral warning should be recorded. The reasons should be given in writing to the employee. Give the employee a timetable for improvement and advise that this is the first stage of the disciplinary procedure.

Written warning (First/second/final written warning.) A written warning that if there is no improvement, dismissal will follow.

Written notice Written notice if the employee fails to meet the requirements stated in the written warnings. The amount of notice should concord with that agreed in the employment contract. The minimum statutory notice required depends upon length of service: <1 month = no notice; 1 month to 2yrs = 1 week; 2–12yrs = 1 week for each complete year worked; >12yrs = 12 weeks.

Instant dismissal Instant dismissal is acceptable where an action is deemed to amount to gross misconduct. Examples of gross misconduct may include theft, breach of confidentiality, and alcohol/drug-related incapacity.

Redundancy Employers must ensure they follow a formal, fair, and transparent process when selecting staff for redundancy. This could, for example, take the form of an assessment sheet for each employee which scores a number of factors, e.g. length of service, qualifications, additional practice responsibilities, etc. with the lowest scoring member(s) of staff being made redundant. Statutory redundancy payments are required for staff who have been employed continuously for >2yrs (full- or part-time). The amount paid depends upon pay, length of service, and age. Employers should provide employees with notice of redundancy in accordance with statutory requirement. Employees are also entitled to paid time off to look for a new job or undergo training.

Appeal The employee must be given the opportunity to appeal any decision relating to discipline/sanction/redundancy/dismissal. Formal procedures must be followed relating to time limits, appeal meetings, and further decisions.

NB: claims for unfair dismissal on grounds of discrimination have no qualification period.

The BDA produce advice sheets on dismissal and redundancy. The Advisory, Conciliation and Arbitration Service (ACAS) will give guidance and have also produced an extensive range of advice sheets, booklets, and online training tools to assist organizations.

Health and safety

- *Hazard*—anything with the potential to cause harm.
- *Risk*—the likelihood that someone will be harmed by a hazard.
- *Risk assessment*—a systematic evaluation of what could cause harm (e.g. equipment, chemicals, work activities) in the workplace, ensuring precautions are in place to minimize these risks, detailed records are kept and regular audits are undertaken.

Health and Safety at Work (HSW) Act 1974

The HSW Act aims to protect employers, employees, self-employed contractors, and the public within the work environment.[2,3] Failure to comply could lead to investigation and prosecution by the Health and Safety Executive (HSE), a statutory body responsible for enforcing the HSW Act. The HSE has the power to enter premises (with or without notice) and carry out an inspection. If required, they can issue an improvement notice (advising when compliance must be achieved) or a prohibition notice (closing the premises until compliance is achieved) ± prosecution. Employees are expected to take reasonable care for their own and other people's safety; refusal to comply may be grounds for dismissal.

Compliance with the HSW Act requires:
- Equipment and systems of work to be safe. Instruction, training, and supervision to be provided as appropriate.
- Maintenance of practice premises, including entrances/exits, in a safe condition.
- Safe handling and storage of potentially harmful and dangerous substances.
- All practices employing more than five members of staff to have a written health and safety policy.
- Legal requirement to either display HSE-approved law poster or provide workers with the equivalent leaflet. Copies of the poster can be obtained online.[4]

Accidents and medical emergencies

A written record should be kept of all accidents and medical emergencies in the practice documenting location, date and time of incident, name of person affected (whether they are staff, patient, contractor), nature of injury, how the event occurred, and how it was managed.

RIDDOR The Reporting of Injuries, Diseases and Dangerous Occurrences Regulations 2013 (RIDDOR 2013)[5] place a legal duty upon employers, the self-employed, and people in control of premises to report:
- Work-related deaths.
- Specified injuries to workers.

---

2 BDA July 2018 Advice sheet: *Health and Safety* (https://bda.org/advice/Pages/Health-and-Safety.aspx).

3 HSE August 2014 *Health and Safety Made Simple: The Basics for Your Business* (⅋ http://www.hse.gov.uk/pubns/indg449.htm).

4 ⅋ http://www.hse.gov.uk/pubns/books/lawposter.htm.

5 RIDDOR 2013 (⅋ http://www.hse.gov.uk/pubns/indg453.htm).

- Injuries to workers resulting in admission to hospital >24h unless for observation or precaution only.
- Injuries causing individual being unable to work >7 days not including the day of injury.
- Injuries to non-workers resulting in being taken to hospital.
- Dangerous occurrences including explosion of, e.g. compressor, inhalation/ingestion of substance requiring medical treatment.
- Acts of non-consensual violence to people at work.

Reporting of such incidents to HSE should be carried out immediately to allow the HSE and local authorities to investigate. For injuries leading to >7 days off work, a report must be made within 15 days. Reports can be made online[6], by post on a standard form, or by phone.

NB: deaths and injuries arising from medical/dental treatment carried out by, or under the direct or indirect supervision of, a dentist are exempt from reporting under RIDDOR.

Adverse incidents involving medical devices should be reported to the MHRA. Reports should be made in writing and can be completed online.[7]

In addition, in England, the Care Quality Commission (CQC) should be notified of deaths that were, or may have resulted, from the carrying out of a regulated activity. Incidents resulting in serious injury to people using the service also need to be notified. Notification forms can be downloaded from the CQC website.

In Northern Ireland, incidents covered by RIDDOR (which differs from the rest of the UK and remains unchanged from the 1997 Act) should be reported to the Health and Safety Executive for Northern Ireland (HSENI).[8]

When notifying any organization about an incident, care must be taken not to disclose confidential information that would be seen to contravene the Data Protection Act 2018.

Medical emergencies GDC Standards state that registrants must follow the Resuscitation Council (UK) guidance on the management of medical emergencies, mandatory equipment, and training (➜ Useful emergency kit, p. 557). Verifiable training must be completed on an annual basis (➜ Continuing professional development, p. 772) as well as regular simulated scenarios within the practice.

First-aid The Health and Safety (First-Aid) Regulations 1981 require all workplaces to have first-aid provisions. The practice should be assessed to ensure compliance based on number of people employed and the risks associated with the work.

Practices with fewer than five employees should have an appointed person in attendance during practice hours. Practices with more than five employees are advised to have a qualified 'first-aider'. Larger practices may consider more than one trained person (either in emergency first aid or first aid at work).

6 🔊 http://www.hse.gov.uk/riddor/.

7 Yellow Card (🔊 https://yellowcard.mhra.gov.uk/).

8 🔊 https://www.hseni.gov.uk/report-incident.

Training needs to be undertaken through an HSE-approved course and renewed as appropriate. First-aid boxes should be appropriate for the number of employees and level of risk.

Needlestick injuries (See ➲ Needlestick injuries, p. 381.) Allow wound to bleed, and wash under warm water. Get advice from occupational health services or local hospital accident and emergency department. If a risk of infection, serological testing of staff and patient may be indicated. An accident report must be completed.

Employers' liability A certificate of insurance must be displayed on the premises.

Control of Substances Hazardous to Health (COSHH) Regulations 2002

The COSHH Regulations require employers to identify all substances (dental materials, cleaning products, blood, etc.) in the workplace which are potentially hazardous, and take steps to prevent or ↓ any risks to health. The following procedure is recommended:

- Carry out a systematic review of each area of the practice workplace.
- Assess the risks to health from hazardous substances and who might be harmed by their use and how.
- Prevent exposure (e.g. don't use substance) or control exposure (if preventing use is not practicable).
- Identify precautions needed e.g. eye/skin protection, ventilation.
- If more than five employees, make and keep a record of the findings of the assessment.
- Ensure all employees are properly trained and supervised.
- Ensure that measures to control exposure are used and safety procedures followed.
- Monitor exposure and carry out health monitoring when indicated by the initial risk assessment.
- Prepare a plan to deal with accidents/emergencies involving hazardous substances.
- Keep records to show regular reviews of risks posed by new and existing substances present in the practice.

NB: product safety data sheets are not a risk assessment in themselves but provide information which should form part of the risk assessment process and should be readily available in case of emergency.

Mercury (Hg) Encapsulated amalgam should be used in preference to non-encapsulated and should be included in a COSHH assessment. Use should be confined to impervious surfaces, ideally a lipped tray lined with foil. Staff should wear gloves when handling Hg-containing substances. ↑ ventilation should be used where possible.

Staff should be trained with dealing with Hg spillage and a policy should be in place. Kits for dealing with spillages should contain a bulb aspirator for collecting large drops of Hg, leak-proof container (ideally with Hg suppressant), mask, and disposable gloves. Proprietary kits are available.

Latex allergy There is now sufficient evidence that healthcare workers and patients are at ↑ risk of latex allergy.[9] More widespread use of latex products has resulted in an ↑ number of the population being sensitive to latex. In order to ↓ the risk:
• Substitute, control, or eliminate latex wherever possible.
• Provide safe and effective latex-free alternatives.
• Limit latex to its most valuable uses.
• Identify sensitized patients.
• ↑ awareness about latex sensitivity.

Chlorhexidine sensitivity Reports of anaphylactic reaction to chlorhexidine have prompted the Medicines and Healthcare products Regulatory Agency (MHRA) to issue an alert. Clinicians are advised to be aware of the risk of anaphylaxis, check for known sensitivity, and report any adverse reactions.[10]

Display screen equipment See ➲ Computers and visual display units (VDUs), p. 766.

Electrical safety
In order to protect both people and property, practices should:
• Carry out a risk assessment to identify where potential electrical hazards exist.
• Ensure all new electrical systems are installed and maintained to suitable standards.
• Ensure staff are properly trained how to use equipment.
• Carry out visual inspections of equipment e.g. cables and plugs, looking for bare wires or checking that the correct fuse is installed.
• Ensure electrical equipment both fixed and portable is periodically inspected and maintained according to a written scheme and that all results are kept.
• Use the lowest voltage equipment suitable for the task.
• Have a safety device, e.g. RCB, to protect and isolate the electrical supply.

The Electricity at Work Regulations 1989 state that equipment should be maintained to prevent danger; however, they do not state what needs to be done, by whom, and how often. Following a risk assessment and reference to manufacturers' recommendations, practices should decide how often to undertake checks and what form these take, e.g. visual by employees, portable appliance testing (PAT), etc. Guidance on intervals for particular categories of equipment can be obtained from the HSE website (🕭 https://www.hse.gov.uk/).

Medical Devices Directive (MDD)
A dental prosthesis or orthodontic appliance is a custom-made device requiring a written prescription from the dentist. Manufacturers of custom-made dental appliances need to register with the MHRA in the UK (or equivalent in other European Union (EU) countries) and comply with legal requirements of the MDD.

---

9 🕭 http://www.hse.gov.uk/healthservices/latex/index.htm.

10 MHRA 2012 *Medical Device Alert MDA/2012/075* (🕭 https://www.mhra.gov.uk/home/groups/dts-bs/documents/medicaldevicealert/con197920.pdf).

The manufacturer of an appliance is legally required to produce a 'Statement of Manufacture' which should contain:

- The name and address of the manufacturer (if outside the EU, the name of the authorized representative).
- Date to allow identification of the device in question.
- The name of the prescribing clinician and practice.
- Specifics of the appliances as indicated by the prescription.
- A statement confirming the device is custom made and intended for the sole use of the named patient.
- Confirmation the appliance conforms to the essential requirements of the MDD.

The person providing the appliance to the patient must make the patient aware of the availability of the statement and offer a copy. Records should document whether the patient takes the statement or not. If declined, the statement should be retained within the patient's record for the lifetime of the appliance.

While contracting the manufacture of dental appliances outside of the UK is permissible, the GDC clarifies that a clinician, who elects to do so, will be held professionally accountable for the safety and quality of the appliance. The clinician would need to ensure appliances manufactured outside the UK satisfy the standards and obligations laid out in the MDD. Prescribing clinicians have a duty to ensure appliances made in the UK are manufactured by a registered technician who is then accountable to the GDC in their own right.[11]

Pressure vessels

The Pressure Systems Safety Regulations 2000[12] cover the safe use of pressure vessels in the workplace, e.g. compressors, autoclaves. Before use, a written scheme of examination should be put in place by a competent person (usually a specialized engineer) stating the periodic examination of the vessel. Records should be kept detailing examination/service/breakdown/repair of the equipment.

Autoclaves require regular checks (daily, weekly, etc.) to ensure that they function within the correct parameters. Details of all cycles and checks should be recorded (notebook, data-logger, etc.) and kept for a minimum of 2yrs and the equipment validated/calibrated periodically by a competent person in line with the manufacturer's instructions.

Cross-infection prevention and control

Requirements for the decontamination of primary care dental practices within the UK are covered by different regulations depending upon region.

- England—Health and Social Care Act 2008: 'Code of practice on the prevention and control of infection and related guidance'; Health Technical Memorandum (HTM) 01-05: 'Decontamination in primary care dental practices'.
- Northern Ireland—HTM 01-05 as amended by PEL 13-13.

---

11 GDC September 2013 *Standards on Commissioning and Manufacturing Dental Appliances* (℘ https://www.gdc-uk.org/).

12 ℘ https://www.legislation.gov.uk/uksi/2000/128/contents/made.

- Scotland—Scottish Dental Clinical Effectiveness Programme— Decontamination into Practice.
- Wales—WHTM 01-05: 'Decontamination in primary care dental practices and community dental services'.

Practices will be assessed on compliance with the relevant code ensuring systems are in place to monitor, prevent, and control infection.

Cross-infection is the transmission of infectious agents between patients and staff within the clinical environment. Potential risks include not only hepatitis and HIV, but also other viruses (e.g. herpes) and bacteria (e.g. methicillin-resistant *Staphylococcus aureus* (MRSA)). Transmission can occur by inoculation or inhalation by direct or indirect contact.

Many patients may be unaware they are carriers of infections and therefore universal precautions are mandatory to ensure a standard cross-infection control policy for all patients. It is unethical to refuse dental care on the grounds that it could expose the dentist to personal risk. Clinicians can be challenged on the grounds of discrimination for declining to treat a patient, or treating a patient differently, on this basis.

All staff should have documented training in cross-infection control and every practice must have a written infection control policy displayed in every surgery to ensure uniformity of procedures. The Infection Prevention Society has produced an infection control audit to allow thorough assessment of all practice systems.[13]

Immunization All new healthcare workers should be tested for, and where appropriate inoculated against, TB and hepatitis B, and those whose post or training requires performance of exposure prone procedures should also be tested for hepatitis C and HIV. Immunization against hepatitis B is with a single booster 5yrs after the primary course. Protection is indicated by HbsAb >100mIU/mL. Antibody levels <10mIU/mL indicate a non-responder. Poor responders have antibody levels of 10–100mIU; it is not clear what protection is afforded by this level of response so consultation with occupational health services is required to determine need for additional blood tests/boosters. Staff should also be immunized against common illnesses and annually against flu. Documentary evidence of immunization and response for all staff should be retained.

Surgery design and equipment Surgeries should include separate areas which are designated 'clean' and 'dirty' zones. Layout and equipment must be planned to allow easy cleaning and to minimize the number of surfaces touched; e.g. taps or lights that can be turned on with infrared light switches or foot controls.

A system of zoning ↑ efficiency as only those areas which are in the contaminated zone need to be disinfected with a suitable disinfectant.

All equipment which has a mains-fed water supply must comply with the Water Fittings Regulations.

---

13 ◌ https://www.gov.uk/government/publications/decontamination-in-primary-care-dental-practices.

Work surfaces During use, instruments should be placed on a sterilizable tray or impervious disposable covering. Care is required to avoid contamination of areas which are difficult to disinfect. Equipment handles, controls, and tubing should be covered by disposable plastic sheeting. Work surfaces should be disinfected using appropriate products between patients. All surfaces should be cleaned at the end of every session, even surfaces apparently uncontaminated.

Personal protective equipment (PPE) and hand hygiene Disposable gloves, eye protection, disposable bibs, and face protection are necessary for clinical procedures. Hand washing/disinfection should occur at the start and end of each session, before and after removing PPE, after washing instruments, on completion of decontamination procedures, and before handling sterilized instruments. In addition, when carrying out decontamination procedures PPE should include heavy-duty gloves and disposable aprons. A poster should be placed above all wash basins to give guidance on best practice and hand-washing techniques. To prevent skin drying out, a water-based cream should be used at the end of each session. Surgery clothing should not be worn outside of the premises and should be laundered daily at the highest temperature the garment will allow.

Instruments Processing of contaminated equipment should ideally take place in a dedicated decontamination room, designed to allow a flow through of instruments from dirty to clean, with ↑ unidirectional ventilation and suitable rinsing, cleaning, sterilizing, inspection, and storage facilities. Disposable instruments and cleaning materials should be used, wherever possible, especially for instruments that are difficult to clean. Reusable items must be cleaned and sterilized after use according to the manufacturer's decontamination instructions. A washer-disinfector is preferred to ultrasonic or manual washing of instruments prior to sterilization, not least because it minimizes the need for manual handling of contaminated instruments, thereby reducing the risk of inoculation injuries being suffered by staff members. Full PPE should be worn during the decontamination process.

Decontamination equipment Guidelines for the selection, installation, maintenance, and daily use of autoclaves, washer-disinfectors, and ultrasonic cleaners are extensive and well documented in HTM 01-05. All equipment must be routinely validated and serviced to demonstrate that it functions to manufacturers' specifications. Records must be kept of all decontamination cycles, periodic tests, and validation for a minimum of 2yrs.

Sharps The Health and Safety (Sharp Instruments in Healthcare) Regulations 2013 require practices to carry out a risk assessment to prevent sharps injuries. The risk assessment should ensure practices have effective arrangements for safe use and disposal of sharps (including using 'safer sharps' where reasonably practicable). New devices may come onto the market to ↓ risks, but care must be taken to ensure alternative devices are suitable for dental use and do not compromise patient care.

Endodontic files/reamers Where endodontic files are designated as being reusable they should be treated as 'single-patient' or 'single-use'. If files are to be retained for use on the same patient, they must be sterilized separately from other instruments and effective measures must be in place to ensure safe storage and exclude any risk of use on another patient in error.

Laboratory items Rinse and disinfect all impressions and appliances according to the manufacturer's recommendations prior to dispatch and on return from the lab. Ensure lab sheet is marked to show appropriate disinfection of laboratory items has been carried out.

Blood spillages Written protocols should be in place. In case of spillage immediately cover with disposable towels; treat with 10,000ppm sodium hypochlorite solution. After 5min dispose of in clinical waste. Use protective clothing and heavy-duty gloves.

Aerosols Minimize these by high-volume suction. PPE should be worn. Flush aspirators and tubing through at the beginning and end of every session with a recommended disinfecting agent. Use of rubber dam reduces splatter and aerosols.

Dental water lines HTM 04-01: 'Safe water in healthcare premises' and HTM 01-05 give guidance on the risks and control of waterborne pathogens, including *Legionella* in dental water lines, building water supply systems, and air conditioning units. Risks must be assessed by a competent person and a written scheme put in place for preventing and controlling any identified risks. All results of periodic testing must be recorded.

Disposal of waste Dental practices produce a wide range of both hazardous and non-hazardous waste. The responsibility for determining if waste is hazardous rests with the practice; however, hazardous waste would typically include amalgam, sharps, radiography developing/fixing fluids, clinical waste, and chemical disinfectants.

HTM 07-01: 'Safe management of healthcare waste' in conjunction with the Hazardous Waste Regulations 2005 details the duties of the dental practice in dealing with all waste. Dentists are responsible for segregating waste, storing it safely, packaging and labelling it appropriately for transport, and arranging for its safe and responsible disposal. Practices should have a policy relating to classification and disposal of waste. Policies should confirm the current procedures for disposal of:
- Clinical waste (contaminated gloves, dressings, etc.) for incineration.
- Non-hazardous waste (gloves, tissues, etc. not contaminated with blood/hazardous substances).
- Sharps (needles, teeth without amalgam, vials, ± medicinal contamination).
- Study models (gypsum).
- X-ray developer and fixer.
- Medicines.
- Amalgam (capsules, amalgam and mercury, teeth with fillings, contents of amalgam separator).
- Lead foil.
- General 'household' waste.

Dental practices are not currently required to register as hazardous waste producers in England, Scotland, or Northern Ireland; however, practices in Wales producing >500kg of waste annually must register with Natural Resources Wales.

While waiting for collection and disposal by a registered collector, all clinical waste must be stored in a secure room or container which cannot be accessed or tampered with by unauthorized persons. Care should be taken that any waste containing patient information is disposed of confidentially. All non-hazardous waste disposal records must be kept for a minimum of 2yrs. All hazardous waste disposal notes must be kept for a minimum of 3yrs.

Extracted teeth HTM 07-01 guidance on 'Safe management of healthcare waste' considers that extracted teeth would be viewed as waste unless a patient has asked to retain it. In this situation, the tooth is then not considered waste as it has not been discarded. However, the guidance states the organization has a duty to ensure items returned to a patient are disinfected/cleaned and instructions given to the patient regarding subsequent disposal (ideally providing suitable packaging for the patient to return it to the practice rather than disposal in domestic waste).

Radiographs—the statutory regulations
Terminology
Legal person
The person responsible for implementing the regulations and good working practice. Usually the practice owner. The legal person must register the practice with the HSE.

Radiation protection supervisor (RPS)
The person appointed by the legal person who is responsible for implementing the local rules. Can be an appropriately trained dentist or DCP.

Radiation protection adviser (RPA)
A person appointed in writing to provide advice on complying with legal obligations, e.g. testing of equipment, staff training, risk assessment, quality assurance programme, etc.

Medical Physics Expert (MPE)
A person to provide advice on techniques and optimum dosage. This person may also be the RPA.

Ionising Radiation (Medical Exposure) Regulations (IR(ME)R) practitioner
The dentist responsible for justifying an exposure and ensuring the benefits outweigh the risks.

Referrer
A dentist who refers a patient to an IR(ME)R practitioner for radiological examination.

Operator
Any person who carries out all or part of the practical aspects associated with a radiological examination, including taking the radiograph, developing films, identifying the patient, etc.

In complying with the regulations,[14,15] the legal person must:
- Complete an inventory of X-ray equipment (including age, manufacturer, model, and serial number) and notify the HSE.
- Complete a risk assessment in consultation with the RPA on exposure of staff and patients. It should be documented and reviewed at least every 5yrs.
- Ensure every IR(ME)R practitioner and operator has appropriate training and undertakes continuing education. Update every 5yrs and keep records of training for inspection.
- Appoint an RPS.
- Complete a radiation protection file. This should include the local rules and other documentation relating to radiation protection within the practice, e.g. written procedures for patient protection, guidelines for referral for radiological examination, quality assurance programmes, records of training, etc.
- Have a set of local rules, which must include the name of the RPS, operating instructions, details of controlled areas, a contingency plan in the event of an equipment malfunction, and the dose investigation levels.
- Identify designated controlled areas. This is usually within a radius of 1.5m, except in the direction of the beam, where it extends until the beam is attenuated.
- Ensure all equipment is regularly serviced and a radiation safety assessment carried out at least every 3yrs. An electrical safety test should be carried out every year.
- Written guidance for exposure settings for all types of radiograph.

A number of requirements are necessary in order to ensure radiation doses are kept 'as low as reasonably practicable':
- Every radiograph taken must be justified (and the justification recorded in the clinical notes).
- Each radiograph taken should be assessed and reported on in the clinical records, so the report can be reviewed a later date.
- Avoid repetition by recording all radiographs taken in patient records. Send radiographs with patient referrals and share radiographs with other colleagues when appropriate.
- Use rectangular collimation for periapical and bitewing radiographs.
- Use a quality assurance programme to ↑ diagnostic yield and ↓ the need for repeat radiographs.
- Digital radiography is the preferred method; however, if unavailable use the fastest film consistent with good diagnostic quality (ISO speed E or faster).
- Routine use of film holders. A patient should only hold a film in position when it is impossible to position the film any other way.
- Where dose levels are displayed, check regularly to ensure diagnostic reference levels (typical dosages for a given exposure type) are not exceeded.

---

14 The Ionizing Radiation Regulations 2017 (✆ https://www.legislation.gov.uk).

15 The Ionizing Radiation (Medical Exposure) Regulations 2017 (IR(ME)R17).

- Where a member of staff is responsible for more than 100 IO or 50 panoramic per week, dose meters should be used and the results recorded and discussed with the RPA. Results should be kept for a minimum of 2yrs.
- Overexposure due to equipment malfunction or procedure should be discussed with the RPA before reporting to the necessary authorities, if appropriate.

Cone beam computed tomography (CBCT) Use of CBCT in dentistry has become increasingly popular in relation to planning treatment for implants and orthodontics. Radiation doses from CBCT (including potential doses to those operating equipment) can be significantly higher than those for conventional radiography equipment. As the existing regulations for conventional dental radiography were not sufficient to cover use of CBCT, specific guidance has been produced by the Health Protection Agency.[16]

Radiographs—practical tips and helpful hints

Practical tips When taking a radiograph, the raised dot on the packet should face the direction of the beam. When the processed film is viewed from the side with the raised dot, the patient's right is shown on the left of the film.

In order of radio-opacity: air, soft tissues, cartilage, immature bone, tooth-coloured fillings, mature bone, dentine and cementum, enamel, metallic restorations.

View films in subdued lighting against an illuminated background.

For soft tissue views (e.g. after trauma), a very short exposure (often below the lowest setting on the X-ray set) is required. A slower occlusal film may be more practical.

The incisive foramen will have a parallax shift in relation to an incisor apex.

Routine use of a lead apron is no longer considered necessary (→ Lead aprons, p. 19).

Dental radiographs are not C/I during pregnancy (→ Lead aprons, p. 19) although the decision whether to proceed rests with the patient.

Processing See Table 19.1 for film faults.

Manual Do this either in a darkroom or a daylight processing tank. It is important to always keep the developer and fixer baths in the same order.

Length of time for each stage of the process varies according to the chemical manufacturer's guidelines and the temperature of the fluids.

Automatic There are several dental types available which can process IO and some EO films. It is more efficient as the operator only needs to place the film in the machine and collect it at the end. As with manual processing the quality of the image can be affected by the temperature and the deterioration of the fluids. A quality assurance programme should be in place to ensure deterioration in quality is prevented. A radiograph of a test object/ guide can be used as a reference and compared to repeat exposures of the same test object taken following replacement of fluids or at regular intervals.

---

16 ♪ https://www.gov.uk/government/publications/radiation-protection-and-safety-guidance-for-dental-cone-beam-ct-equipment.

Table 19.1 Film faults

Film dark	Fogged film: out-of-date or poorly stored film
	Overexposure
	Overdevelopment
	Temperature too high
Film pale	Underexposed
	Underdeveloped: impatience, exhausted chemicals
	Temperature too low
Poor contrast	Overdevelopment
	Developer contaminated with fix
	Inadequate fixation &/or washing
Poor definition	Patient movement
Blotches	Dark blotches are due to developer splashes, and white blotches to fixer splashes
Marks on film	Deterioration of digital film
	Damage during processing—clips, scratches, films stuck together

Self-developing film The developer and fixer are contained within a sachet, which also contains the film. Following exposure, tabs are pulled which release first developer and then fixer onto the film. The film is then removed and rinsed. Although this method obviates the need for processing equipment, the results tend to be inferior.

Digital detectors These allow an image to be viewed and stored on a computer.

Advantages
- Processing time is ↓.
- Image can be enhanced to ↑ diagnostic yield.
- Reduced exposure; settings should be ↓ to the minimum compatible with the diagnostic quality required of the image.
- Elimination of chemical processing.

Disadvantages
- Cost.
- Hardware/software problems.
- Rigid sensors can be difficult for patients to tolerate resulting in holders not being positioned correctly.
- Film plates can become damaged over time resulting in artefacts on the images.
- Images need to be securely stored and back-up undertaken as for clinical records (● Wise precautions or how to avoid litigation, p. 710).

Financial management

A good accountant and a friendly bank manager are invaluable and may be best recruited on recommendation from another practitioner.

It is advisable to develop a structured system for dealing with fees and estimates, tailored to the individual practice, which is understood and adhered to by all staff.

Delegating Delegating many aspects of calculating and collecting fees (to appropriately trained and motivated staff) should make the practice more cost-effective. However, failure to monitor the situation adequately can, at best, result in a false sense of security.

Book-keeping This is time-consuming but necessary. Many book-keeping tasks can be performed by computer, either with an integrated practice management system or stand-alone software. Suggested minimum:
• Fees due and fees received.
• Bank deposits.
• Patient lists.
• Record units of activity performed compared to monthly targets. Monitor practice and individual performance and address any imbalance early.
• Income/expenditure. Every month compile an income/expenditure record to develop a feel for the financial situation. It is wise to seek the advice of your accountant as to the methodology—accurate accounts will make their job easier (and cheaper).
• Petty cash transactions should be recorded, together with all relevant receipts. Float money (<£50) is best stored in a separate locked box.
• Wages and pension contributions.
• Staff absences and sickness records.

NB: the Inland Revenue has powers allowing it to inspect documents relating to accounting/tax. Financial transactions should be recorded separately to patient records to avoid risk of confidentiality being breached.

Banking It is helpful to bank all monies at the end of each day, as the bank statement then indicates the daily takings. To encourage settlement of fees, it is wise to accept payment in any form, i.e. cash, cheque, or debit/credit card. It is good policy to negotiate overdraft facilities in advance to cover those occasions where cash-flow problems arise.

Organizations that store, transmit, or process card holder data should comply with PCI DSS (Payment Card Industry Data Security Standards) to prevent fraud/theft.

Budgeting An annual forecast and budget should be prepared jointly with the accountant. This simple form of management control helps you to monitor the practice's income and expenditure and to identify any variations quickly so that you can act upon them if necessary.

Bad debts These can often be prevented by having a practice payment policy which is clearly advertised to patients and adhered to; e.g. payment in part at the beginning of treatment and the balance on completion; or payment in full, up front.

At the examination appointment patients should be given a written estimate and advised when payment is due. If a patient forgets, at the last visit they should be asked to sign a form confirming that the treatment has been satisfactorily completed and that they agree to pay (£x) within 7 days. If payment is still not forthcoming, reminders should be sent out at 7, 14, and 28 days. If there is still no joy, consider using debt collectors, but beware of a counter claim of negligence. It is preferable to find out why the patient has not paid before making a further decision.

Tax This is really where a good accountant comes in. By providing them with information on income and expenditure on a monthly basis, they will be able to provide advice on what to do before the end of the financial year to minimize the taxman's percentage.

Insurance Essential for property, contents, equipment, indemnity, staff, loss of income, and personal insurance.

Credit Offering patients the opportunity to pay in instalments can greatly ↑ the uptake of more costly treatments, e.g. implants. The Consumer Credit Act 1974 requires those extending credit to the public by allowing them to pay for goods/service in instalments, to obtain a licence. Financial Services and Markets Act 2000 (Miscellaneous Provisions) (No. 2) Order 2015 allows a business to be exempt from a licence if it allows customers to pay bills in no more than 12 instalments within 1yr. These loans must be interest free and have no charges. Practices should obtain legal advice to assess whether a licence is required.

Running late

Running late happens occasionally to everyone, usually when you were hoping to finish early and rush off to do something else. Time pressures can create the risk of clinicians trying to 'cut corners', a strategy which can misfire and, at best, result in even more time being wasted at a later stage. There is also evidence that practitioners who habitually work under time pressures and run late have a greater risk from complaints and litigation.

If running late becomes a regular problem, stop and reassess/audit your working practices. Identify why the clinic runs late: ? unplanned emergencies, ? insufficient appointment length, ? incorrect appointment booking, ? patients attending late, ? clinic not starting on time (staff and colleagues may be able to help provide a more objective view of the reasons).

Once identified, ensure steps are taken to deal with causes of delays. Some additional hints to ↓ everyday stress:

- Divide appointments into 5min blocks to provide maximum flexibility.
- Ensure appointment times are realistic and allow time for setting and clearing up.
- Within reason do not try to carry out treatment that wasn't planned for that appointment.
- Ensure patients in reception are fully informed of any delays and given the opportunity to rearrange their appointments if they wish.
- If another member of staff is free, e.g. hygienist or dental nurse, you may be able to delegate some simple tasks.
- A working day comprising a longer morning and a shorter afternoon may be more productive.
- If you are so busy that longer procedures have to be booked well in advance, designate some specific sessions for them each month (thus ↓ the temptation to squeeze them in).
- Schedule complex work for the morning and less stressful work (e.g. check-ups) for the end of sessions. Errors are more likely to occur when you are tired.
- For last-minute cancellations, have a list of patients who are willing to come in at short notice.
- Define the working day and try not to extend beyond this.
- Coffee breaks and lunchtime should not always be used to catch up on other work; have a rest occasionally.
- After holidays, book out extra time for dealing with more urgent treatments/emergencies. Then you will be able to cope with fitting in urgent patients on your return and not feel stressed.
- Allocate time each day for 'emergency appointments'.

Emergencies A patient who simply demands to be seen immediately or at a stipulated time may not be a true emergency. Patients with a genuine need for urgent care are more likely to be willing to attend at any time available. Ensure staff understand which conditions need to be seen as an emergency and should not be delayed.

Buffer zones built into day-lists should ensure dealing with emergencies is not a problem. Out-of-hours arrangements should be in place so patients can access advice and treatment if appropriate.

Marketing

As consumers of healthcare, patients have a choice as to where they go for their treatment. Whether NHS, private, or independent, the success or otherwise of a practice is going to depend on its ability to attract and keep patients. Marketing involves identifying and defining needs/desires of potential clients. Advertising is the means by which we communicate with these potential and existing clients.

Advertising Advertising does not need to be brash; after all, it is merely a means of letting the public know about the existence of a practice and the services that are available. Previously, advertising in the 'yellow pages' may have been the limit of practice advertising; however, a wealth of alternative resources may now be more effective:

- Practice information leaflets (➲ Practice leaflets, p. 764). These can be distributed to existing patients and possible sources of new recruits, e.g. nurseries, doctors' waiting rooms.
- Open days. These allow apprehensive patients to find out more about modern dentistry and facilities without the need to have an examination or treatment.
- Practice website. With the increasing popularity of the Internet this can be an efficient and dynamic medium for practice promotion. The practice website can additionally be linked to other sites, e.g. 'find a dentist', 'local services'.
- Social media. This is becoming an increasingly popular way for practices and individual dentists to advertise, allowing information, photographs, and links to further advice to be made available to a larger audience. GDC regulations require that dentists make it clear that photographs or descriptions of treatment advertised may not be appropriate for every patient and that it is conditional on a satisfactory assessment being carried out.[17]
- Adverts in local publications: remember to follow GDC guidelines regarding all forms of advertisement. The best advert is often a satisfied patient who will recommend you by word of mouth.

First appearances count This starts before the patient arrives at the surgery as most patients will make their initial enquiry by phone.

The phone should always be answered promptly, in person. Many patients are frustrated by being left on hold or receiving an answerphone message, particularly if their enquiry is not then dealt with promptly.

When the prospective patient arrives at the surgery the external and internal decor, together with the welcome they receive, will play a role in determining a patient's impression of the professionalism of the practice. Ensure non-dental areas are well maintained and that the exterior of the premises looks well cared for. Dentists providing care at the practice should be clearly identified.

---

17 GDC 2013 *Standards for the Dental Team* (🔊 https://www.gdc-uk.org).

The reception should be as relaxing as possible. A small area for children to play or, if possible, a crèche, are good practice-builders. A range of interesting magazines and practice leaflets on different aspects of dental care/health should be available.

Staff The receptionist must be friendly and helpful (even on Monday mornings). It is worth spending some time with the reception team, deciding on stock responses to some of the more common problems that arise (e.g. dealing with the angry patient). Care should be taken that receptionists are not seen to provide clinical advice; however, ↑ their knowledge of dental techniques is helpful so patient queries can be answered appropriately.

It is also helpful to find out how patients heard about the practice, so as to better target future marketing strategies. The presentation and attitude of all the staff is of vital importance. An attractive and functional uniform in the practice colour or bearing the practice logo helps to invoke an image of professionalism.

Emergencies Although it is tempting to exclude non-registered patients from receiving out-of-hours emergency treatment, it is a good practice-builder to consider seeing anybody in pain, as some of them will become regular patients.

Market research It is vital to know your patient base. Is there a significant group which may need special attention (e.g. elderly or young families)? What extra services would your patients like to see (e.g. implants, a crèche)? What do they feel about your opening times—is there another group of patients who might attend if the opening times were amended?

Remember, the most important marketing aid is without doubt the personal touch.

Patient satisfaction surveys As well as attracting new patients, it is even more important to retain existing patients. The use of questionnaires is a great way of ensuring that the practice is meeting expectations and maintaining standards. Well-chosen questions can address specific areas that the practice may require feedback on and giving patients the chance to voice their opinions (and show they have been listened to and acted on) is a great practice-builder.

Data protection Dental practices must be sure they give patients clear guidance on the use of their personal information and seek consent to send marketing information in any format, allowing patients to opt out at any time. Dentists wishing to post photographs of patients and/or their teeth on websites or social media, for example, will need explicit written consent (⊃ Data Protection Act, p. 766).

Practice leaflets

What information to include?

Dentists providing NHS services in England/Wales contractually must ensure a practice information leaflet is available and reviewed every 12 months. The contract requires specific information to be included, which is a useful starting point for all practices irrespective of jurisdiction or whether private or NHS:

- Name of the contractor/partners/providers, or for corporate practices, the names of directors.
- Full name of each person providing care, date of registration with the GDC, and their registered qualifications.
- Whether any teaching/training is carried out or likely to be carried out by the contractor.
- Address of each of the practice premises.
- Practice phone/fax/website details (if applicable).
- Details of how to request services and what services are available.
- The rights of the patient to express a preference for which practitioner they wish to see.
- If practice premises have disabled access and alternative arrangements where this is not the case.
- Normal surgery hours for each clinician and days of opening.
- Arrangements for out-of-hours care.
- Telephone number/web address of NHS 111 (or equivalent).
- Complaint procedure details (➔ Complaints, p. 690).
- Rights/responsibilities of the patient, e.g. to keep appointments.
- Policy on violent/abusive patients.
- Information regarding who has access to patient information and patient rights regarding disclosure of information.
- Name, address, telephone number, and website of commissioning body.
- The name, telephone number, postal and website address of the CQC (or equivalent).

Further optional information can be included:

- Practice philosophy.
- Map showing the location of the practice.
- Information on the interests of the dentists, both dental and non-dental.
- Illustrations of the practice and photos of staff and facilities.
- Details of charges for broken private appointments if applicable.
- Methods of payment accepted.
- Special facilities and treatment available, e.g. sedation, crèche.

How to set about producing a leaflet

Broadly speaking, there are two approaches: either get professional help (e.g. designer, photographer, printer) or DIY, using a desk-top printing package on the practice computer. The two are not mutually exclusive and all practices should consider taking advice from a designer. Before seeking help, it is important to have some idea of what you want.

- What is your potential market (young families with small children, older professionals and their families)?
- Black/white or two or more colours?

- Glossy booklet or a folded A4 sheet?
- Cost?
- Number of copies required, bearing in mind leaflets may need to be updated (avoid being led astray by the bulk discounts)?
- How is the leaflet to be distributed?

It is wise to shop around and examine the work of several professionals before choosing.

Design and layout

As well as providing information, aim to create the impression of a caring practice. The key to success is simplicity. Use of a practice logo ± house style (or colours) helps reinforce practice image. This idea of a corporate image is not new, but has worked well in the business world. A designer will be able to suggest styles and layouts best suited to your projected market, as well as help with the text wording. Photos and illustrations will ↑ the cost, but also the impact, as will using more than one colour.

Also see ➔ Websites, p. 767.

Points to watch

- Registrants should ensure information about themselves in any promotion is factually correct and not misleading. Registrants will be answerable to the GDC if details about themselves are incorrect—even if they had no input in the wording of a leaflet.
- Don't refer to a dentist as being a specialist unless registered on a relevant specialist list with the GDC. Similarly, avoid the term 'specialize' unless you are actually a specialist.
- Don't advertise other services or goods.
- Be legal, decent, honest, and truthful.
- Do not use patient photographs/case studies without obtaining the express consent of the patient ensuring they understand how images will be used. Patients must be made aware of their right to withdraw their consent at any stage.
- Professional designers may not be aware of professional/ethical obligations. It is important that the wording of any promotional material is carefully checked.

Computers and IT

The majority of practices now use computers in some form, whether solely to assist with practice administration or as a fully integrated reception/surgery system. It is important that a backup of all information is carried out daily and the backup data stored off-site securely. An audit trail must be present within the software to allow any alterations made to clinical records to be identified.

Computers and visual display units (VDUs)

The Health and Safety (Display Screen Equipment) Regulations 1992 require employers to minimize risks arising from working with VDUs/monitors/display screen equipment. Employers should assess the work area, furniture and equipment, the nature of the work being carried out, and any special needs of individual staff. The following should be addressed:

- Chairs should be adjustable, so a comfortable working height is achieved.
- Workspace should be sufficient to allow keyboard/mouse and screen to be positioned and used comfortably.
- Lighting should be optimal with minimal reflection on the VDU. The brightness of the VDU should be adjustable.
- Breaks/change of activity should be allowed to prevent long periods of VDU work.
- Eye tests should be provided and paid for by the employer if requested by an employee. If glasses are prescribed specifically for working with the VDU (and normal glasses cannot be used), the employer must also pay for these.
- Training should be given to ensure employees use the VDU and workstation comfortably and safely to minimize health risks.

Data Protection Act

The Data Protection Act (2018)[18,19] which encompasses the European General Data Protection Rules (2018) places strict controls upon businesses with regard to the way they collect, use, store, and dispose of patient information. It is designed for the computer age and allows patients to take more control of their data. Under the terms of the Act, data must be:

- Obtained fairly and used only for a specific and lawful purpose.
- Not excessive but accurate, adequate, and relevant.
- Only disclosed to certain recipients.
- Protected and held securely.
- Accessible to patients on request.
- Not kept for longer than necessary.
- Only transferred outside the EU with adequate protection.

Dental practices must:

- Appoint a controller (usually the practice owner) and register with the Information Commissioner's Office (and pay a fee).

---

18 BDA Advice sheet 'Protecting Personal Information: Data Protection including GDPR 2018' (⅍ https://www.bda.org).

19 ⅍ https://ico.org.uk/for-organisations/guide-to-the-general-data-protection-regulation-gdpr/.

- Appoint a data protection officer and comply with the requirements of the NHS Information Governance toolkit if they carry out NHS treatment.
- Have a data protection policy.
- Carry out a risk assessment to ascertain if there are weaknesses in their systems (e.g. computer security, policies, etc.) and action the findings.
- Give patients a copy of the practice privacy notice when information is first collected and ensure they understand what that information will be used for and how to withdraw their consent or ask for deletion or amendment of information.
- Give privacy notices to staff and self-employed contractors.
- Ensure all information (digital, manual, audio-visual) is stored securely. Keep up to date with anti-virus software.
- Protect computer passwords and consider encrypting any personal data stored electronically or transferred via email.
- Train staff and ensure terms of employment or contracts of self-employment include a confidentiality clause.
- Report data breaches to the Information Commissioner's Office within 72h of becoming aware of them. If the practice feels it does not warrant notification it must be able to justify that decision.
- Give individuals the right to access their personal information (e.g. dental records).
- Provide a copy of any information requested within 1 month (up to 3 months if the request is complex) and do so free of charge. A request should be made in writing to the data controller. In situations where a request is made for disclosure without a patient's authority, advice should be sought from an indemnity provider.

Websites
Most patients now expect to be able to find information out about a practice through a website. Websites, however, may also come under scrutiny from commissioning bodies, regulatory bodies, and other colleagues. Registrants must ensure information about themselves and the practice is factually correct and not misleading (➲ Points to watch, p. 765). Websites must comply with GDC guidance on ethical advertising and confirm:
- Professional qualifications of all registrants providing care at the practice and the country from which qualifications were derived.
- GDC registration number.
- Name and address at which the dental service is provided.
- Contact details including email and telephone number.
- GDC address and contact details, or a link to the GDC website.
- Details of the practice complaints procedure and information of who to contact if not satisfied with the response (➲ Complaints, p. 690).
- The date the website was last updated.

Independent and private practice

'Independent' is the term preferred by many for private practice, perhaps as it sounds less avaricious. An increasing proportion of dentists are turning to other methods of remuneration than the NHS; indeed, the pace of change is so fast that it is difficult to provide information that will necessarily be relevant in the future. These pages are limited to discussing general principles.

Researching the market To develop the potential of a practice it is necessary first to fully evaluate its present position. An appreciation of the existing patient base can be gained simply by going through the manual or computer records and looking at the geographical spread and socio-economic groups. If most patients are part of a family group, then future developments need to provide advantages for parents and children; e.g. if changing to independent practice, then a family-based capitation scheme might be more applicable.

Also, the potential for attracting new patients to the practice, and the competition from other practices in the area for those and existing patients, should be assessed.

It is also important to research and take into consideration staff views about any changes to be made to the practice. Ensure staff are informed about the reasons and advantages these changes will bring.

Business planning To be successful, a business needs to understand its strengths and weaknesses as well as having a sense of direction and purpose. This can be done through a 'SWOT' analysis (identifies Strengths, Weaknesses, Opportunities, and Threats).

If the financial basis of a practice is to be changed, a business plan will need to be drawn up and discussed with the practice's accountants and bankers.

A marketing plan should involve:
• What you want to achieve with the practice.
• A step-by-step strategy to reach the endpoint.
• Investing in and implementing the plan.
• Gathering feedback.
• Reviewing the plan and repeating the process.[20]

Fee setting This difficult exercise should be carried out in conjunction with the advice of the practice accountant. The following will need to be calculated:
• Practice overheads.
• Profit desired (be realistic).
• Inflation.
• Number of sessions worked per week (considering holidays and attendance at courses).

From this the target hourly rate can be calculated. Local market conditions need to be considered, which may necessitate a little rounding down of

20 R. Rattan & G. Manolescue 2002 *The Business of Dentistry, Vol. 8*, Quintessence Publishing.

the profits desired, or a ↓ in overheads if that is possible. Once a realistic hourly rate has been calculated, either fees can then be determined for each procedure by the average amount of time taken, to give a set price list, or patients charged according to the time taken. Laboratory charges and hygienist fees, as indicated, should be additional.

Types of practice There are basically four different approaches:
- A combination of independent and NHS practice. This may be affected by contractual obligations to a commissioning body regarding availability of NHS services and mixing with private treatment.
- Low-cost independent practice.
- Traditional private practice.
- Insurance-based schemes.

Private dental schemes Types of approaches that may be considered:
- *Capitation-based*—patients pay a monthly fee to the company. The practice receives the fee from the company minus an administration fee. Patient's fees may take into account pre-existing dental status ± practice overheads. The dentist provides treatment as covered by the agreement but certain items, e.g. orthodontics and laboratory fees, may be excluded. Providers of capitation schemes may assist with marketing schemes and training in setting fees.
- *Insurance schemes*—patients pay a monthly fee and treatment costs are reimbursed up to a set amount.
- *Practice membership schemes*—patients may receive a number of examination/hygiene appointments per year for a set fee. Items of service are discounted. Additional insurance for trauma, out-of-hours emergency treatment, etc. may be offered.
- *Fee per item.*

Prescribing for private and independent patients When a private patient requires medicines as part of a course of private dental treatment, a private prescription should be provided. Dentists can also supply or sell medicines to any patient, but need to take into account dispensing rules. Alternatively, common drugs can be given as required and their cost included in the overall fee.

Complaints Patients may contact the Dental Complaints Service (**Ɔ** Dental Complaints Service, p. 691) for assistance with a complaint about private treatment.

Dental Foundation Training

Dental Foundation Training is designed to give a supervised and mentored introduction into general dental practice and is an obligatory requirement for new graduates working within NHS general practice. Obtaining a DFT position requires application through the national recruitment process; in England/Wales/Northern Ireland via ℗ https://www.copdend.org/ and in Scotland via the NES portal at ℗ https://nes.scot.nhs.uk/. Application is open to graduates from the UK, the EU, and eligible candidates from outside the EU.

Dental Foundation Trainees Dental Foundation Trainees work as salaried practitioners thereby reducing pressure to achieve a high-volume turnover. Each trainee should receive on-the-job training and supervision from their trainer, as well as tutorials on a weekly basis. Trainers and trainees must complete an online e-portfolio to allow a continual process for assessment of knowledge and practical skills to be recorded leading to a Certificate of Satisfactory Completion of Dental Foundation Training.

Trainees are members of the NHS superannuation scheme and their contribution is deducted at source. On completion of DFT a training number is awarded which enables a dentist to apply to provide NHS dental services in their own right.

Trainers To be accepted, a practice needs to satisfy the criteria set by the Foundation Training committee. GDPs with suitable experience are eligible to become either sole or joint trainers. They are selected after an assessment and interview as well as a visit to the practice to check suitability as a training environment and compliance with clinical governance and wider legislation.

Trainers receive training for their teaching and assessment roles with many achieving postgraduate qualifications in clinical or healthcare education. A grant is paid and the trainees' salary is reimbursed in full.

Contract A standard contract, which both parties are required to sign, is available from the BDA and scheme organizers. The contract runs for 12 months, at the end of which each party is free to make their own arrangements. It normally includes a binding-out clause which prevents the trainee subsequently accepting as a patient someone he or she has treated at the practice, should they move to another practice.

Dental Core Training (DCT) DCT is additional structured training which provides further professional development. 2yr training schemes have been implemented across a number of deaneries which combine DFT and DCT1, this is currently known as DFT/DCT or longitudinal training. A second year period of post-graduate training would typically involve working in community/hospital/dental school. A smaller number of more senior training posts are also envisaged (DCT2/3) allowing dentists to obtain additional skills which may form part of a pathway to specialty training.

National recruitment Applications are submitted through an on-line portal where all jobs for each stage (e.g. DFT, DCT1, DCT2, etc.) are listed. Candidates complete an online Situational Judgement Test (SJT) in advance of the formal interviews. The interview assessment centres that follow the SJT involve a combination of panels during which candidates are assessed on their communication skills, understanding of clinical scenarios, professionalism, and management and leadership abilities. For some levels of training a portfolio is also required, which is currently scored using a checklist and specifically allocated points for each section.

Clinical governance, continuing professional development, clinical audit, and peer review

Clinical governance

Dental practices in the UK must comply with clinical governance and quality assurance frameworks. Periodic and, where there is deemed to be cause for concern, urgent practice inspections take place to ensure that services are being delivered in a safe, caring, and effective manner. The quality of care provided in dental practices comes under scrutiny from the relevant statutory body (England, CQC; Wales, Health Inspectorate Wales; Scotland, NHS Scotland; Northern Ireland, Regulation and Quality Improvement Authority).

Based on the Health and Social Care Act 2008 (Regulated Activities) Regulations 2014 the CQC (England) assesses practices using five key questions:

- *Is it safe?* Systems for safeguarding from abuse. Assessing and managing risks. Safe care and treatment. Medicines management. Track record. Learning when things go wrong and improving.
- *Is it effective?* Assessing needs and care and delivering evidence-based treatment. Monitoring outcomes and comparing with similar services. Staff skills, knowledge, and experience. How staff, teams, and services work together. Supporting patients emotionally. Consent to care and treatment.
- *Is it caring?* Kindness, respect, and compassion. Involving people in decisions about their care. Privacy and dignity.
- *Is it responsive?* Person-centred care. Taking account of the needs of different people. Access to care and treatment in a timely way. Listening and responding to concerns and complaints.
- *Is it well led?* Leadership capacity and capability. Clear vision and strategy. Culture of the organization. Governance and management of risk and performance. Management of information. Engagement and involvement. Learning, improvement, and innovation.[21]

During an inspection practices must make all documentation available to demonstrate that they are meeting requirements. Inspectors may also interview dentists, staff, and patients.

Continuing professional development

CPD is mandatory for all dental professionals in order to continue their registration. GDC *Enhanced CPD Guidance*[22] sets out the statutory requirements for learning and personal development over the 5yr cycle. All dental professionals must:

- Carry out the required amount of CPD. Dentists 100h; dental therapists, dental hygienists, orthodontic therapists, and clinical dental technicians 75h; dental nurses and dental technicians 50h.

---

21 ॐ https://www.cqc.org.uk/guidance-providers/healthcare/key-lines-enquiry-healthcare-services.

22 ॐ https://www.gdc-uk.org/professionals/cpd/enhanced-cpd.

- Produce a personal development plan (PDP) to set out learning requirements at the start of the cycle. This must cover the relevant field of practice, be adaptable to reflect changing needs (e.g. new techniques), and ideally be based on the findings of appraisal, audit, or peer review. It must have clear anticipated outcomes linked to each activity and an expected timeframe.
- Keep a CPD log including date of learning, number of hours, evidence, e.g. certificate, title, provider, content, development outcome (communication, management, clinical knowledge, behaviour/ethics), and benefit to career/everyday practice.
- Keep evidence of the activity for the period of the cycle plus 5yrs after the cycle ends, e.g. certificate (which must show delegate's name and GDC number, date, hours of CPD undertaken, subject, learning content, aims and objectives, anticipated GDC development outcomes, CPD quality assurance with the name of the person or body providing the quality assurance, and confirmation from the provider that the information contained in it is full and accurate).
- Complete an annual CPD statement on the eGDC account which comprises a declaration of the number of hours of CPD completed during the CPD year; a declaration that a CPD record has been kept; a declaration of a PDP; a declaration that the CPD is relevant to the current or intended field of practice; and a declaration that the statement is full and accurate.
- Complete an end of cycle statement on the eGDC account which comprises a declaration of the total number of hours of CPD undertaken in the 5yr cycle; a declaration that a CPD record has been kept; a declaration of a PDP; a declaration that the CPD is relevant to the current or intended field of practice; and a declaration that the statement is full and accurate.

Enhanced regulations for CPD came into force on 1 January 2018 for dentists and 1 August 2018 for dental care professionals. There may be a transition period for some registrants up to 2022 where the 5yr cycle is made up partly from the 2008 regulations and partly from the 2018 regulations.

Peer review
The aim of peer review is to improve the quality of care provided in dental practice by encouraging groups of dentists, either within the same or different practices, to review and then discuss all aspects of their work and to identify areas in which change can be made. This could be by informal gatherings, e.g. over lunch, visits to each other's practices, or as study groups with set agendas, well-defined projects, or guest speakers.

Clinical audit
What it is Clinical audit is a quality improvement cycle that involves measurement of the effectiveness of healthcare against agreed and proven standards for high quality, and taking action to bring practice in line with these standards so as to improve the quality of care and health outcomes.[23]

23 HQIP 2011 *New Principles of Best Practice in Clinical Audit*, Radcliffe Publishing.

The aim is to encourage clinicians to self-assess different aspects of their practice, implement changes, and monitor them with a view to improving service and patient care. While a rolling cycle of audits may be in place, specific audits may be prompted by an adverse incident or complaint.

Aims and objectives Improvement of the quality of care provided. This is achieved by identifying less-than-adequate care and raising it to the standard of the agreed best.

General principles Audits can be retrospective or prospective.[24] Retrospective audit may be particularly useful to review practice following, e.g. a patient complaint/significant event. Prospective audit looks at future care. The basis of all audits should be frank and open discussion without fear of criticism.

The quality of care provided should be objectively assessed against an agreed standard of care. Standards should not be fixed and immutable, so as to allow evolutionary change. It is imperative that the results of such discussion should lead to changes in practice when indicated. Confidentiality is an absolute prerequisite.

Audit can involve all the dental team. Examples of areas that can be subject to audit include compliance with radiography requirements (e.g. justification/reporting), record keeping, cross infection, and time keeping. With all audit crucial requirements are genuine motivation and interest among the participating staff, objectivity, honesty, and adequate data.

An 'audit cycle' is illustrated in Fig. 19.1.

24 R. Rattan 2007 *Quality Matters: From Clinical Care to Customer Services*, Quintessence Publishing.

Meeting to agree a 'gold standard' of care for a
specific condition. Decide 'what needs to be achieved'
↓
Collection of data (retrospective or prospective) and analysis
↓
Review meeting to compare actual standard with 'gold standard'.
Where standard not achieved, identify reasons why
↓
Propose changes to address any deficiency and implement
↓
Prospective analysis of care following implementation of
new recommendations.
↓
Meeting to compare actual standard with 'gold standard'.
↓
'Gold standard' not met → re-enter cycle.
'Gold standard' met → is 'gold standard' good enough?
If yes—recognize, and set date for periodic review
If no—agree new standard and re-enter cycle.

Fig. 19.1 Audit cycle.

Evidence-based practice

Evidence-based dentistry This allows the examination and application of current scientific evidence (e.g. research, epidemiology, audit) to guide the clinical decision-making processes involved in providing dental treatment.

Hierarchy of evidence
- Systematic review and meta-analysis (strongest).
- Randomized controlled clinical trial (RCCT).
- Cohort studies.
- Case–control studies.
- Cross-sectional surveys.
- Case series/case reports and expert opinion (weakest).

The 'gold standard' for clinical studies is a well-planned RCCT as these minimize the risk of bias. But in many areas of clinical practice evidence from such trials is yet not available. In the meantime, clinicians should continue to evaluate carefully the techniques they use and the results of studies reported in the literature, although the sheer volume of scientific literature makes keeping up to date a difficult task.

Systematic review This is a method of collating and assessing the results of research on a particular topic. This implies that a thorough search for suitable articles and indeed unpublished work has been made, and explicit criteria used to decide whether an article should be included or rejected.

Meta-analysis This is a systematic review which uses special statistical methods to combine the results of several studies. Only RCCTs should be included. By considering a number of studies the effects (and side effects) of a treatment are magnified as the sum total of subjects is effectively ↑. Whether the findings are consistent for different population groups or treatment variations can also be evaluated. For example, if this technique had been used to evaluate the results of research into the use of streptokinase in the treatment of myocardial infarction a positive benefit would have been demonstrated almost 20yrs before it became apparent from the individual studies.

Cochrane Cochrane aims to collate the results of systematic reviews in all areas of healthcare and ensure that the findings are kept up to date. The results can be accessed electronically via the Cochrane Library, on CD-ROM, and the Internet (➲ Useful websites, p. 804).

Clinical guidelines Defined as 'systematically developed statements which assist clinicians and patients in making decisions about appropriate treatment for specific conditions'.[25] They may be developed nationally or locally, but should always be seen as guidance and are not a substitute for clinical judgement. To be effective, clinical guidelines should be brief, practical, and based on the results of sound research. They should be reviewed regularly in the light of new research and their effectiveness audited.

Clinical guidelines can be drawn up by any group of clinicians; in dentistry this approach is mainly being coordinated nationally by the royal colleges &/ or specialist societies.

NICE refers to the National Institute for Clinical Excellence, a government based body which on 1 April 2013 changed its name (but not the acronym by which it continues to be referred to) to the National Institute for Health and Care Excellence. One of the roles is to investigate the effectiveness of different treatment modalities. Of relevance to dentistry are the guidelines relating to the removal of wisdom teeth, dental recall interval, and antibiotic prophylaxis.

25 T. Mann 1996 *Clinical Guidelines*, NHS Executive.

Chapter 20

Syndromes of the head and neck

Principal sources and further reading R. C. M. Hennekam et al. (eds) 2010 *Gorlin's Syndromes of the Head and Neck* (5e), OUP. Although this book is a few years old now, it is still one of the best resources relating to head and neck syndromes.

Introduction

The aim of this chapter is neither to bemuse the reader nor to demonstrate esoteric knowledge, although both may appear to occur. The real importance behind the learning of names associated with conditions which may be of relevance to, or be picked up by, clinical examination of the head and neck, is that, once learned, some difficult diagnostic problems can be quickly solved and appropriate Rx instituted. We have retained eponyms where relevant. Examiners have a tendency to remember their favourite eponymous syndrome and it helps to at least agree on the name. We have, however, mainly avoided the use of the possessive when using eponyms because invariably others were involved in describing or elucidating the condition and the syndrome does not belong to the individual(s) associated with it. The following list is in no way comprehensive but takes you through conditions met by the authors either in their clinical practice or in examinations, and which could therefore be considered worth knowing about.

Definitions

Malformation A 1° structural defect resulting from a localized error of morphogenesis.

Anomalad A malformation *and* its subsequently derived structural changes.

Syndrome A recognized pattern of malformation, presumed to have the same aetiology but not interpreted as the result of a single localized error in morphogenesis.

Association A recognized pattern of malformation not considered to be a syndrome or an anomalad, *at the present time*.

Syndromes

Albright syndrome (McCune–Albright syndrome) Consists of polyostotic fibrous dysplasia (multiple bones affected), patchy skin pigmentation (referred to as café-au-lait spots), and an endocrine abnormality (usually precocious puberty in girls). Facial asymmetry affects up to 25% of cases.

Apert syndrome A rare developmental deformity consisting of a craniosynostosis (premature fusion of cranial sutures) and syndactyly (fusion of fingers or toes). Severe mid-face retrusion leads to exophthalmos of varying severity. Early surgical intervention may be indicated for raised intracranial pressure or to prevent blindness from subluxation of the globe of the eye.

Beckwith–Wiedemann syndrome Consists of exomphalos, macroglossia, gigantism, and adrenal and renal anomalies. May have profound hypoglycaemia. Tongue reduction is sometimes required.

Behçet's disease (Pronounced behh-chet, after Turkish doctor Hulusi Behçet.) Oral ulcers with two of skin lesions, uveitis, genital ulcers, or blistering of skin when cannulated. Clinical Δ only. No tests, associated with HLA-B51. It is, in fact, a multisystem disease of immunological origin—need to recognize and refer for multidisciplinary care. It has a different sex predilection depending on the geographical region studied. M:F—Mediterranean 8:1, Far East 2:1, Europe 1:1. Azathioprine, ciclosporin, and thalidomide are in use to treat it. See also ➔ Behçet's disease, p. 440.

Binder syndrome Maxillonasal dysplasia, severe mid-facial retrusion, and absent or hypoplastic frontal sinuses are the main features. There is no associated intellectual defect.

Castleman syndrome A rare cause of massive cervical swelling which resembles lymphoma but with no identifiable malignant cells. Some variants are benign, others are considered premalignant. Benign giant lymph node hyperplasia is another name and says it all.

Chediak–Higashi syndrome A combination of defective neutrophil function, abnormal skin pigmentation, and ↑ susceptibility to infection (→ severe gingivitis, periodontitis, and aphthae in young children). It is a genetic disease.

Cleidocranial dysostosis (cleidocranial dysplasia) An autosomal dominant inherited condition consisting of hypoplasia or aplasia of the clavicles, delayed ossification of the cranial fontanelles, and a large, short skull. Associated features are shortness of stature, frontal and parietal bossing, failure to pneumatize the air sinuses, a high-arched palate &/or clefting, mid-face hypoplasia, and failure of tooth eruption with multiple supernumerary teeth. Many of the teeth present have inherent abnormalities such as dilaceration of roots or crown gemination. Hypoplasia of 2° cementum may occur. The condition mainly, though *not* exclusively, affects membranous bone.

'Cri du chat' syndrome A chromosomal abnormality caused by deletion of part of the short arm of chromosome 5, resulting in microcephaly, hypertelorism, and a round face with a broad nasal bridge and malformed ears. Associated laryngeal hypoplasia causes a characteristic shrill cry. There is associated severe intellectual disability.

Crouzon syndrome The commonest of the craniosynostoses. It is an autosomal dominant condition consisting of premature fusion of cranial sutures, mid-face hypoplasia, and, due to this, shallow orbits with proptosis of the globe of the eye. Radiographically, the appearance of a 'beaten copper skull' is characteristic. The enlarging brain is entrapped by the prematurely fused sutures and ↑ intracranial pressure can lead to cerebral damage and resulting intellectual deficiency. This and the risk of blindness justify early craniofacial surgery to correct the deformity.

Down syndrome (trisomy 21) The commonest of all malformation syndromes, affecting up to 1:600 births. Risk ↑ with maternal age. Children with Down syndrome account for one-third of severely mentally handicapped children. Facial appearance is characteristic with brachycephaly, mid-face retrusion, small nose with flattened nasal bridge, and upward sloping palpebral fissures (formerly known as 'mongoloid slant'). There is relative macroglossia and delayed eruption of teeth. Major relevant associations are heart defects, atlanto-axial subluxation, anaemia, and an ↑ risk of leukaemia. Most children and adults with Down syndrome are extremely friendly and cooperative.

Eagle syndrome Dysphagia and pain on chewing and turning the head. It has been proposed that this is due to an elongated styloid process.

Ehlers–Danlos syndrome A group of disorders characterized by hyperflexibility of joints, ↑ bleeding and bruising, and hyperextensible skin. There appears to be an underlying molecular abnormality of collagen in this inherited disorder. Bleeding is commoner in type IV, early-onset periodontal disease in type VIII. Pulp stones may be seen in all types.

Frey syndrome (Lucie Frey, a Polish physician.) A condition in which gustatory sweating and flushing of skin occur. It follows trauma to skin overlying a salivary gland and is thought to be due to post-traumatic crossover of sympathetic and parasympathetic innervation to the gland and skin, respectively. Its frequency following superficial parotidectomy ranges from 0% to 100% depending on which surgeon you are talking to, but is almost certainly present in all cases to some degree if looked for carefully enough (use starch–iodine test).

Gardener syndrome This comprises multiple osteomas (particularly of the jaws and facial bones), multiple polyps of the large intestine, epidermoid cysts, and fibromas of the skin. It shows autosomal dominant inheritance. The discovery on clinical or X-ray examination of facial osteomas mandates examination of the lower gastrointestinal tract, as these polyps have a tendency to rapid malignant change. This is a highly 'worthwhile' syndrome.

Goldenhar syndrome A variant of hemifacial microsomia and consists of microtia (small ears), macrostomia, agenesis of the mandibular ramus and condyle, vertebral abnormalities (e.g. hemivertebrae), and epibulbar dermoids. Also, cardiac, renal, or skeletal abnormalities can occur. Up to 10% of patients may have an intellectual disability—in other words, 90% do not.

Gorlin–Goltz syndrome (multiple basal cell naevi syndrome) (➲ Skin neoplasms, p. 550.) Consists of multiple BCCs (epitheliomas), multiple jaw cysts (odontogenic keratocysts), vertebral and rib anomalies (usually bifid ribs), and calcification of the falx cerebri. Frontal bossing, mandibular prognathism, hypertelorism, hydrocephalus, and eye and endocrine abnormalities have also been noted.

Graves disease Autoantibodies to thyroid-stimulating hormone cause hyperthyroidism with ophthalmopathy; women aged 30–50yrs are commonly affected; exophthalmos can be helped by craniofacial approach to orbital decompression.

Heerfordt syndrome (uveoparotid fever) Sarcoidosis with associated lacrimal and salivary (especially parotid) swelling, uveitis, and fever. Sometimes there are associated neuropathies, e.g. facial palsy.

Hemifacial microsomia Prevalence: 1:5000 births. Bilateral in 20% of cases. Congenital defect characterized by lack of hard and soft tissue on affected side(s), usually in the region of the ramus and external ear (i.e. first and second branchial arches). Wide spectrum of ear and cranial deformities found.

'Histiocytosis-X' Really three broad groups of diseases with the histological feature of tissue infiltration by tumour-like aggregates of macrophages (histiocytes) and eosinophils.
- *Solitary eosinophilic granuloma.* Mainly affects males <20yrs. Mandible is a common site. Responds to local Rx.
- *Hand–Schüller–Christian disease.* Multifocal eosinophilic granuloma causing skull lesions, exophthalmos, and diabetes insipidus. Affects younger group. May respond to cytotoxic chemotherapy.
- *Letterer–Siwe disease.* Rapidly progressive, disseminated histiocytosis. Associated pancytopenia and multisystem disease; can be fatal.

Horner syndrome Consists of a constricted pupil (miosis), drooping eyelid (ptosis), unilateral loss of sweating (anhidrosis) on the face, and occasionally sunken eye (enophthalmos). It is caused by interruption of sympathetic nerve fibres at the cervical ganglion 2° to, e.g. bronchogenic carcinoma, invading the ganglion or neck trauma. Scores high on the 'worthwhile' rating.

Hurler syndrome A mucopolysaccharidosis causing growth failure and intellectual disability. A large head, frontal bossing, hypertelorism, and coarse features give it its classical appearance. Multiple skeletal abnormalities (dysostosis multiplex), corneal clouding, and serum and urinary acid mucopolysaccharide abnormalities also occur.

Hypohydrotic ectodermal dysplasia Hypodontia found in association with lack of hair, sweating, and saddle nose.

Kawasaki disease Usually affects children <5yrs with pyrexia, rash, cervical lymphadenopathy, dry cracked lips, red eyes, and red fingers and toes. Arteritis is the most serious complication. Immunoglobulin and aspirin in hospital is the mainstay of Rx.

Kikuchi syndrome This is really Kikuchi disease, histiocytic necrotizing lymphadenitis. Increasing cause of cervical lymphadenopathy. Associations with SLE and haemophagocytic syndrome.

Klippel–Feil anomalad The association of cervical vertebral fusion, short neck, and low-lying posterior hairline. A number of neurological anomalies have been noted, and unilateral renal agenesis is frequent. Cardiac anomalies sometimes occur.

Larsen syndrome A mainly autosomal dominant condition, with a predilection for females, consisting of cleft palate, flattened facies, multiple congenital dislocations, and deformities of the feet. Sufferers are usually of short stature. Larynx may be affected.

Lesch–Nyhan syndrome A defect of purine metabolism causing intellectual disability, spastic cerebral palsy, choreoathetosis, and aggressive self-mutilating behaviour (particularly involving the lips).

MAGIC syndrome Stands for Mouth And Genital ulcers and Interstitial Chondritis and is a variant of the Behçet's disease group.

Marcus Gunn syndrome Aka 'jaw wink syndrome'. It is unilateral ptosis which opens (not winks) on moving the jaw to the contralateral side. Odd.

Marfan syndrome An autosomal dominant condition characterized by tall, thin stature and arachnodactyly (long, thin, spider-like hands), dislocation of the lens, dissecting aneurysms of the thoracic aorta, aortic regurgitation, floppy mitral valve, and high-arched palate. Joint laxity is also common. This condition is highly prevalent among top-class basketball and volleyball players, for obvious reasons.

Melkerson–Rosenthal syndrome Consists of facial paralysis, facial oedema, and fissured tongue. It is probably a variant of the group of conditions now known as orofacial granulomatosis.

Multiple endocrine neoplasia A group of conditions affecting the endocrine glands. MEN IIb is of particular relevance as it consists of multiple mucosal neuromas which have a characteristic histopathology, phaeochromocytoma, medullary thyroid carcinoma, and a thin wasted appearance. Calcitonin levels are elevated if medullary thyroid carcinoma is present. Index of suspicion should be high in tall, thin, wasted-looking children and young adults presenting with lumps in the mouth. Biopsy is mandatory and if histopathology is suggestive the thyroid must be adequately investigated. This is another 'worthwhile' syndrome.

Orofacial–digital syndrome One of the many CLP syndromes, all of which are associated with hypodontia (laterals especially) and super-numeraries. This one has finger abnormalities as well.

Papillon–Lefèvre syndrome Palmoplantar hyperkeratosis and juvenile periodontitis, which affects both 1° and 2° dentition. Normal dental development occurs until the appearance of the hyperkeratosis of the palms and soles, then simultaneously an aggressive gingivitis and periodontitis begin. The mechanism is not well understood.

Patterson–Brown–Kelly syndrome (Plummer–Vinson syndrome) The occurrence of dysphagia, microcytic hypochromic anaemia, koilonychia (spoon-shaped nails), and angular cheilitis. The dysphagia is due to a post-cricoid web, usually a membrane on the anterior oesophageal wall, which is premalignant. The koilonychia and angular cheilitis are 2° to the anaemia but may be presenting symptoms. The main affected group is middle-aged women, and correction of the anaemia may both relieve symptoms and prevent malignant progression of the web.

Peutz–Jeghers syndrome An autosomal dominant condition of melanotic pigmentation of skin (especially peri-oral skin) and mucosa, and intestinal polyposis. These polyps, unlike those of Gardener syndrome, have no particular propensity to malignant change, being hamartomatous, and are found in the small intestine. They may, however, cause intussusception or other forms of gut obstruction. Ovarian tumours are sometimes associated with the condition (10% of woman with Peutz–Jeghers syndrome).

Progeria Probably a collagen abnormality. It causes dwarfism and premature ageing. Characteristic facial appearance occurs due to a disproportionately small face with mandibular retrognathia and a beak-like nose, creating an unforgettable appearance; death occurs in the mid-teens.

Pycnodysostosis Micrognathia with hypoplasia of the mandibular angle, exophthalmos, dwarfism, short fingers, and osteopetrosis. Rarely present for orthognathic/orthodontic Rx. Be aware of the osteopetrosis.

Ramsay Hunt syndrome Lower motor neurone facial palsy, with vesicles on the same side in the pharynx, external auditory canal, and on the face. It is thought to be due to herpes zoster of the geniculate ganglion.

Reiter syndrome Consists of arthritis, urethritis, and conjunctivitis. There are frequently oral lesions, which resemble benign migratory glossitis in appearance but affect other parts of the mouth. The condition is probably an unwanted effect of an immune response to a low-grade pathogen; however, some still believe it to be a sexually transmitted disease, although there is no hard evidence for this.

Reyes syndrome Not a head and neck syndrome but encephalopathy and fatty degeneration of the liver which can be lethal. Probable association with aspirin and viral illness in children and the reason you don't give aspirin to those aged <16.

Robin sequence Named after Pierre Robin (and mistakenly called Pierre Robin syndrome at times). This is micrognathia, cleft palate, and glossoptosis. Huge number of associated anomalies.

Romberg syndrome (hemifacial atrophy) Consists of progressive atrophy of the soft tissues of half the face, associated with contralateral Jacksonian epilepsy and trigeminal neuralgia. Rarely, half the body may be affected. It starts in the first decade and lasts ~3yrs before it becomes quiescent.

Sicca syndrome (primary Sjögren syndrome) Xerostomia and keratoconjunctivitis sicca, i.e. dry mouth and dry eyes. There is an ↑ risk of developing parotid lymphoma with this condition. Interestingly, although Sicca syndrome has certain serological abnormalities in common with systemic connective tissue disorders such as rheumatoid arthritis, it does not have any of the symptomatology (unlike Sjögren syndrome).

Silent sinus syndrome Can cause painless facial asymmetry, diplopia, and enophthalmos. It is a spontaneous collapse of the maxillary sinus (and hence orbital floor which is its roof) associated with negative sinus pressure presumed to be due to failure of ventilation at the osteomeatal complex which needs to be surgically opened.

Sjögren syndrome (secondary Sjögren syndrome) In addition to dry eyes and dry mouth this has both the serology and symptomatology of an autoimmune condition, usually rheumatoid arthritis, but sometimes SLE, systemic sclerosis, or 1° biliary cholangitis. Actual swelling of the salivary glands is relatively uncommon and late-onset swelling of the parotids may herald the presence of a lymphoma.

Stevens–Johnson syndrome A severe version of erythema multiforme, a mucocutaneous condition that is probably autoimmune in nature and precipitated particularly by drugs. Classical signs are the target lesions, concentric red rings which especially affect the hands and feet. Stevens–Johnson syndrome is said to be present when the condition is particularly severe, and is associated with fever and multiple mucosal involvement. Viral infections, e.g. herpes simplex, are the second commonest cause.

Stickler syndrome Perhaps the commonest syndrome associated with cleft palate (20%). Consists of flat mid-face, cleft palate, myopia, retinal detachment, hearing loss (80%), and arthropathy. About 30% of Robin sequence patients have Stickler syndrome, therefore examine eyes.

Sturge–Weber anomalad This is due to a hamartomatous angioma affecting the upper part of the face, which may extend intracranially. There may be associated convulsions, hemiplegia (on the contralateral side of the body), or intellectual impairment. The risks of surgery are obvious.

Treacher Collins syndrome (mandibulofacial dysostosis)
This basically involves defects in structures derived from the first bran-chial arch. It is inherited as an autosomal dominant trait with variable ex-pressivity, and consists of downward-sloping palpebral fissures (formerly known as 'antimongoloid slant'), hypoplastic malar complexes, mandibular retrognathia with a high gonial angle, deformed pinnas, hypoplastic air sinuses, colobomas in the outer third of the eye, and middle and inner ear hypoplasia (and hence deafness). About 30% have cleft palates and 25% have an unusual tongue-like projection of hair pointing towards the cheek. Most have *completely normal intellectual* function, which may be missed be-cause they are deaf and 'funny-looking kids' (how would you like to be called a funny-looking dentist/doctor?). These people may well miss out on fulfilling their potential because of society's (and some professionals') attitude to deformity. This syndrome is a prime indication for corrective craniofacial surgery.

Trotter syndrome Unilateral deafness, pain in the mandibular division of the trigeminal nerve, ipsilateral immobility of the palate, and trismus, due to invasion of the lateral wall of the nasopharynx by malignant tumour. Pterygopalatine fossa syndrome is a similar condition where the first and second divisions of the trigeminal are affected.

Van der Woude syndrome Present in 1–2% of cleft patients, lip pits (which are actually small sinuses to minor salivary glands) associated with cleft lip &/or palate. Autosomal dominant with variable penetrance. Second premolars are missing in 10–20%.

Von Recklinghausen neurofibromatosis/syndrome Multiple neurofibromas with skin pigmentation, skeletal abnormalities, CNS involve-ment, and a predisposition to malignancy are the basics of this syndrome. It undergoes autosomal dominant transmission and has a large and varied number of manifestations. Lesions of the face can be particularly disfiguring.

Useful information and addresses

Tooth notation

Because of the difficulties of putting the grid notation (Fig. 21.1 and Fig. 21.2) in word processed documents, it is common practice to indicate the quadrant by abbreviating the arch and side. Thus, the upper right second premolar is UR5 and the lower left second deciduous molar is LLE.

FDI
Permanent teeth

$$R \frac{18 \ 17 \ 16 \ 15 \ 14 \ 13 \ 12 \ 11 \mid 21 \ 22 \ 23 \ 24 \ 25 \ 26 \ 27 \ 28}{48 \ 47 \ 46 \ 45 \ 44 \ 43 \ 42 \ 41 \mid 31 \ 32 \ 33 \ 34 \ 35 \ 36 \ 37 \ 38} L$$

Deciduous teeth

$$R \frac{55 \ 54 \ 53 \ 52 \ 51 \mid 61 \ 62 \ 63 \ 64 \ 65}{85 \ 84 \ 83 \ 82 \ 81 \mid 71 \ 72 \ 73 \ 74 \ 75} L$$

Zsigmondy–Palmer, Chevron, or Set Square system
Permanent teeth

$$R \frac{8 \ 7 \ 6 \ 5 \ 4 \ 3 \ 2 \ 1 \mid 1 \ 2 \ 3 \ 4 \ 5 \ 6 \ 7 \ 8}{8 \ 7 \ 6 \ 5 \ 4 \ 3 \ 2 \ 1 \mid 1 \ 2 \ 3 \ 4 \ 5 \ 6 \ 7 \ 8} L$$

Deciduous teeth

$$R \frac{e \ d \ c \ b \ a \mid a \ b \ c \ d \ e}{e \ d \ c \ b \ a \mid a \ b \ c \ d \ e} L$$

Fig. 21.1 Tooth notation systems.

European
Permanent teeth

$$R \frac{8+ \ 7+ \ 6+ \ 5+ \ 4+ \ 3+ \ 2+ \ 1+ \mid +1 \ +2 \ +3 \ +4 \ +5 \ +6 \ +7 \ +8}{8- \ 7- \ 6- \ 5- \ 4- \ 3- \ 2- \ 1- \mid -1 \ -2 \ -3 \ -4 \ -5 \ -6 \ -7 \ -8} L$$

Deciduous teeth

$$R \frac{05+ \ 04+ \ 03+ \ 02+ \ 01+ \mid +01 \ +02 \ +03 \ +04 \ +05}{05- \ 04- \ 03- \ 02- \ 01- \mid -01 \ -02 \ -03 \ -04 \ -05} L$$

American
Permanent teeth

$$R \frac{1 \ 2 \ 3 \ 4 \ 5 \ 6 \ 7 \ 8 \mid 9 \ 10 \ 11 \ 12 \ 13 \ 14 \ 15 \ 16}{32 \ 31 \ 30 \ 29 \ 28 \ 27 \ 26 \ 25 \mid 24 \ 23 \ 22 \ 21 \ 20 \ 19 \ 18 \ 17} L$$

Deciduous teeth

$$R \frac{A \ B \ C \ D \ E \mid F \ G \ H \ I \ J}{T \ S \ R \ Q \ P \mid O \ N \ M \ L \ K} L$$

Fig. 21.2 European and US tooth notation.

Some qualifications in medicine and dentistry

BA	Bachelor of Arts
BC/BCh/BS	Bachelor of Surgery
BChD/BDS	Bachelor of Dental Surgery
BM	Bachelor of Medicine
DDPH	Diploma in Dental Public Health
DDR	Diploma in Dental Radiology
DDS/DDSc	Doctor of Dental Surgery/Science
DGDP	Diploma in General Dental Practice
DOrth	Diploma in Orthodontic
DOT	Diploma in Orthodontic Therapy
DPCO	Diploma in Primary Care Orthodontics
DPDS	Diploma Postgraduate Dental Studies
DPhil	Doctor of Philosophy
DRD	Diploma in Restorative Dentistry
DSc	Doctor of Science
DSCD	Diploma in Special Care Dentistry
FDS	Fellowship in Dental Surgery
FFD	Fellow in Faculty of Dental Surgery
FFGDP	Diploma of Fellowship in General Dental Practice
FRCGP	Fellow of Royal College of General Practitioners
FRCP	Fellow of Royal College of Physicians
FRCS	Fellow of Royal College of Surgeons
LDS	Licentiate in Dental Surgery
MBBCh/MBChB	Bachelor of Medicine and Bachelor of Surgery
MCCD	Membership in Clinical Community Dentistry
MCDH	Master of Community Dental Health
MD	Doctor of Medicine
MDentSci/MDSc	Master of Dental Science
MDS	Master of Dental Surgery
MFDS	Member of the Faculty of Dental Surgery
MFGDP	Diploma of Membership of Faculty of General Dental Practitioners (UK)

MGDS	Diploma of Membership in General Dental Surgery
MJDF	Diploma of Membership of the Joint Dental Faculties at the Royal College of Surgeons of England
MOralSurg	Membership in Oral Surgery
MOrth	Membership in Orthodontics
MPaedDent	Membership in Paediatric Dentistry
MPhil	Master of Philosophy
MRCGP	Member of Royal College of General Practitioners
MRCS	Member of Royal College of Surgeons
MSc	Master of Science
MSpecDent	Membership in Special Care Dentistry
NVQ	National Vocational Qualification
PhD	Doctor of Philosophy

File sizes for endodontic therapy

See Table 21.1 and Table 21.2.

Table 21.1 File sizes for endodontic therapy

Size	Tip diameter	ISO colour
08	0.08	Grey
10	0.10	Purple
15	0.15	White
20	0.20	Yellow
25	0.25	Red
30	0.30	Blue
35	0.35	Green
40	0.40	Black
45	0.45	White
50	0.50	Yellow
55	0.55	Red
60	0.60	Blue
70	0.70	Green
80	0.80	Black
90	0.90	White
100	1.00	Yellow
110	1.10	Red
120	1.20	Blue
130	1.30	Green
140	1.40	Black

Table 21.2 ProTaper® system

Shaping files	Finishing files	Colour
SX 3–4Ncm		Orange
S1 3–4Ncm		Purple
S2 1–1.5Ncm		White
	F1 1.5–2Ncm	Yellow
	F2 2–3Ncm	Red
	F3 2–3Ncm	Blue
	F4 2–3Ncm	Green
	F5 2–3Ncm	Yellow

Ncm, newton centimetre.

What's your poison?

Large numbers of patients (and colleagues) use drugs (including alcohol, nicotine, and caffeine) both prescription and illegal for self-treatment and recreational purposes.

Society varies internationally in its view of the use of these substances, e.g. alcohol is widely available and legally consumed internationally but is illegal in many Islamic countries.

In the UK, the BMA regards excessive drug use, including alcohol, as a health issue rather than a criminal one in both patients and professionals. The emphasis is on harm reduction. A basic awareness of the nature and effects of the commonly used intoxicants will be valuable to all dentists.

Here are the commonly used intoxicants and some pros and cons:

Alcohol The legal, huge income-generating intoxicant of choice for most. A sedative and disinhibitor which accounts for both its attraction and much of the social havoc it can wreak. This is the only drug to have a highly educated, refined culture and industry built around it. Prohibition remains the classic example of why criminalizing intoxicants will never work. Biochemically and psychologically addictive, the long-term results of abuse can be worse than that with opioids. In low quantities, alcohol has a small evidence base to support health-promoting effects. Weekly recommended 'dose' is not more than 14 units for men and women. More than 6 units in one sitting is considered to be 'binge drinking'.

Amphetamine Legally prescribed for narcolepsy and widely used by all military forces since World War II, this stimulant ↑ dopamine and noradrenaline levels. Can deliver an intense sense of energy, euphoria, and arousal. Problems are paradoxical impotence, paranoia, panic, and serious cardiac effects. Related drugs used to treat attention deficit hyperactivity disorder are used as alternative low-grade stimulants and intelligence enhancers. Freebase 'crystal meth' methamphetamine is a more powerful version which is smoked. Snorting regularly can destroy the nasal septum; injecting ↑ cardiac risks and viral contamination. Post-use comedowns are severe; schizoaffective disorders are a well-recognized problem.

Anabolics Steroids can induce extreme mood swings ('roid rage'), acne, testicular atrophy, osteoporosis, and liver and cardiac damage. *EPO*—popular and topical drug of abuse in endurance sports ('Edgar')—can cause clots. There is little doubt they can enhance physical performance in a variety of competitive sports, but they do so at a devastating cost to the athlete.

Caffeine As well as the universally available drinks containing caffeine, it is also sold as tablets as a stimulant. Historically a feared stimulant drug as the choice of intellectuals (who may foment revolution under its influence), this is now universally legal but can cause insomnia and palpitations up to atrial fibrillation.

Cannabis Plant derivative usually smoked although as tetrahydrocanna-binol (the active ingredient) is fat soluble it can be used in food (cake and chocolate are popular). Medicinal uses are widespread as an antiemetic, analgesic, and in a wide range of conditions but most particularly multiple sclerosis. Sedative, anxiolytic, and disinhibitory it can be hallucinogenic, particularly in intensively produced methods such as 'skunk'. Good evidence of negative psychological effects in younger regular users, especially cognitive impairment, disassociation, and depression.

Cocaine Another plant derivative, this stimulant drug has a number of myths about it. It is relatively short-acting and stimulating but less over-whelmingly so than many of the other stimulants. Associated with wealth and glamour by its accoutrements (silver straws, rolled banknotes to snort it) it is not as addictive as many other drugs but tolerance develops rapidly. It is a powerful vasoconstrictor (which can lead to destruction of the nasal septum) and topical analgesic. The freebase concentrate of cocaine 'crack' delivers an intense, overwhelming stimulant high with an equally overwhelming comedown. This leads to it being used with an opioid to reduce the comedown (speedballing). This is altogether more addictive and dangerous, inducing violent panic attacks and a powerful sense of paranoia.

Ecstasy 3,4-Methylenedioxy-*N*-methylamphetamine (MDMA) is a de-rivative of amphetamine with a fascinating history.[1] A stimulant with mild hallucinogenic properties which ↑ serotonin levels. Minimally addictive with a slow development of tolerance and a tendency to make people want to dance and hug, its dangers come from activity-induced hyperthermia and hyponatraemia induced by overconsumption of water. A moderate comedown lowers mood. In the long term the effects on artificially raised serotonin are unknown but it seems intuitive to expect an ↑ in depressive illnesses. Very little pure MDMA is now available, the vast majority being adulterated with other frankly less safe constituents.

Gamma-hydroxybutyrate (GHB, GB) A sedative anaesthetic and one of the original 'legal highs', this is an odourless, colourless, salty, al-cohol substitute with zero calories but similar effect (sedation, disinhibition, arousal). A reputation as a 'date rape' drug (as it could be easily added to spike drinks) saw its popularity wane. Other than sudden unconsciousness and memory loss (or fitting in severe cases) after overdose, this drug has less in the way of long- and short-term unwanted effects. Its use is limited to small, specific club scenes.

---

1 A. Shulgin & A. Shulgin 1995 *PIHKAL: A Chemical Love Story*, Transform Press.

Hallucinogens (LSD, PCP, DMX, mescaline, mushrooms) Although lysergic acid diethylamide ('acid') is the best known of these drugs due to the hippy culture of the 1960s, the CIA's experimentation with the US military, and latterly its re-emergence in some 'ecstasy' tablets, it was predated by several thousand years by many cultures who used shamanic hallucinogenic experiences powered by peyote, mescaline, and psilocybin in mushrooms as a quasi-religious event. Not physically addictive, the experience is very variable between people and doses. Contrary to myth, visual reality is rarely altered but all the senses are significantly distorted—sometimes pleasantly, sometimes not. Unlike amphetamine the military found no great use for it.[2]

Inhalants Nitrous oxide and ether were the original recreational inhalants but quickly became useful medical drugs. Both, particularly nitrous oxide, continue to be abused by a small number of professionals with access. Solvents, glue, petrol, and lighter fluid tend to be the province of the very young. These have a dangerous sedative intoxication with associated risk of convulsions and myocardial sensitization.

Ketamine A genuine anaesthetic drug. Medical and veterinary use is IM or IV as a useful bronchodilating GA agent. Sold illegally as a white powder for snorting, it produces a dissociative state, body and mind appearing separate, with jerking moments as if returning from sleep. Some experience the well-recognized anaesthetic 'emergence phenomena' with vivid hallucinations. The majority of ketamine is probably consumed in adulterated MDMA tablets where it would be a disappointment if the consumers could remember ever trying genuine MDMA.

Mephedrone and naphyrone These emerged as 'legal highs' in the continuing effort to produce drugs with a similar effect to the old, illegal but popular stimulants, cocaine and ecstasy. Produced as powder to be snorted or in tablet form, they can produce a euphoric stimulant effect but with powerful unwanted psychological, disorientating, and cardiovascular effects. Both are now illegal and further generations of 'poor man's ecstasy' are being worked on.

Nicotine Tobacco in all forms is the other great legal intoxicant of addiction. Users describe its use as being anxiolytic and appetite suppressing. There are no known medical uses or benefits. Harm is legion. The number of deaths caused by addiction to nicotine and the effects of the by-products of this addiction vastly outnumber those of all the illegal drugs added together.

Nitrates (amyl-, butyl-, and isopropyl) Known as 'poppers' and legal if sold as 'room odorizers' or 'CD cleaner' these are popular in some clubs and sex shops. They cause profound vasodilatation when inhaled along with smooth muscle relaxation and a short, profound period of arousal. Dangerous if used in conjunction with sildenafil/tadalafil as profound hypotension and collapse can occur. Headache is very common.

2 S. Walton 2001. *Out of It: A Cultural History of Intoxication*, Penguin.

Opioids Although heroin (diamorphine) is perhaps the best known of the opioids, derived from the opium poppy, they are a wide, diverse group ranging through morphine, methadone, to codeine with long- and short-acting versions (oxycodone to remifentanil). All act on opioid receptors in the brain, all produce a sedative euphoria to a greater or lesser degree, and all have well-recognized beneficial medical effects. All produce a degree of physical and psychological addiction although this is rarely seen in those using opioids for genuine analgesia. Reversal by naloxone is one important way of categorizing these drugs (partial agonists such as meptazinol, pentazocine, and buprenorphine are not fully reversed). Constricted pupils, depressed respiration, and general intoxication with anxiolysis are characteristics. Codeine is a particular problem as it is widely available, quietly addictive, and withdrawal presents as a headache (which responds to codeine, the classical 'analgesic headache'). Interestingly even non-opioid analgesics such as pregabalin have found a market for misuse.

Spice A synthetic cannabinoid (often sprayed on to dried herbs giving it the appearance of cannabis), developed to have an effect like tetrahydro-cannabinol, the main psychoactive chemical in cannabis. Spice is mostly consumed by smoking it. In the UK, it is illegal to produce, sell, or import spice.

Tranquillizers Originally barbiturates were the major problem in this area but these have largely vanished from both the legal and the black markets, being replaced by benzodiazepines and the Z-drugs (zopiclone, zolpidem). Both of the latter act on the gamma-aminobutyric acid pathway, creating a feeling of sedation and relaxation. The dealing of prescription drugs on the black market is vast and varies from country to country. In the US 'Xanax®' (alprazolam) is ubiquitous but unknown in the UK where temazepam is regarded as a partially controlled drug. The Z-drugs were introduced as non-addicted alternatives to benzodiazepines (themselves introduced to be a better drug than barbiturates). None are advisable in the long term as both tolerance and dependence can develop.

Passing exams

Preparation   First, there is unfortunately no substitute for the sheer hard work of revising, and to have a chance of being adequate this should start well before the exam. Beware of those who try to impress by saying they have passed every exam, first time, having only started revising the night before. These people are not super-intelligent (in fact, their behaviour suggests the reverse), they have possibly been lucky, or more likely they are lying.

Equally, the human brain is not a computer and revising for hours, day in day out, could result in 'burn-out'. Each person needs to find their own method, but a break of 5–10min every hour and a complete hour off after 3h of work, has succeeded for others. It is important to figure out what works best for you, another advantage of starting early.

It is important to be sure that you are revising the correct material in sufficient depth. One way of ensuring this is to go over past questions. If some are tackled under exam conditions, this also gives practice in exam technique.

If your nerve is strong enough, it is probably wise to stop working 2–3 days before the exams start and have a rest, doing something that you enjoy. Most people baulk at this suggestion, but see the logic as of a marathon runner resting before an important race. Studying the night before is akin to an elite runner going out the night before the Olympic marathon and running 26.2 miles just to make sure they can cover the distance.

Written exams   It is important to know beforehand how many questions you have to answer and whether they all have to be tackled or if there is a choice. If essay style—work out how long should be spent on each question and, if a choice is permitted, take a few minutes to decide which to answer and in what order. It is better to tackle your best question second, thus allowing the butterflies to settle. Read each question carefully, and periodically stop to check that you are answering the question set, not the one you'd like to answer. A rough plan helps to produce a more logical essay and provides an aide-memoire in case of panic halfway through. Write neatly.

Multiple choice exams   These are popular with educationalists because they are 'reliable', can be marked by computer, and can be 'number-crunched'. Extended matching questions are a variation on the theme.
- Do the necessary revision; it is impossible to waffle hopefully round the subject in a multiple choice exam.
- Remember that your first instinct is often right so consider carefully before revising your answer to any question.

Objective structured clinical examinations (OSCEs)   These should be:
- *Objective*—independent and competent examiners should have agreed what skills are being examined, with agreed marking scales.
- *Structured*—have agreed criteria (in advance) for the correct answer for each element of the exam.
- *Clinical*—to test clinical and practical competence, including communication and problem-solving skills.
- *Examination*—this may include evaluation of written responses &/or observation by an examiner.

They usually comprise a series of stations, which test a different skill, often interspersed with rest stations. A set time is allocated to each station. The clinical proficiencies tested may include taking a history from a 'patient' (usually actors are used rather than actual patients) and establishing a diagnosis, communication, and psychomotor skills. Students may be evaluated by an examiner, who observes and marks their responses and actions at a particular station.

Logbooks These are increasingly used to evaluate clinical experience and competencies and often include a reflective learning log.

GOOD LUCK!

Dentistry and the Internet

The World Wide Web has permeated all areas of our lives and is a great resource, not only for social networking, but also for finding information and gaining knowledge.

e-learning e-learning is 'the use of electronic technology and media to deliver, support, and enhance teaching and learning'. It is one type of distance education that removes the barriers of time and space—'anytime, anywhere learning'.

It links geographically distant learners and teachers, facilitating didactic teaching, discussion forums, and live seminars and lectures. The use of hyperlinks facilitates access to other useful pages on the Internet. However, newer technologies are not necessarily better (or worse) for teaching or learning than older technologies, just different. Therefore, it is necessary to pick and choose to find what suits your learning style.

Internet searching The Web is a fantastic way of finding information quickly and easily. However, the downside is that skill is required to ensure that your search yields a manageable number of relevant sites/pages. Structuring your search using 'rules' that are used by the major search engines will help:

- Search boxes are not case sensitive.
- Using **AND** will include both words/terms.
- Using **OR** will include either the word before or the word after.
- Placing a **+** sign directly in front of a word means it must be included.
- Placing a **−** sign directly in front of a word means it will be excluded.
- Using quotation marks around a group of words will ensure that phrase is included.
- Using a 'wildcard' symbol will include any words with the same stem, e.g. dent* will yield dental, dentistry, dentist, etc.
- Using **:site** will limit the search to a named domain.
- Using **:link** will yield pages that link to the specified web address.

Social media We acknowledge that this is an area where our Internet-savvy readers will have greater knowledge than this short section provides; however, hopefully it will be of help to those who are less familiar. Social media includes blogs and microblogs (e.g. Twitter), content communities (e.g. Youtube), social networking sites (e.g. Facebook, Instagram, LinkedIn, and Google+), and Internet forums.

Blog Short for web log, an online diary or commentary.

Twitter Online messages are limited to 280 characters. You can opt to 'follow' another user and receive their tweets. Also used for seeking answers to queries. 'Re-tweeting' is forwarding another user's tweet. Good netiquette to credit originator.

YouTube Website where you can upload, watch, and rate videos. Content includes humorous home videos, promotional short films, and also surgical and dental procedures. With regard to the latter, be aware that there is no quality control on the content of the clips.

Instagram A social network site for sharing photos and videos launched in 2010, owned by Facebook. The platform allows users to edit photos using pre-set 'filters' and content can be shared publicly or to pre-approved 'followers'. There are also options to post live videos, direct message, and organize posts with information about location or tags.

Facebook Massively popular online community of profiles. Originally individuals, but now brands, institutions, dental practices, etc. have got involved. You can permit 'friends' to access your personal profile, which means they can add content—potentially a minefield for a professional.

LinkedIn Essentially a business/professional version of Facebook where profile = CV.

Trolls Individuals who use the anonymity of the Internet to post unkind comments.

ResearchGate Scientific online community. Users can record their publications and obtain an impact factor rating.

Social media has potential benefits and risks for healthcare. On the plus side it can help drive awareness, provide accurate information, build professional networks, and host patient support groups.

Risks for professionals The General Medical Council has recently published guidance which can be found on their website (see URL in ➲ Useful websites, p. 804). Although the following may seem obvious, they have tripped up the unwary:
- Keep separate professional and personal profiles.
- Maintain patient confidentiality.
- Avoid posting images that you would not wish your patients to see.
- Avoid your friends posting images of you that you would not wish your patients to see.
- Avoid conducting professional disagreements via social media.
- Be aware of the potential audience—this may include your Regulator if sent on to them.
- Constantly review your privacy settings.
- Don't reply/post in anger—sleep on it.
- If you are the subject of defamatory comment or criticism online, contact your defence organization before responding.

NB: if you have a practice website that uses cookies (data from a website that is stored on your computer to facilitate future visits to that site), you need to have a system to gain users' content.

The BBC has a very good glossary: ॐ http://www.bbc.co.uk/webwise/a-z.

Useful websites

The Internet plays an ↑ role as a source of information, however, some caution is required as there is little guidance as to which sites are reputable and reliable—a fact which patients sometimes need to be reminded of. The following are, at best, a sampler of interesting websites (we take no responsibility for their content). Please also see the 'Useful addresses' section (◑ Useful addresses, p. 806). If you have any suggestions for future editions then please let us know.

Acronyms: ℅ http://www.ada.org/sections/professionalResources/pdfs/dentalpractice_abbreviations.pdf
American Dental Association: ℅ http://www.ada.org
British Association of Dental Nurses: ℅ http://www.badn.org.uk
British Association of Dental Therapists: ℅ http://www.badt.org.uk
British Association of Oral and Maxillofacial Surgeons:
℅ http://www.baoms.org.uk
British Association for the Study of Community Dentistry:
℅ http://www.bascd.org
British Dental Practice Managers Association:
℅ http://www.adam-aspire.co.uk
British Endodontic Society: ℅ http://www.britishendodonticsociety.org.uk
British National Formulary: ℅ http://www.bnf.org
British Orthodontic Society: ℅ http://www.bos.org.uk
British Society of Dental Hygiene and Therapy:
℅ http://www.bsdht.org.uk
British Society for Disability and Oral Health (BSDH):
℅ http://www.bsdh.org.uk
British Society for Oral Medicine: ℅ http://www.bsom.org.uk
British Society for Paediatric Dentistry (BSPD): ℅ http://www.bspd.co.uk
British Society of Periodontology: ℅ http://www.bsperio.org.uk
British Society of Restorative Dentistry: ℅ http://www.bsrd.org.uk
Care Quality Commission: ℅ http://www.cqc.org.uk
Centre for Evidenced Based Dentistry: ℅ http://www.cebd.org
Centre for Reviews and Dissemination: ℅ http://www.york.ac.uk/inst/crd
Chief Dental Officer: ℅ http://www.dh.gov.uk/cdo
Chief Medical Officer: ℅ http://www.dh.gov.uk/cmo
Clinical Dental Technicians Association: ℅ http://www.bacdt.org.uk
Clinical evidence (a compendium of research findings on clinical questions): ℅ http://www.clinicalevidence.org
Cochrane Collaboration: ℅ http://www.cochrane.co.uk
Cochrane Oral Health group: ℅ http://www.ohg.cochrane.org
Committee of Postgraduate Dental Deans and Directors:
℅ http://www.copdend.org.uk
Confederation of Dental Employers (CODE):
℅ http://www.codeuk.com
Conference of Postgraduate Medical Deans:
℅ http://www.copmed.org.uk
CONSORT (Consolidated Standards of Reporting Trials Statement):
℅ http://www.consort-statement.org

Contact a Family (provides information on a wide range of disabilities and syndromes): ✍ http://www.cafamily.org.uk
Deafblind UK: ✍ http://www.deafblind.org.uk
Dental Professionals Association: ✍ http://www.uk-dentistry.org
Dental Technologists Association: ✍ http://www.dta-uk.org
Dental Trauma Guide: ✍ http://www.dentaltraumaguide.org
Dentanet: ✍ http://www.dentanet.org.uk
Dentinal Tubules: ✍ http://www.dentinaltubules.com
Department of Health: ✍ http://www.dh.gov.uk
Equator Network Resource Centre for Research reporting:
✍ http://www.equator-network.org
European Collaboration on Craniofacial Anomalies:
✍ http://www.eurocran.org
Faculty of Medical Leadership and Management:
✍ http://www.fmlm.ac.uk
General Medical Council (GMC): ✍ http://www.gmc-uk.org
GMC medical education and training glossary:
✍ http://www.gmc-uk.org/GMC_glossary_for_medical_education_and_
training_1.1.pdf_48186236.pdf
Health Protection Agency: ✍ http://www.hpa.org.uk
Institute of Healthcare Management: ✍ http://www.ihm.org.uk
International Organization for Standardization (ISO): ✍ http://www.iso.org
Kings Fund: ✍ http://www.kingsfund.org.uk
Latex Allergy Support Group: ✍ http://www.lasg.org.uk/guidance
National Institute for Health and Care Excellence:
✍ http://www.nice.org.uk
National Library for Health: ✍ http://www.library.nhs.uk
National Oral Health Promotion Group: ✍ http://www.nohpg.org
NHS Education for Scotland: ✍ http://www.nes.scot.nhs.uk
NHS Employers: ✍ http://www.nhsemployers.org/Pages/home.aspx
NHS Evidence: ✍ http://www.evidence.nhs.uk
Patient information: ✍ http://www.informedhealthonline.org
PubMed: ✍ http://www.pubmedcentral.nih.gov
Scottish Intercollegiate Guidelines Network (SIGN):
✍ http://www.sign.ac.uk
TRIP database: ✍ http://www.tripdatabase.com
Voluntary Services Overseas: ✍ http://www.vso.org.uk

NB: all these addresses were correct at the time of going to press.

Useful addresses

Aberdeen University School of Medicine and Dentistry, Polwarth Building, Foresterhill, Aberdeen, AB25 2ZD.
☎ 01224 437972. ℘ http://www.abdn.ac.uk/medicine-dentistry
Barts and the London Dental School, Garrod Building, Turner Street, Whitechapel, London E1 2AD.
☎ 020 7882 8478. ℘ http://www.smd.qmul.ac.uk
Birmingham Dental School, St Chad's Queensway, Birmingham B4 6NN.
☎ 0121 466 5579. ℘ http://www.dentistry.bham.ac.uk/home
British Dental Association, 64 Wimpole Street, London W1G 8YS.
☎ 020 7935 0875. ℘ http://www.bda.org
British Dental Health Foundation, Smile House, 2 East Union Street, Rugby CV22 6AJ. ☎ 01788 546365. ℘ http://www.dentalhealth.org.uk
Bristol Dental School, Lower Maudlin Street, Bristol BS1 2LY.
☎ 0117 928 9000. ℘ http://www.bristol.ac.uk/dental
British Library, 96 Euston Road, London NW1 2DB.
☎ 0843 2081144. ℘ http://www.bl.uk
British Medical Association, BMA House, Tavistock Square, London WC1H 9JP. ☎ 020 7387 4499. ℘ http://www.bma.org.uk
Cardiff Dental School, Heath Park, Cardiff CF14 4XY.
☎ 029 2074 2470. ℘ http://www.cardiff.ac.uk/dentl
Cork Dental School, Wilton, Cork, Eire.
☎ 00 353 21 490 1100. ℘ http://www.ucc.ie/en/dentalschool
Dental Defence Union, 230 Blackfriars Road, London SE1 8PJ.
☎ 0800 716376. ℘ http://www.themdu.com/index-dental.asp
Dental Protection, 33 Cavendish Square, London W1G OPS.
☎ 0845 608 4000. ℘ http://www.dentalprotection.org
Dublin Dental School, Dublin University, Trinity College, Dublin 2, Eire.
☎ 00 353 1612 7200. ℘ http://web1.dental.tcd.ie/index.php
Dundee Dental School, Park Place, Dundee DD1 4HN.
☎ 01382 660111. ℘ http://www.dundee.ac.uk/dentalschool
Edinburgh Dental Institute, 4th Floor, Lauriston Building, Lauriston Place, Edinburgh EH3 9HA. ☎ 0131 536 4970. ℘ http://www.dentistry.ed.ac.uk
Faculty of Dental Surgery, The Royal College of Surgeons of England, 35–43 Lincoln's Inn Fields, London WC1A 3PE.
☎ 020 7869 6810. ℘ http://www.rcseng.ac.uk/fds
Faculty of General Dental Practice (UK), The Royal College of Surgeons of England, 35–43 Lincoln's Inn Fields, London WC2A 3PE.
☎ 020 7869 6765. ℘ http://www.fgdp.org.uk
FDI World Dental Federation, Tour de Cointrin, Avenue Louis Casai 84, Case Postale 3, 1216 Geneve-Cointrin, Switzerland.
☎ +41 22 560 8150. ℘ http://www.fdiworldental.org
Fluoridation Society, PO Box 18, Uppermill, Oldham OL3 6WU.
☎ 01457 238507. ℘ http://www.bfsweb.org
General Dental Council, 37 Wimpole Street, London W1G 8DQ.
☎ 020 7887 3800. ℘ http://www.gdc-uk.org
Glasgow Dental School, 378 Sauchiehall Street, Glasgow G2 3JX.
☎ 0141 211 9600. ℘ http://www.gla.ac.uk/schools/dental

Kings College London Dental Institute, 1st Floor, Hodgkin Building, London Bridge, London SE1 1UL.
☎ 020 7848 6512. 🖰 http://www.kcl.ac.uk/dentistry/index.aspx
Leeds Dental Institute, Leeds Dental Institute, University of Leeds, Clarendon Way, Leeds LS2 9LU.
☎ 0113 343 6199. 🖰 http://www.dentistry.leeds.ac.uk
Liverpool Dental School, School of Dentistry, University of Liverpool, Pembroke Place, Liverpool L69 3BX.
☎ 0151 706 5298. 🖰 http://www.liv.ac.uk/dentistry
London School of Hygiene and Tropical Medicine, Keppel Street, London WC1E 7HT. ☎ 020 7636 8636. 🖰 http://www.lshtm.ac.uk
Manchester Dental School, University Dental Hospital of Manchester, Cambridge Street, Manchester M15 6FH.
☎ 0161 306 0239. 🖰 http://www.dentistry.manchester.ac.uk
Medical and Dental Defence Union of Scotland, 120 Blythswood Street, Glasgow G2 4EA.
☎ 0845 270 2034. 🖰 http://www.mddus.com/mddus/home.aspx
National Advice Centre for Postgraduate Dental Education, The Royal College of Surgeons of England, 35–43 Lincoln's Inn Fields, London WC2A 3PE. ☎ 020 7869 6804. 🖰 http://www.rcseng.ac.uk/fds/nacpde
Newcastle upon Tyne School of Dental Sciences, Framlington Place, Newcastle upon Tyne NE2 4BW.
☎ 0191 222 8347. 🖰 http://www.ncl.ac.uk/dental
Peninsula Dental School, The John Bull Building, Tamar Science Park, Research Way, Plymouth PL6 8BU.
☎ 01752 437444. 🖰 http://www.pcmd.ac.uk/dentistry.php
Queens University of Belfast, Centre for Dental Education, Grosvenor Road, Royal Victoria Hospital, Belfast BT12 6NP.
☎ 02890 632733. 🖰 http://www.qub.ac.uk/schools/mdbs/dentistry
Royal College of Physicians and Surgeons of Glasgow, 234–242 St Vincent Street, Glasgow G2 5RJ. ☎ 0141 221 6072. 🖰 http://www.rcpsg.ac.uk
Royal College of Surgeons of Edinburgh, Nicolson Street, Edinburgh EH8 9DW. ☎ 0131 527 1600. 🖰 http://www.rcsed.ac.uk
Royal College of Surgeons of England, 35–43 Lincoln's Inn Fields, London WC2A 3PE. ☎ 020 7405 3474. 🖰 http://www.rcseng.ac.uk
Royal College of Surgeons of Ireland, 123 St Stephen's Green, Dublin 2, Eire. ☎ 00 353 1402 2100. 🖰 http://www.rcsi.ie
Royal Society of Medicine, 1 Wimpole Street, London W1G 0AE.
☎ 020 7290 2900. 🖰 http://www.rsm.ac.uk
Sheffield School of Clinical Dentistry, University of Sheffield, 19 Claremont Crescent, Sheffield S10 2TA.
☎ 0114 271 7801. 🖰 http://www.shef.ac.uk/dentalschool
UCL Eastman Dental Institute, 256 Gray's Inn Road, London WC1X 8LD.
☎ 020 3456 7899. 🖰 http://www.ucl.ac.uk/eastman
University of Central Lancashire (UCLan), Preston, Lancashire PR1 2HE.
☎ 01772 201201. 🖰 http://www.uclan.ac.uk
World Health Organization, Avenue Appia 20, 1211, Geneva 27, Switzerland. ☎ +41 22 791 2111. 🖰 http://www.who.int

All details were correct at the time of going to press.

Index

Tables, figures and boxes are indicated by *t*, *f* and *b* following the page number